Orthopaedic Medicine:
A Practical Approach

For Butterworth-Heinemann:

Senior Commissioning Editor: Heidi Harrison
Development Editor: Siobhan Campbell
Production Manager: Cheryl Brant
Design: George Ajayi

Orthopaedic Medicine:
A Practical Approach

SECOND EDITION

Monica Kesson MSc MCSP Cert Ed Cert FE

Elaine Atkins DProf MA MCSP Cert FE

With a Foreword by
Patsy Cyriax

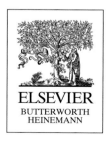

ELSEVIER
BUTTERWORTH
HEINEMANN

EDINBURGH LONDON NEW YORK OXFORD PHILADELPHIA ST LOUIS SYDNEY TORONTO 2005

ELSEVIER
BUTTERWORTH
HEINEMANN

ISBN 0 7506 5563 1

British Library Cataloguing in Publication Data
A catalogue record for this book is available from the British Library

Library of Congress Cataloging in Publication Data
A catalog record for this book is available from the Library of Congress

Note
Medical knowledge is constantly changing. As new information becomes
available, changes in treatment, procedures, equipment and the use of drugs
become necessary. The authors/contributors and the publishers have taken great
care to ensure that the information given in this text is accurate and up to date.
However, readers are strongly advised to confirm that the information, especially
with regard to drug usage, complies with the latest legislation and standards of
practice.   *The Publisher*

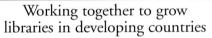

Working together to grow
libraries in developing countries

www.elsevier.com | www.bookaid.org | www.sabre.org

ELSEVIER   BOOK AID   Sabre Foundation
            International

your source for books,
journals and multimedia
in the health sciences

www.elsevierhealth.com

Printed in Italy

Contents

About the authors

Monica Kesson MSc MCSP Cert Ed Cert FE
Elaine Atkins DProf MA MCSP Cert FE

The authors studied physiotherapy together at St Thomas' Hospital, London, where the methods of Dr James Cyriax were taught. From that original inspiration they have continued to develop their clinical practice encompassing a wider scope of physiotherapy skills but always building on the solid, logical base provided by orthopaedic medicine.

Both authors now work in private practice and combine this with a teaching commitment to the Society of Orthopaedic Medicine, supporting the development of collaborative partnerships with higher education institutions and multidisciplinary working. As course principals they are involved in advancing education in orthopaedic medicine and are particularly interested in empowering students to learn through clinical reasoning and reflective practice.

Foreword to the second edition

Almost in their first paragraph, authors Monica Kesson and Elaine Atkins note how James Cyriax was, at the start of his career, 'intrigued' by an influx of patients with soft-tissue pain presenting with normal X-rays.

A fuller account of those early days may help to put this splendid new edition of *Orthopaedic Medicine: A Practical Approach* in its historical context. In 1926, when Dr Cyriax began as an orthopaedic house surgeon at St Thomas' Hospital, he noticed that a significant element of the outpatients department caseload – those lacking 'bony abnormalities' – were referred to the massage department with a diagnosis no more specific than say, 'painful shoulder'. His curiosity was piqued.

Dr Cyriax's diagnostic and physical journey from surgery to orthopaedic medicine is the mainspring of this book. In the late 1920s he followed these patients down St Thomas' long corridor to the massage department to find them in rows, still with not a diagnosis among them, receiving diffuse heat and diffuse superficial massage to the area of skin where their pain was perceived. Treatment, it transpired, was not on the basis of need but, as it were, on the basis of traditional supply.

He decided there and then to devise somehow a way of pinpointing the source of these pains so that treatment could be diverted from the symptom to the source. He did not know what he was looking for, nor how he would do the looking. His only tool was clinical examination.

It took several years before St Thomas' set up a dedicated clinic in the massage department (later the Department of Physical Medicine). Here, month after month, Dr Cyriax systematically subjected each tissue which could be a source of pain to a variety of stimuli and tensions, seeking stimuli that would create or aggravate the patient's pain, and coherent patterns of positive and negative responses which would incriminate an individual structure.

To the best of my recollection, his central insight came on a London bus. The thought abruptly crystallized that a strongly resisted contraction would aggravate pain emanating from contractile tissues – without involving inert tissues; and that passive stretching put significant additional load not upon tissues which were contractile but on those which were inert. Diagnosis by selective tension was born; the conditions of an entire branch of medicine became amenable to diagnosis and treatment.

By 1942, when I joined the department, things were moving fast. New diagnoses emerged in rapid succession. Accurate transverse friction massage was tried and its success or failure was used to confirm tentative diagnoses. We students sat in at the clinics. We learned to monitor progress by re-testing the patient's physical signs before and after each treatment. With growing *esprit de corps*, we realized that our ideas and suggestions commanded respect. Perhaps best of all, our patients were discharged, pain-free, in as little as 2–3 weeks. During those years a new medical discipline came into being.

Since the 1940s a host of new conditions – and new treatments – have been added to the canon of musculoskeletal lesions. The contribution of physiotherapy to the establishment of orthopaedic medicine has been enormous; it is a fitting provenance for the authors of this scholarly and practical work. This beautifully organized volume, with its many advances, would have been greatly admired by my late husband, and I commend it without hesitation to a new generation.

Patsy Cyriax MCSP
October 2004

Preface

Orthopaedic medicine is a specialism in medicine that is dedicated to the examination, diagnosis and non-surgical treatment of disorders of the musculoskeletal system (i.e. disorders of joints, ligaments, muscles and tendons; the means by which we move). The specialism is founded on the life's work of Dr James Cyriax MRCP (1904–1985), for many years Honorary Consultant Physician to the Department of Physical Medicine, St Thomas' Hospital, London, and is acknowledged as the bedrock of musculoskeletal medicine and therapy.

The Society of Orthopaedic Medicine (SOM), an educational charity, was established in 1979 to continue to promote the theory and practice of orthopaedic medicine – 'the Cyriax approach' – chiefly through its educational courses. The courses contribute to postgraduate programmes in medicine and physiotherapy and take place throughout the year at a variety of different venues, both nationally and internationally. The over-arching aim of the SOM is to continue to develop and integrate the specialism into medical and physiotherapy practice.

Cyriax was prolific in his writing and produced several editions of his key texts (Cyriax 1984a, 1984b; Cyriax & Cyriax 1983). Following his death in 1985 there was concern that his writings might not be advanced in the light of continuing research. With the first edition of *Orthopaedic Medicine: A Practical Approach* our aim was to compile a text that would both complement and update the existing texts in orthopaedic medicine and we set out to trawl the more recent research findings to support, or refute, the tenets established by Cyriax.

The content of both the first and second editions is structured to link to the scheme of the SOM's educational course and the book is designed as a tool to enable postgraduate medical practitioners and chartered physiotherapists, primarily, to develop their skills in the management of musculoskeletal lesions.

The target audience for the first edition of this text comprised medical practitioners and physiotherapists who were past and present course students, in addition to those with a general interest in the specialism and undergraduate students. However, the healthcare world is constantly developing and expanding in line with social and political developments, and extended practice and a framework for multidisciplinary working are now in place. The theory and practice of orthopaedic medicine now extends into allied professions such as podiatry, osteopathy and specialist nursing and the widening audience has been kept in mind in the preparation of this second edition.

Cyriax set high standards for innovative and reflective thinking in clinical practice and promoted the development of clinical experience underpinned by current evidence. The growth of the evidence base of orthopaedic medicine has gathered momentum and professionals have become more aware of the requirement to become both research minded and research active to be able to justify practice.

With this second edition of *Orthopaedic Medicine* we have persisted with the challenge to support the specialism with evidence. None the less, areas remain where there is neither evidence to support nor evidence to refute the approach. All those who practise in the musculoskeletal field are encouraged to continue to search and communicate the work of others, and to disseminate their own findings, to be able to substantiate further the original work of Cyriax and to promote enhanced patient care.

Monica Kesson and Elaine Atkins

References

Cyriax J 1984a Textbook of orthopaedic medicine, 8th edn. Baillière Tindall, London, vol 1
Cyriax J 1984b Textbook of orthopaedic medicine, 11th edn. Baillière Tindall, London, vol 2
Cyriax J, Cyriax P 1983 Illustrated manual of orthopaedic medicine. Butterworths, London

DEDICATION

To Dr James Cyriax

This book is dedicated to the memory of Dr James Cyriax. His devotion to the development of orthopaedic medicine and his commitment to a multidisciplinary approach to the assessment, diagnosis and management of musculoskeletal lesions has had a significant influence on the advancing model of collaborative working towards increased patient benefit.

Dr Cyriax provided the original inspiration to both of us, from our earliest days within our profession and throughout our careers. Through his writing he set a standard for orthopaedic medicine education which we have aimed to maintain and we are indebted to him for his example and influence.

'One life – a gleam of time between two eternities'

Anon

Acknowledgements

The following anatomy texts were invaluable and deserve special mention:

Backhouse K M, Hutchings R T 1986 A Colour Atlas of Surface Anatomy. Wolfe Medcial Publications, London

Keogh B, Ebbs S 1984 Normal Surface Anatomy. William Heinemann Medical Books, London

McMinn R M H, Gaddum-Rosse P, Hutchings R T et al 1995 McMinn's Functional and Clinical Anatomy. Times Mirror International

Palastanga N, Field D, Soames R 1994 Anatomy and Human Movement. Butterworth Heinemann, Oxford

Williams P 1998 Gray's Antatomy, 38th edn. Churchill Livingstone, Edinburgh

We are grateful to the following people, all of whom have been unstinting in their support and patience: Dr Ian Davies, for his major contribution to the injections; Robert Edwards of Elsevier, for this edition, who has been patient, encouraging and both a rock and a brick throughout; Heidi Harrison and Caroline Makepeace, his predecessors, who have also spurred us on with wit and wisdom from the early days of the first and second editions; the early reviewers from the Council of the Society of Orthopaedic Medicine whose excellent suggestions for improvement have seen it through to the second edition: Marilou Argote, Dr Ian Davies, Dr Philip Knowles, Jose Marcelino, Margaret Rees and Dr Andrew Watson; all our colleagues in the Society of Orthopaedic Medicine for giving us valuable feedback on the first edition and supporting our endeavours for the second; Paul Rees for setting us straight on the movements at the ankle and foot; Sue Cover and her staff at the library at the Canterbury Centre for Health and Clinical Sciences – nothing was too much trouble; all our colleagues within our respective practices, especially Barbara Johnson, a wonderful prop; our friends, who have continued to provide welcome social breaks; Stephanie Saunders, whose modifications to some examination and treatment techniques and Grades A, B and C for mobilizations have continued to be useful in clinical orthopaedic medicine practice. They are specially acknowledged where they are included throughout.

We continue to acknowledge the early icons of orthopaedic medicine who through their enthusiastic example provided such inspiration: Jackie Caldow, Anne Crofts, Liz Edwards, Jenny Hickling, Stephanie Saunders and of course, Dr James Cyriax himself, to whom we dedicate this edition.

Our immediate families continue to 'understand' all that it takes to see our project through and our gratitude and love are extended to them as always: thank you Rod, Andrew and Denise, Clive, Kate and Tess.

SECTION 1

Principles of orthopaedic medicine

INTRODUCTION TO SECTION 1

The aim of this book is to provide principles of diagnosis and treatment that can be applied to any of the soft tissue lesions encountered in clinical practice.

This first section presents the theory behind the principles and practice of orthopaedic medicine, beginning with the theory underpinning the assessment procedure towards clinical diagnosis. Clinical diagnosis involves the development of a hypothesis through the consideration of both subjective and objective findings and each is discussed.

The histology and biomechanics of the soft tissues follow, with a review of the healing process, aiming towards an understanding of the effects of injury on the soft tissues. This should enable the application of appropriate treatment to the different phases of healing to achieve the restoration of full, painless function.

Building on the theory of the first chapters, the first section ends with a presentation of the principles of treatment as applied in orthopaedic medicine and discusses the techniques of mobilization and injection, aims and application and indications for use.

Clinical tips are provided throughout Section 1 to emphasize clinical application and indications for use.

In December 1995 injections were declared to be within the scope of physiotherapy practice. Since then physiotherapists working as rheumatology or orthopaedic practitioners, as seniors in hospital clinics or in private practice have risen to the challenge, taking care to comply with stringent protocols. The Chartered Society of Physiotherapy (CSP) has endorsed *A Clinical Guideline for the Use of Injection Therapy by Physiotherapists* that was originally prepared by the Association of Chartered Physiotherapists in Orthopaedic Medicine (ACPOM), a clinical interest group of the CSP (Chartered Society of Physiotherapy 1999).

Courses in orthopaedic medicine (see Appendix) provide an excellent grounding in the theory and practice of injections, particularly since the modules are attended by both doctors and physiotherapists in an atmosphere of shared experience. Separate courses in injection therapy have now been developed that include supervised practice in the clinical setting to allow the demonstration of competence. More relevant, however, is the development of confidence in performing the techniques, facilitated by continued application and evaluation of practice.

At the time of writing, limited prescribing rights for physiotherapists, including those applicable for musculoskeletal injections, are still under discussion. Clearly a close relationship must be maintained with the medical profession, but physiotherapy autonomy should also be supported.

Within this text, injections must therefore be considered to be as pertinent to the physiotherapist reader as to the doctor. A brief presentation of relevant pharmacology and general considerations is presented here. However, in view of the scant pharmacology taught at undergraduate level, the physiotherapist may find it beneficial to explore some additional reading in this area. The relevant chapters of the companion text *Musculoskeletal Injection Skills* have been written with this shortfall in mind (Kesson et al 2003).

References

Chartered Society of Physiotherapy 1999 Clinical guideline for the use of injection therapy by physiotherapists. Chartered Society of Physiotherapy, London

Kesson M, Atkins E, Davies I 2003 Musculoskeletal injection skills. Butterworth Heinemann, Oxford.

Chapter **1**

Clinical diagnosis

SUMMARY

Orthopaedic medicine is based on the life's work of the late Dr James Cyriax (1904–1985). He developed a method of assessing the soft tissues of the musculoskeletal system, employing a process of diagnosis by selective tension, which uses passive movements to test the inert structures and resisted movements to test the contractile structures.

This chapter describes the theory behind his logical method of subjective and objective examination, which, by reasoned elimination, leads to the incrimination of the tissue in which the lesion lies.

Dr Cyriax's starting point in the development of orthopaedic medicine was the premise that all pain has a source. It was a simple extension of that logic that, to be effective, all treatment must reach the source and all treatment must benefit the lesion.

Cyriax was intrigued by the number of patients passing through orthopaedic clinics who presented with normal X-ray findings, and acknowledged the soft tissues as the source of the complaints. He devised a mechanism of clinical examination to establish the source of the pain which was logical and methodical, and was deliberately pared to the minimum procedure in order to discover in which tissue the lesion lay. His style of assessment conformed to the claim of Sir Robert Hutchinson in 1897, that 'every good method of case taking should be both comprehensive and concise' (Hunter & Bomford 1963).

An important emphasis of Cyriax's examination procedure is that negative findings are as significant as positive, eliminating from the enquiry those structures which are *not* at fault. The systematic approach he devised produces a set of findings that can be interpreted through logical reasoning towards eventual clinical diagnosis. The term 'diagnosis' at this stage implies the hypothesis against which we all work, which becomes proven or disproved in light of the patient's subsequent response.

In recent years, much work has been devoted to developing areas of specialist assessment. However, the orthopaedic medicine examination procedure gives clinicians a sound framework from which to start and any special examination techniques can be superimposed upon it. For example, once a basic spinal assessment has been carried out, extra tests can be included to search for aspects of neural tension, repeated or combined movements can be included, or localized joint palpation can be applied.

A further aim of the examination is to establish whether or not the lesion is suitable for the treatments offered in orthopaedic medicine or other allied treatment modalities, or whether the patient would more suitably be referred on for appropriate specialist opinion. More detailed tests such as blood tests, X-rays, computed tomography (CT) and magnetic resonance imaging (MRI) scans can be employed as necessary but do not form part of the basic examination procedure.

The orthopaedic medicine assessment procedure follows a set model for the collection of clinical data. It contains the following elements:

- Observation, noting face, gait and posture
- A detailed history
- Inspection for bony deformity, colour changes, muscle wasting and swelling
- Palpation for heat, swelling and synovial thickening
- State at rest
- Examination by selective tension, assessing active, passive and resisted movements
- Palpation for the site of the lesion, once the causative structure has been identified

OBSERVATION

Observation
■ Face
■ Gait
■ Posture

Note the patient's *face*, *gait* and *posture*.

A general observation is made as the patient is met, or even before the meeting without the patient's knowledge, for example when the patient is walking across the car park or approaching reception. Observe the patient's face for any signs of sleeplessness and pain. Serious disease accompanied by unrelenting pain is usually indicated in the patient's overall demeanour.

Certain postures indicate specific conditions. An antalgic posture (one assumed by the patient to avoid pain) is often adopted in neck pain as a wry neck, or as a lateral shift when associated with a lumbar lesion.

In the upper limb, note any apparent guarding, perhaps with an altered arm swing associated with a painful shoulder, elbow or even wrist.

The patient's gait pattern may be altered, with a limp indicating pain or a leg length discrepancy. An altered stride may be due to limitation of movement at a joint, or protection from weight-bearing. The use of an aid such as a stick or crutches provides an obvious clue to the need for extra support to avoid or to assist with weight-bearing. As part of the overall observation, a check may also be made on whether such aids are being used correctly.

HISTORY

History or subjective examination
- Age, occupation, sports, hobbies and lifestyle
- Onset and duration
- Site and spread
- Symptoms and behaviour
- Past medical history
- Other joint involvement
- Medications

A complete history is taken from the patient to ascertain as much information as possible about the condition. At some joints the history is more relevant than at others with respect to diagnosis. The history of the spinal joints and knee joint, for instance, may give many clues to diagnosis whereas with many of the commonly encountered conditions of the shoulder or elbow, such as capsulitis or tennis elbow, the history gives almost no clues at all.

The term 'history' implies a chronological account of how the condition has progressed but this forms part of a broader compass that includes other aspects, such as aggravating and alleviating factors or past medical history. The history-taking is really the subjective part of the examination procedure and it is traditional in medical and physiotherapy practice to use a model for the collection of clinical data from the patient (Beckman & Frankel 1984).

Most models, including the model used in orthopaedic medicine, involve the categorizing of the subjective examination under different headings to ensure that all information is collected. However, if this pattern is adhered to too rigidly it can be restricting for the patient. The use of closed questions to steer patients' responses results in interviews being physician/physiotherapist-led and constant interruptions may restrict the fluency of patients' accounts such that they are prevented from presenting the true nature of the problem (Beckman & Frankel 1984, Blau 1989).

Studies on the process of history-taking revealed that physicians interrupted and took control of the interview on average 18 s into the consultation, and that by asking specific closed questions they halted the spontaneous flow of information (Beckman & Frankel 1984). However, if allowed to continue uninterrupted and with no specific guidance, patients talked on average for less than 2 min, during which time most of the information required by the physician was disclosed (Blau 1989). This study was repeated by Wilkinson (1989) who found the time taken to be even shorter, with 89 of the 100 patients surveyed speaking for less than $1\frac{1}{2}$ min and 41 of those for less than 30 s.

Bearing the previous points in mind, while consideration of the various categories adopted in orthopaedic medicine is necessary, in clinical practice it is better to begin the patient interview with an open question such as 'What can I do for you?' or 'What brings you to me?' and then to allow the history to be expressed in the patient's own words. Anything not mentioned can be searched for after the patient has finished speaking.

Of course, not all patients will obligingly reveal their history and some guidance will be required to keep to the relevant. Nonetheless, a balance should still be sought between allowing the patient time to speak and controlling the interview to prevent irrelevant deviation (Blau 1989).

The model for history-taking in orthopaedic medicine will now be described. The clinician should note the relevant details from the history on the patient's record card for subsequent interpretation while accepting that the process of clinical reasoning continues throughout the interview and that the 'rambling thoughts of a clinician' cannot – and should not – be impeded.

AGE, OCCUPATION, SPORTS, HOBBIES AND LIFESTYLE

The age of the patient may be relevant as certain conditions predominantly affect certain age groups. For example, children may suffer from Perthes disease or slipped epiphysis in the hip, pulled elbow, or loose bodies associated with osteochondritis dissecans in the knee. Adolescents may suffer from Osgood–Schlatter's disease or maltracking problems in the knee. Mechanical lumbar lesions, ligament or tendon injuries are common in the middle-aged and degenerative osteoarthrosis is usually suffered by the elderly.

Occupation may be relevant in terms of the postures adopted while at work and the activities involved in the patient's job. In this respect, it is important to explore the job's requirements rather than merely to note the job title.

An overview of the patient's general lifestyle may give clues to the cause of the problem and, relating to treatment, can provide an indication of the requirements for rehabilitation back to full activity. For example, tendon or muscle belly lesions frequently occur in sports requiring explosive activity, as in tennis and squash.

SITE AND SPREAD

Patients usually complain of pain but there may be other symptoms that cause them to seek advice, such as stiffness, weakness and pins and needles, for example. Whatever the symptoms, much information can be gained towards diagnosis by establishing where the symptoms are and their overall spread. For instance, it is important to know not just where the symptoms are now but where they have been. A low back pain often travels into the leg but usually becomes less apparent in the back as it does so, a typical presentation of nerve root irritation of mechanical origin. A low back pain moving into the leg without remission in the back implies a spreading lesion and requires a different interpretation.

Since pain is the most usual complaint, it will form the main basis of the discussion in this section. Whether right or wrong in their assessment, patients usually localize their pain as coming from a certain point and can describe the area of its spread, although sometimes only vaguely. Cyriax considered that all pain is referred and explored the pattern of referred pain to try and establish some rules which would help in its interpretation towards establishing the true source of the pain (Cyriax & Cyriax 1983).

The study of pain itself is a vast topic, most of which is outside the scope of this book, and the reader is referred for a detailed account to the many other sources which confine themselves to the in-depth study of this field. Nevertheless, pain and its behaviour are relevant to orthopaedic medicine, particularly in the assessment procedures, both towards the achievement of an accurate clinical diagnosis and as a guide to the effectiveness of the treatment techniques applied.

To be able to identify the source of the pain, a thorough knowledge of applied and functional anatomy is essential, coupled with an understanding of the behaviour of pain, particularly in relation to its ability to be referred to areas other than the causative site. It is acknowledged that other influences can affect the perception of pain and within this chapter *referred pain* will be discussed, with a brief consideration of *psychosocial* factors.

It is commonly found in clinical practice that pain of visceral origin can mimic that of somatic origin ('pain arising from noxious stimulation of one of the musculoskeletal components of the body', Bogduk 1997) and vice versa. Pain arising from pathology in the heart, for example, may produce a spread of pain into the arm imitating the pain of nerve root sleeve compression from a cervical lesion. Similarly, mid-thoracic back pain may arise from a stomach lesion.

There have been several suggestions put forward for the mechanism of referred pain and the more significant ones are discussed here. McMahon et al (1995) cite Sinclair who suggested that primary sensory neurons have bifurcating axons which innervate both somatic and visceral structures. Some evidence was found for this theory, but some of the findings were challenged, particularly as such axons had failed to be demonstrated in appreciable numbers. While unable to find neurons with visceral and somatic fields, McMahon et al mention that Mense and colleagues did find a few single sensory neurons with receptive fields in two tissues, in both skin and muscle in the tail of a cat, but overall there was scant support for Sinclair's suggestion. More recently, Sameda et al (2003) have demonstrated peripheral axons dichotomizing (branching into two) into both the L5, L6 disc and groin skin in rats. This could provide a possible explanation for pain referred to the groin area from damage to the L5 and S1 nerve roots from L4–L5 and L5–S1 disc herniation in man, in spite of the nerve supply of the groin area arising from the higher lumbar spinal nerves.

More evidence has been provided for the mechanism that visceral and somatic primary sensory neurons converge onto common spinal neurons, causing a confusion in the ascending spinal pathways and leading to misinterpretation of the origin of the pain. The message from the primary lesion could be wrongly interpreted as coming from the area of pain referral (Vecchiet & Giamberardino 1997). This has been dubbed the convergence–projection theory.

A side-track from the convergence–projection theory is the convergence–facilitation theory, attributed to McKenzie (cited in McMahon et al 1995) that claims that the viscera are insensitive and that visceral afferent activity did not directly give rise to pain. It was suggested that an irritable focus was produced within the spinal cord, where somatic inputs would take over to produce abnormal referred pain in the appropriate segmental distribution. This theory was not generally accepted, however, since it denied that true visceral pain could exist. However, it did provide an explanation for heightened referred sensations, including that of secondary hyperalgesia (Vecchiet & Giamberardino 1997). Its basic concepts were also developed in the early 1990s under the descriptor of 'central sensitization' that attempts to explain hyperalgesia and the prolongation of chronic pain.

Referred pain does not only present itself for misinterpretation between visceral and somatic structures but is also a phenomenon which may prevent accurate localization among the musculoskeletal tissues. Cyriax & Cyriax (1983) suggested that the misinterpretation of pain occurs at cortical level where stimuli arriving at certain cortical cells from the skin can be accurately localized to that area. When stimuli from other deeper tissues of the same segmental derivation reach those same cells, the sensory cortex makes assumptions on the basis of past experience and attributes the source of the pain to that same area of skin. This accounts for the dermatomal reference of pain but the theory can be extended to include the referral of other symptoms.

Knowledge of the nerve supply of soft tissue structures, coupled with factors affecting dermatomal reference and the general rules of referred pain, is a useful aid to diagnosis. It will help to direct the clinician to the true source of the patient's pain and so facilitate the application of effective treatment.

Several workers have tried to establish patterns of referred pain by examining the dermatomes. However, the dermatomes appear to vary according to the different methods for defining them. These mainly derive from embryonic development, observation of herpetic eruptions, areas of vasodilatation resulting from nerve root stimulation and the areas of tactile sensation remaining after rhizotomy (surgical severance) of spinal nerve roots, as described below. These dermatomes are referred to as embryonic, herpetic, vasodilatation and tactile, respectively.

Sir Henry Head (1900) laid the foundations for the mapping of dermatomes by analysing herpetic eruptions. Herpes zoster is an inflammatory lesion of the spinal ganglia which produces an eruption on the skin in the corresponding segmental cutaneous area. By defining the dermatomes in this way, little overlap was found and there was only slight variation between subjects studied.

Stricker and Bayliss, as described by Foerster (1933), used faradic stimulation of the distal part of a divided posterior root to produce vasodilatation. This produced a clearly defined area similar to the dermatomes defined in the isolation method, but slightly smaller in size.

The skin is supplied by both ventral and dorsal nerve roots. Foerster (1933) examined the areas of skin supplied by the dorsal roots which carry the afferent sensory fibres and efferent fibres producing vasodilatation. He described two methods of isolating the area of skin supplied by the dorsal nerve roots, using the terms *anatomical* and *physiological*.

The anatomical method, attributed to Herringham & Bolk (Foerster 1933), involved the isolation of fibres arising from a single nerve root by dissection through the plexus and the peripheral nerves into the skin. It was impossible to follow the finest ramifications by this method but it largely demonstrated that there was little or no overlap of dermatomes classified in this way.

Within the physiological method of differentiation, Foerster (1933) describes how Sherrington divided the nerve roots above and below a single nerve root to map the area supplied by the intervening intact root in the monkey. There was such overlap of different dermatomes identified by this method that division of a single root produced no loss of sensibility. He used the same technique in humans and found the same pattern of overlap in the tactile dermatomes.

Despite the experimental findings, the extent of individual dermatomes, especially in the limbs, is largely based on clinical evidence. This leads to a wide variation between the opinions of different disciplines (Williams 1998). The dermatomes given in this book are drawn mainly from the clinical experience of Cyriax and are different from those given in *Gray's Anatomy* (Williams 1998), for example. In the authors' experience, they provide a sound basic guide for clinical practice and are presented as shown in Figure 1.1.

Nerve root dermatomes

(Conesa & Argote 1976, Cyriax 1982, Cyriax & Cyriax 1983) (Fig. 1.1)

C1: top of head (Fig. 1.1a)

C2: side and back of the head, upper half of the ear, cheek and upper lip, nape of the neck (Fig. 1.1b)

C3: entire neck, lower mandible, chin, lower half of the ear (Fig. 1.1c)

C4: epaulette area of the shoulder (Fig. 1.1d)

C5: anterolateral aspect of the arm and forearm as far as the base of the thumb (Fig. 1.1e)

C6: anterolateral aspect of the arm and forearm, thenar eminence, thumb and index finger (Fig. 1.1f)

C7: posterior aspect of the arm and forearm, index, middle and ring fingers (Fig. 1.1g)

C8: medial aspect of the forearm medial half of the hand, middle, ring and little fingers (Fig. 1.1h)

T1: medial aspect of the forearm, upper boundary uncertain (Fig. 1.1i)

T2: Y-shaped dermatome, medial condyle of humerus to axilla, branch to sternum and branch to scapula (Fig. 1.1j)

T3: area at front of chest, patch in axilla (Fig. 1.1k)

T4, 5, 6: circling trunk above, at and below the nipple area (Fig. 1.1l)

T7, 8: circling trunk at lower costal margin (Fig. 1.1l)

T9–11: circling the trunk, reaching the level of the umbilicus (Fig. 1.1l)

T12: margins uncertain, extends into groin, covers greater trochanter and the iliac crest (Fig. 1.1l)

L1: lower abdomen and groin, lumbar region between levels L2 and L4, upper, outer aspect of the buttock (Fig. 1.1m)

L2: two separate areas: lower lumbar region and upper buttock whole of the front of the thigh (Fig. 1.1n)

L3: two separate areas: upper buttock, medial aspect and front of the thigh and leg as far as the medial malleolus (Fig. 1.1o)

L4: lateral aspect of the thigh, front of the leg crossing to the medial aspect of the foot, big toe only (Fig. 1.1p)

Figure 1.1   Dermatomes.

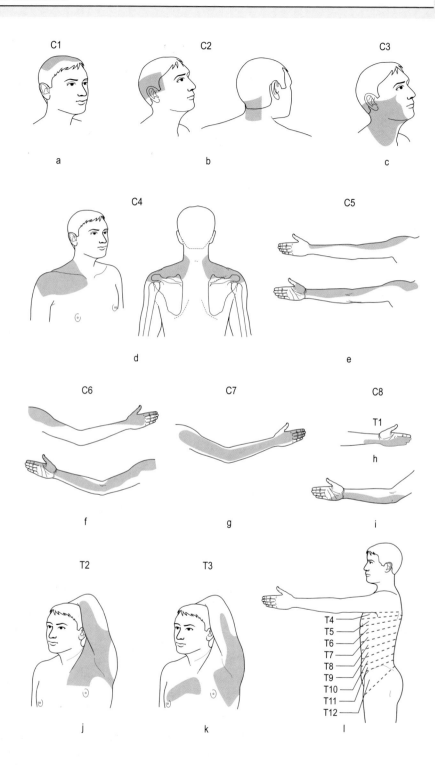

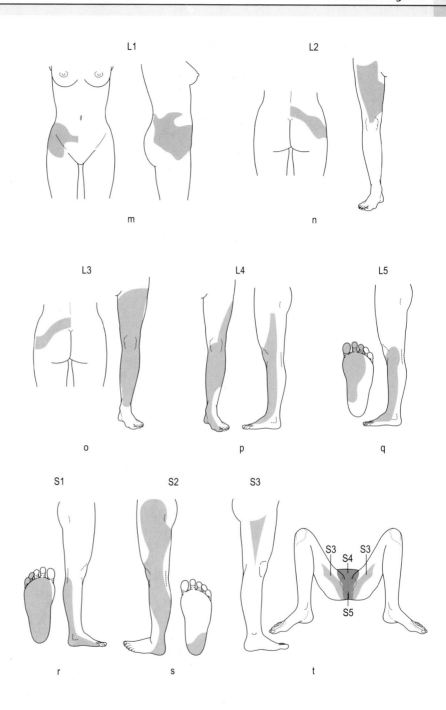

L5: lateral aspect of the leg, dorsum of the whole foot first, second and
   third toes, inner half of the sole of the foot (Fig. 1.1q)

S1: sole of the foot, lateral two toes, lower half of the posterior aspect of
   the leg (Fig. 1.1r)

S2: posterior aspect of the whole thigh and leg, plantar aspect of the heel (Fig. 1.1s)

S3: circular area around the anus, medial aspect of the thigh (Fig. 1.1t)

S4: saddle area: anus, perineum, genitals, medial upper thigh (Fig. 1.1t)

S5: coccygeal area (Fig. 1.1t)

In general the muscle groups lie under the dermatome which shares the same nerve supply. However, the dermatome and myotome may not overlie each other and there are some apparent exceptions to this rule. This can cause confusion in the consideration of referred pain, in that a lesion in the relevant muscle may appear to refer pain to an unrelated site. The most commonly encountered discrepancies are as follows:

- Scapular muscles are supplied by C4–C7, but underlie thoracic dermatomes
- Latissimus dorsi is supplied by C6–C8, but underlies thoracic and lumbar dermatomes
- Pectoralis major is supplied by C5–T1 but underlies thoracic dermatomes
- The heart, a thoracic structure, is supplied by C8–T4 and may refer pain into the arm, axilla and chest
- The diaphragm is supplied by C3–C5 and diaphragmatic irritation may lead to pain being felt in the epaulette region of the shoulder
- The gluteal muscles are supplied by L5, S1–S2 but underlie L1–L3 dermatomes
- The testicle is supplied by T11–T12, L1, but underlies the S4 dermatome where pain may be felt locally or can be referred to the lower thoracic or upper lumbar regions

Cyriax (1982) and Cyriax & Cyriax (1983) identified several factors that influence the referral of pain:

- Strength of the stimulus
- Position of the structure in the dermatome
- Depth of the structure
- Type or nature of the structure

Strength of the stimulus

The more acutely inflamed or irritable the lesion (i.e. the greater the stimulus), the further into the dermatome will the symptoms be referred (Inman & Saunders 1944). For example, an acutely inflamed subacromial bursitis may refer its pain to the wrist, the distal extent of the C5 dermatome, and a lumbar lesion involving compression and inflammation of the L4 nerve root may refer pain and associated symptoms to the big toe, at the distal end of the L4 dermatome.

Position in the dermatome

Pain and tenderness tend to refer distally. Therefore a structure placed more proximally in the dermatome may be capable of referring its symptoms over a greater distance to the end of the dermatome.

The length or distance of dermatomal referral is particularly obvious in the limbs, where the dermatomes tend to be long. However, if the dermatome is short, even with an acutely inflamed or irritable lesion, the reference will halt at the end of its dermatome, or most distal dermatome in the event of more than one nerve supply.

Structures within the hand and forefoot are already at the distal end of their relevant dermatome. Referral of symptoms is therefore less and such lesions are easier to localize (Inman & Saunders 1944).

Depth of the structure

Cyriax (1982) proposed that lesions in the more deeply placed structures tended to give greater reference of pain, which was also the finding of Kellgren (1939) and Inman & Saunders (1944). The deeper structures therefore give rise to greater misunderstanding in terms of clinical diagnosis.

Joint, ligament and bursa lesions tend to conform to this assumption but a notable exception is provided by lesions within bone. Pain and tenderness arising from fractures or involvement of the cortical bone tend to be well-localized, even though bone itself is the most deeply placed tissue in musculoskeletal terms. Lesions involving the cancellous part of bone may give the more typical pattern of referred pain.

Segmental pain arising from lesions in the deeply sited viscera can also be misleading.

Nature of the tissue

The factor of depth of the structure should perhaps be considered alongside that of the nature of the tissue, since studies to observe the effect of lesions in tissues of different nature and site on patterns of referred pain are hard to dissociate.

Kellgren (1938, 1939) observed patterns of referred pain induced by the injection of 6% hypertonic saline into deeply placed structures including muscle, tendon sheaths, fascia, periosteum and interspinous ligaments. On injection of muscle, diffuse referred pain was produced which appeared to follow a segmental pattern and was associated with deep tenderness rather than hyperaesthetic skin. Witting et al (2000) compared local and referred pain following intramuscular capsaicin injection into the brachioradialis muscle and intradermal injection in the skin above the muscle. Intradermal injection produced more intense but localized pain whereas referred pain was more marked after the intramuscular injection and was deeply located as well as referring to skin. Kellgren also observed that pain arising from the limb muscles tended to refer to the region of the joints moved by these muscles, where it could easily be confused as arising from the joint itself.

Tendon sheath and fascia gave sharply localized pain. Stimuli did not produce pain from articular cartilage or compact bone but when applied to cancellous bone a deep diffuse pain was produced. Stimulation of the interspinous ligaments gave rise to segmentally referred pain which, as in muscle, was associated with tenderness in the deeply placed structures.

Inman & Saunders (1944) noted a variability of sensitivity to the different structures beneath the skin, creating a 'league table' of those tissues with the highest sensitivity to those with the least, as follows: bone, ligaments, fibrous capsules of joints, tendons, fascia and muscle. These findings were supported in part by Kuslich et al (1991), who investigated tissues in the lumbar spine as potential sources of low back pain using progressive local anaesthetic during operative exploration of the spine. Their emphasis too was that muscles, fascia and the periosteum and compact layer of bone (they did not test cancellous bone) were relatively insensitive. In contrast, in the work of Travell & Simons (1996) trigger points in muscle have been identified as a focus of hyperirritability which gives rise to referred pain and tenderness.

It had been particularly noted by Inman & Saunders (1944) that capsules and ligaments were most sensitive close to their bony attachments, and therefore most likely to be pain-producing on trauma to these commonly injured sites.

Controversy has existed for many years as to whether the disc or the zygapophyseal joint is the primary source of back pain, especially when associated with pain in the limb. Aprill et al (1989) studied the reference of pain from the cervical zygapophyseal joints to establish whether each joint had a specific area of reference of pain in a segmental distribution. They found reasonably distinct and consistent segmental patterns of pain referral associated with joints between each of the levels of C2–C7, but there was no referral of pain into the arm from any of the tested levels. The paper acknowledged that the study had not set out to distinguish the pain arising from zygapophyseal joints from other potential sources.

Two pain syndromes of somatic and radicular origin have been described associated with the spinal joints (Bogduk 1997). In *somatic pain syndromes* it is proposed that the source of the pain could be in any structure in the spine that receives a nerve supply, i.e. muscles, ligaments, zygapophyseal joints, intervertebral discs, dura mater and dural nerve root sleeve. Somatic pain is not associated with neurological abnormalities and does not involve nerve root compression. The quality of somatic pain is described as dull, diffuse and difficult to localize.

The source of pain in *radicular pain syndromes* is proposed to be compression of the nerve root, but how compression causes pain remains unresolved (see Ch. 13). Experimental compression of dorsal root ganglia or previously damaged nerve root has been shown to cause pain. The clinical experiments of Smyth & Wright (cited in Bogduk 1997), show this neuralgic pain to be produced in a particular form, namely lancinating and shooting in quality and referred in relatively narrow bands. However, a lesion cannot selectively compress nociceptive axons, therefore for compression to be the source of radicular pain, other neurological abnormalities should be present, for example paraesthesia, numbness, muscle weakness and loss of reflexes (Bogduk 1997).

Kidd & Richardson (2002) further clarify that somatic referred pain is nociceptive, being initiated by stimulation of receptors on peripheral terminals of sensory fibres, either by damage or inflammation within somatic structures. In contrast, radicular pain is neuropathic and arises as a result of sensory fibres being abnormally stimulated along their course, i.e. when nerves themselves are damaged or inflamed.

Kellgren (1939), in charting the distribution of pain, demonstrated that injection of the interspinous ligaments of L2–S2 produced pain in the leg. However, Kuslich et al (1991) found that sciatica could only be produced by stretching or direct pressure on an already inflamed nerve root.

In the same study, the zygapophyseal joint capsule was found to be tender in some instances but the pain was never referred to the leg. The zygapophyseal joint's main significance in the production of low back pain was its ability to compress or irritate other local sensitive tissues, particularly with osteophyte formation, including the annulus fibrosus. The annulus fibrosus was demonstrated to be the tissue of origin in most cases of low back pain without pain or symptom referral into the limb. It should be noted that the sacroiliac joint was not included in either study to be able to establish its ability to produce leg pain.

More recently, O'Neill et al (2002) demonstrated that noxious stimulation of the intervertebral disc can give rise to low back and referred extremity pain, with the distal extent of pain produced depending on the intensity of stimulation. Nociceptors within the discal tissue may have become more sensitized in patients presenting with non-radicular leg pain allowing provocation of peripheral symptoms at lower thresholds of stimulation. They suggest that Kuslich et al (1991), discussed above, would have observed a similar pattern of pain referral on stimulation of the annulus if they had applied a stimulus of sufficient intensity.

O'Neill et al support Bogduk (1997) in describing referred leg pain from the somatic lumbar annulus fibrosus as being poorly localized, dull and aching, adding that it is usually less troublesome than the patient's low back pain. They warn that it is important to be able to differentiate between referred pain arising from somatic structures and radicular pain associated with nerve root compression from disc herniation, because the two types of pain have different causal mechanisms and may therefore require different treatment. They add that the traditional description 'pain radiating below the knee' as representing radicular pain rather than referred somatic pain is unreliable.

Bogduk (1994), however, proposed that somatic and radicular pain syndromes can coexist. For example, the annulus fibrosus of the disc may be a source of somatic low back pain but may also cause secondary compression by a posterolateral displacement causing compression of the nerve root leading to radicular pain.

As mentioned above, there are no separate ascending spinal pathways for the transmission of *visceral pain* and sensations from the viscera are represented within the somatosensory pathways that also transfer sensations from somatic structures (Galea 2002). This can lead to confusion in differential diagnosis between pain arising from visceral lesions and that arising from musculoskeletal lesions. Galea describes how the level of the spinal cord to which visceral afferent fibres project depends on their embryonic innervation and notes that many viscera migrate well away from their embryonic derivation during development, such that visceral referred pain may be perceived at remote sites.

Specific consideration of visceral referred pain is provided within the appropriate chapters as part of differential diagnosis. However, Vecciet & Giamberardino (1997) describe general aspects of visceral pain that can be borne in mind, particularly for those conditions requiring more urgent referral. Initially, the pain is usually felt in the same site along the midline of the chest or abdomen, mainly in the lower sternal area and the epigastric region, regardless of the viscera affected. It is generally perceived as a deep, dull, vague sensation that is poorly defined and may not be able to be described. It can vary from a sense of discomfort to one of oppression or heaviness and may be associated with autonomic signs such as pallor, sweating, nausea, vomiting and changes in heart rate, blood pressure and temperature. Strong emotional reactions are also often present and include anxiety, anguish and sometimes even feelings of impending death.

Other common features of segmentally referred pain were identified by Cyriax as 'rules' of referred pain (Cyriax 1982, Cyriax & Cyriax 1983). As with all pronounced rules exceptions may be noted, but nonetheless they act as a general guideline in assessing pain behaviour and locating the causative lesion.

A notable exception to the rules of referred pain is provided by the dura mater which, as a centrally placed structure, produces so called *'multisegmental reference'* on compression or irritation.

> **Rules of referred pain from unilateral structures**
> - It does not cross the midline.
> - It refers distally.
> - It refers segmentally.
> - It occupies part or all of its dermatome.

Multisegmental reference of pain

Throughout his writing Cyriax refers to the phenomenon of 'extrasegmental' reference of pain (Cyriax 1982, Cyriax & Cyriax 1983). He uses the term to explain the observation that symptoms arising from the dura mater do not obey the rules of referred pain, in terms of referring segmentally, but rather that a pattern of reference is produced which is 'outside' or 'extra' to that of the segment. With another interpretation, the terminology falls short of being ideal since it implies that the pain is not experienced within the segment in which the causative lesion is housed. This is not so and *multisegmental* would perhaps be a more correct term.

The ventral aspect of the dura mater, the annulus fibrosus and other central spinal structures are innervated by the sinuvertebral nerve which sends branches to segments above and below its level of origin (Bogduk 1997). This could account for the multisegmental reference of pain arising from compression of central structures.

Multisegmentally referred pain is felt diffusely across several segments, usually as a dull background ache, and is often associated with tenderness or trigger spots (Fig. 1.2). Other unilateral symptoms might be superimposed upon it, as in lesions involving pressure on both the dura and the dural nerve root sleeve.

Mention of the effect of compression of the dura mater leads into the general observation that lesions associated with compression of neural tissue produce varying patterns and nature of symptoms, according to the tissue involved. These will be listed as follows, beginning with the dura mater itself:

Figure 1.2   Multisegmental
pain. CSP= cervical spine pain;
TSP=thoracic spine .pain;
LSP=lumbar spine pain.

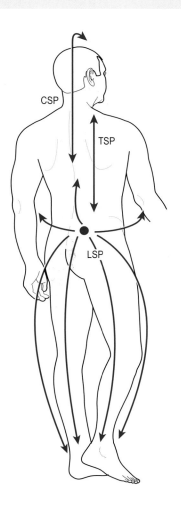

CSP

TSP

LSP

Dura mater

- Multisegmental reference of pain and
  tenderness (Fig. 1.2).

Spinal cord

- No pain, multisegmental reference of
  paraesthesia, i.e. in both feet, or all extremities
  if associated with cervical lesions.
- May produce upper motor neuron lesion with
  spastic muscle weakness.
- May produce a spastic gait.

- May produce an extensor plantar response.

Dural nerve root sleeve

- Pain produced on compression of the tissue, i.e.
  the pressure or 'compression phenomenon'
  (Cyriax 1982).
- Segmental reference of pain in all or part of the
  dermatome.
- Difficult to ascribe an aspect to the pain, e.g.
  anterior or lateral.
- Difficult to define an edge to the pain.

Nerve root

- Neurological signs and symptoms produced on compression:
  - segmental reference of paraesthesia felt at the distal end of the dermatome
  - lower motor neuron lesion with flaccid muscle weakness
  - absent or reduced reflexes
- May become pain-sensitive.

Nerve trunk

- Symptoms produced on release of pressure, i.e. the 'release phenomenon' (Cyriax 1982), e.g. after sitting on a hard gate with pressure placed on the sciatic nerve trunk for a period of time, a shower of 'painful pins and needles' will be experienced in the leg until the nerve recovers.
- Sensation of deep painful paraesthesia in the cutaneous distribution of the nerve trunk.

- Some aspect, no edge to the symptoms.
- The longer the compression, the greater the length of time before the onset of pins and needles, e.g. the thoracic outlet syndrome produces diffuse pins and needles in all five digits of one or both hands after going to bed at night, several hours after the compression has been released from the brachial plexus.

Peripheral nerve

- Compression produces paraesthesia and numbness.
- Clear edge and aspect to the symptoms, e.g. carpal tunnel syndrome producing paraesthesia and/or numbness in the cutaneous distribution of the lateral three and a half digits on the palmar aspect of the hand, or meralgia paraesthetica involving compression of the lateral cutaneous nerve of the thigh, which is associated with a clearly demarcated area of paraesthesia and/or numbness in the anterolateral aspect of the thigh.

Psychosocial factors

Whenever pain itself is the central focus for information towards clinical diagnosis, consideration needs to be given to both its sensory and affective aspects. Thus discussion within this section on the characteristics of referred pain has been based on the sensory component of pain, addressing the mechanism and factors of referred pain, particularly relating to its dermatomal distribution.

Consideration has been given to the concept of 'central pain', arising from changes within the central nervous system (Butler 1995, Mendelson 1995). However, notwithstanding the contribution of central pain to the chronic state, attention needs to be given to the affective aspects of pain as an emotional experience rather than as a pure sensation (Butler 1995). The so-called psychosocial (involving aspects of both social and psychological behaviour) factors can have varying effects on the patient's perception of pain as well as distorting the account given to the clinician.

In addressing this issue in orthopaedic medicine, the term *psychogenic pain* has traditionally been used. The term has survived the controversy on whether or not it exists and, according to the literature review of Mendelson (1995), the work of Engel, Walters and Merskey has led to a general acceptance that pain can be amplified or evoked by psychological factors. However, the term *psychosocial* is currently more commonly used and several studies provide evidence that certain personality traits and experiences of individuals have predisposed them to the persisting cycle of chronic pain (Waddell 1998).

Identification of a significant psychological influence will allow for modification in the treatment approach adopted and certainly may provide a contraindication for some of the techniques used in orthopaedic medicine, most notably the manipulative treatments used for spinal pain.

Cyriax (1982) presented characteristics which, if recognized in patients, give an indication that affective influences are a predominant feature of the complaint and should be taken into account in arriving at a diagnosis, as well as in subsequent treatment selection or appropriate referral.

He suggested that any or all of the following features might be present:

- No recognizable pattern of symptoms or signs in the subjective or objective examination
- Poor cooperation in both sections of the examination
- Overenthusiastic assistance from the patient, often accompanied by an element of 'triumph' if the clinical diagnosis remains obscure
- Patients may seek the answer expected of them
- Mutually contradictory signs through an incomplete knowledge of the condition

Juddering is a response occasionally noted on resisted testing but there is no evidence for any neurological condition which allows muscles to work in spasms of effort to produce such a juddering pattern. This is not the cogwheel resistance to movement encountered in parkinsonism. Severe pain usually produces an 'all-or-nothing' effort where resistance is lost completely as a result of pain, e.g. in resisted wrist extension as a test for tennis elbow where the wrist 'breaks' due to the sharp pain elicited.

Active movements are cited later in this chapter as a useful means of establishing the patient's willingness to perform the movement. This can relate to the psychosocial influence as well as allowing consideration of any unwillingness caused by actual pain, or fear of producing it.

Waddell (1992, 1998), after extensive study in the field of problematic back pain, describes behavioural symptoms and signs that provide information and raise awareness of illness behaviour. In contrast, Adams et al (2002) suggest that the balance of back pain research has swung too far towards psychosocial issues to the neglect of the physical. However, Waddell has traditionally emphasized the need for careful assessment, warning that a 'galaxy of signs does not exclude a remediable condition'. On orthopaedic medicine courses, students are cautioned against the misinterpretation of unusual signs and symptoms by the statement: 'beware of the bizarre but consistent patient', whose behaviour could be indicative of underlying serious pathology.

Several effective approaches have been devised in the treatment of chronic pain, often based on the concept of increasing activity and fitness levels and promoting the maxim that 'hurt does not equate to harm'. Skilled counselling may also be required. This book has set out to acknowledge the possible influence of psychosocial factors but does not intend to expand further on its management. The interested reader is referred to appropriate texts relating to this work.

ONSET AND DURATION

The mode of onset of the lesion can provide indicators which lead to a clinical diagnosis and can also contribute to the treatment selection and overall prognosis of the condition. Was the onset sudden or gradual? Meniscal tears and acute muscle belly lesions come on suddenly whereas overuse tendon and bursa problems and nuclear disc lesions have a gradual onset. Fractures usually have a sudden onset associated with trauma but systemic conditions or serious pathology such as tumours have an insidious onset. None of these latter conditions are suitable for treatment within the specialism of orthopaedic medicine.

In the lumbar spine the mode of onset leads towards a particular hypothesis with regard to pathology, which then provides a guideline for treatment selection. For example, a gradual onset may respond more effectively to treatment with traction, while, in the absence of any contraindications, a sudden onset may require manipulative treatment.

The duration of the symptoms is important as an indicator of the acute or chronic stage in healing which in itself gives guidance for the treatment approach to be adopted, as well as indicating the likely effectiveness and progress of treatment applied. For example, the acutely sprained ligament will require a gentle approach to treatment aiming to reduce swelling, promote healing and to prevent adverse scar tissue formation. In contrast, the chronic ligamentous lesion will require a more aggressive approach to treatment aiming to restore function by breaking down any adverse adhesion formation with stretching and manipulative techniques as appropriate. A lumbar lesion of gradual onset is less likely to respond to treatment if it has been present for 3 months than if it has been present for 1 month.

SYMPTOMS AND BEHAVIOUR

The way the pain behaves will assist diagnosis. Mechanical joint lesions are usually better for rest and worse on activity. Also, changing posture can alter the pain. Ligamentous lesions like movement and are usually worse after a period of resting. Serious pathology may present with unrelenting pain and night pain is likely to be a feature. Generally speaking, benign musculoskeletal lesions do not present with constant, unremitting pain and there is usually some position of rest which eases pain, or some periods when the pain is easier or even absent. In distinguishing between serious pathology and an irritable musculoskeletal lesion it can be helpful to note whether the pain prevents sleep or disturbs sleep.

There will be special questions at each joint which are relevant to the patient's symptoms. For example, how do stairs affect knee pain? How does a cough or sneeze affect back pain? Does the patient with neck pain experience any dizziness? Pertinent questions asked at each joint region will aid diagnosis and, importantly, will also rule out any contraindications to treatment.

The clinician will also wish to investigate if there have been any previous episodes of similar complaints. Spinal pain may be a progression of the same condition and a lumbar disc lesion may characteristically present as increasing episodes of worsening pain.

PAST MEDICAL HISTORY

Asking about the existence of serious illness, operations or accidents gives insight into the patient's past medical history. Past trauma or serious illness may be relevant to current diagnosis, e.g. old fracture of the tibia leading to degenerative changes in the ankle joint, or mastectomy for carcinoma followed by the formation of bony secondaries in the spine.

OTHER JOINT INVOLVEMENT

This particularly gives clues to the patient's pain being associated with systemic joint disease. It will alert the examiner to the presence of inflammatory arthritis, such as rheumatoid arthritis and ankylosing spondylitis, or degenerative osteoarthrosis, all of which have a distinctive pattern of onset and joints affected. Inflammatory joint disease provides a contraindication to manipulative treatment.

MEDICATIONS

These give a clue to past or underlying disease, e.g. the use of tamoxifen indicates a history of breast cancer, long-term steroids may indicate inflammatory joint disease. Anticoagulants are in themselves a contraindication for manipulation since manipulation may cause disruption of capillaries and the prolonged bleeding time induced by anticoagulant therapy may lead to haematoma formation. Steroids may not be so much a contraindication in themselves but consideration needs to be given to the underlying pathology which necessitates their prescription.

The quantity and regularity of the dose of analgesic and non-steroidal anti-inflammatory drugs provide an indication of the level of pain being experienced by the patient and can be used as an objective marker to monitor the progress of treatment in terms of any change in their requirement.

INSPECTION

Inspection
■ Bony deformity
■ Colour changes
■ Muscle wasting
■ Swelling

Having completed the history, the patient is inspected, suitably undressed and in a good light, paying particular attention to any *bony deformity*, *colour changes*, *muscle wasting* or *swelling*.

BONY DEFORMITY

This may include spinal asymmetry, leg length discrepancy, excessive valgus or varus deformity at joints, bony lumps or exostoses. Obvious distortion of bony or joint contours following trauma could indicate fracture or dislocation.

COLOUR CHANGES

Redness may indicate the presence of acute inflammation as one of the four cardinal signs of inflammation: redness, heat, swelling and pain. There may be signs of bruising following trauma or pallor or reddening associated with circulatory or sympathetic involvement. The presence of scars and rashes may also be indicative of relevant pathology.

MUSCLE WASTING

Any obvious muscle wasting is noted which may have origin in a neurological condition, usually from nerve root compression at the relevant spinal level, as a result of reflex muscle inhibition associated with joint effusion (de Andrade et al 1965), or as a consequence of disuse.

SWELLING

Swelling is indicative of the presence of inflammation resulting from trauma or overuse, as in tenosynovitis and bursitis or arthritis. Swelling which presents immediately indicates bleeding in the area. Other swellings may include ganglia, lipomata and soft tissue nodules.

PALPATION

> **Palpate a peripheral joint**
> - Heat
> - Swelling
> - Synovial thickening

At this stage of the objective examination, peripheral joints are palpated for signs of inflammatory activity in the form of *heat*, *swelling* and *synovial thickening*. The area is not palpated for tenderness – this must wait until the end of the examination when the structure at fault has been identified through the rest of the examination procedure. It may also be necessary to palpate for peripheral pulses at this stage if circulatory disturbance is suspected.

HEAT

The joint is palpated for heat using the back of the hand and comparing the same aspect on each side. The same hand is used throughout since the dominant hand may be a few degrees warmer than the nondominant. Any bandaging or support that the patient has been wearing which could have warmed the area should be taken into account.

SWELLING

Swelling is often apparent on inspection alone but may be palpated for, particularly to detect minor swelling, in the knee, for example.

SYNOVIAL THICKENING

Synovial thickening has a 'boggy' feel to it and indicates the presence and level of inflammation in a joint. It is particularly evident in rheumatoid arthritis at the wrist, ankle and knee.

STATE AT REST

The state at rest must be established before any examination requiring joint movement or muscle activity takes place, in order to provide a baseline against which to note the effect of any such movements. Comparison can then be made with subsequent movements which may make the symptoms better or worse.

An open question such as 'How do you feel as you are standing/sitting there?' usually elicits the status quo and avoids the leading use of the word 'pain'.

Based on the observation that normal tissue functions painlessly whereas abnormal tissue does not, Cyriax devised a method of applying appropriate stress to the structures surrounding each joint in order to test their function. Passive movements were employed to test the so-called inert structures such as joint capsules and ligaments, whereas resisted tests were used to test the contractile structures incorporating muscle, tendon and attachments to bone. This then was the method of applying selective tension to tissues (Cyriax 1982, Cyriax & Cyriax 1983) and the movements he propounded will now be described.

EXAMINATION BY SELECTIVE TENSION

ACTIVE MOVEMENTS

Active movements
- Range
- Pain
- Power
- Willingness
- Painful arc

Active movements give an idea of the *range* of movement available in the joint, the *pain* experienced by the patient and the *power* in the muscle groups. They are not carried out routinely at all joints, since they are non-selective and employ both inert and contractile tissues.

They are useful in establishing the *willingness* of the patient to perform the movements as an indicator of the level of pain being experienced within each range. In this role they can act as a guide to the range of movement available before applying passive stresses to the joint.

Active movements can also be used to eliminate neighbouring joints as a potential source of pain. For example, as part of the shoulder examination, six active neck movements are performed. If the patient's pain is not elicited then the cervical spine is eliminated from the enquiry at that initial stage.

They are also most important in illustrating how willing the patient is to move, with respect to the patient's pain tolerance and particularly noting any unusual or bizarre responses. The appropriateness of the patient's response can be significant in the subsequent selection of treatment techniques. This is helpful when assessing the so-called 'emotional' joints, i.e. the joints which are prone to an exaggeration of symptoms and which include all spinal areas, the shoulders and, to a lesser extent, the hips.

A particular sign known as the *painful arc* is demonstrated by active movement. By definition, a painful arc is an arc of pain with pain-free movement on either side. It implies that a structure is being pinched or compressed at that point of the movement and is a useful finding towards diagnosis. For example, a painful arc may be found on active abduction at the shoulder if a lesion lies in the subacromial bursa, or the supraspinatus, infraspinatus or subscapularis teno-osseous attachments, where it may be pinched as it passes under the coracoacromial arch before passing beyond and beneath it, out of harm's way. The painful arc is not usually found in isolation and positive findings on other tests will further incriminate the causative structure.

PASSIVE MOVEMENTS

Passive movements
■ Pain
■ Range
■ End-feel

Passive movements test the *inert structures* which include the joint capsule, joint menisci, ligaments, fascia, bursae, dura mater and the dural nerve root sleeve. Relaxed muscle and tendon can act as inert structures when they are stretched by their opposite passive movement. Passive movements principally give information on *pain, range* and *end-feel*.

The observation of pain and range of movement will be familiar to all clinicians working with soft tissue lesions. However, the notion of end-feel may be a new concept which is particularly valuable in the assessment of the soft tissues and is inherent in the orthopaedic medicine approach.

End-feel is the specific sensation imparted through the examiner's hands at the extreme of passive movement (Cyriax 1982, Cyriax & Cyriax 1983).

Normal end-feel

Normal end-feel
■ Hard
■ Soft
■ Elastic

Normal end-feel is divided into three categories: hard, soft and elastic. Normal bone-to-bone approximation, as in extension of the elbow, gives a characteristic *hard end-feel* to passive movement. A *soft end-feel* is characteristic of a stop to the movement brought about by approximation of tissue, as in passive knee or elbow flexion. An *elastic end-feel* is felt when the tissues are placed on a passive stretch and is the elastic resistance produced in the inert tissues at the end of range in normal joints. Examples are provided in stretching the end of range of lateral rotation at the shoulder or hip.

There may be a range of end-feels within the 'elastic' group, but all are indicative of normal tissue tension, such as the 'leathery' end-feel of passive pronation and supination of the forearm, or the even tighter 'rubbery' end-feel of ankle plantarflexion and wrist flexion where the resistance to the movement is in part provided by the tendons spanning the joint.

Pain is also a component at the end of range of normal movements, acting as a protection in preventing continuation of movement to the point of producing tissue damage.

Abnormal end-feel

Abnormal end-feel
■ Hard
■ Springy
■ Spasm
■ Empty

The sensation imparted in the abnormal end-feel falls into four categories: hard, springy, spasm and empty.

The cause of the abnormal *'hard'* end-feel is different from that of the normal hard bone-to-bone end-feel and it is a particular feature of the movements limited in arthritis.

In early arthritis, joint movement is initially limited by pain and involuntary muscle spasm halts the movement (Cyriax 1982). This involuntary muscle spasm provides a brake to the movement and feels 'hard' to the examiner. Certainly the end-feel feels harder than expected, but in the early stages some elasticity is preserved. Early arthritis of the hip, for example, may produce a 'hard' end-feel on either passive flexion or medial rotation but it should be emphasized that this is not caused by bony degenerative change blocking the joint movement. This difference is important as it aids the clinician in the selection of treatment techniques.

In more advanced arthritis, the 'hard' end-feel is also due to capsular contracture (Cyriax 1982). The capsular resistance together with the involuntary muscle spasm may still allow some 'give' at the end of range, but it will not feel as elastic as the earlier stage. In late arthritis, bony changes may occur, leading to a genuine hard end-feel and crepitus associated with advanced arthritis, as well as that arising from involuntary muscle spasm and capsular contracture.

An abnormal *springy end-feel* is associated with mechanical joint displacement, usually a loose body. The sensation imparted to the examiner is one of not quite getting to the end of range, with the joint springing or bouncing back. It is similar to the sensation of trying to close a door with a small piece of rubber or grit caught in the hinge which causes the door to spring back.

The abnormal end-feel associated with involuntary muscle spasm is different from that produced by voluntary muscle spasm. Voluntary muscle spasm comes in abruptly to halt the movement and indicates acute pain or serious pathology. If the pain is very severe it may also be associated with an empty end-feel.

An *empty end-feel* occurs where the examiner does not have the opportunity to appreciate the true end-feel because the patient calls a halt to the movement prematurely and urgently because of pain, often raising a hand to prevent further movement. The sensation imparted to the examiner is empty, as described, in that the complaint of serious pain comes on before any spasm or tissue resistance.

The empty end-feel is associated with serious pathology such as fracture, neoplasm or septic arthritis. A further cause may be a highly irritably lesion such as acute subacromial bursitis where the empty end-feel is instantly apparent on passive abduction of the shoulder.

The assessment of end-feel together with the restriction of movement at each joint produces a particular pattern which is either capsular or non-capsular.

The capsular pattern

> **Capsular pattern**
> - Indicates arthritis.
> - Varies from joint to joint.
> - Is limitation of movement in a fixed proportion.

The capsular pattern is a limitation of movement in a defined pattern which is specific to each joint and indicates the presence of an arthritis. The pattern varies from joint to joint and is characterized by limitation of movement in a fixed proportion. It is the same whatever the cause of the arthritis (Cyriax 1982, Cyriax & Cyriax 1983) and the history will suggest the form of arthritis, be it degenerative, inflammatory or traumatic (Table 1.1).

Characteristically, the movements restricted in the capsular pattern take on the 'hard' end-feel of arthritis, different from the expected normal elastic capsular resistance.

Table 1.1 Capsular pattern

Joint	Capsular pattern
The movements which become limited in the capsular pattern take on a characteristically 'hard' end-feel	
Shoulder joint	Most limitation of lateral rotation Less limitation of abduction Least limitation of medial rotation
Elbow joint	More limitation of flexion than extension
Radioulnar joints	Pain at end of range of both rotations
Wrist joint	Equal limitation of flexion and extension Eventual fixation in the mid-position
Trapezio-first metacarpal joint	Most limitation of extension
Metacarpophalangeal joints	Limitation of radial deviation and extension Joints fix in flexion and drift into ulnar deviation
Interphalangeal joints	Slightly more limitation of flexion than extension
Cervical spine	*Demonstrated by the cervical spine as a whole:* Equal limitation of side flexions Equal limitation of rotations Some limitation of extension Usually full flexion
Thoracic spine	*Demonstrated by the thoracic spine as a whole:* Equal limitation of rotations Equal limitation of side flexions Some limitation of extension Usually full flexion
Hip joint	Most limitation of medial rotation Less limitation of flexion and abduction Least limitation of extension
Knee joint	More limitation of flexion than extension
Ankle joint	More limitation of plantarflexion than dorsiflexion
Subtalar joint	Increasing limitation of supination Eventual fixation in pronation
Mid-tarsal joint	Limitation of adduction and supination Forefoot fixes in abduction and pronation
First metatarsophalangeal joint	Marked limitation of extension Some limitation of flexion
Other metatarsophalangeal joints	*May vary:* Tend to fix in extension
Interphalangeal joints	Fix in flexion
Lumbar spine	*Demonstrated by the lumbar spine as a whole:* Limitation of extension Equal limitation of side flexions Usually full flexion

The reason for the development of the capsular pattern could be the presence of joint effusion, causing the joint to assume the position of ease and/or protective muscle spasm (Eyring & Murray 1964). An effusion is often present in an arthritis and the acuteness of the condition determines the quantity of the effusion. Joints with symptomatic effusions are held in the position of ease mentioned above and movements out of this position produce pain.

Eyring & Murray (1964) noted a possible relationship between intra-articular pressure and pain. Experiments were conducted to determine the position of minimum pressure in various joints and it was observed that symptomatic joints with effusion spontaneously assume a position of minimum pressure, which coincides with that of minimum pain.

The involuntary muscle spasm, in protecting the painful, inflamed joint, prevents the use of the painful range of movement and if the range of movement is underused it will become limited. In arthritis, the individual joints resent some movements more than others, hence the capsule contracts disproportionately, making some movements more limited than others and giving rise to the characteristic pattern of limitation. For example, in the study conducted by Eyring & Murray the position of minimum pressure for the elbow was found to be between 30° and 70° of flexion. The pressure was not influenced by either pronation or supination. The capsular pattern of the elbow joint is proportionally more limitation of flexion than extension but without involvement of pronation or supination.

The capsular patterns described in Table 1.1 provide a useful guide to diagnosis of arthritis but research support is mixed. Pellecchia et al (1996) established that the Cyriax evaluation scheme was highly reliable in assessing patients with shoulder pain. Fritz et al (1998) found evidence to support the concept of the capsular pattern in the inflamed or osteoarthritic knee whereas although they established some support for the capsular pattern in the knee, Bijl et al (1998) were unable to recommend it as a valid test. No support for the capsular pattern at the hip was provided by the studies of Bijl et al (1998) and Klässbo et al (2003) and it is questioned by Sims (1999).

Non-capsular pattern

Non-capsular pattern
- Intra-articular displacement
- Ligamentous lesion
- Extra-articular lesion

The non-capsular pattern of a joint is, quite simply, anything other than the capsular pattern. That is, it is a limitation of movement that does not conform to the capsular pattern and occurs as a result of a component or part of the joint being affected rather than the whole joint.

A mechanical lesion such as an intra-articular displacement produces the non-capsular pattern which may be evident at the spinal joints with a herniation of discal material or locking of a zygapophyseal joint, and in a loose body at the elbow joint or a meniscal tear at the knee. A mechanical lesion in a degenerative joint may produce a non-capsular pattern superimposed on the capsular pattern.

A ligamentous lesion will give pain and possible limitation of the movement which stretches the structure. However, sprains of ligaments which form an integral part of the capsule itself, such as the anterior talofibular ligament of the ankle and the medial collateral ligament of the knee, cause a secondary capsulitis and hence a non-capsular pattern is superimposed on the capsular pattern.

Since a contractile unit can be stretched by passive movement, the unit may respond as an inert structure when relaxed, producing pain when it is stretched by the passive movement in opposition to its functional movement. For example, the subscapularis muscle and tendon which produce medial rotation at the shoulder will be stretched by passive lateral rotation. This is also particularly evident in acute tenosynovitis when the involved tendon is pulled through its inflamed synovial sheath. In acute tenosynovitis at the wrist, for example, pain will be produced on the appropriate resisted test and the opposite passive movement.

An extra-articular lesion such as a bursitis produces a non-capsular pattern and commonly presents as a 'muddle' of signs involving passive and resisted tests, when any movement which squeezes or stretches the inflamed bursa will produce positive signs.

RESISTED TESTS

> **Resisted tests**
> ■ Pain
> ■ Power

Resisted isometric muscle tests assess the *contractile unit* – comprising the muscle, musculotendinous junction, tendon and the teno-osseous attachment to bone – for *pain* and *power*. The tendon is not strictly a contractile structure but is tested as part of the functional contractile unit. When assessing the resisted tests it is important to look for reproduction of the patient's presenting pain and there are specific points to bear in mind which ensure that, as far as possible, only the contractile unit is being tested rather than the inert structures. It is accepted that, although joint movement may not be seen to occur, isometric muscle contraction will cause compression and joint shearing and, in the spinal joints, a rise in intradiscal pressure (Lamb 1994).

The joint should be placed in the mid-position with the inert structures relaxed so that no stress falls upon them. The muscle group is tested isometrically, as strongly as possible, so encouraging maximal voluntary contraction but without allowing movement to occur at the joint. This also ensures that minor lesions will be detected. Patient and examiner's body positioning should be such that all muscles not being tested are eliminated from the testing procedure.

Resisted tests may produce any of several findings, each of which has a different implication. The test may be:

- Strong and painless – normal
- Strong and painful – contractile lesion
- Weak and painless – neurological weakness
- Weak and painful – partial rupture or serious pathology such as fracture or bone tumour
- Painful on repetition – claudication or provocation of overuse injury
- All resisted tests about the joint painful or juddering – serious pathology, or marked psychosocial component

In addition to the active, passive and resisted tests, a brief neurological examination is included as part of the routine examination for a spinal joint, testing for root signs.

Having completed the subjective and objective examination sequence the causative structure, if not its pathology, will, in almost all cases, have been identified (Cyriax 1982, Cyriax & Cyriax 1983).

PALPATION

At this stage palpation of the structure determined to be at fault may be made to identify the site of the lesion to which appropriate treatment can be applied.

If the diagnosis is still unclear further tests may be added either mechanically, for example using techniques of neural tension tests, combined, repeated or accessory movements, or with the use of blood tests, X-rays, electromyograph (EMG) or scanning techniques, as mentioned above.

References

Adams M, Bogduk N, Burton K et al 2002 The biomechanics of back pain. Churchill Livingstone, Edinburgh

Aprill C, Dwyer A, Bogduk N 1989 Cervical apophyseal joint pain patterns II: a clinical evaluation. Spine 15:458–461

Beckman H B, Frankel R M 1984 The effect of physician behaviour on the collection of data. Annals of Internal Medicine 101:692–696

Bijl D, van Baar M E, Oostendorp R A B et al 1998 Validity of Cyriax's concept capsular pattern for the diagnosis of osteoarthritis of hip and/or knee. Scandinavian Journal of Rheumatology 27:347–351

Blau J N 1989 Time to let the patient speak. British Medical Journal 298:39

Bogduk N 1994 Innervation, pain patterns and mechanisms of pain production. In: Twomey L T (ed) Clinics in physical therapy, physical therapy of the low back, 2nd edn. Churchill Livingstone, Edinburgh, p 93–109

Bogduk N 1997 Clinical anatomy of the lumbar spine and sacrum, 3rd edn. Churchill Livingstone, Edinburgh

Butler D 1995 Moving in on pain. In: Shacklock M (ed) Moving in on pain. Butterworth Heinemann, Oxford p 8–12

Conesa S H, Argote M L 1976 A visual aid to the examination of nerve roots. Baillière Tindall, London

Cyriax J 1982 Textbook of orthopaedic medicine, 8th edn. Baillière Tindall, London, vol 1

Cyriax J, Cyriax P 1983 Illustrated manual of orthopaedic medicine. Butterworths, London

de Andrade J R, Grant C, Dixon A St J 1965 Joint distension and reflex muscle inhibition in the knee. Journal of Bone and Joint Surgery 47A: 313–322

Eyring E J, Murray W R 1964 The effect of joint position on the pressure of intraarticular effusion. Journal of Bone and Joint Surgery 46A:1235–1241

Foerster O 1933 The dermatomes in man. Brain 56:1–39

Fritz J M, Delitto A, Erhard R E et al 1998 An examination of the selective tissue tension scheme, with evidence for the concept of the capsular pattern at the knee. Physical Therapy 10:1046–1056

Galea M 2002 Neuroanatomy of the nociceptive system. In: Strong J, Unruh A M, Wright A et al (eds) Pain: a textbook for therapists. Churchill Livingstone, Edinburgh

Head H 1900 The pathology of herpes zoster and its bearing on sensory localization. Brain 16:353–523

Hunter D, Bomford R R 1963 Hutchison's Clinical methods, 14th edn. Baillière Tindall & Cassell, London

Inman V T, Saunders J B 1944 Referred pain from skeletal structures. Journal of Nervous and Mental Disease 99:660–667

Kellgren J H 1938 Observations on referred pain from muscle. Clinical Science 3:175–190

Kellgren J H 1939 On the distribution of pain arising from deep somatic structures with charts of segmental pain areas. Clinical Science 4:35–46

Kidd B L, Richardson P M 2002 How does neuropathophysiology affect the signs and symptoms of spinal disease? Best Practice and Research – Clinical Rheumatology 16(1):31–42

Klässbo M, Harms-Ringdahl K, Larsson G 2003 Examination of passive ROM and capsular patterns of the hip. Physiotherapy Research International 8(1):1–12

Kuslich S D, Ulstrom C L, Michael C J 1991 The tissue origin of low back pain and sciatica. Orthopaedic Clinics of North America 22:181–187

Lamb D W 1994 A review of manual therapy for spinal pain. In: Boyling J D, Palastanga N (eds) Grieve's Modern manual therapy, 2nd edn. Churchill Livingstone, Edinburgh

McMahon S B, Dmitrieva N, Koltzenburg M 1995 Visceral pain. British Journal of Anaesthesia 75:132–144

Mendelson G 1995 Psychological and psychiatric aspects of pain. In: Shacklock M (ed) Moving in on pain. Butterworth Heinemann, Oxford, p 66–89

O'Neill C W, Kurganky M E, Derby R et al 2002 Disc stimulation and patterns of referred pain. Spine 27(24): 2776–2781

Pellecchia G L, Paolino J, Connell J 1996 Intertester reliability of the Cyriax evaluation in assessing patients with shoulder pain. Journal of Orthopaedic and Sports Physical Therapy 23:34–38

Sameda H, Takahashi K, Takahashi T et al 2003 Dorsal root ganglion neurons with dichotomising afferent fibres to both the lumbar disc and groin skin: a possible neuronal mechanism underlying referred groin pain in lower lumbar disc diseases. Journal of Bone and Joint Surgery 85B(4):600–603

Sims K 1999 Assessment and treatment of hip osteoarthritis. Manual Therapy 4(3):136–144

Smyth M J, Wright V 1959 Sciatica and the intervertebral disc: an experimental study. Journal of Bone and Joint Surgery 40A:1401–1418

Travell J G, Simons D G 1996 Trigger point flipcharts. Lippincott, Williams & Wilkins, Philadelphia

Vecciet L, Giamberardino M A 1997 Referred pain: clinical significance, pathophysiology, and treatment. Physical Medicine and Rehabilitation Clinics of North America 8(1):119–136

Waddell G 1992 Understanding the patient with back pain. In: Jayson M (ed) The lumbar spine and back pain, 4th edn. Churchill Livingstone, Edinburgh, p 469–485

Waddell G 1998 The back pain revolution. Churchill Livingstone, Edinburgh

Wilkinson C 1989 Time to let the patient speak [letter]. British Medical Journal 298: 389

Williams P L 1998 Gray's Anatomy: the anatomical basis of medicine and surgery, 38th edn. Churchill Livingstone, Edinburgh

Witting N, Svensson P, Gottrup H et al 2000 Intramuscular and intradermal injection of capsaicin: a comparison of local and referred pain. Pain 84: 407–412

Chapter 2

Soft tissues of the musculoskeletal system

SUMMARY

Orthopaedic medicine is concerned with the examination, diagnosis and treatment of soft tissue lesions. In order to understand the relevant mechanisms of injury and repair and the rationale for treatment of soft tissue lesions, the soft tissues themselves need to be defined and examined. The principal soft tissues of orthopaedic medicine encompass the connective tissues, muscle tissue and nervous tissue. Within this chapter, basic histology and biomechanics of the soft tissues relevant to orthopaedic medicine will be studied to provide background knowledge for clinical practice.

CONNECTIVE TISSUE

The connective tissues form a large class of tissues responsible for providing tensile strength, substance, elasticity and density to the body, as well as facilitating nourishment and defence. Connective tissue has a major role in repair following trauma and a mechanical role in providing connection and leverage for movement, as well as preventing friction, pressure and shock between mobile structures. Connective tissue is the main focus of treatment procedures in orthopaedic medicine.

Connective tissue consists primarily of cells embedded in an extracellular matrix which is composed of fibres and an interfibrillar component – the amorphous ground substance (Fig. 2.1).

Not all types of connective tissue cell are found in each tissue, and the cell content can alter, with some cells being resident in the tissue and others brought to specific areas at times of need. Generally, the cells make up approximately 20% of the tissue volume and mainly consist of fibroblasts, macrophages and mast cells.

CONNECTIVE TISSUE CELLS

Fibroblasts

Fibroblasts, usually the most abundant of the connective tissue cells, are responsible for producing the contents of the extracellular matrix, namely fibres and amorphous ground substance. They are found lying close to the bundles of fibres they produce and are closely related to chondroblasts and osteoblasts, the cells responsible for producing

Figure 2.1 Irregular connective tissue, cellular and fibre content. Adapted from Cormack D 'Ham's Histology' © Lippincott Williams & Wilkins (1987) with permission.

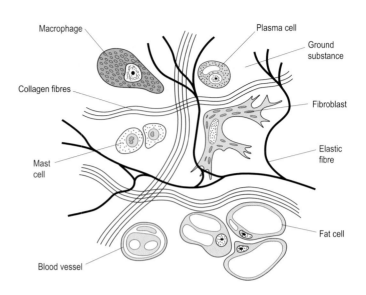

cartilage and bone matrix. The less active mature fibroblasts are known as fibrocytes.

Since fibroblasts produce the contents of the extracellular matrix, they play a key role in the repair process after injury. Stearns (1940b) observed that once fibre formation was initiated the fibroblast was able to produce an extensive network of fibrils in a remarkably short time.

Myofibroblasts are specialized cells which contain contractile filaments producing similar properties to smooth-muscle cells. They assist wound closure after injury.

Macrophages (histiocytes)

Macrophages may be resident in the connective tissues or circulating as monocytes which migrate to an area of injury and modulate into tissue macrophages (Fowler 1989). They are large cells that have two important roles. The first is phagocytosis and the second is to act as director cells, in which role they have a considerable influence on scar formation (Hardy 1989).

As a phagocyte, the macrophage acts as a housekeeper to the wound, ingesting cellular debris and subjecting it to lysosomal hydrolysis, thus debriding the wound in preparation for the fibroblasts to begin the repair process. Matter such as bacteria and cellular debris is engulfed by the phagocyte on contact.

As a director cell, the macrophage chemically activates the number of fibroblasts required for the repair process. Corticosteroids can inhibit the function of the macrophage in the early inflammatory stage, resulting in a delay in fibre production (Dingman 1973, Leibovich & Ross 1974, Fowler 1989). This should be taken into consideration when exploring treatment options in the early stage.

Clinical tip
Treatment techniques that agitate tissue fluid increase the chance contact of the macrophage with debris and can be applied during the early stages of inflammation to promote phagocytosis (Evans 1980), e.g. gentle transverse frictions and grade A mobilization (see Ch. 4) as well as heat, ice, ultrasound, pulsed electromagnetic energy, etc.

Mast cells

Mast cells are large, round cells containing secretory granules that manufacture a number of active ingredients including heparin, histamine and possibly serotonin. The contents of the mast cell granules are released in response to mechanical or chemical trauma and they therefore play a role in the early stages of inflammation. Heparin temporarily prevents coagulation of the excess tissue fluid and blood components in the injured area while histamine causes a brief vasodilatation in the neighbouring non-injured area (Wilkerson 1985, Hardy 1989). Serotonins are internal nociceptive substances released during platelet aggregation in response to tissue damage. They cause contraction of blood vessels and activate pain signals (Kapit et al 1987).

EXTRACELLULAR MATRIX

The extracellular matrix accounts for about 80% of the total tissue volume, with approximately 30% of its substance being solids and the remaining 70% being water. It consists of fibres and the interfibrillar amorphous ground substance, the substances responsible for supporting and nourishing the cells. The amorphous ground substance also determines the connective tissue's compliance, mobility and integrity.

The fibrous portion of connective tissue is responsible for determining the tissue's biomechanical properties. Two major groups of fibres exist: collagen fibres and elastic fibres.

Collagen fibres

Collagen is a protein in the form of fibre and is the body's 'glue'. It possesses two major properties, great tensile strength and relative inextensibility, and forms the major fibrous component of connective tissue structures, i.e. tendons, ligaments, fascia, sheaths, bursae, bone and cartilage.

Individual collagen fibres are normally mobile within the amorphous ground substance, producing discrete shear and gliding movement as well as dealing with compression and tension. Collagen is also the main constituent of scar tissue, in which it demonstrates its great versatility by attempting to mimic the structure it replaces.

Collagen fibres are large in diameter and appear to be white in colour. They are arranged in bundles and do not branch or anastomose. They are flexible but inelastic individually. The arrangement and weave of individual collagen fibres and collagen fibre bundles give the connective tissue structure elastic qualities; for example, an individual piece of nylon thread is inelastic, but when woven to produce tights, the weave gives the material elasticity (Peacock 1966). Collagen fibre bundles elongate under tension to their physiological length and recoil when tension is released.

The bundles of fibres are laid down parallel to the lines of the main mechanical stress, often in a wavy, sinusoidal or undulating configuration. This gives the tissue an element of crimp when not under tension. Crimp provides a buffer so that longitudinal elongation can occur without damage, as well as acting as a shock absorber along the length of the tissue, to control tension (Amiel et al 1990).

Collagen fibres are strong under tensile loading but weak under compressive forces, when they have a tendency to buckle. The orientation of the collagen fibres determines the properties that a structure will have. Crimp patterns are dependent upon function and therefore differ in different tissues, i.e. the arrangement of collagen fibres perpendicular to the surface in articular cartilage provides a cushioning force for weight-bearing while the parallel arrangement in tendons provides great tensile strength for transmitting loads and resisting pull. Crimp patterns may also vary between different ligaments and different tendons.

Production and structure of collagen fibres and collagen cross–linking

Procollagen, the first step in collagen fibre formation, is produced intracellularly by the fibroblast. Amino acids are assembled to form polypeptide chains, which are attracted and held together by weak intramolecular hydrogen bonds known as *cross-links* (Fig. 2.2). Three polypeptide chains bond to form a procollagen molecule in the form of a triple helix which is exocytosed by the fibroblast into the extracellular space.

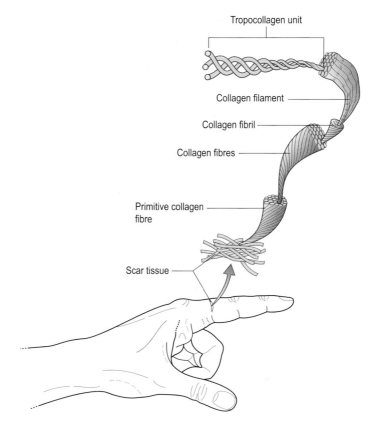

Figure 2.2   Collagen aggregation. Reprinted from Hardy M The Biology of Scar Formation. Physical Therapy (1989) 69 (12): 1014–1024, with permission.

Tropocollagen unit

Collagen filament

Collagen fibril

Collagen fibres

Primitive collagen fibre

Scar tissue

Figure 2.3   Intramolecular cross-links. Reprinted from Hardy M The Biology of Scar Formation. Physical Therapy (1989) 69 (12): 1014–1024, with permission.

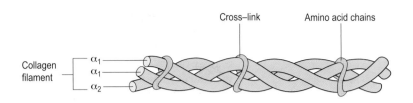

Figure 2.4   Intermolecular cross-links. Reprinted from Hardy M The Biology of Scar Formation. Physical Therapy (1989) 69 (12): 1014–1024, with permission.

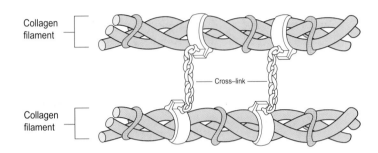

Clinical tip
Transverse frictions and mobilization techniques used in orthopaedic medicine aim to mobilize the reducible and mature scar tissue cross-links.

Once outside the cell the chains are known as tropocollagen molecules and several tropocollagen molecules become bonded by intermolecular cross-links to form a filament or microfibril (Fig. 2.3). With the maturation into tropocollagen, the cross-links are stronger covalent bonds and occur at specific nodal intercept points, making the structure more stable (Nimni 1980, Donatelli & Owens-Burkhart 1981, Hardy 1989). Cross-links exist at every level of organization of collagen acting to weld the units together into a rope-like structure (Fig. 2.4). Intermolecular cross-linking in particular gives collagen its great tensile strength as it matures. The greater the intermolecular cross-linking the stronger the collagen structure, with bone being considered to be the most highly cross-linked tissue (Hardy 1989).

Collagen turnover, the dynamic state of the tissue, may be related to the number of cross-links with fibres being continuously and simultaneously produced and broken down. When collagen production exceeds breakdown, more cross-links develop and the structure resists stretching. If collagen breakdown exceeds production there is a reduction in the number of cross-links and the structure stretches more easily (Alter 2000). Immature collagen tissue possesses reducible cross-links and as collagen matures these reducible links stabilize to form stronger non-reducible cross-links. Excessive cross-link formation can be prevented in immature scar tissue by the application of transverse frictions and graded mobilization techniques. Established cross-links in adhesive scar tissue are mobilized by transverse frictions before the longitudinal orientation of the fibres can be encouraged through the application of graded stress. In some instances manipulative rupture of adhesive scar tissue is indicated (see Ch. 3).

Many microfibrils make up a collagen fibril and many collagen fibrils make up a collagen fibre. Collagen fibres continue to aggregate together into larger and larger bundles and the production, aggregation and orientation of collagen are strongly influenced by mechanical tension and stress. Bundles of collagen are arranged in a specific pattern to accommodate to the function of each individual connective tissue structure (Chamberlain 1982).

It has been shown that when fibroblasts grown in tissue culture are subjected to regional tension, the cells exposed to the tensile forces multiply more rapidly and orient themselves in parallel lines in the direction of the tension (Le Gros Clark 1965).

Stearns (1940a, 1940b) identified that internal and external mechanical factors influence fibre orientation. Cell movement and occasional cytoplasmic retraction produced early local orientation of fibres, while a period of secondary orientation of fibres into heavy parallel layers was probably the result of external mechanical factors. This secondary orientation of fibres appeared to take place during the remodelling phase of wound healing and is the way in which soft tissue structures develop in response to intermittent stress and mechanical tension.

Immobilization produces rapid changes of collagen tissue as it adapts to its new resting length. Collagen which develops in the absence of mechanical stress (i.e. in the absence of movement) has a random orientation, a change in the numbers and thickness of the fibres and loss of ground substance. This reduction in the lubricating interfibular gel allows greater adherence at the fibre–fibre interface (Hardy & Woodall 1998).

Collagen takes on many forms and functions. In tendons it is tough and inelastic, in cartilage it is resilient, while in bone it is hard. This difference in structure is related to the diameter, orientation and concentration of the fibres. Collagen fibres have been classified into groups (Nimni 1980). The most common form is type I collagen consisting of large diameter fibres, found abundantly in structures subjected to tensile forces. Type II collagen consists of a mixture of large and narrow diameter fibres and is abundant in structures subjected to pressure or compressive forces. Reticulin is considered to be a delicate supporting network of fragile type III collagen fibres; it may be present in the earliest stages of soft tissue repair.

Clinical tip
The influence of mechanical stress and tension on collagen alignment can be used to advantage in orthopaedic medicine during the repair process, when collagen fibres are initially laid down in the early repair phase and in the later remodelling phase of healing. In order to promote tissue gliding and to regain tissue length the use of graded mobilization techniques are advocated.

Elastic fibres

Elastic fibres, consisting of the protein elastin, are yellow in colour and much thinner and less wavy than collagen fibres. Elastic fibres run singly, never in bundles, and freely branch and anastomose.

Elastic fibres provide the tissue with extensibility so that it can be extended in all directions but if tension is constantly exerted in one direction the elastic fibres may be laid down in sheets known as lamellae, e.g. ligamentum flavum (the 'yellow ligament'). Elastic fibres make up some of the connective tissue fibres of ligaments, joint capsules, fascia and connective tissue sheaths.

Amorphous ground substance

The interfibrillar amorphous ground substance with its fibrous content comprises the connective tissue extracellular matrix. As well as maintaining the mobility and integrity of the tissue structure at a macrostructural level, it is responsible for nourishing the living cells by facilitating the diffusion of gases, nutrients and waste products between the cells and capillaries.

It contains carbohydrate bound to protein (Williams 1998). The carbohydrate is in the form of polysaccharides, hexuronic acid and amino sugars, alternately linked to form long-chain molecules called glycosaminoglycans (GAGs). The main GAGs in connective tissue matrix are hyaluronic acid, chondroitin-4-sulphate, chondroitin-6-sulphate and dermatan sulphate (Donatelli & Owens-Burkhart 1981).

When GAGs are covalently bonded to proteins, the molecules are called proteoglycans (Cormack 1987). These proteoglycan molecules have the property of attracting and retaining water (Bogduk 1997). This hydration of structures depends on the proportion of proteoglycans and the flow of water into the extracellular matrix. Increased hydration creates rigidity in the extracellular matrix, allowing it to exist as a semisolid substance or gel, which improves the tissue's ability to resist compressive forces. Therefore tissues which are subjected to high compressive forces, such as bone and articular cartilage, have a high proteoglycan content. The proteoglycans also form a supporting substance for the fibre and cellular components. Decreased hydration allows it to exist as a viscous semisolution or sol, which improves the tissue's ability to resist tensile forces. Therefore tissues which are subjected to high tensile forces, such as tendons and ligaments, have a low proteoglycan concentration (Levangie & Norkin 2001).

The concentration of GAGs present in tissues is related to their function and gives connective tissue structures viscous properties. More water is associated with a higher GAG concentration and rabbit ligamentous tissue has a significantly greater water content than that in rabbit tendinous tissue (Amiel et al 1982). This increase in GAG and water content alters the viscoelastic properties and may provide the ligament with an additional shock-absorbing feature that is unnecessary in most tendons.

The amorphous ground substance forms a lubricant, filler and spacing buffer system between collagen fibres, fibrils, microfibrils and the intercellular spaces (Akeson et al 1980). It reduces friction and maintains distance between fibres as well as facilitating the discrete shear and gliding movement of individual collagen fibres and fibrils. It is the lubrication and spacing at the fibre–fibre interface that are crucial to the gliding function at nodal intercept points where the fibres cross in the tissue matrices (Amiel et al 1982). If the tissues are allowed to adopt a stationary attitude (i.e. becoming immobile), anomalous cross-links form at the nodal intercept points.

A balance between the cross-link formation relative to the tissue's tensile strength and mobility is important to normal connective tissue function. Excessive cross-linking and loss of GAGs and water volume results in loss of the critical distance between the fibres. The fibres come

Clinical tip

The aim in orthopaedic medicine is to maintain normal connective tissue mobility through the phases of acute inflammation, repair and remodeling, and to regain mobility in the chronic inflammatory situation. This mobility is essential to function and the bias of orthopaedic medicine treatment techniques is towards preserving the mobility of connective tissue structures.

into contact with each other and stick together leading to altered tissue function and pain resulting from loss of extensibility and increased stiffness.

The elasticity of connective tissue fibres together with the viscosity of the amorphous ground substance gives connective tissue structures viscoelastic properties that ensure that normal connective tissues are mobile.

The biomechanical properties of connective tissue depend on the number and orientation of collagen fibres and the proportion of amorphous ground substance present. Each connective tissue structure is specifically designed for function but the tissues can be grouped simply into irregular and regular connective tissue.

IRREGULAR CONNECTIVE TISSUE

Irregular connective tissue consists of a mixture of collagen and elastic fibres interwoven to form a loose meshwork that can withstand stress in any direction. Its main function is to support and protect regular connective tissue structures.

The following examples of irregular connective tissue are commonly encountered in orthopaedic medicine.

The *dura mater* is the outermost of three irregular connective tissue sleeves which enclose the brain and the spinal cord. It is extended to form the dural nerve root sleeve that invests the nerve roots within the intervertebral foramen. At or just beyond the intervertebral foramen the dural nerve root sleeve fuses with the epineurium of the nerve root. The dura mater and dural nerve root sleeve extensions are formed of sheets of collagen and elastic fibres providing a tough but loose fibrous tube. The dura mater is separated from the bony margins of the vertebral canal by the epidural space that contains fat, loose connective tissue and a venous plexus. These structures are mobile in a non-pathological state and can accommodate normal movement (Netter 1987, Williams 1998, Palastanga et al 2002). Adhesions may develop in the dura mater and dural nerve root sleeve, compromising this mobility and giving rise to clinical symptoms.

An *aponeurosis* is a sheet of fibrous tissue that increases the tendinous attachment to bone. It distributes the tendon forces, increasing the tendon's mechanical advantage, and needs to retain mobility in its attachment to perform its function.

The *epimysium* is a layer of irregular connective tissue surrounding the whole muscle; the *perimysium* surrounds the fascicles within the muscle; and the *endomysium* surrounds each individual muscle fibre. In a similar arrangement, a fibrous sheath, the *epineurium*, surrounds each nerve; the *perineurium* surrounds each fascicle; and each individual nerve fibre is invested in a delicate sheath of vascular loose connective tissue, the *endoneurium*. Since connective tissue mobility is important to the function of muscle, its arrangement in nerve structure implies that it is also important to the function of nervous tissue.

The *paratenon* is an irregular connective tissue fibroelastic sheath, adherent to the outer surface of all tendons. It is composed of relatively large amounts of proteoglycans to provide a gliding surface around the tendon, allowing it to move freely among other tissues with a minimum of drag (Merrilees & Flint 1980). True tendon synovial sheaths are found most commonly in the hand and foot where they act to reduce friction between the tendon and surrounding tissues. The synovial sheath consists of two layers, an outer fibrotic sheath and an inner synovial sheath which has parietal and visceral layers. Between these two layers is an enclosed space containing a thin film of synovial fluid. The synovial sheath may also assist in tendon nutrition (Józsa & Kannus 1997).

Like the synovial tendon sheaths, *bursae*, flat synovial sacs, also prevent friction and pressure and facilitate movement between adjacent connective tissue structures. Bursae can be subcutaneous (e.g. the olecranon bursa), subtendinous (e.g. psoas bursa), sub- or intermuscular (e.g. gluteal bursa), or adventitious – developing in response to trauma or pressure (e.g. subcutaneous Achilles bursa).

Fascia lies in sheets to facilitate movement between the various tissue planes. *Deep fascia* has a more regular formation as it forms a tight sleeve to retain structures, adds to the contours of the limbs and is extended to form the intermuscular septa. It provides a compressive force which facilitates venous return and may act as a mechanical barrier preventing the spread of infection.

Fascia may develop *retinacula* which hold tendons in place, preventing a bowstring effect on movement, e.g. the retinacula at the ankle. It may produce thickenings forming protective layers such as the *palmar* and *plantar aponeuroses*, or it may form envelopes to enclose and protect major neurovascular bundles, e.g. the femoral sheath in the femoral triangle.

> *Clinical tip*
> Tissue injury involves the surrounding and supporting irregular connective tissue as well as the regular connective tissue structure itself. It is therefore important to recognize the extensive nature of irregular connective tissue and its close relationship with the regular connective tissue structures encountered in orthopaedic medicine.

REGULAR CONNECTIVE TISSUE

In contrast to irregular connective tissue, this group of tissues has a highly organized structure with fibres running in the same linear direction in a precise arrangement that is related to function. The main collagen fibre bundles will be aligned parallel to the line of major mechanical stress, which functionally suits such structures as tendons and ligaments that are mainly subjected to unidirectional stress (Donatelli & Owens-Burkhart 1981).

The following examples of regular connective tissue are commonly encountered in orthopaedic medicine.

TENDONS

Muscles and tendons are distinct tissues, although they functionally act as one structure, the contractile unit. The tendon cells are derived from the embryonic mesenchyme, the tissue occupying the areas between the embryonic layers, classifying tendon as a connective tissue (Williams 1998).

Functions of tendons
- To attach a muscle to bone.
- To transmit the force of muscle contraction to the bone to produce functional movement.
- To set the muscle belly in the optimum position for functional movement and to affect the direction of muscle pull.
- To be able to glide within the surrounding tissues, accepting stress and tensile forces with minimal drag.

Muscle cells are derived from mesoderm, the intermediate embryonic layer, such that muscle itself belongs to a separate tissue group.

The tendon is an inert structure which does not contract, but as part of the contractile unit it is directly involved in muscle action. Therefore the tendon is assessed by resisted testing via the muscle belly. Active movement does not produce transverse movement within the tendon but its fibrous structure may be moved passively by transverse frictions, to prevent or to mobilize adhesions.

Tendons are exposed to strong, unidirectional forces and to function they require great tensile strength and inelastic properties. They are able to withstand much greater tensile forces than ligaments and are composed of closely packed parallel bundles of collagen microfibrils, fibrils and fibres, bound together by irregular connective tissue sheaths into larger bundles (Fig. 2.5). Most fibres are orientated in one direction, parallel to the long axis, which is the direction of normal physiological stress (Alter 2000). Tendons do not usually contain any elastic fibres since their muscle belly acts as an energy damper such that elastic fibres are not required (Akeson 1990).

The fibres are large-diameter type I collagen, well-suited to accept tensile forces. The proteoglycans are packed in between the fibres and because the tendon is so compact, there is little room for the tendon cells or an adequate blood supply. The tendon's blood vessels lie in the epitenon (adherent to the surface of the tendon) and the endotenon (a division between collagen fibre bundles) (Gelberman et al 1983).

As mentioned above, tendons are surrounded by a fibroelastic paratenon functioning as an elastic sleeve to facilitate their gliding properties and permitting free movement in the surrounding tissues. Under the paratenon, the entire tendon is surrounded by the thin connective tissue sheath of the epitenon; the two together are sometimes referred to as the peritendon. On its inner surface the epitenon is continuous with the endotenon which invests each tendon fibre (Józsa & Kannus 1997).

The *musculotendinous junction* is the area where tension generated in the muscle fibres is transmitted from intracellular contractile proteins to extracellular connective tissue proteins. It is a relatively weak area making it susceptible to injury (Józsa & Kannus 1997).

The *teno-osseous junction* is the point of insertion of the tendon into the bone where the viscoelastic tendon transmits force to the rigid bone.

Figure 2.5   Structure of a tendon.

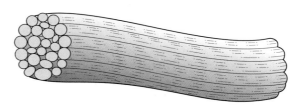

At this point the tendon goes though a transition from tendon to fibrocartilage, mineralized fibrocartilage and finally bone. The mechanism of overuse injuries involving the teno-osseous junction is not well understood. Repetitive strain reduces the ability of the tendon to endure further tension disrupting the microscopic and macroscopic structure of the tendon. Inflammation (i.e. tendinopathy or peritendinitis) may be the initial clinical finding of tendon overuse and if this progresses, focal degeneration (i.e. tendinosis), partial and complete tears may follow (Józsa & Kannus 1997). However, Khan & Cook (2000) and Cook et al (2000) critically reviewed the inflammatory model of tendon pain and found that it does not withstand scrutiny. Instead the pathology is thought to be degenerative – i.e. tendinosis, with collagen fibre breakdown, increased ground substance and neovascularization in the absence of inflammation. The term 'tendinopathy' is suggested to indicate painful overuse tendon conditions without implying pathology, reserving the terms 'tendinosis', 'paratendinitis' and 'tendinitis' as histopathological labels. For this reason *tendinopathy* will be used throughout this text to indicate painful overuse tendon lesions.

Tenosynovitis occurs in ensheathed tendons and involves the synovium rather than the tendon itself. Inflammation of the synovium can produce adhesions between the two layers of the sheath which may produce a palpable crepitus (Cyriax 1982). Adhesion formation interferes with the normal function of the tendon sheath, which is to allow controlled movement of the sheath around the tendon and to facilitate nutrition by forcing synovial fluid into the tendon (Barlow & Willoughby 1992).

Tenovaginitis is a term used to describe thickening of the synovial sheath (Cyriax 1982) and is associated with chronic tenosynovitis, e.g. de Quervain's stenosing tenosynovitis of the sheath containing the abductor pollicis longus and extensor pollicis brevis tendons.

As with all other connective tissues structures, tendons remodel in response to mechanical demand and they are sensitive and responsive to changes in physical load, a property which may be demonstrated by a difference in structure within one tendon unit. Merrilees & Flint (1980) looked at the macrostructural features of different regions of the flexor digitorum profundus tendon in the rat. This tendon, in common with most tendons, is subjected to longitudinal stress throughout its length, but it also possesses a sesamoid-like area as it passes under the calcaneum and talus. In this area the tendon is subjected to compressive forces, as well as to the normal longitudinal stress.

In the zone subjected to tension, the collagen fibres were arranged in longitudinal bundles, but in the zone subjected to pressure, the sesamoid-like area took on a form similar to that of fibrocartilage, i.e. a loose weave of collagen fibres and chondrocyte-like cells arranged in columns perpendicular to the main fibre axis.

This illustrates the ability of connective tissue structures to adapt to different functions and to changes in physical loads in a normal situation. In abnormal situations, such as a period of immobility when physical demand is reduced, adaptations in collagen turnover occur. When physical demand is increased, collagen production increases. The

Clinical tip

In order to maintain or restore the gliding properties of the tendon within its synovial sheath, transverse frictions are applied with the tendon on the stretch. This position allows the therapist to roll the sheath over a firm tendon base, imitating the function of the tendon sheath.

turnover (synthesis and lysis) of collagen is a continuing process allowing the remodelling and adaptation of structures to suit demand.

LIGAMENTS AND JOINT CAPSULES

> **Properties of ligaments and joint capsules**
> - Flexibility, requiring elastic properties, to allow normal movement to occur at a joint.
> - Resilience, requiring tensile strength, to be tough and unyielding to excessive movement at a joint.

The joint capsule and its supporting ligaments are similar in function, both allowing and restraining movement at the joints. Ligaments can be considered to be a reinforcement of the joint capsule in an area of special stress. As inert tissue structures they are assessed by passive movements which should be applied at the extremes of range to test function.

The ligaments, together with the fibrous capsule, guide and stabilize the articular surfaces. When excessive stresses are applied to a joint, proprioceptive impulses recruit a muscle response so that the passive stabilizing effect of the ligament is reinforced by dynamic muscle stabilization (Akeson et al 1987).

To meet its functional requirements of resisting shear as well as tensile and compressive forces, the structure of a ligament will be different from that of a tendon. The main ligamentous fibres are 70–80% collagen laid down in bundles, which assume a wavy configuration providing an element of elongation and recoil to facilitate movement (Fig. 2.6). Interwoven with these main fibre bundles are 3–5% elastic fibres, to enhance extensibility and elasticity (Akeson et al 1987). When ligaments are put under longitudinal tensile stress the parallel wavy bundles of

Figure 2.6 Structure of a ligament. Adapted from Nordin M & Frankel V H 'Basic Biomechanics of the Musculoskeletal System' © Lippincott Williams & Wilkins (1989) with permission.

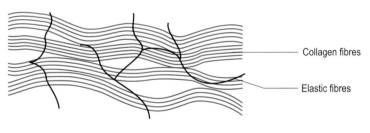

Collagen fibres

Elastic fibres

Crimp pattern in a relaxed ligament

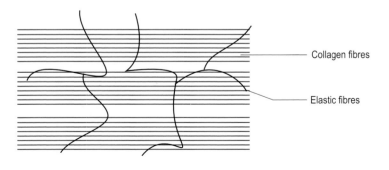

Collagen fibres

Elastic fibres

Crimp straightened under tension

collagen straighten out to prevent excessive movement and to provide tensile strength.

Although the joint capsule is similar in function to ligaments, its structure is slightly different. The capsule consists of sheets of collagen fibres which form a fibrous cuff joining opposing bony surfaces. The fibrous structure is predominantly collagen but, rather than a parallel array of fibres, its pattern is more a criss-cross weave, with the fibres becoming more parallel as the capsule is loaded (Fig. 2.7) (Amiel et al 1990, Woo et al 1990). The ability of the fibres to change and straighten depends on them being mobile and able to slide independently of one another. Capsular contractures in the form of disorganized collagen will prevent independent fibre gliding at the nodal intercept points, considerably reducing function and causing pain.

The joint capsule has two layers: an outer fibrous capsule and an internal synovial membrane. The outer fibrous capsule is strong and flexible but relatively inelastic. It is supported functionally by its ligaments which may be intrinsic, forming an integral part of the joint capsule (e.g. coronary and medial collateral ligaments of the knee), or accessory, being either intracapsular (e.g. the cruciate ligaments) or extracapsular (e.g. lateral collateral ligaments of the knee). The fibrous

Figure 2.7   Structure of the joint capsule.

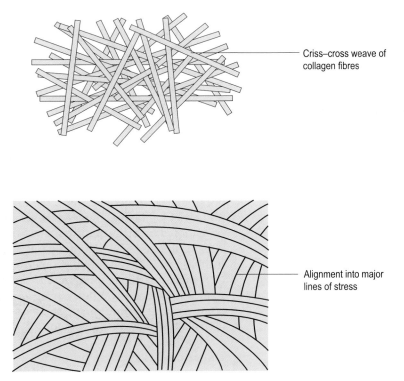

Criss–cross weave of collagen fibres

Alignment into major lines of stress

capsule is perforated by vessels and nerves and contains afferent sensory nerve endings, including mechanoreceptors and nociceptors.

The synovial membrane is mainly a loose connective tissue membrane with a degree of elasticity to prevent its folds and villi becoming nipped during movement. It covers all surfaces within the joint except the articular surfaces themselves and menisci. Adipose fat pads may exist in the joint, acting as shock absorbers, and distinct fringes of synovium may be present, e.g. the plicae of the knee joint. These folds, fringes and villi allow the joints to accommodate to movement.

The synovium is a highly cellular membrane containing synoviocytes, i.e. the synovium-producing cells, and collagen fibres. It has a rich nerve, blood and lymphatic supply. A capillary network is situated on the inner surface of the synovium to produce synovial fluid. Synovial fluid is pale yellow and viscous. It lubricates the ligamentous structures of the joint and nourishes cartilage and menisci through a mechanism of transsynovial flow aided by movement (Akeson et al 1987).

In an arthritis of a joint, the inflammation causes pain and involuntary muscle spasm which prevents full range of movement. The relative immobility causes changes to occur in the connective tissue which lead to capsular contracture, further loss of function and pain. This will be seen clinically as the capsular pattern.

> *Clinical tip*
> Trauma can cause a haemarthrosis and the difference between this and a trauma-induced synovial effusion is indicated clinically by the immediate onset of swelling as a result of bleeding into the joint, as opposed to the more slowly developing synovial effusion, sometimes over several hours.

CARTILAGE

Cartilage is a weight-bearing connective tissue displaying a combination of rigidity, which is resistant to compression, resilience and some elasticity. It is relatively avascular and relies on tissue fluid for nourishment. There are three main types:

1. Elastic cartilage
2. Fibrocartilage
3. Hyaline cartilage.

Elastic cartilage consists of a matrix of yellow elastic fibres and is very resilient. It is found in the external ear, the epiglottis and the larynx.

Fibrocartilage has a large proportion of type I collagen fibres in its matrix, providing it with great tensile strength. Examples are the annulus fibrosus of the intervertebral discs, the menisci of the knee joint, the acetabular and glenoid labra, the articular disc of the acromioclavicular and wrist joints, the lining of the grooves which house tendons, and as a transitional cartilage at the teno-osseous junction of the tendons (Cormack 1987, Williams 1998, Palastanga et al 2002). The annulus fibrosus in the lumbar spine has a unique geometrical pattern of collagen fibres.

Hyaline cartilage is *articular cartilage*. Its relatively solid gel-like matrix provides a weight-bearing surface which is elastic and resistant to compression. It moulds to the shape of the bones, presenting a smooth articular surface for movement.

Hyaline articular cartilage is composed of scantily deposited chondroblasts and chondrocytes which produce the gel extracellular matrix consisting of type II collagen fibres and amorphous ground substance. The extracellular matrix contains distinctive large

Figure 2.8   Proteoglycan complex of hyaline cartilage. Adapted from 'Gray's Anatomy' by P L Williams by permission of Elsevier Ltd.

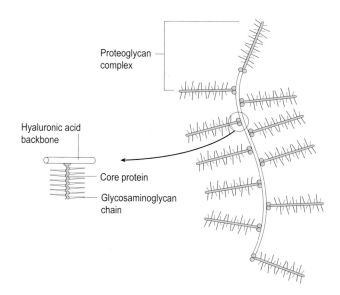

Proteoglycan complex

Hyaluronic acid backbone

Core protein

Glycosaminoglycan chain

supermolecular proteoglycan aggregates which resemble bottle brushes (Fig. 2.8). These provide a network for trapping and retaining water which significantly contributes to the resilience of cartilage (Cormack 1987). The collagen fibres themselves are relatively weak under compression, therefore the water-enhanced matrix compensates for this by providing a resilient weight-bearing surface.

Three separate structural zones exist in hyaline articular cartilage which contribute to its biomechanical functions (Nordin & Frankel 2001). A superficial zone is approximately 10–20% of the total thickness of the cartilage and helps to prevent friction between the joint surfaces and to distribute the compressive forces. It consists of fine, tangential, densely packed fibres lying in a plane parallel to the articular surface (Fig. 2.9). A middle, vertical zone is approximately 40–60% of the total thickness with the cells arranged in vertical columns, perpendicular to the surface, with scattered collagen fibres. The middle layer allows deformation of the collagen fibres absorbing some of the compressive forces. The deep zone is approximately 30% of the total thickness and forms a transition between the articular cartilage and the underlying calcified cartilage layer. The fibres are arranged in radial bundles. Hyaline articular cartilage has no blood vessels and depends on fluid flow through compressive forces for nutrition. This fluid flow depends on the magnitude and duration of the compressive force and a balance of weight-bearing and non-weight-bearing is important to its health (Levangie & Norkin 2001).

The zonal arrangement of cartilage provides a 'well-sprung mattress' arrangement to cope with compression forces. The variation in collagen fibre orientation in each zone enables the articular cartilage to vary its material property with direction of the load.

Figure 2.9   Zonal arrangement of articular cartilage. Adapted from Nordin and Frankel (1989).

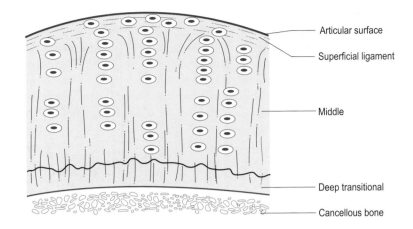

Articular surface

Superficial ligament

Middle

Deep transitional

Cancellous bone

Clinical tip
Articular cartilage requires movement for nutrition and to maintain fluid levels within its matrix in order to withstand compressive forces. Prolonged loading reduces fluid levels in the matrix through the action of tissue creep which may lead to degenerative changes. It is essential therefore to maintain mobilization of inflamed or degenerate joints.

The fluid content of articular cartilage is responsible for its nutrition as well as its mechanical properties, allowing diffusion of nutrients and products between the cells and the synovial fluid. When cartilage is loaded, the fluid in the 'sponge' moves, which is important for the mechanical properties of the cartilage as well as for joint lubrication. Intermittent loading creates a pumping effect but prolonged loading will eventually press fluid out of the cartilage without allowing new fluid to be taken up, leading to degeneration.

MUSCLE

Clinical tip
Connective tissue mobility is important to normal muscle function. Although skeletal muscles have some regenerating properties, healing of large muscle belly lesions is largely through the formation of scar tissue. Disorganized scar tissue alters function and acts as a physical barrier to regenerating muscle fibres.

Muscle tissue is a separate tissue group responsible for contraction and functional movement. It consists of cells known as muscle fibres due to their long, narrow shape.

Muscle has a large connective tissue component which supplies its nutrients for its metabolism and facilitates contraction by providing a continuous connective tissue harness. This continuous harness consists of the epimysium, perimysium and endomysium (Fig. 2.10). Each end of the harness is continuous with strong connective tissue structures which anchor it to its attachments.

Skeletal muscle is of obvious concern in orthopaedic medicine and following trauma it is capable of some regenerating properties. However, large muscle belly lesions due to major trauma will be filled with a mixture of disorganized scar tissue and new muscle fibres.

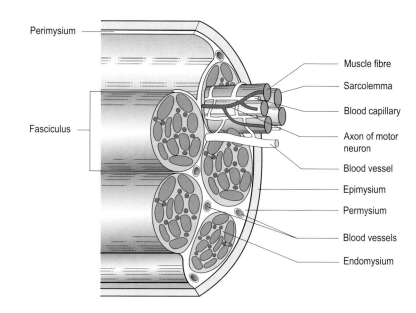

Figure 2.10   Connective tissue component of skeletal muscle. From Anatomy and Human Movement by N Palastanga D Field and R Soames. Reprinted by permission of Elsevier Ltd.

Perimysium

Fasciculus

Muscle fibre

Sarcolemma

Blood capillary

Axon of motor neuron

Blood vessel

Epimysium

Permysium

Blood vessels

Endomysium

NERVOUS TISSUE

Clinical tip
Connective tissue mobility is essential to the normal function of the central and peripheral nervous systems. Compression of any part of the system or reduction in connective tissue mobility will compromise function.

Nervous tissue is designed for the conduction of nerve impulses and initiation of function. The central nervous system is largely devoid of connective tissue, being made up of specialized tissue held together by neuroglia. Three connective tissue meninges (pia mater, arachnoid mater and dura mater) and the cerebrospinal fluid protect the system inside its bony framework.

The peripheral nervous system is not as delicate, with connective tissue constituting part of the nerves, providing strength and resilience. The epineurium is an outer connective tissue sheath enclosing large nerves. The perineurium surrounds each fascicle or bundle of nerve fibres and the endoneurium invests each individual nerve fibre.

BEHAVIOUR OF CONNECTIVE TISSUES TO MECHANICAL STRESS

Excessive mechanical stress is responsible for connective tissue injury and manual techniques utilize mechanical stresses to mobilize, permanently elongate or rupture scar tissue, where the adhesions formed are preventing full painless function. Understanding the mechanical response of connective tissue structures to stress is helpful in interpreting mechanisms of injury and rationalizing treatment programmes. However, it should be appreciated that most experimental evidence has been derived from animal and cadaveric specimens in the laboratory setting, and the physical principles have been adapted in order to explain the mechanical properties demonstrated. Connective tissue can change its structure and function in response to applied forces by altering the composition of the extracellular matrix, demonstrating its dynamic nature and the relationship between form and function (Levangie & Norkin 2001).

The *stress*, or *load*, is the mechanical force applied to the tissue. The *strain* is the resultant deformation produced by the applied stress.

The *stress–strain curve* is a way of illustrating the reaction of connective tissue structures to loading (Fig. 2.11). Experimentally, a tensile stress is applied to collagen until it ruptures. The applied stress or elongating force is plotted on the *y* axis and the strain, the extent to which collagen elongates, measured as a percentage of its original length, is plotted along the *x* axis.

Collagen at rest is crimped; as stress is applied, the fibres straighten initially, responding with an elastic type of elongation and the crimp pattern is lost (Akeson et al 1987, Bogduk 1997, Hardy & Woodall 1998). The straightening out of the fibres is represented by the first part of the

Figure 2.11   Stress-strain curve. Adapted from Bogduk 1997, Nordin & Frankel 2001, Keir 1991, Kisner & Colby in Sports Injuries by C Norris. Reprinted by permission of Elsevier Ltd.

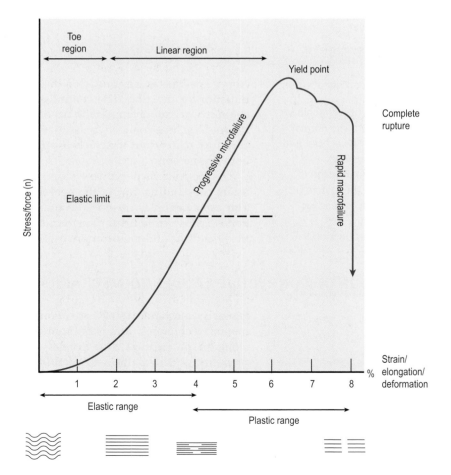

curve, known as the *toe region*. Crimp straightens easily and there is little or no resistance to the applied stress. At the end of the toe region some of the elongation may be due to sliding of the collagen fibres in the interfibrillar gel (Nordin & Frankel 2001). The capacity of the tissues to lengthen is initially determined by their structural weave; the more regularly oriented the collagen fibres, the shorter the toe region, for example a ligament displays a shorter toe region than the more loosely woven joint capsule but a longer toe region than the more regularly arranged tendon (Threlkeld 1992, Hardy & Woodall 1998).

The second part of the curve is known as the *linear region*. The straightened fibres realign in the linear direction of the applied stress and the structure becomes longer and thinner. Water and proteoglycans are displaced and the chemical cross-links between fibres and fibrils are strained, producing a resistance or stiffness in the tissue, so that a progressively greater stress is required to produce equivalent amounts of elongation. The steeper the stress–strain curve, the stiffer the tissue.

If the deforming stress is removed at this point, the elastic properties of the collagen tissue allow the structure to return to its original resting length. In the early part of the linear region a point is reached at which slack is taken up in connective tissue and this represents the end of passive range.

In the second half of the linear region, stress causes some of the strained cross-links to break and *microfailure* begins to occur in a few overstretched fibres. Microfailure is said to occur somewhere after 4% of elongation has been achieved (Bogduk 1997), at which point the collagen is said to have reached its *elastic limit*. A traumatic stress applied at this stage produces minor pain and swelling but no clinical laxity (equivalent to a Grade I injury – see Ch. 11 for definitions of the grades of injury as applied to the medial collateral ligament of the knee).

Once the elastic limit of collagen has been exceeded, collagen exhibits *plastic properties*, the property of the tissue to deform permanently when loaded beyond its elastic limit, and progressive microfailure produces permanent elongation once the deforming stress is removed. A traumatic stress applied within the plastic range produces more pain and swelling, together with some clinical laxity (equivalent to a Grade II injury – see Ch. 11 for definitions of the grades of injury as applied to the medial collateral ligament of the knee).

A further increase in stress causes major collagen fibre failure and the *yield point* is reached, represented by the peak of the stress–strain curve, where a large number of cross-links are irreversibly broken. The stress–strain curve drops rapidly, indicating *macrofailure* or complete rupture, where the structure is unable to sustain further stress even though it may remain physically intact. Threlkeld (1992), reporting Noyes et al, stated that the estimated macrofailure of connective tissue occurs at approximately 8% of elongation. A traumatic stress that produces complete rupture causes severe pain initially which is followed by less pain and gross clinical laxity (equivalent to a Grade III injury – see Ch. 11 for definitions of the grades of injury as applied to the medial collateral ligament of the knee).

Clinical tip
Passive movements applied during clinical examination represent the stress applied to take up the slack. The strain is represented by the range of movement observed and the end-feel of the movement.

The stress applied to tissues can be divided into several categories (Bogduk 1997, Norris 1998):

- *Tensile stress* – a pulling or elongating force applied longitudinally parallel to the long axis of the structure
- *Compressive stress* – a pushing or squashing force applied perpendicular to the long axis of the structure
- *Shear stress* – a sliding force applied across the long axis of the structure
- *Torsional stress* – a twisting force or torque applied in opposite directions about an axis of rotation

Collagen, however, does not have pure elastic properties and the presence of the amorphous ground substance provides a viscous fluid factor. Therefore the viscoelastic properties of collagen may be affected by the type of stress applied and the speed of application, influencing the outcome of the different mobilization techniques used in orthopaedic medicine as discussed in Chapter 4.

The *stiffness* of a structure is its resistance to deformation under the applied stress. A stiff structure displays reduced elastic properties and a shorter toe phase. Scar tissue, which forms within a connective tissue structure, is not as elastic as the surrounding normal tissue. Therefore, slack will be taken up sooner in the adherent scar tissue and mobilization techniques can be applied to produce elongation or rupture. Tough scar tissue requires considerable force or stress to deform it, and it does not easily resume its original shape. Once the failure point of scar tissue is reached it ruptures relatively quickly (Norris 1998).

The *viscoelastic properties* of connective tissue structures cause them to behave differently under different loading rates. If the structure is loaded quickly it behaves more stiffly than the same tissue loaded at a slower rate (Threlkeld 1992). Higher force, short duration stretching at normal or lower temperatures favours recoverable elastic tissue deformation whereas low force, long duration stretching at higher temperatures favours permanent plastic deformation (Warren et al and Leban, cited in Alter 2000). This behaviour of the tissue is utilized in tissue mobilization techniques. Adhesions may be ruptured by a quickly applied shear stress, or stretched by a slow sustained tensile stress. Increasing the temperature of a structure allows lower sustained loads to achieve greater elongation (Warren et al 1971).

Creep is a property of viscous structures which occurs when a prolonged stress is applied in the linear phase. Creep, or elongation of the tissue, is inversely proportional to the velocity of the stress and the slower the applied stress, the greater the lengthening (Hardy & Woodall 1998). Deformation occurs through a gradual rearrangement of the collagen fibres, proteoglycan gel and water and/or through straining and perhaps breaking some of the collagen fibre cross-links (Bogduk 1997). When the stress is released, resumption of the original length of the structure occurs at a slower rate than its deformation and this mechanical behaviour is known as *hysteresis* – i.e. the loading and unloading stress–strain curves are not identical as would be demonstrated in a purely elastic structure.

The original length may not be achieved and the difference between the two lengths is known as *set*.

Repeated or cyclical loading may achieve an increment of elongation with each loading cycle. This may lead to eventual failure of the structure through accumulated fatigue. A larger load requires fewer repetitions to produce failure, but a certain minimum load (the endurance limit) must be applied to achieve this effect (Norris 1998).

The aim of mobilization is to maintain or regain the gliding function and length of the tissues, allowing or restoring full painless function. Mobilization to maintain tissue function is conducted within the elastic range, while mobilization aimed at elongating or rupturing established scar tissue adhesions occurs by applying appropriate stress at the end of the linear region and within the plastic range of the tissue. Timing of application of the mobilization stresses is important and is determined by the grade of the injury and resultant irritability of the tissues. Young scar tissue is 'ripe' for mobilization and can be altered by stress parameters that do not affect older scar tissue. The tensile strength limitations of the healing tissues should be respected and uncontrolled or overaggressive mobilization avoided (Madden cited in Hardy & Woodall 1998).

References

Akeson W 1990 The response of ligaments to stress modulation and overview of the ligament healing response. In: Daniel D, Akeson W H, O'Connor J J (eds) Knee ligaments: structure, function, injury and repair. Lippincott, Williams & Wilkins, Philadelphia, p 315–327

Akeson W, Amiel D, Woo S L-Y 1980 Immobility effects on synovial joints, the pathomechanics of joint contracture. Biorheology 17:95–110

Akeson W, Amiel D, Abel M F et al 1987 Effects of immobilisation on joints. Clinical Orthopaedics and Related Research 219:28—37

Alter M J 2000 Science of flexibility, 2nd edn. Human Kinetics, Champaign, Illinois

Amiel D, Woo S L-Y, Harwood L, Akeson W H 1982 The effect of immobilization on collagen turnover in connective tissue: a biochemical–biomechanical correlation. Acta Orthopaedica Scandinavica 53:325–332

Amiel D, Billings E, Akeson W 1990 Ligament structure, chemistry and physiology. In: Daniel D, Akeson W H, O'Connor J J (eds) Knee ligaments: structure, function, injury and repair. Lippincott, Williams & Wilkins, Philadelphia, p 77–90

Barlow Y, Willoughby J 1992 Pathophysiology of soft tissue repair. British Medical Bulletin 48:698–711

Bogduk N 1997 Clinical anatomy of the lumbar spine and sacrum. Churchill Livingstone, Edinburgh

Chamberlain G J 1982 Cyriax's friction massage: a review. Journal of Orthopaedic and Sports Physical Therapy 4:16–22

Cook J L, Khan K M, Maffulli N et al 2000 Overuse tendinosis, not tendinopathy, part 2: applying the new approach to patellar tendinopathy. Physician and Sports Medicine 28(6):31–41

Cormack D H 1987 Ham's Histology, 9th edn. J B Lippincott, Philadelphia

Cyriax J 1982 Textbook of orthopaedic medicine, 8th edn. Baillière Tindall, London, vol 1

Dingman R O 1973 Factors of clinical significance affecting wound healing. Laryngoscope 83(9):1540–1555

Donatelli R, Owens-Burkhart H 1981 Effects of immobilisation on the extensibility of periarticular connective tissue. Journal of Orthopaedic and Sports Physical Therapy 3:67–72

Evans P 1980 The healing process at cellular level: a review. Physiotherapy 66:256–259

Fowler J D 1989 Wound healing: an overview. Seminars in Veterinary Medicine and Surgery 4:256–262

Gelberman R H, Vande Berg J S, Lundberg G N et al 1983 Flexor tendon healing and restoration of the gliding surface. Journal of Bone and Joint Surgery 65A:70–83

Hardy M A 1989 The biology of scar formation. Physical Therapy 69:1014–1023

Hardy M, Woodall W 1998 Therapeutic effects of heat, cold and stretch on connective tissue. Journal of Hand Therapy 11(2):148–152

Józsa L, Kannus P 1997 Human tendons: anatomy, physiology and pathology. Human Kinetics, Champaign, Illinois

Kapit W, Macey R, Meisami E 1987 The physiology coloring book. Harper Collins, USA

Khan K M, Cook J L (2000) Overuse tendon injuries: where does the pain come from? Sports Medicine and Arthroscopic Review 8:17–31

Le Gros Clark W E 1965 The tissues of the body, 5th edn. Oxford University Press, Oxford

Leibovich S J, Ross R 1974 The role of the macrophage in wound repair. American Journal of Pathology 78:71–91

Levangie P K, Norkin C C 2001 Joint structure and function: a comprehensive analysis, 3rd edn. F A Davis, Philadelphia

Merrilees M J, Flint M H 1980 Ultrastructural study of tension and pressure zones in a rabbit flexor tendon. American Journal of Anatomy 157:87–106

Netter F H 1987 Musculoskeletal system, part 1. Ciba Collection of Medical Illustrations, vol 8. Ciba-Geigy, Summit, New Jersey

Nimni M E 1980 The molecular organisation of collagen and its role in determining the biophysical properties of the connective tissues. Biorheology 17:51–82

Nordin M, Frankel V H 2001 Basic biomechanics of the musculoskeletal system, 3rd edn. Lippincott, Williams & Wilkins, Philadelphia

Norris C M 1998 Sports injuries: diagnosis and management for physiotherapists, 2nd edn. Butterworth Heinemann, Oxford

Palastanga N, Field D, Soames R 2002 Anatomy and human movement, 4th edn. Butterworth Heinemann, Oxford

Peacock E E 1966 Some biochemical and biophysical aspects of joint stiffness. Annals of Surgery 164:1–12

Stearns M L 1940a Studies on the development of connective tissue in transparent chambers in the rabbit's ear, I. American Journal of Anatomy 66:133–176

Stearns M L 1940b Studies on the development of connective tissue in transparent chambers in the rabbit's ear, II. American Journal of Anatomy 67:55–97

Threlkeld A J 1992 The effects of manual therapy on connective tissue. Physical Therapy 72:893–902

Warren C G, Lehmann J F, Koblanski J N 1971 Elongation of the rat tail tendon: effect of load and temperature. Physical Medicine and Rehabilitation 52:465–474

Wilkerson G B 1985 Inflammation in connective tissue: etiology and management Athletic Training Winter:298–301

Williams P L 1998 Gray's Anatomy: the anatomical basis of medicine and surgery, 38th edn. Churchill Livingstone, Edinburgh

Woo S L-Y, Wang C W, Newton P O et al 1990 The response of ligaments to stress deprivation and stress enhancement. In: Daniel D, Akeson W H, O'Connor J J (eds) Knee ligaments: structure, function, injury and repair. Lippincott, Williams & Wilkins, Philadelphia, p 337–349

Chapter 3

Connective tissue inflammation, repair and remodelling

SUMMARY

An injury causes disruption of connective tissue unity. The body's response to this is generally thought to be one of inflammation, repair and remodelling ultimately to restore anatomical structure and normal function to the damaged tissue. However, recent studies have questioned the presence of inflammatory changes in chronic overuse tendon lesions and the inflammatory model has been challenged.

This chapter examines the different phases of healing and explores the process of scar tissue formation and its implication in restoring or preventing pain-free function. General principles of treatment are applied to each phase, aiming to facilitate healing, and the factors which promote or impede healing are considered.

The different phases of connective tissue healing are not separate and each is overlapped by the other, with one response signalling another until the wound is bridged by scar tissue. The inflammatory phase prepares the area for healing, the repair phase rebuilds the structure and the remodelling phase provides the final form of the tissue (Hardy 1989).

The degree of inflammation in response to injury depends on the degree of trauma. A minor injury causes a minimal response whereas a major injury will produce a significant inflammatory response which will pass through acute, subacute and chronic phases.

Lesions encountered in orthopaedic medicine include acute and chronic muscle belly lesions, ligamentous lesions, overuse tendinopathy, tenosynovitis, arthritis, bursitis and mechanical joint displacements.

Acute inflammation is significant and the patient can usually recall the precise time and mode of onset. Following injury the inflammatory response is rapid with noticeable pain and swelling, which can last for hours or days. With chronic inflammation, the patient cannot usually recollect the onset and the reaction is low-grade with less noticeable pain and swelling. Chronic inflammation may occur as a progression from acute inflammation or as a result of overuse, and can last for weeks, months or even years. As mentioned above, the inflammatory model in chronic tendinopathy has been challenged and the pathological process may involve degenerative rather than inflammatory changes (Khan & Cook 2000, Cook et al 2000).

THE INFLAMMATORY PHASE

The initial inflammatory reaction involves vascular and cellular changes. Injury is rapidly followed by transient vasoconstriction, lasting for 5–10 min, and is succeeded by vasodilatation which may result in haemorrhage. If the lesion is still bleeding at the time of treatment this will necessitate careful management.

In the early stage of inflammation the blood vessel walls become more permeable and plasma and leukocytes leak into the surrounding tissues as inflammatory exudate or oedema. Swelling may take a few hours to develop and the amount of swelling is determined by the type of tissue involved in the injury. For example, muscle bellies may produce considerable swelling and bleeding but the structure of tendons prevents the collection of fluid and they do not easily swell. Similarly, ligaments themselves do not usually show dramatic swelling but intrinsic joint ligaments (e.g. the medial collateral ligament of the knee) may provoke a traumatic arthritis of the joint causing considerable pain and swelling. Swelling may also be restricted physically by fascial bands and intermuscular septa.

The vascular response is directly due to damage of blood vessel walls and indirectly due to the influence of chemical mediators. These chemical mediators include heparin and histamine, released by the mast cells, bradykinin originating from plasma and plasma proteins, serotonin from platelets and prostaglandins, which are hormone-like compounds, produced by all cells in the body.

Heparin temporarily prevents coagulation of the excess tissue fluid and blood in the area. Bradykinins have multiple effects. They are potent mediators of the inflammatory response, can directly cause pain and vasodilatation, can activate the production of substance P and can enhance prostaglandin release. Substance P promotes vasodilatation, increases vascular permeability and stimulates phagocytosis and mast cell degranulation, with the subsequent release of histamine and serotonin. Prostaglandins may provoke or inhibit the inflammatory response. Histamine and serotonin produce a short-lived vascular effect whereas both bradykinins and prostaglandins promote more long-term vasodilatation. The overall vascular activity is responsible for the gross signs of inflammation: heat (*calor*), redness (*rubor*), swelling (*tumor*), pain and tenderness (*dolor*) and disturbed function (*functio laesa*) (Peery & Miller 1971).

Inflammation causes pain and tenderness. Mechanical pain is due to mechanical stress, tissue damage, muscle spasm and the accumulated oedema causing excess pressure on surrounding tissues. Chemical pain arises through chemosensitive nerve receptors which are sensitive to histamine, serotonin, bradykinins and prostaglandins which are released into the tissues during this inflammatory phase. However, most nociceptors (pain receptors) are sensitive to more than one type of stimulus. The inflammatory substances may cause extreme stimulation of nerve fibres without necessarily causing them damage.

The nociceptors become progressively more sensitive the longer the pain stimulus is maintained and proinflammatory prostaglandins are believed to sensitize nociceptors leading to a state of hyperalgesia, an increased response to a painful stimulus (Wilkerson 1985, Kloth & Miller 1990).

If the tissue is still haemorrhaging, attempts must be made to stop this as blood is a strong irritant and will cause chemical and mechanical pain, as well as prolonging the inflammatory process (Dingman 1973, Evans 1980). This is particularly true of a haemarthrosis which, if present, should be aspirated immediately.

In the first few hours of the early inflammatory phase fibronectin, a structural glycoprotein which acts as a tissue 'glue', appears in the wound, deposited along strands of fibrin in the clot (Williams 1998). This fibrin–fibronectin meshwork is associated with immature fibroblasts, which are thought to deposit type III collagen fibres to provide a scaffold for platelet adhesion and anchorage for further invading fibroblasts (Nimni 1980, Lehto et al 1985).

In minor injury, the inflammatory process is short and the scar tissue produced is minimal. The red blood cells break down into cellular debris and haemoglobin pigment, and the platelets release thrombin, an enzyme which changes fibrinogen into fibrin. The fibrin forms a meshwork of fibres which trap the blood clot and an early scar is formed.

If the injury is significant, the next stage of the inflammatory phase is phagocytic. Circulating monocytes modulate into macrophages (Fowler 1989) and join the resident macrophage population to clear the debris from the site of injury through phagocytic action (Leibovich & Ross 1974). The macrophages increase in great numbers during the first 3 or 4 days (Dingman 1973). They engulf any matter with which they come into contact, clearing the wound environment and preparing it for subsequent repair. As well as performing a phagocytic role, the macrophage acts as a director cell, directing the repair process by chemically influencing an appropriate number of fibroblast cells activated in the area.

A stage of neovascularization is also reached, with capillaries starting to develop after about 12 h and continuing to develop for a further 2 or 3 days (Daly 1990). The new vessels supply oxygen and nourishment to the injured tissues, but are delicate and easily disrupted. Relative immobilization is necessary at this stage and heat is contraindicated as it will cause increased bleeding from the fragile vessels (Hardy 1989).

Inflammation is a normal response to either trauma or infection and to have no inflammatory response would mean that healing would not occur. Too little inflammation will delay healing and too much inflammation will lead to excessive scarring. The so-called PRICE principle of employing protection, relative rest, ice, compression and elevation in the early stages can help to control heat, swelling and pain and to reduce, but not abolish, inflammation.

Clinical tip
The principles of protection, rest, ice, compression and elevation (PRICE) are applied in acute injuries, the irritability of the tissues, usually indicated by the level of pain on movement, providing a guide for when mobilization techniques are appropriate.

The control of swelling is important towards regaining function since the greater the amount of inflammatory exudate, the more fibrin will be found in the area which becomes organized into scar tissue (Evans 1980). Although pain inhibits normal movement, graded mobilization should be encouraged as early as possible to promote healing and to avert adverse scar tissue formation.

Pain itself can be further reduced by analgesic drugs. Nonsteroidal anti-inflammatory drugs (NSAIDs) modify the inflammatory response, reduce chemical pain and reduce temperature by inhibiting the production of prostaglandins. There are exponents of the so-called 'NICE' principle, adding in the prescription of non-steroidal drugs to the usual first-line after-care of injury. However, a counter view is that these should not be prescribed for the first 2 or 3 days after injury since they will tend to delay healing (Boruta et al 1990). It may be more appropriate to allow the body's natural inflammatory response to proceed with analgesics such as paracetamol and/or physical measures such as mobilization, massage and electrotherapy as appropriate methods of pain control.

Corticosteroids are contraindicated in the acute inflammatory phase as they inhibit macrophage activity which delays debridement of the wound and scar tissue production by delaying the onset and proliferation of the fibroblasts (Leibovich & Ross 1974, Hardy 1989). Each stage of the inflammatory phase is essential to the repair process and suppression in the early stages will delay healing.

Gentle transverse frictions and controlled mobilization can be initiated early to allow healing in the presence of movement, as guided by the irritability of the tissues. Mobilization is initiated very gently, to start moving the injured connective tissue towards regaining painless function, but without unduly stressing the healing breach. Overstressing the healing tissue would disrupt the early fragile scar and set up a secondary inflammatory response, leading to excess scar tissue formation. Mobilization also has an effect on the mechanoreceptors which is thought to reduce pain.

> *Clinical tip*
> Gentle frictions together with gentle mobilization will agitate tissue fluid and increase the chance contact of the macrophage with cellular debris, so promoting healing (Evans 1980).

REPAIR PHASE

The repair phase is simultaneous with the inflammatory phase and overlaps the remodelling phase.

Some tissues, e.g. the synovial lining of the joints, bone and skeletal muscle, are capable of direct regeneration. All other connective tissues are incapable of regeneration, and repair of these structures involves a reconstruction process of the damaged tissue by collagen fibre or scar tissue formation. Scar tissue does not have exactly the same properties or tensile strength as the tissue it is rebuilding, but its structure comes to resemble that tissue closely to ensure that normal function is regained (Douglas et al 1969, Hardy 1989).

Once the wound has been prepared by phagocytosis, the macrophage becomes the director of repair and signals an appropriate number of fibroblasts to the area. As the inflammatory phase subsides the fibroblast becomes the dominant cell in the repair phase and synthesizes the connective tissue matrix, comprising the amorphous ground substance and collagen. Fibroblasts may appear in the wound during the first 24 h after injury, but maximum numbers are not achieved until day 5–10 (Bryant 1977, Chamberlain 1982, Fowler 1989). They do not decrease in number until 3 weeks after the injury (Chamberlain 1982).

Fibroblasts secrete the amorphous ground substance which provides the cross-linking mechanism for the collagen fibres it also synthesizes. This arrangement 'glues' the wound together, with cross-links forming at appropriate nodal intersect points. Once the fibroblasts are stimulated to produce collagen there is rapid closure of the healing breach. Collagen fibres proper are laid down approximately 5–10 days after injury and the repair process continues as they arrange themselves into larger units or bundles (Stearns 1940b, Chamberlain 1982).

The rate of repair is directly related to the size of the wound (Stearns 1940a, 1940b). A small wound with approximated edges will heal quickly with a minimal inflammatory response and collagen fibres will be laid down early to bind the edges together, providing that the edges remain in apposition. Consider a clean, stitched skin wound, when the stitches are usually safely removed after 7 days and the wound has sufficient tensile strength to withstand movement.

Large, unapproximated wounds are deep as well as wide and healing initially requires the formation of granulation tissue. It may be several days after injury before the fibroblasts initiate fibre formation and several weeks before there is sufficient collagen to provide enough tensile strength for the wound to withstand normal movement. Therefore all timings mentioned above are approximate and the clinician will conduct a thorough assessment. The level of irritability of the tissues is a guide to the time for application of the appropriate graded mobilization.

During the early part of the repair process, a stage of wound contraction occurs assisted by the contractile action of myofibroblasts (Gabbiani et al 1971, Daly 1990). Linear wounds contract rapidly while circular or rectangular wounds contract relatively slowly (Grillo et al 1958, Fowler 1989, Hardy 1989, Daly 1990, Williams 1998). Wound contracture, as distinct from contraction, results from fibrosis or adhesion formation and this will be discussed later in this chapter.

Initial collagen fibre formation is random. The number of collagen fibres and the tensile strength of the wound increase substantially during the first 3 weeks after injury to become approximately 15–20% of the normal strength of the tissue (Hardy 1989, Daly 1990, Hardy & Woodall 1998). However, the tensile strength does not depend entirely on the number of fibres, since after this time the number of collagen fibres stabilizes but the tensile strength of the wound continues to increase. Tensile strength is related to a balance between the synthesis and lysis of collagen (the production and breakdown of collagen, a continuous, dynamic process), the development of collagen cross-links and the orientation of collagen fibres into the existing weave. This process of maturation is known as the remodelling phase (van der Meulen 1982, Williams 1998).

Clinical tip
The level of irritability is a guide to the application of the appropriate graded mobilization.

REMODELLING PHASE

The remodelling phase sees the new collagen or scar tissue attempt to take on the physical characteristics of the tissue it is replacing. It begins in earnest approximately 21 days after injury and continues for 6 months or more, possibly even for years. Remodelling is responsible for the final structural orientation and arrangement of the fibres as well as its tensile strength.

Initial, immature scar tissue is weak and the fibres are oriented in all directions through several planes. Remodelling allows these randomly arranged fibres to become rearranged in both a linear and a lateral orientation. The orientation of collagen fibres occurs in two ways: through induction and through tension.

Normal tissue adjacent to the wound induces structure in the replacement scar tissue. Thus dense tissue induces dense, highly cross-linked scar tissue while pliable tissue induces loose, less cross-linked scar tissue (Hardy 1989). The final physical weave of the collagen so formed is responsible for the functional behaviour of the wound within the connective tissue it is replacing.

Internal and external stresses apply tension to the wound during the remodelling phase, e.g. muscle tension, joint movement, passive gliding of fascial planes, connective tissue loading and unloading, temperature changes and mobilization (Hardy 1989). It is recognized that both mobilization and immobilization can strongly influence the structural orientation of collagen fibres (Stearns 1940a, 1940b; Akeson et al 1987).

During the maturation phase of scar formation, immature scar tissue is converted to mature scar tissue and the cross-linking system changes from weak hydrogen bonding to strong covalent bonding (Price 1990). While the scar tissue is relatively immature the weak electrostatic bonding forms reducible cross-links which allow scar tissue to be mobilized with a gentle, steady stress. During this stage transverse frictions and mobilization within the limits of pain are appropriate to maintain the mobility of immature scar tissue with graded mobilization promoting the alignment of fibres.

Remodelling involves the reorganization of scar while it matures with fibres being absorbed, replaced and reoriented. When stresses arising from mobilization are applied to collagen fibres, the resultant piezo-electric effect (generation of small voltages called streaming potentials) is believed to be responsible for the production, maintenance, alignment and absorption of collagen fibrils (Price 1990, Williams 1998).

Cross-linking is responsible for the tensile strength of new, desirable scar tissue, but if the cross-linking becomes excessive it will be responsible for the toughness and lack of resilience of unwanted fibrous adhesions (Kloth & Miller 1990). Immobilization causes loss of the ground substance, which reduces the interfibrillar distance and causes friction between the collagen subunits, facilitating the formation of excessive cross-links (Akeson et al 1967, Akeson 1990).

Clinical tip
The application of appropriate stress by graded mobilization ensures that collagen fibre orientation occurs throughout the tissue and matches its function.

Collagen fibre formation and orientation conform to lines of stress within connective tissue, and are similar in this respect to osseous alignment (Le Gros Clark 1965, Price 1990, Williams 1998).

Ligaments require strong scar tissue fibres within their parallel wavy weave to be capable of resisting excessive joint stresses as well as being able to relax and fold when the tension is removed. The scar tissue formed between the ligament and bone must mimic the normal weave to allow normal movement of the joint (Hardy 1989). Scar tissue formed within a muscle belly needs to be flexible to allow the muscle fibres to broaden as the muscle contracts and extensible enough to allow the muscle to lengthen when stretched. Scar tissue within tendons must be oriented in a parallel weave along the lines of mechanical stress to ensure maximum tensile strength of the tendon while also maintaining the gliding properties of the tendon.

Collagen synthesis and remodelling continue in the 6 months following injury with the tissue returning to its normal state of activity 6–12 months after injury under normal conditions (Daly 1990). However, the increase in tensile strength in fascia and other dense connective tissues is thought to take much longer (Dingman 1973). Fully repaired skin wounds eventually achieve only approximately 70% of their original strength (Douglas et al 1969, Bryant 1977, Daly 1990).

As the scar matures, it becomes dense, tough and less resilient than immature scar tissue. The developing stable cross-links become more prolific and the stronger covalent bonds which form do not yield as readily to applied stresses (Price 1990).

An increasing depth of transverse frictions provides pressure and lateral stretch to the mature scar. Deeper transverse frictions and a greater range of mobilization are required to mobilize mature scar tissue compared with immature scar tissue.

> **Clinical tip**
> To avoid adverse scar tissue formation, gentle transverse frictions and a progressively increasing range of mobilization should be continued until a full pain-free range of movement is restored. This aims to prevent excessive cross-links occurring between individual fibres and encourages fibre alignment. Applying appropriate stress to restore length should avoid the necessity to stretch.

ADHESION FORMATION AND CONTRACTURE

Synthesis and lysis, together with orientation of the collagen fibres (i.e. remodelling), ensure the final form of scar tissue. A balance is needed between collagen synthesis and lysis for an appropriate turnover of collagen and sufficient stresses should be applied to the tissue to stimulate fibre orientation but without disrupting the healing breach. This has implications for the grade of mobilization applied and is discussed in Chapter 4.

Increasing the size of the healing breach would set up secondary inflammatory changes, leading to excessive scar tissue formation and eventual contracture, adhesions and fibrosis. Excessive scar tissue, adhesions or contracture within any soft tissue structure will impede function and cause pain. Pain itself, as a characteristic of inflammation, acts as an inhibitor to normal function and, if a state of chronic inflammation is maintained, the function of the tissue will continue to deteriorate. This self-perpetuating inflammation presents an ongoing chronic functional problem which may be difficult to treat.

An abnormal excessive production of scar tissue may result in hypertrophic or keloid scars (Daly 1990, Price 1990). Hypertrophic scars develop when excessive collagen is deposited within the original wound site while keloid scarring involves excessive collagen deposits in the tissues surrounding the scar. In the connective tissue structures important to orthopaedic medicine, this excessive production of scar tissue may be seen as adhesion formation and contracture either within the healing structure or within the surrounding tissues.

In the treatment of hypertrophic scarring, prolonged pressure has been used to restore the balance between collagen synthesis and lysis (Hardy 1989). In a chronically inflamed wound where excessive scar tissue has been produced, the technique of deep transverse frictions applies pressure to the area of scar tissue as well as providing a lateral stress to mobilize adhesions.

The use of intralesional corticosteroid is said to produce keloid regression through its multiple steroid effects, which include inhibition of fibroblast migration, decreased collagen synthesis and increased collagenase activity (Carrico et al 1984). This effect may be transferred to the use of intralesional steroid for chronic inflammation in chronic connective tissue lesions such as tendinopathy, bursitis and some chronic ligament strains.

> *Clinical tip*
> In chronic lesions, deep transverse frictions and graded mobilization techniques are applied to mobilize the existing scar tissue. Alternatively, an intralesional injection of corticosteroid may be given.

FACTORS WHICH MAY AFFECT WOUND HEALING

Chronic trauma can cause excessive movement or tension on devitalized tissues, promoting unwanted scarring. This may be the mechanism of chronic overuse syndromes in which repetitive trauma disrupts tissue unity.

Haematoma formation retards the healing process by acting as an irritant, producing a mechanical blockage which separates the torn edges and provides a medium for infection (Dingman 1973).

Infection of the injured tissue presents a serious complication which delays the healing process.

Age, according to Mulder (1990), can delay cell migration and proliferation, wound contracture and collagen remodelling, and decrease the tensile strength of the wound, so increasing the chance of wound dehiscence or splitting. Experimental wounds in young rats showed better mechanical properties in terms of greater strength, elastic stiffness and energy absorption than those in older rats. The fibre organization was more complex and better organized in the young rats and healing was observed to be faster (Holm-Pedersen & Viidik 1971).

Changes in the gel–fibre ratio occurring with age are consistent with the changes occurring with immobilization. Contractures tend to occur more frequently, after less trauma and after shorter periods of time in the relatively immobile joints of the elderly. Chemical changes in the gel–fibre ratio have been noted in such tissues as the skin and the nucleus pulposus of older individuals (Akeson et al 1968).

The following medications, therapies and conditions may also affect wound healing.

While anti-inflammatory medication may not be the most appropriate treatment for acute inflammation, its use in chronic lesions is most appropriate for suppressing inflammation and relieving pain. NSAIDs, either taken orally or topically applied, may be used in conjunction with physical measures (PRICE). NSAIDs do not cause a significant change in collagen synthesis; they inhibit production of histamine, serotonin and prostaglandins (Wilkerson 1985). However, aspirin, in addition to its anti-inflammatory function, inhibits platelet aggregation and may prolong bleeding (Rang et al 2003).

The oral intake of corticosteroids inhibits collagen synthesis, reduces tensile strength and delays wound healing (Dingman 1973, Ahonen et al 1980, Mulder 1990). Corticosteroids administered in the acute inflammatory phase interfere with macrophage migration but if delivered after the macrophage invasion, i.e. after 3 days, their effect on wound healing is much less severe (Fowler 1989).

Anticoagulants, e.g. heparin and warfarin, prolong bleeding and delay wound healing.

The effect of chemotherapy depends on the drugs used and their dosage, but fibroblast proliferation may be affected and subsequently collagen synthesis is delayed (Carrico et al 1984).

Radiotherapy radiation can damage fibroblasts, cause vascular damage and decrease collagen production, but it depends on the dose, frequency and location of the irradiated area in relation to the injury site (Mulder 1990).

Acquired immunodeficiency syndrome (AIDS) patients are in a state of immunosuppression and this will delay the healing process.

Diabetes appears to affect the inflammatory stage rather than collagen synthesis, implying that insulin is important in the early phase of healing (Carrico et al 1984).

Other factors which could affect healing include vitamin A and C deficiency, protein deprivation, systemic vascular disorders and systemic connective tissue disorders.

References

Ahonen J, Jiborn H, Zederfeldt B 1980 Hormone influence on wound healing. In: Hunt T K (ed) wound healing and wound infection: theory and surgical practice. Appleton Century Croft, New York, p 95–105

Akeson W 1990 The response of ligaments to stress modulation and overview of the ligament healing response. In: Daniel D, Akeson W H, O'Connor J J (eds) Knee ligaments: structure, function, injury and repair. Lippincott, Williams & Wilkins, Philadelphia, p 315–327

Akeson W, Amiel D, La Violette D 1967 The connective tissue response to immobility: a study of chondroitin-4 and 6-sulfate and dermatan sulfate changes in periarticular connective tissue of control and immobilised knees of dogs. Clinical Orthopaedics 51:183–197

Akeson W, Amiel D, LaViolette D et al 1968 The connective tissue response to immobility: an accelerated ageing response? Experimental Gerontology 3:289–301

Akeson W, Amiel D, Abel M F et al 1987 Effects of immobilisation on joints. Clinical Orthopaedics and Related Research 219:28–37

Boruta P M, Bishop J O, Braly W G et al 1990 Acute lateral ankle ligament injuries: literature review. Foot and Ankle 11:107–113

Bryant W 1977 Wound healing. Clinical Symposia 29:2–28

Carrico T J, Mehrhof A I, Cohen I K 1984 Biology of wound healing. Surgical Clinics of North America 64:721–731

Chamberlain G J 1982 Cyriax's friction massage: a review. Journal of Orthopaedic and Sports Physical Therapy 4:16–22

Cook J L, Khan K M, Maffulli N et al 2000 Overuse tendinosis, not tendinopathy, part 2: applying the new approach to patellar tendinopathy. Physician and Sports Medicine 28(6):31–41

Daly T J 1990 The repair phase of wound healing – re-epithelialization and contraction. In: Kloth L C, McCullock J M, Feedar J A (eds) Wound healing: alternatives in management. F A Davis, Philadelphia, p 14–29

Dingman R O 1973 Factors of clinical significance affecting wound healing. Laryngoscope 83:1540–1554

Douglas D M, Forrester J C, Ogilvie R R 1969 Physical characteristics of collagen in the later stages of wound healing. British Journal of Surgery 56:219–222

Evans P 1980 The healing process at cellular level: a review. Physiotherapy 66:256–259

Fowler J D 1989 Wound healing: an overview. Seminars in Veterinary Medicine and Surgery 4:256–262

Gabbiani G, Ryan G B, Majno G 1971 Presence of modified fibroblasts in granulation tissue and their possible role in wound contraction. Experientia 27:549–550

Grillo H C, Watts G T, Gross J 1958 Studies in wound healing: I. Contraction and the wound contents. Annals of Surgery 148:145–152

Hardy M A 1989 The biology of scar formation. Physical Therapy 69:1014–1023

Hardy M, Woodall W 1998 Therapeutic effects of heat, cold and stretch on connective tissue. Journal of Hand Therapy 11(2):148–152

Holm-Pedersen P, Viidik A 1971 Tensile properties and morphology of healing wounds in young and old rats. Scandinavian Journal of Plastic Reconstructive Surgery 6:24–35

Khan K M, Cook J L 2000 Overuse tendon injuries: where does the pain come from? Sports Medicine and Arthroscopic Review 8:17–31

Kloth L C, Miller K H 1990 The inflammatory response to wounding. In: Kloth L C, McCullock J M, Feedar J (eds) Wound healing: alternatives in management. F A Davis, Philadelphia, p 3–13

Le Gros Clark W E 1965 The tissues of the body, 5th edn. Oxford University Press, Oxford

Lehto M, Duance V C, Restall D 1985 Collagen and fibronectin in a healing skeletal muscle injury. Journal of Bone and Joint Surgery 67B:820–827

Leibovich S J, Ross R 1974 The role of the macrophage in wound repair. American Journal of Pathology 78:71–91

Mulder G D 1990 Factors complicating wound repair. In: Kloth L C, McCullock J M, Feedar J (eds) Wound healing: alternatives in management. F A Davis, Philadelphia, p 43–51

Nimni M E 1980 The molecular organisation of collagen and its role in determining the biophysical properties of the connective tissues. Biorheology 17:51–82

Peery T M, Miller F N 1971 Pathology: a dynamic introduction to medicine and surgery, 2nd edn. Little, Brown, Boston

Price H 1990 Connective tissue in wound healing. In: Kloth L C, McCullock J M, Feedar J (eds) Wound healing: alternatives in management. F A Davis, Philadelphia, p 31–41

Rang H P, Dale M M, Ritter J M et al 2003 Pharmacology, 5th edn. Churchill Livingstone, Edinburgh

Stearns M L 1940a Studies on the development of connective tissue in transparent chambers in the rabbit's ear, I. American Journal of Anatomy 66:133–176

Stearns M L 1940b Studies on the development of connective tissue in transparent chambers in the rabbit's ear, II. American Journal of Anatomy 67:55–97

van der Meulen J H C 1982 Present state of knowledge on processes of healing in collagen structures. International Journal of Sports Medicine 3:4–8

Wilkerson G B 1985 Inflammation in connective tissue: etiology and management. Athletic Training Winter:298–301

Williams P L 1998 Gray's Anatomy: the anatomical basis of medicine and surgery, 38th edn. Churchill Livingstone, Edinburgh

Chapter 4

Orthopaedic medicine treatment techniques

SUMMARY

Over the years, the emphasis of treatment for musculoskeletal lesions has moved from one of total immobilization to one of early mobilization. The benefits of early mobilization have become clear and, while a short period of immobilization may still be necessary, the overall aim of orthopaedic medicine treatment techniques is to restore full painless function to the connective tissues through appropriate mobilization.

The selection of techniques depends on several factors that include the stage the lesion has reached in the healing cycle with particular attention to the overall irritability. An accurate assessment and clinical diagnosis allows the effective application of the selected treatment techniques and the development of a carefully rationalized treatment programme.

The treatment techniques used in orthopaedic medicine fall into two broad categories of mobilization and injection, and within this chapter the techniques will be considered in turn, on the basis of the theory presented in the preceding chapters, with notes on their application.

Treatment techniques used in orthopaedic medicine may be categorized as follows:

Mobilization
- Transverse frictions
- Grade A mobilization
- Grade B mobilization
- Grade C mobilization (manipulation)
- Traction

Injection
- Corticosteroid and local anaesthetic
- Sclerosant therapy

MOBILIZATION

Connective tissue structures are more responsive to a decrease in mechanical demand than they are to progressive increases (Tipton et al 1986). Therefore, depriving the healing soft tissues of motion and stress can lead to a number of structural changes within the articular and periarticular connective tissues that may be difficult to reverse. These changes may include all or some of the following:

- Disorganized fibre orientation
- Adhesion formation at the fibre–fibre interface (Fig. 4.1)
- Adhesion formation between ligaments, tendons and their surrounding connective tissue
- Reduced tensile strength of ligaments, tendons and muscles
- Loss of the gliding capacity of connective tissue, especially tendons
- Weakening of ligament and tendon insertion points
- Inhibition of muscle fibre regeneration by scar tissue
- Proliferation of fibrofatty tissue into the joint space and adherence to cartilage surfaces
- Decrease in the volume of synovial fluid with adhesion formation between synovial folds
- Cartilage erosion and osteophyte formation

(Burke-Evans et al 1960; Enneking & Horowitz 1972; Akeson et al 1973, 1980, 1986; Videman 1986; Hardy 1989; Järvinen & Lehto 1993.)

It is noticeable that these connective tissue changes, associated with immobilization, are similar to the changes seen with the degenerative ageing process.

The length of connective tissue structures tends to adapt to the shortest distance between origin and insertion, which produces the

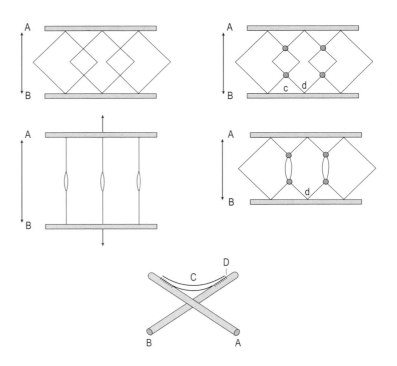

Figure 4.1   Adhesion formation at the fibre–fibre interface. From Woo S L., Mathews J V, Akeson W H et al 1975 Connective tissue response to immobility. Arthritis and Rheumatism. 18: 257–264. This material is used by permission of Wiley-Liss, Inc., a subsidiary of John Wiley and Sons, Inc.

consequences of immobilization that can lead to pain and long-term loss of function (Videman 1986).

Several authors have discussed the effects of stress and motion deprivation on healing connective tissues in animal experiments (Akeson et al 1967, 1973, 1986; Woo et al 1975, 1990; Arem & Madden 1976; Woo 1982; Akeson 1990). During a 9-week period of immobilization, dysfunction was not simply due to connective tissue atrophy, as there was no statistical difference in the quantity of collagen fibres, but due to an increase in collagen turnover and to other changes within the connective tissue matrix (Amiel et al 1982). Loitz et al (1988) noticed similar changes within a 3-week period of immobilization. The changes noted were:

- Development of anomalous cross-linking of existing and new collagen fibres (Fig. 4.2)
- Alteration of the dynamics of collagen turnover (synthesis/lysis)
- Random deposition of new collagen fibres within the existing collagen weave

In explanation of the changes a difference was noted in the quantity and quality of the amorphous ground substance, consistent in all connective tissue structures, which amounted to a reduced concentration of water and glycosaminoglycans (GAGs). As a result, the critical distance and separating effects between adjacent collagen fibres were reduced and the interfibrillar lubrication was lost. Friction developed at the fibre–fibre interface leading to the development of anomalous cross-links which altered the gliding function of the collagen fibres. This formation of cross-links was observed to be time-dependent and occurred when fibres remained stationary for a period of time, i.e. assumed a stationary attitude.

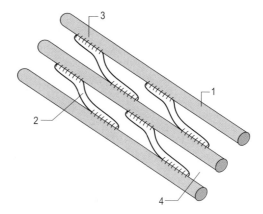

Figure 4.2 The anomalous cross-link formation within existing collagen fibres. 1=Existing fibre; 2=newly synthesized fibril; 3=cross-links created as the fibril becomes incorporated into the fibre; 4=fibres normally move freely past one another (ligament, tendon, muscle) or separate (muscle belly). Adapted from Woo S L, Mathews J V, Akeson W H et al 1975 Connective tissue response to immobility. Arthritis and Rheumatism. 18: 257–264. This material is used by permission of Wiley-Liss, Inc., a subsidiary of John Wiley and Sons, Inc.

The incorporation of new, disorganized collagen fibres into the existing collagen weave physically restrains mobility. Overall this has an effect of altering the elasticity, plasticity and pliability of the connective tissue structures. It is important to note that adhesion formation is a normal part of the repair process and it cannot be prevented entirely. However, it may be possible to prevent excessive or unwanted adhesions, or to mobilize them if they develop unwittingly. Treatment aims to maintain or regain the anatomy and biomechanical function of collagen fibres, enabling them to deal with tension, compression, shear and glide.

Collagen turnover (synthesis/lysis) is a normal, dynamic process that is influenced by stress and motion. When deprived of these physical forces through immobilization, the balance of collagen turnover is lost and a greater ratio of immature collagen fibres is present with a potential for the formation of increased anomalous, reducible cross-links. Pliable young scar tissue is ripe for early mobilization techniques that will reduce the formation of anomalous cross-links.

Stress and motion deprivation is also responsible for the random, disorganized deposition of new collagen fibres within the existing weave that results in an overall reduction in tensile strength. Collagen tissue has elastic properties, mainly by virtue of the weave of its collagen subunits, and it will become relatively inelastic if that weave is altered (Peacock 1966). The careful, controlled application of normal stress and motion will stimulate new collagen to be laid down in parallel with the existing weave and the collagen tissue will maintain its elasticity, plasticity and tensile strength. Wolff's law, relating to laying down of trabeculae in cancellous bone along the lines of stress, could be broadened to encompass the response of the musculoskeletal system to stress as a whole (Akeson 1990).

Immobilization affects the gliding function of tendons and ligaments by virtue of the restricting adhesions failing to elongate to permit painfree function (Weiner & Peacock 1971). In orthopaedic medicine the principles of mobilization, including transverse frictions, can be applied to healing tendons in tendinopathy, and tenosynovitis. The application of manipulation to rupture adhesions to permit normal gliding function may be necessary in lesions of tennis elbow and some chronic ligamentous strains.

In muscle lesions, collagen or scar tissue formation provides a necessary framework for muscle fibre regeneration. However, excessive scar tissue may form a physical barrier and hinder the progress of the regenerating muscle fibres. The connective tissue component of muscles is subject to the usual deleterious changes of immobilization. An adequate period of relative rest, depending on the injury and irritability of the lesion, is required to allow the muscle to regenerate sufficiently to combat the mechanical forces of mobilization (Lehto et al 1985, Järvinen & Lehto 1993). The early application of graded mobilization, including transverse frictions, will maintain muscle function and stimulate structural orientation without the excessive formation of scar tissue.

Articular changes during periods of immobilization depend on the restriction of the movement, the length of the immobilization period and the amount of contact, pressure and friction between the joint surfaces. The amount of synovial fluid is reduced, which renders the articular cartilage more vulnerable to injury by friction and pressure. Longer periods of immobilization of 45–60 days have shown cartilage erosion, subchondral cyst and osteophyte formation, consistent with the changes observed clinically in joints affected by osteoarthrosis and age-related changes. Studies involving the immobilization of rat knee joints showed that if immobilization did not exceed 30 days, the changes due to immobilization were reversible but the longer the joints were immobilized, the longer it took to remobilize them, irrespective of the method used (Burke-Evans et al 1960). Degenerative changes occurring during immobilization can be partly inhibited by traction and continuous passive motion (Videman 1986).

The beneficial effects of intermittent and continuous passive motion have been well-documented (Loitz et al 1988, Takai et al 1991). The original concept of continuous passive motion was developed by Salter in 1970 to reduce the harmful effects of immobilization (Salter 1989). Joints were moved continuously through a predetermined range of movement. This application of cyclical tensile loading facilitates the orientation of collagen fibres, providing tensile strength and a stronger functional and structural repair of connective tissue, including articular cartilage.

General principles of orthopaedic medicine treatment techniques

Soft tissue injury involves all tissues in the injured area to varying degrees and can be classified into three degrees of severity (CSP 1998):

- Grade I or mild injury involves overstretching of the structures with minimal swelling and bruising, mild pain, no joint instability, minimal muscle spasm and minimal loss of function
- Grade II or moderate injury involves some tearing of fibres with moderate swelling and bruising, moderate pain on movement, moderate muscle spasm, some loss of function and possible joint instability
- Grade III or severe injury involves a complete tear of the injured structure with significant swelling and bruising, severe pain at rest and severe disturbance of function

Injury also reduces the tissue's ability to accept tensile stress, the extent of which is proportional to the degree of tissue damage. Rather than consider an injury acute in terms of days since onset, it is wiser to consider acuteness in terms of the irritability of the lesion. In approaching the application of treatment in this way, the clinician makes a judgment on the amount of intervention and the appropriate time to apply it. In 1998 the Chartered Society of Physiotherapy, the professional body of physiotherapy in the UK, endorsed the *Guidelines for the Management of Soft Tissue Injury with Protection, Rest, Ice, Compression and Elevation (PRICE) During the First 72 Hours* that were prepared by the clinical interest group the Association of Chartered Physiotherapists in Sports Medicine (ACPSM) (CSP 1998). The principles of **PRICE** are applicable to any acute injury.

Protection is applied according to the severity of the injury and pain. Based on animal studies, the ACPSM Guidelines (CSP 1998) suggest that a moderate, second degree injury requires 3–5 days protection, while a mild or first degree injury requires a shorter period and a severe or third degree injury requires longer. *Rest* is required following acute injury to reduce metabolic demand and blood flow. However, a balance must be achieved with sufficient controlled movement of the injured and surrounding structures while avoiding any undue stress of the healing breach. Once it has been judged, based on irritability, that the newly formed fibrous tissue can withstand some controlled stress, increased movement is encouraged to stimulate the alignment of fibres. Healing within the presence of movement ensures the development of a strong mobile scar. *Ice, compression* and *elevation* can be applied in conjunction with the suggested treatment regimes given below.

Until recently, it has generally been assumed that there is an inflammatory component involved in chronic overuse tendon lesions, hence the term 'tendinopathy'. The work of Khan & Cook (2000) and Cook et al (2000) has challenged this thinking based on the evidence of numerous studies which show few or no inflammatory cells associated with such lesions. Instead changes consistent with the degenerative process (tendinosis) have been noted together with a poor healing response. Hence the term *tendinopathy* has been adopted to describe chronic overuse tendon lesions where the pathology has not been histologically confirmed.

This raises several issues, not least, how can corticosteroid injection, a known anti-inflammatory treatment, resolve pain in tendinopathy if there is no inflammatory component to the lesion? Khan & Cook (2000) highlight clinical experience together with reference to a number of studies which show corticosteroid injection to provide at least short-term pain relief, but the mechanism of that pain relief remains unknown.

Another issue involves the patient's prognosis. Based on an inflammatory model, it is commonly suggested that the tennis elbow patient or the Achilles tendon patient will recover with treatment such as those suggested below delivered 2–3 times per week for 2–3 weeks. However, clinical experience shows such lesions to be generally resistant to treatment and the following offers a plausible explanation. If the pathological process of such lesions is degeneration rather than inflammation, this may alter the view on prognosis, with the patient being more likely to take many months to fully recover. The application of deep transverse frictions to chronic lesions clinically produces tenderness in the region, which takes time to settle. The work of Gregory et al (2003), discussed below, suggests that ultrastructural changes as a result of transverse frictions may take up to 6 days to resolve (although the study mentioned is an animal model) and this may have implications for considering the application of the technique on a weekly basis, for example.

In summary, the aim of mobilization treatment techniques applied in orthopaedic medicine, including transverse frictions, is to prevent or to reverse the connective tissue changes associated with a period of immobilization. It is important to recognize that stress deprivation causes rapid structural changes and recovery is much slower, which must be taken into account when preparing treatment programmes.

Careful consideration should be given to the application of other treatment modalities, either simultaneously or consecutively with the application of appropriate mobilization. Abusive use of movement can produce mechanical forces sufficient to stretch or disrupt the healing breach, producing excessive scar tissue formation. Additional soft tissue trauma leads to secondary inflammation and the vicious circle of chronic inflammation (Noyes 1977). The correct amount of movement applied at the appropriate time is the key.

Mobilization should be used at optimum levels, with appropriate grade, range, force, direction, speed and duration to achieve the specific treatment aims (Arem & Madden 1976). Hunter (1994), however, correctly points out that, although soft tissue mobilization techniques are known to be clinically effective, no research has been conducted to establish the grade of mobilization required for each stage of the healing process. Orthopaedic medicine mobilization techniques (transverse frictions and the specific mobilization techniques, Grades A, B and C) are graded on the basis of patient feedback and observation against the under-pinning knowledge of the different phases of healing and the experience of the clinician. The appropriate depth and grade of mobilization technique is applied according to the severity of the lesion and this is determined in part by assessment of irritability, rather than in terms of length of time from the onset.

TRANSVERSE FRICTIONS

Massage is the manipulation of the soft tissues of the body with the hands using varying degrees of force (Carreck 1994) and a dominant theme in the literature shows massage to be a therapeutic art lacking scientific support. It involves the laying-on of hands and mimics natural gestures such as rubbing a painful area or soothing a child's injury by kissing it better. As one of the oldest forms of analgesia, it conveys feelings of caring, touch and relaxation which indicate that both physical and psychological factors are relevant (Huebscher 1998, Braverman & Schulman 1999). Hemmings et al (2000) demonstrated a high patient satisfaction rate associated with massage. Techniques include effleurage (gliding movements), petrissage (kneading) and tapotement (striking), all of which are generally accepted to have their effects in the superficial tissues such as the skin. Mennell (cited in Chamberlain 1982) first introduced specific massage movements called 'friction' in the early 1900s. Cyriax further developed this technique, adding movement for the treatment of pain due to inflammation caused by trauma. He described 'deep' friction massage which reaches deep structures of the body such as ligaments, muscles and tendons, to distinguish it from the general massage described above (Cyriax 1984). The technique of transverse frictions has been further refined in recent years to allow the grading of the technique according to the irritability of the lesion and patient feedback.

Transverse frictions, therefore, are a specific type of connective tissue massage applied precisely to move the target tissue – of tendons, muscles and ligaments – for a specific purpose. It is applied prior to and in conjunction with specific mobilization techniques to gain its effects.

The term 'deep' transverse frictions has been deliberately avoided as the blanket term to prevent the abuse of this technique. Unfortunately, deep transverse friction has been taught to many therapists as just that, and the technique has not been adapted or graded to suit the lesion to gain specific purpose. Consequently, it has developed a reputation for being very painful for the patient and tiring for the therapist, often being abandoned for these reasons (Ingham 1981, Woodman & Pare 1982, Cyriax & Cyriax 1983, de Bruijn 1984). It is an underrated modality at our fingertips (pun intended) and, when applied correctly, it is an extremely useful technique.

Transverse frictions can be graded in depth and duration of application for acute and chronic lesions. If correctly applied, an analgesic effect is achieved and it does not have to be a painful experience for the patient. In this text, the terms *gentle transverse frictions* (for acute irritable lesions) and *deep transverse frictions* (for chronic non-irritable lesions) will be used to give an indication of the grade required for specific treatments. However, no attempts have been made to quantify this grade and it should be developed in response to patient feedback and according to the experience of the therapist.

The evidence base to support the use of transverse frictions needs urgent development, but a number of studies exist which suggest plausible reasons for the effects of the technique, paving the way for future research. With one exception, most studies use a small sample of 17–46 subjects, making it difficult to generalize results to a wider population, and several involve animal models. No one treatment modality has been shown to be significantly better than another, and some studies use subjective terms such as 'traditional' and 'standard physiotherapy' to indicate the use of combined modalities. There is no consensus on a standardized method of application, with techniques varying from three 1-min applications to a 10-min continuous application in one session.

Stratford et al (1989) evaluated the use of phonophoresis (the delivery of drugs via the skin using ultrasound) and transverse frictions for tennis elbow but the lack of statistical power was deemed to be due to the small sample size. Vasseljen (1992) demonstrated that 'traditional physiotherapy' methods of transverse frictions and ultrasound performed better than laser in tennis elbow under subjective, but not objective, testing. However, the subjective interpretation in this study may have been more reliably evaluated using qualitative research methods.

Assessing the effect of the addition of transverse frictions to a 'standard' physiotherapy programme, Schwellnus et al (1992) showed no significant difference between comparison groups in the treatment of iliotibial band friction syndrome. This study was identified for the Cochrane Library by Brosseau et al (2002) as the only randomized controlled trial to meet investigation criteria. In providing a rationale for their research, Schwellnus et al suggest that the effect of transverse frictions is to realign fibres without detaching them from their origins. However, this is inconsistent with current physiological evidence which shows fibre alignment to occur along the lines of the applied stress. Therefore it is the applied mobilization technique following the application of transverse frictions which is important for realignment of fibres.

Verhaar et al (1996) conducted the only study to investigate the use of transverse frictions combined with mobilization, in this case a manipulation for tennis elbow. A prospective randomized controlled trial was conducted with 106 patients divided into two groups, one receiving transverse frictions and Mill's manipulation (see Ch. 6) and the other corticosteroid injection. Short- term follow-up showed significant improvement in both groups, with the injection group faring better than the transverse frictions group, while long- term follow-up showed no statistical difference between the two groups. An honest evaluation of the limits of this study is included by the authors, citing reasons such as failing to eliminate observer bias together with blinding and organizational difficulties. They suggest that as the conclusion of the study identified all methods of treatment as effective, then the least invasive, least expensive and most time-efficient should be used, in this case injection. However, injection is an invasive technique and the number of patients requiring surgery in the injection group in the long term was not addressed in the study.

Pellecchia et al (1994) demonstrate some support for 'combined modalities' including transverse frictions when compared with iontophoresis (delivery of drugs via the skin using electrical energy), but conclude that iontophoresis may be more effective and efficient. The study is limited by its small sample size of 26 subjects, scant discussion on how randomization and blinding occurred and a lack of analysis on the six subjects who dropped out. The authors discuss the limitations of their study, explaining that ethical considerations resulted in decisions which favoured the interests of the patients over a stronger experimental design. This study clearly illustrates the difficulties experienced in developing good experimental evidence.

Drechsler et al (1997) provide a clear rationale for an experiment to compare two treatment regimes for tennis elbow, while also adding to the current debate on the deficiencies of treatment regimes which address inflammatory rather than degenerative causes of tendinopathy. A 'standard' treatment group was exposed to several interventions including transverse frictions while a neural tension group was exposed to mobilization of the radial nerve. Results showed no significant difference for any variable tested; nevertheless, it is concluded that neural and joint mobilizations together were superior to the 'standard' treatment techniques.

In contrast to the above studies, Davidson et al (1997) and Gehlsen et al (1998) used animal studies to provide support for the application of augmented soft tissue mobilizations, applied parallel to the fibre direction, to promote the healing process in tendinopathy. These soft tissue pressures could be considered to be similar to the pressures delivered by deep transverse frictions. Controlled application of microtrauma through pressure in this way promoted fibroblastic proliferation and activation, dependent upon the depth of the pressure applied, leading to repair in the absence of inflammation.

Parallels could be drawn with a study conducted by Gregory et al (2003) who used an animal model to demonstrate the ultrastructural changes occurring in previously normal muscle tissue following 10 min deep transverse frictions. Obvious reddening of the skin was present immediately after deep transverse frictions, with inflammation and changes in myofibre morphology still apparent 24 h later. However, the ultrastructural changes described after 6 days were not those routinely associated with regeneration of muscle tissue after injury, such as haemorrhage, inflammation and macrophage activity, but more consistent with the repair process. It was also clear that the ultrastructural changes occurred locally under the area to which treatment had been directed. What the study was unable to clarify was whether or not these changes are potentially beneficial and would facilitate the healing process, or would aggravate the injury if present.

Kelly (1997) conducted a study to specifically test transverse frictions as a single modality, although this involved normal volunteers rather than symptomatic patients. The gastrocnemius muscle in 46 subjects received 5 min deep transverse frictions. An increase in the range of movement (dorsiflexion) and force of isometric muscle contraction (plantarflexion) occurred, indicating that transverse frictions may promote improved muscle function. Credit in this study was also given to motivational and psychological factors arising from the hands-on treatment; this has further implications for external validity. Iwatsuki et al (2001) seem to corroborate the work of Kelly in an investigation into the biting force of the masticatory muscles in subjects diagnosed with cerebrovascular accident before and after transverse frictions. Improved function due to an increase in the biting force of these muscles was demonstrated. The reason for the result was deemed to be due to relaxation of muscle spasm, although once again the sample size was small.

Despite the paucity of evidence, good clinical results have been observed following transverse frictions and until proven ineffective, its use is advocated according to certain principles discussed below. The above studies suggest that possible beneficial effects include improved muscle function, stimulation of an inflammatory reaction and repair due to proliferation and activation of fibroblasts in the absence of inflammation. If ultrastructural changes occur local to the applied pressure and take time to subside, this has implications for ensuring that the technique is delivered to the target tissue and for the timing of subsequent applications of the technique.

AIMS OF TRANSVERSE FRICTIONS

To induce pain relief

An in-depth discussion of the pain-relieving effects of manual therapy techniques is outside the scope of this book and the reader is referred to the work of Vicenzino & Wright (2002), who provide an account of the current evidence. Pain relief following the application of transverse frictions has been clinically observed and a number of working hypotheses are proposed to substantiate this.

Aims of transverse frictions

- To induce pain relief.
- To produce therapeutic movement.
- To produce a traumatic hyperaemia in chronic lesions.
- To improve function.

The reduction in pain is experienced as a numbing or analgesic effect, i.e. a decrease in pain perceived by the patient who will often acknowledge this by saying you have 'gone off the spot'. However, with faith in diagnosis and accurate knowledge of anatomy, this should be the signal to grade the friction more deeply to apply beneficial treatment appropriate to the lesion. Following treatment the comparable signs can be reassessed and a reduction in pain and increase in strength is usually noted. This induced analgesia is utilized to allow the application of graded mobilization techniques in acute lesions. In chronic lesions, an initial analgesic effect is required through the application of a gentler grade of transverse frictions before the technique is applied with increasing depth to produce the traumatic hyperaemia discussed below, and to allow graded mobilization to be applied.

The traumatic hyperaemia induced by the application of deeper graded transverse frictions over a longer period of time in chronic lesions may produce analgesia through changes in the local microenvironment of the tissues via an increased blow flow. These changes may include removal of the chemical irritants which sensitize or excite local nociceptors, a decrease in local oedema and pressure, the production of local heat and facilitation of the repair process.

Pain modulation may be induced through several complex phenomena, including spinal and central nervous system mechanisms acting individually or in combination, to produce desired effects. The gate control theory proposed by Melzack & Wall in 1965 is a theory of pain modulation that affects the passage of sensory information at spinal cord level, especially nociceptive impulses. Within the spinal cord there are mechanisms which 'open the gate' to impulses provoked by noxious stimuli, and mechanisms which 'close the gate', thus reducing the awareness of noxious stimuli. Pressure stimulates low-threshold mechanoreceptors, the A-beta fibres, that reduce the excitability of the nociceptor terminals by presynaptic inhibition, effectively 'closing the gate' on the pain. The A-beta fibres are myelinated, fast conducting fibres which basically 'overtake' the slow conducting fibres to reach the gating mechanism, closing it to incoming painful stimuli. The greater the mechanoreceptor stimulation, the greater the level of pain suppression (Bowsher 1994, Wells 1994). Put simply, rubbing a painful spot reduces pain, enabling the transverse frictions to be graded in depth, specific to individual lesions, and thus to produce their beneficial effects.

The reduction in pain achieved seems to be fairly long-lasting, possibly longer than expected. Transverse frictions, like rubbing or scratching the skin, are considered to be a form of noxious counterirritation that leads to a desired analgesic effect (de Bruijn 1984). Inhibition, which produces lasting pain relief, is believed to be through the descending inhibitory control systems via the periaqueductal grey area – the key centre for endogenous opioid analgesic mechanisms. Endogenous opioids are inhibitory neurotransmitters which diminish the intensity of the pain transmitted to higher centres (de Bruijn 1984, Melzack & Wall 1988, Goats 1994).

De Bruijn (1984) treated 13 patients with deep transverse frictions to various soft tissue lesions. The time required to produce analgesia during the application of deep transverse frictions was noted to be 0.4–5.1 min (mean 2.1 min) while the post-massage analgesic effect lasted 0.3 min–48 h (mean 26 h).

Carreck (1994) evaluated the effect of a 15-min general lower limb massage (effléurage and pétrissage) on pain perception threshold in 20 healthy volunteers and showed that the massage significantly increased the pain perception threshold for experimentally induced pain. Conversely, Kelly (1997), using deep transverse frictions on normal volunteers, reported no significant change in the pain pressure threshold, although there was an improvement in function that will be discussed below.

Massage in its various forms is considered to be a placebo, having a therapeutic effect on the psychological aspects of pain. There is no doubt that a professional attitude, including a thorough patient assessment and diagnosis, an explanation of the problem and the beneficial effects of the proposed treatment intervention, together with involvement of patients in their own recovery, has great effect. Transverse frictions as a form of massage may also have a placebo effect.

To produce therapeutic movement

Transverse friction aims to achieve a transverse sweeping movement of the target tissues – muscles, tendons and ligaments. This transverse movement, together with graded mobilization, discourages the stationary attitude of fibres that promotes anomalous cross-link formation. The therapeutic movement may facilitate the shear and gliding properties of collagen, allowing subsequent longitudinally applied stresses, through graded mobilization techniques, to stimulate fibre orientation towards enhanced tensile strength. In this way adhesion formation is prevented in acute situations and mobilized in chronic situations.

Friction potentially exists whenever two objects come into contact with each other, which is why it is important that the depth of application of transverse frictions should ensure that the therapist's finger makes contact with the target tissue, albeit via the skin and superficial tissues. A shear force is one that attempts to move one object over or against another and is applied parallel to the contacting surfaces in the direction of the attempted movement. The greater the contact force via the therapist's finger on the target tissue and/or the rougher the contacting surfaces, the greater the force of friction. Imagine rubbing your hands together; the harder you press, the greater the contact force and the greater the friction generated (Levangie & Norkin 2001). Friction generates heat and may therefore promote movement of the tissues by reducing pain and viscosity.

A therapeutic to-and-fro movement aims to mimic the function of the target tissue to prevent adhesive scar tissue formation in acute lesions and to mobilize established scarring in chronic lesions. For this reason, muscle bellies are placed into a shortened position to facilitate broadening of the muscle fibres and ligaments are moved across the underlying bone. In the case of tendons, transverse frictions aim to passively move the structures, either within the surrounding connective tissue or between a tendon and its sheath. Tendons in sheaths are therefore put on the stretch to allow mobilization of the sheath around the solid base of the underlying tendon.

When applied in the early inflammatory phase, gentle transverse frictions – approximately half a dozen sweeps – cause an agitation of tissue fluid that may increase the rate of phagocytosis by chance contact with the macrophages (Evans 1980). It is a useful treatment to apply in the acute inflammatory stage following injury, depending upon the irritability of the condition. It is applied in this 'gentle' manner before scar tissue formation has truly begun, but should be graded appropriately to avoid increased bleeding or disruption of the healing breach.

In an experiment to evaluate pain and range of movement in acute lateral ligament sprain of the ankle, the effect of transverse frictions together with Grade A mobilization was compared to Grade A mobilization alone (Kesson & Rees, unpublished work, 2002). The experimental group received transverse frictions and Grade A mobilization, while the comparison group received Grade A mobilization alone. The sample size of 16 was too small to allow statistical significance or generalization but the experimental group showed a greater overall increase in range of movement and a greater overall decrease in pain on single leg standing than the comparison group. However, it was noted that two subjects experienced a decreased range of movement and four experienced increased pain on single leg standing in the experimental group. The mean number of days post injury for the experimental group was 4.4 and if this trend were upheld in a larger trial it could have implications for assessing the appropriate time to apply transverse frictions in terms of assessment of irritability. The suggestion is that the appropriate time for applying transverse frictions and Grade A mobilization cannot be determined in terms of number of days post injury, but should be assessed in terms of the injury sustained and the irritability of the lesion.

In the chronic inflammatory phase, deep transverse frictions produce therapeutic movement, increasing frictional forces and generating heat to soften and mobilize adhesive scar tissue. This prepares the structure for other graded mobilizations that aim to apply longitudinal stress or selectively rupture the unwanted adhesions.

To produce a traumatic hyperaemia in chronic lesions

Increasing the depth of transverse frictions, i.e. the contact between the therapist's finger and the target tissue, together with an increase in time of the application of the technique to approximately 10 min produces a controlled traumatic hyperaemia and is used exclusively for chronic lesions.

A superficial erythema (redness) develops in the skin through dilatation of the arterioles and it is assumed that the same reaction is occurring in the deeper tissues where the effect is required (Winter 1968). The area of redness that develops under the finger may also be slightly raised and warm (a wheal), indicating increased permeability of the capillary walls that allows tissue fluid to pass into the surrounding area (Norris 1998). Massage, which increases blood flow in this way, changes the microenvironment of the tissues, producing local heat and decreasing pain by facilitating the removal of chemical irritants which sensitize or excite local nociceptors. This may also produce a decrease in pain by facilitating the transportation of endogenous opiates.

The work of Gregory et al (2003), described above, indicated that transverse frictions applied for 10 min produced ultrastructural changes in skeletal muscle initially consistent with the inflammatory process and ultimately with the reparative process. The observation of the redness and the wheal following the application of 10 min transverse frictions may be sufficient to stimulate a controlled inflammatory reaction which may be responsible for boosting the repair process in chronic lesions. Applying appropriate graded mobilizations after the friction technique aims to ensure healing within the presence of movement and the production of a strong mobile scar.

Although no clinical evidence exists to support the exact timing of 10 min after achieving an analgesic effect, it is the approximate time taken to induce and observe the skin changes described. However, tenderness in the target and overlying tissues may be a product of the induced inflammatory response, therefore at least 48 h (possibly 6 days, see the work by Gregory et al described above) is recommended between the treatment sessions in chronic lesions, in order for the tenderness to subside. The work of Davidson et al (1997) and Gehlsen et al (1998) suggests that in chronic tendinopathy (i.e. a degenerative process) repair may occur in the absence of inflammation by increasing the number and activity of the fibroblasts. Their work suggests that greater fibroblastic proliferation and activity occur with deeper pressures, indicating the appropriateness of deeper graded transverse frictions in chronic lesions.

Although the traumatic hyperaemia may be desirable in chronic lesions, this is not the case in acute lesions where the response is already excessive. Gentle transverse frictions applied to acute lesions for approximately six sweeps after achieving an analgesic effect are performed with reduced depth and time to avoid producing this traumatic hyperaemia. Such patients are treated ideally on a daily basis, or as often as possible, to ensure healing within the presence of movement and to encourage the formation of strong mobile scar tissue.

To improve function

> **Clinical tip**
> The exact grade of transverse frictions is determined by the irritability of the lesion and through feedback from the patient, but to be effective, they must be deep enough to reach the target tissue.

The therapeutic movement achieved and pain relief induced by transverse frictions produce an immediate clinical improvement in function of the structure treated. This can be demonstrated by reassessment of the comparable signs immediately after treatment and provides an optimum situation for the application of other graded mobilizing techniques.

As discussed above, Kelly (1997) and Iwatsuki et al (2001) conducted studies which demonstrated improved muscle function in terms of strength of contraction, with Kelly also demonstrating increased range of movement.

**PRINCIPLES OF
APPLICATION OF
TRANSVERSE
FRICTIONS**

Transverse frictions should be applied to the exact site of the lesion. This relies on clinical diagnosis and palpation of the lesion, based on anatomical knowledge and the structural organization of the tissue. Tenderness is not necessarily an accurate localizing sign, therefore palpation must reproduce the patient's pain and be different in comparison with the other limb.

Transverse frictions are always applied transversely across the longitudinal fibre orientation of the structure (Fig. 4.3). This aims to prevent or mobilize adhesion formation between individual fibres and between fibres and the surrounding connective tissues. Application of the technique in this manner deters a stationary attitude of fibres and aims to

Figure 4.3   Transverse friction massage of: (a) a tendon (supraspinatus); (b) a tendon in sheath (peronei); (c) a ligament (medial collateral) in flexion and extension; (d) muscle belly (hamstring).

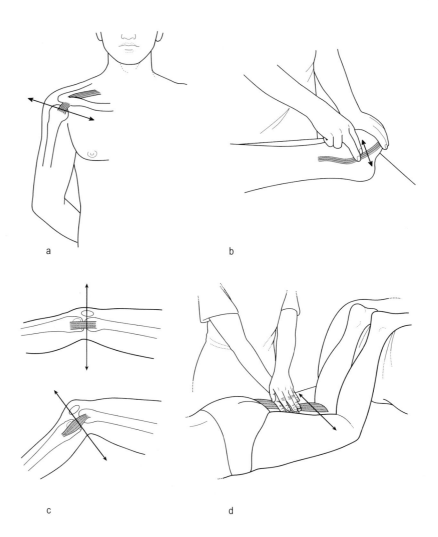

prevent or mobilize anomalous cross-links. The longitudinal stress applied in accompanying graded mobilization techniques, stimulates fibre orientation within the collagen weave and increases tensile strength.

Transverse frictions are applied with sufficient sweep or amplitude theoretically aiming to move the connective tissue fibres of the affected structure. The therapist must be positioned to ensure that this sweep is maintained through the application of body weight.

Transverse frictions are applied with effective depth, aiming to reach and benefit the target tissue. Knowledge of anatomy is paramount. The depth is maintained by applying the technique slowly and deliberately, but it is the shear force between the superficial tissues and the underlying target tissue which generates friction and produces heat, as mentioned above. While this latter effect is desirable, care must be taken to maintain the depth of the technique, as to increase speed tends to lift the effect towards the more superficial tissues.

The grading and duration of application of transverse frictions is intended as a clinical guide, the depth of technique being dependent upon the irritability of the lesion and feedback from the patient. The depth of the initial sweeps should always be gentle to gain an analgesic effect before proceeding with the effective frictions. Application in this way will dispel the myth that transverse frictions are a painful treatment technique.

The patient is positioned taking into account the situation in which the structure is most accessible and the degree of stretch or relaxation appropriate:

- Tendons in a sheath are placed on the stretch to allow the transverse frictions to roll the sheath around the firm base of the tendon, facilitating functional movement between the tendon and its sheath
- Tendons are placed into a position of accessibility, with the lesion commonly lying at the teno-osseous junction. Consideration is given to anatomy
- Muscle bellies are placed in a shortened, relaxed position to facilitate broadening of the muscle fibres, imitating function
- Ligaments are put under a small degree of tension to tighten the overlying soft tissues, allowing the target tissue to be reached
- Transverse frictions or corticosteroid injection are alternative treatment techniques for the teno-osseous junctions of tendons; musculotendinous junctions usually respond well to transverse frictions

The therapist should adopt a position that utilizes body weight to an optimum, ensuring sufficient sweep and depth. Sitting is possible, but the most effective position to apply body weight is with the patient situated on a plane lower than the therapist. Consideration should be given to the variety of ways the hands can be used to avoid fatigue and overuse (Fig. 4.4). The therapist's finger and the patient's skin and superficial tissues should move simultaneously to avoid raising a blister and to ensure that the superficial tissues are moving over the underlying target tissue, generating a friction force between them. The most efficient way of achieving this is to apply the technique in two directions. Pressure is first

Figure 4.4   Hand positions for transverse friction massage. (a) Index finger reinforced by middle finger; (b) middle finger reinforced by index finger; (c) thumbs; (d) ring finger; (e) pinch grip; (f) hands; (g) hand guiding the flat of the elbow.

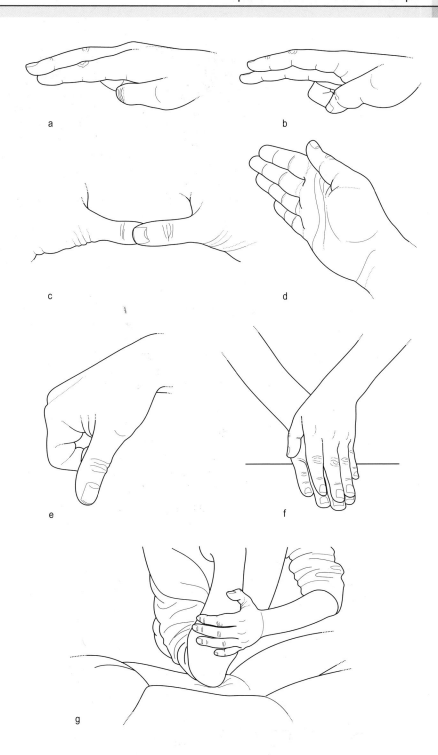

directed against the structure and then maintained while the transverse sweep is applied.

As a general guideline, transverse frictions are applied for an appropriate time to achieve the desired effects. For chronic lesions, 10 min after the analgesic effect has been achieved is suggested. However, due to the induced traumatic hyperaemia or local inflammatory response, treatment is repeated at a suggested minimum interval of 48 h to allow the tenderness generated in the target and overlying tissues to subside. It is suggested that gentle transverse frictions are applied to acute lesions for six effective sweeps once some analgesia is achieved and the target tissue reached. Treatment can be on a daily basis, if practically possible, to promote pain relief and therapeutic movement. These guidelines are largely based on expert clinical opinion and, as discussed above, no clinical evidence has been found to support them. From the practical aspect, the duration of application fits in with appointment times and allows for both reassessment and the application of other modalities of treatment judged to be appropriate.

Absolute contraindications to transverse frictions are few. The technique is never applied to active conditions, e.g. areas of active infection such as a boil or pimple or active inflammatory arthritis in which the connective tissue structures are too irritable. Care is required if there is fragile skin or the patient is currently undergoing anticoagulant therapy.

GRADED MOBILIZATION TECHNIQUES

Grade A, B and C mobilizations (Saunders 2000) are specific mobilization techniques applied to achieve a particular purpose. Each mobilization described below is an individual technique aiming to achieve specific effects and they are not intended to be a progression of each other.

GRADE A MOBILIZATION

Grade A mobilization is a passive, active or active/assisted mobilization performed within the patient's pain-free range of movement, aiming to provide or maintain mobility. It is applied within the elastic range. In peripheral lesions it is usually applied to irritable, acutely inflamed or painful lesions and it may be facilitated by the previous application of transverse frictions. At the spinal joints, the term 'Grade A' is used to indicate that the mobilization technique is applied in the mid-range, a pain-free mobilization for an acute, irritable spinal lesion to reduce pain and facilitate movement.

AIMS OF GRADE A MOBILIZATION

To promote tissue fluid agitation

In peripheral lesions, Grade A mobilization, either active or passive, produces a gentle soft tissue movement agitating tissue fluid in the acute inflammatory phase and facilitating the phagocytic action of the macrophages (Evans 1980). The movements are of small amplitude, slow, pain-free, without force and repeated often.

To prevent a stationary attitude of fibres

Grade A mobilization will promote movement within connective tissue structures to prevent a stationary attitude of fibres. In the acute phase of inflammation, the movement should occur without stress or disruption of the healing breach. The patient is instructed to exercise up to the point of discomfort, but not into or through pain, and must understand the importance of this controlled, precise movement. In this way a critical amount of movement is applied to encourage function but not to delay healing.

The function of a muscle belly is maintained by performing active inner-range, isometric, pain-free contractions aiming to broaden muscle fibres. The function of a ligament is promoted by performing active isotonic pain-free movement, maintaining the ligament's ability to glide over the underlying bone. In overuse lesions, e.g. tendinopathy, the patient maintains normal function by performing movement within the pain-free range and avoiding the painful movements.

To apply a longitudinal stress to connective tissue structures

Grade A+ mobilization (i.e. a Grade A mobilization which begins to 'nudge' the pain) aims to impart sufficient longitudinal stress to promote orientation of collagen fibres within the existing parallel collagen weave. In acute lesions, once it is judged that there is sufficient tensile strength in the wound, the patient may begin to 'nudge' pain to provide longitudinal stress but without disrupting the healing breach. The Grade A+ mobilizations are of short duration, are not forceful and are repeated often. This form of mobilization is appropriate for the repair phase of connective tissue injuries, and as progress is made an increasing range of movement is encouraged. In this way the developing scar tissue is stressed, not stretched, aiming to restore full functional range. Tissues which heal within the presence of movement in this way should not require 'traditional' stretching into the painful range.

To promote normal function

Grade A mobilization is applied early in the inflammatory phase to ensure that function is rapidly regained. Healing within the presence of movement promotes a return to function, i.e. form follows function. The range of movement is gradually increased, applying sufficient stress to the wound to promote orientation of fibres. Controlled mobilization of acute lesions should prevent the need for stretching tissue.

In chronic injuries, once the lesion is rendered pain-free by transverse frictions or corticosteroid injection, normal movement will promote remodelling and alignment of fibres and restoration of function. However, until signs and symptoms subside, it is suggested that overuse activity should be avoided in lesions aggravated by repetitive movements, and resisted exercise and stretching postponed until the scar tissue is fully mobilized and the selective tension tests pain-free.

To reduce a loose body or bony subluxation in a peripheral joint

To reduce a peripheral joint loose body (e.g. in the hip, knee or elbow) or a bony subluxation (e.g. carpal bone), a Grade A mobilization is performed under strong traction, the principal component of this technique, giving the fragment space to move.

GRADE B MOBILIZATION

A Grade B mobilization is a mobilization performed at the end of available range. In peripheral lesions it is a specific sustained stretching technique that aims to facilitate permanent elongation of connective tissue. At the spinal joints, the term 'Grade B' is used to indicate that the mobilization technique is applied at the end of available range.

AIMS OF GRADE B MOBILIZATION

To stretch capsular adhesions in peripheral joints

In the early stages of arthritis, pain causes the joint to be held in a position of ease, restricting movement of some parts of the joint capsule. This promotes a disordered deposition of collagen fibres and the normal flexibility of the joint capsule is impeded by anomalous cross-link formation. The changes in the capsule contribute to contracture and the capsular adhesions severely restrict the range of movement, causing pain and altered function. The aim of treatment by Grade B mobilization is to lengthen the capsular contracture permanently, to restore normal movement.

Adhesions that develop within the capsule of the synovial joint tend to be tough and unyielding. The shoulder and hip joints commonly demonstrate this gross loss of function and respond well to Grade B mobilization, providing the joints are in a non-irritable state. However, the technique could be applied to any non-irritable capsulitis in which pain and loss of movement are clinical features. Characteristically the joint is limited in the capsular pattern, with the restricted movements demonstrating a 'hard' end-feel (see Ch. 1). Grade B mobilization is aimed at restoring the movements limited in the capsular pattern.

Grade B mobilization is applied at the end of available range, appreciating the end-feel and the patient's pain response. To be successful, the end-feel should still have some elastic quality, but the sensation of muscle spasm may also be apparent as the technique is applied within a painful range. The technique is a slow, sustained and repeated stretch, performed at the end of available range for the duration of the patient's pain tolerance. As soon as the end range position is released, an immediate relief of pain should be felt. If pain lingers at this stage, the joint may be too irritable and the technique may not be appropriate. Successful treatment is dependent upon patient compliance as the management of the condition is long-term. Theoretically the tissue to be stretched needs to be taken into the plastic range to achieve permanent lengthening, with sufficient force applied to strain and break some of the collagen cross-links in the adhesive scar tissue, producing microfailure. However, as the capsular tissue possesses viscoelastic properties, this can be utilized to gain increased range of movement. The following factors relating to the behaviour of connective tissue under mechanical stress (see Ch. 2) can be applied to this mobilization that is suggested for tough, unyielding capsular adhesions.

A static stretch of slow, sustained, lower load force, applied towards the end of the elastic limit of the scar tissue, utilizes the viscous flow phenomenon which enables the contracted scar tissue to gradually *creep* or lengthen (Amis 1985, Hardy & Woodall 1998). The Grade B mobilization is a static stretch applied to the patient's pain threshold point. The increased length achieved is apparently due to cross-link disruption, fibre slippage and eventual structural changes (Hardy & Woodall 1998). Lengthening, under these circumstances, is inversely proportional to the velocity of the applied stretch with a slowly applied force meeting with less resistance or stiffness (it is easier to move slowly through a viscous medium). *Hysteresis* (the slower rate at which the structure recovers from the elongating force) may also play a role and can be linked to cyclical loading where subsequent applications of Grade B mobilization achieve a modest increment of increased length with each mobilization applied.

The structural changes occurring in the mobilized tissue may produce a low grade inflammatory response and the patient should be warned about post treatment soreness. The importance of continued movement to maintain the elongation achieved cannot be stressed enough, and the patient must be given an appropriate exercise programme to maintain the range achieved.

The optimum duration and frequency of the static stretch has yet to be determined, but the work of Brandy & Irion (1994) and Brandy et al (1997) suggests that in order to achieve an increase in range of knee flexion, a static stretch of 30 seconds applied to the hamstring muscles is sufficient. However, their studies fall short of determining how long the increased flexibility in the muscles lasted.

The application of heat relieves pain and lowers the viscosity of collagen tissue, allowing a greater elongation of collagen tissues for less force. Warren et al (1971) considered the effect of temperature and load on elongation of the collagen fibre structure of rat tail tendon. Heat and load were applied at selected temperatures of 39, 41, 43 and 45°C. The greatest elongation with least microdamage was achieved with lower loads at the higher therapeutic temperatures. The mechanism of a combined application of temperature and load affected the viscous flow properties of collagen.

Raising local temperature to between 40 and 45°C (40°C is the temperature of a very hot bath) achieves this useful therapeutic effect. Ultrasound can be applied to produce this thermal effect as it has a preference for heating collagen tissue (Low & Reed 1994). To achieve its best effects, heat should be applied concurrently with the Grade B mobilization; however, for practical purposes it is usually applied before.

To reduce pain   In arthritis, the inflammatory changes involve both the synovial lining of the joint and the fibrous capsule. The capsule develops small lesions that undergo scar tissue formation, producing adhesions or capsular thickenings. The adhesions are affected by joint movement which through abnormal tension, stimulates the free nerve endings lying in the capsule, producing mechanical pain. The nerve endings also respond to the chemical products of inflammation – histamine, kinins and prostaglandins. Impulses are transported in the non-myelinated C fibres and a 'slow', aching, throbbing pain is produced which is poorly defined, i.e. chemical pain (Norris 1998). The pain and associated involuntary muscle spasm reduce movement, allowing healing to occur in a shortened position and resulting in reduced function.

Sustained or repetitive passive joint movement may modify the firing responses in large diameter mechanoreceptor joint afferents, particularly when the capsular stretch is maintained at or near the end of range. This presents an explanation that accounts for the pain-relieving effects of end range mobilization, including passive Grade B stretching techniques as well as manipulation.

The permanent lengthening achieved by Grade B mobilization reduces the mechanical stress and therefore inflammation, which in turn relieves pain. Normal movement patterns are restored. This provides a stimulus to fibre alignment and orientation within the collagen weave.

> *Clinical tip*
> Grade B mobilization produces some treatment soreness. This gives a guide to irritability of the lesion and progression of treatment.

To improve function

The increase in joint range and pain relief achieved by Grade B mobilization improves overall function. However, the gradual onset of loss of movement through capsular contraction can considerably alter movement patterns. Careful assessment of the patient is necessary and a treatment programme planned which considers all components of the dysfunction, including altered biomechanics, muscle imbalance and neural tension.

Grade B mobilization is not used exclusively for capsular contractures. In chronic muscle, tendon and ligament lesions, adaptive shortening may be part of an overall dysfunction. The shortened tissues can be stretched by applying the principles of Grade B mobilization, both by the therapist and as a home treatment regime. Grade B mobilization is applied once the structure has been rendered functionally pain-free by deep transverse frictions and negative findings are established on examination by selective tension. Contracted tissue has an influence on neural structures; however, neural tension techniques fall outside the scope of this text.

GRADE C MOBILIZATION

Grade C mobilization is a manipulative technique and will be referred to as such. It is a passive movement performed at the end of range, i.e. once all the slack has been taken up, and is a minimal-amplitude, high velocity thrust. Most importantly, its principles of application are different in spinal and peripheral lesions.

Spinal manipulation can produce an immediate reduction in pain and a dramatic restoration of range of movement, but the mechanism by which manipulation achieves this is not well understood. Clinicians must work to the current best models in attempting to provide an explanation for their manual treatment interventions to both professional colleagues and patients alike. The benefit of manipulation may come from many interrelated factors rather than a single mechanism. A major factor towards successful manipulation is in the selection of appropriate patients with uncomplicated back pain of recent onset.

By strict definition, to *manipulate* is defined as 'to work with one's hands, to treat by manipulation' (Chambers 1998). Historically the term was applied to describe any technique that was applied using the hands. More recently, the term *manipulation* has come to mean 'a minimal amplitude high velocity movement performed at the end of range'. The essence of this definition has been adopted by all practitioners of manipulation, and may also commonly be termed 'Grade C', 'high velocity thrust' or 'Grade V' technique, etc.

A key point of an applied manipulation is that it is passive, i.e. out of the patient's control, and aims to move beyond the end of the passive range of the joint into the 'paraphysiological space', described by Sandoz (1976) as existing after the end of the passive limit but before the limit of anatomical integrity is reached where damage can occur. This section will briefly address the evidence to support the application of manipulation as part of the management of back pain and will then discuss the theories that relate to its proposed effects.

Many authors have reviewed clinical manipulation trials (Abenhaim & Bergeron 1992, LaBan & Taylor 1992, Barker 1994, O'Donaghue 1994, Shekelle 1994, Koes et al 1996, van Tulder & Koes 2002). These are often part of an overview of evidence to support the wide range of available treatment approaches in, for example, the management of low back pain (Waddell et al 1996, van Tulder et al 1997). Most of the trials reviewed tend to fall short of the ideal scientific criteria necessary for good quality research (Koes et al 1995). Harvey et al (2003) acknowledge that one of the confounders of research has been the different definitions of the therapeutic procedures involved. They describe a spinal manipulation 'package' that was agreed by the professional bodies representing chiropractors, osteopaths and physiotherapist in the United Kingdom (UK). The package was used in the UK Back pain Exercise And Manipulation (UK BEAM) trial, a national study of physical treatments in primary care.

It is generally accepted from the scientific data produced to date that spinal manipulation has shown short-term benefits of improvement in pain, movement and functional ability. Waddell et al (1996) reviewed the evidence relating to low back pain for the Royal College of General Practitioners which guided the Clinical Standards Advisory Group (CSAG) audit towards the development of guidelines for the management of acute low back pain. A system of diagnostic triage was introduced on which to base management. The guidelines have continued to be presented as a patient booklet, *The Back Book* (Roland et al 1996), to promote the recommendations of the guidelines on a wider scale. For simple acute back pain, the advice is given to avoid bed rest and to stay active, and manipulation is upheld as providing short-term improvement in pain and activity levels.

The long-term benefits of manipulation remain unknown although, if the aim of manipulation is to expedite recovery, these are of little significance. There is insufficient evidence to support or to refute the use of manipulation for chronic low back pain but manipulation is particularly appropriate for patients with uncomplicated acute back pain with symptoms of short duration (Shekelle 1994, Waddell et al 1996).

Several studies have focused on a comparison of manipulation with other conservative approaches and from this perspective there is little evidence to support the effectiveness of manipulation over modalities such as massage, exercise, back schools etc. or the administration of analgesics (Hsieh et al 2002, Assendelft et al 2003, Cherkin et al 2003).

However, for selected patients, when manipulation works it works quickly, which may have positive implications for reducing the overall cost of the management of acute back pain. Until soundly disproved, the authors endorse the benefit of Cyriax manipulation techniques, based on many years of clinical experience.

A step on from the consideration of the effectiveness of manipulation in the management of low back pain is the examination of its effects. The effects of manipulation on the soft tissues are still to be definitely established but moves have been made towards developing a 'theory of manipulation' to explain treatment outcomes. Drawn from the consensus of opinion of many authors, the broad effects of manipulation are the relief of pain, relief of muscle spasm and the restoration of movement and function.

Twomey (1992) draws together and generally dismisses the traditional theories that manipulation reduces subluxations, corrects vertebral alignment, adjusts nuclear prolapse or tears joint adhesions. Shekelle (1994) modifies these theories, however, suggesting that manipulation releases entrapped synovial folds or plicae, 'unbuckles' displaced motion segments, relaxes hypertonic muscle by sudden stretching, or disrupts articular or periarticular adhesions.

With respect to the first hypothesis listed above, synovial fringes are described within the facet joint (Bogduk 1997) but theories suggesting that they may present as a primary or secondary source of pain through entrapment are unsubstantiated. Twomey (1992) has already described the synovial fringes as 'slippery' structures that are unlikely to be trapped.

Earlier, Taylor & Twomey (1986) presented the hypothesis that rather than implicating the synovial fringes, the 'acute locked back' arises from impaction of a tag of articular cartilage within the apophyseal space, rather as a torn meniscus in the knee that, being connected to a well innervated capsule, can be a sudden cause of pain. 'Gapping' of the joint surfaces could allow the tag to return to its normal position so relieving the load on the capsule, allowing normal movement to return and a subsequent reduction in pain. This model depends on the demonstration that 'gapping' of the apophyseal joint does indeed occur with manipulation which will now be explored.

The relative movements between the target and other vertebrae are difficult to demonstrate and several studies rely only on mathematical predictions based on the forces applied. Dolan & Adams (2001) support that moderately flexed postures tend to unload the apophyseal joints. This is also supported by Punjabi et al cited in Lee & Evans (2001), who note that flexion increases the size of the intervertebral foramina. Gal et al (1995) performed a series of lower thoracic manipulative thrusts on two unenbalmed post rigor mortis human cadavers and recorded significant relative movements, primarily between the targeted vertebra and immediately adjacent vertebrae, during thrusts. Vertebral pairs remained slightly hyperextended after the thrusts, even when the posteroanterior forces had returned to preload levels. The link to the in vivo situation is probably unreliable but Gal et al concluded that their findings might be a useful step towards understanding the deformation behaviour of the vertebral column during manipulation.

Solinger (1996) set out to develop an analytical theory to describe the dynamics of small movement impulses applied to vertebrae in manipulation. He noted an initial passive oscillatory response to the thrust, governed by ligamentous and discogenic forces, and a subsequent less regular motion that he postulated was caused by muscular reflex contractions. He also measured relative separations of the L2, L3 vertebrae in vivo following high speed manipulative thrusts and demonstrated that both force and speed or duration of the thrust are important to optimize the efficacy of manipulation.

Zusman (1994) corroborates the suggestion that manipulation moves or frees the impediment, permitting movement and halting nociceptive input and associated muscle spasm. He also highlights the need for this to be demonstrated and suggests that magnetic resonance imaging (MRI) will hold the key to demonstrating what is happening at spinal level as manipulation is applied.

Cramer et al (2000) performed a small randomized trial on 16 healthy subjects comparing the effects of side-posture with rotation positioning and side-posture with rotation adjusting (manipulation) on the lumbar zygapophyseal joints, as evaluated by before and after measurements of MRI scans. Two other small groups in the study were measured in the neutral position, both before and after manipulation. The side-posture with rotation position itself produced some separation that was apparently increased following manipulation. This comparative increase was less than 1 mm. Both groups measured in neutral remained unchanged. The authors of the study acknowledge that a larger clinical trial is needed to further define their results.

The technology for producing moving MRI images (interventional MRI) has now been developed and McGregor et al (2001) used this method to observe the effects of Grade I and Grade IV posteroanterior mobilization in the cervical spine to assess for any movement at individual spinal levels. The scans demonstrated clear deformation of the overlying soft tissues and some angulation of the spine as a whole but minimal, if any, intervertebral movement (Fig. 4.5).

The expression 'unbuckles displaced motion segments' satisfies a variety of theoretical frameworks relating to the target structures or suggested mechanisms for the production of low back pain.

Twomey (1992) noted the common belief at the time that the disc was not the primary cause of back pain and that the zygapophyseal joint was more likely to be the source of the problem. Adams & Hutton (1981) and Adams et al (2002) have examined the biomechanical behaviour of the disc under different stresses, supporting the shift of evidence towards internal derangements within the outer annulus of the disc as the primary cause of back pain. Bogduk (1997) describes common theories of discal pathology that he terms 'internal disc disruption' where the internal architecture of the disc is disrupted with degradation of the nucleus pulposus and the presence of radial fissures in the lumbar spine that may reach the outer third of the annulus. The outer annulus is known to have a nerve supply and may therefore present as a primary cause of back pain. In internal disc disruption, the external surface remains essentially

Figure 4.5   Sagittal images obtained during (a) grade 1 PA mobilisation of 6th cervical vertebra; (b) grade 4 PA mobilisation of 6th cervical vertebra. From McGregor A, Wragg P, Gedroyc W M W (2001) Can interventional MRI provide an insight into the mechanics of a posterior-anterior mobilisation? Clinical Biomechanics 16:926–929. Reprinted by permission of Elsevier Ltd.

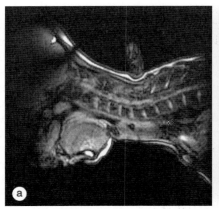
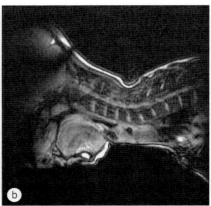

normal but the nucleus may bulge, as a bulge or protrusion, into the outer layers of the disc, where it may also produce pain.

Mixter & Barr (1934) were the first to suggest that rupture of the intervertebral disc could be a causal factor in sciatica, and Cyriax was one of the first clinicians to propound that in nuclear prolapse, discal material ruptures through the outer annulus into the vertebral canal, where it can have a secondary effect on pain-sensitive structures. Cyriax (1982), Twomey (1992) and Zusman (1994) all suggest that manipulation is unlikely to change or benefit a nuclear disc prolapse and there is little support from the literature that manipulation is – or is not – effective with this underlying pathology. The model of spontaneous recovery (Bush et al 1992) (see below) may provide a more plausible explanation for resolution of disc prolapse.

Several earlier and more recent studies have aimed to examine the effect of forces on the spine to explain disc degeneration (Farfan et al 1970, Adams & Hutton 1981, Noren et al 1991, Krismer et al 1996, Adams et al 2002) that may provide the groundwork towards the development of a hypothesis for the mechanism of treatment effects, particularly on the application of rotational manipulation techniques. Bogduk (1997) describes torsion injuries that can strain the collagen fibres of the annulus fibrosus, comparable to a ligament sprain. He warns that the condition has yet to be demonstrated in vivo but offers a feasible model (discussed below) for the pathology acquired on injury and for the effect of manipulation in relieving symptoms.

The reflex response to manipulation has invited study towards clarification of the therapeutic benefits of manipulation. Hertzog et al (1999) demonstrated consistent EMG reflex responses following manipulation. Collaca & Keller (2001) and Keller & Collaca (2000) studied the EMG reflex responses to manipulation and found that patients with frequent to constant low back pain tended to have more marked responses than patients with occasional or intermittent back pain. Evans (2002) discusses mechanisms for the relaxation of hypertonic muscle, describing both reduction in paraspinal spontaneous electromyography activity and reduction in hyperalgesia of paraspinal myofascial trigger points. Since hypertonic muscle, i.e. muscle spasm, would tend to be protective, he suggests that the emphasis should be on the creation of post-manipulative hypoalgesia that may lead in itself to relaxation of hypertonic muscle, the mechanisms of which are still being investigated.

Lehman et al (2001) applied a painful mechanical stimulus above the spinous process in 17 subjects with chronic low back pain and found that manipulation weakened the ensuing electromyography response. Although there was no statistical significance in the results and the effects were short term, the possibility of these responses causing some of the clinically observed beneficial effects, including reduction of pain and decrease in hypertonicity of muscles, has been put forward.

Wyke's work on the neurology of joints was pivotal in providing a model to explain the reflex relaxation of periarticular muscles following sudden stretching of the capsule, periarticular ligaments and tendons (Wyke 1967, Wyke 1979, Wyke 1980). Wyke (1979) and Zusman (1994) suggested that passive movements may activate the mechanoreceptors within capsular and other tissues. In addition, Katavich (1998) concludes that the deformation of joint capsule can modify reflex motor responses, leading to changes in muscle tone. The author notes the work of Clarke where sustained or repetitive passive joint movement, or indeed pressure over the joint, has been shown to modify firing responses in large diameter mechanoreceptor joint afferents, particularly when the capsular stretch is maintained at or near the end of range. This presents an explanation that accounts for the pain-relieving effects of end-range mobilization, including passive Grade B stretching techniques (see above) as well as manipulation.

If these observations are put together, mobilization and manipulation may stimulate mechanoreceptors to modify neural activity within the central nervous system, altering reflex pathways that affect the voluntary and involuntary activation of muscles and leading to relief of muscle spasm, increased movement and reduction in pain (Wright 1995).

The general rule is that manipulation should not be applied through spasm and that other techniques or modalities, such as graded mobilizations, heat or electrotherapy, may need to be applied to achieve reflex relaxation of this protective mechanism. It was the opinion of Brodeur (1995), however, that the high velocity thrust of manipulation had a split second's chance to affect the capsule and the Golgi organs within the periarticular contractile structures before any reflex spasm could resist the movement.

Cyriax, in 1984, and for at least 50 years before, did not shirk from his opinion that 'when minor ligamentous adhesions limit movement and cause pain they should be manipulatively ruptured'. His statement referred mainly to peripheral joints, and in spinal lesions he tended to refer to the effects of manipulation on what he termed 'small cartilaginous displacements'. He put forward these disruptions of the annulus fibrosus as a primary cause of low back pain of sudden onset, a theory that is supported by Bogduk (1997) (See below).

Lamb (1994) says that manipulation 'releases minor adhesions' and Zusman (1994) acknowledges the formation of fragile collagen fibrils in the early stages of repair, suggesting that graduated or 'abrupt' alteration in the length or location of undesirable and restrictive scar tissue is the most logical means by which ranges of movement might be improved with manually delivered passive movements: the 'abrupt' presumably describing manipulation.

Cramer et al (2000) present a theoretical model of manipulation breaking adhesions within the zygapophyseal joints and Bogduk (1997) describes torsion injuries that can strain the collagen fibres of the annulus fibrosus, comparable to a ligament sprain. If the fibres can be injured by torsion, the implication is that they can be affected by manipulative techniques, particularly those applied with rotation.

Dolan & Adams (2001) comment on the mathematical models that are often used to quantify the overall forces and moments acting on the lumbar spine, and explain that in order to describe how spinal tissues can be injured, it is necessary to distribute these forces between and within different spinal structures. They emphasize that it is the concentration of the force which causes injury and elicits pain. It may be reasonable, therefore, to extrapolate that opinion to propose that it is also the concentration of force within different spinal structures that affects the injured tissue and different spinal structures to lead to the relief of pain.

Scientific evidence is perhaps lacking in terms of knowing exactly what does happen to adverse adhesions, if they are implicated in joint hypomobility, but biomechanical models are useful towards the development of hypotheses.

Threlkeld (1992) expands on the viscous properties of connective tissue and describes how when the tissue is loaded more quickly, it behaves more stiffly than the same tissues loaded more slowly. Thus adhesions may be ruptured more readily by stress applied quickly, as in manipulation. If the concentration of forces applied in manipulation tends to fall selectively on the resisting scar tissue within the annulus, before the normal tissue is affected (Threlkeld 1992) (see Ch. 2), this can provide a sound model for the achievement of increased movement and pain relief with particular presentations of back pain.

Manipulation is often associated with an audible 'crack', said to be due to cavitation of the joints and a small diversion onto the subject of cavitation is pertinent at this stage. The forces applied on manipulation increase the joint volume, with a corresponding decrease in fluid partial pressure, creating a gas bubble as the intra-articular gases are drawn out of the solution. As the fluid rushes into the area of low pressure volume, the gas bubble collapses, producing the 'crack' (Herzog et al 1993).

Gibbons & Tehan (2001) propose that it is the cavitation that distinguishes manipulative techniques from other manual modalities and many clinicians judge the success of a manipulation by whether or not cavitation occurs (Conway et al 1993). Gibbon & Tehan focus on appropriate positioning to be able to localize forces to achieve cavitation, with the implication that it is a necessary component, although they do not specify why.

Brodeur (1995) provides a comprehensive review of the 'audible release' associated with joint manipulation. He cites an early study by Roston & Haines which demonstrated with serial X-rays of the third metacarpal joint that if the distraction force was high enough in the third metacarpophalangeal joint to produce a crack, there was dramatic increase in joint space of up to 3 mm. Cavitation was not achieved in lax or overly tight articular capsules but there was a more steady increase in the joint space nonetheless.

Gibbons & Collins (2001) aimed to determine whether high velocity thrust manipulation of the atlanto-axial joint improved pre-existing atlanto-axial rotation asymmetry in asymptomatic subjects, and then to compare this with the effects of a sham thrust without cavitation. The results indicated that while there was a trend towards improvement of the more restricted rotation in both the cavitation and non-cavitation groups, neither reached significance and no evidence was provided that the noiseless manipulation is or is not as effective as the manipulation with cavitation.

Evans (2002) provides an interesting discussion of the effects of manipulation but appears to misrepresent that Cyriax suggested that manipulation could benefit nuclear herniation. As discussed in Chapter 13, Cyriax (1982, 1984) did attribute presentations of low back pain to discal pathology but produced models of 'cartilaginous' and 'nuclear' displacements, devising associated sets of signs and symptoms to guide treatment choice. The cartilaginous presentation was linked to disruption of the annulus of the disc, often, perhaps erroneously, called 'fragments' of cartilage, and was suggested as being suitable for manipulation where changes could be effected within the collagen structure of the annulus, with a consequent sudden reduction in pain. The 'nuclear' presentation was designated by Cyriax as being more suitably treated with traction, in line with the more progressive or prolonged positions more appropriate for inducing movement in the viscoelastic nucleus, as Evans suggests.

Evans's theories relating to structures within the zygapophyseal joint as a possible cause of the 'locked back', and as discussed above, are indeed feasible but they are no more proven than theories relating to symptoms associated with torn fibres within the collagen structure of the annulus, as put forward by Bogduk (1997) and less explicitly by Cyriax himself. Thus, in the meantime, the model of disruption of fibres within the outer annular layers can provide a possible effect of manipulation in breaking down adhesions in the outer annulus.

While the debate on the pathology of back pain and the effects of manipulation will no doubt continue, the reader of this text will be encouraged to devise treatment programmes based on models of presentation and patient selection with careful consideration of patients' history and presenting signs and symptoms, and thorough screening for possible contraindications to treatment.

As a final consideration, Lee et al (1996) draw attention to the many variations in technique that may affect the movements at the spine. They can be summarized as: the magnitude of the applied force, the rate of increase of the force, the duration of loading and the accuracy and specificity of the application of the force. Other variations in the patient, the clinician and the treatment couch should also be considered, all of which need to be considered within the clinical reasoning process and can confound efforts to develop an ultimate theory of spinal manipulation.

SPINAL AND SACROILIAC JOINT MANIPULATION

To restore movement

In the spinal or sacroiliac joints in which a non-capsular pattern exists, indicating internal derangement limiting the range of movement in some, but not all directions, manipulation aims to 'unlock' the joint, possibly reducing the internal derangement and relieving compression to restore full, painless function. As suggested above, the effects of mobilization and manipulation may not be that simple and are probably multifactorial, involving all adjacent tissues.

To relieve pain

Manipulation-induced hypoalgesia – pain relief – is well documented (Wright 1995, Vernon 2000). Restoration of functional movement may in itself lead to reduction in pain but, arguably, relief of pain may be required to achieve this. Pain relief may also occur through stimulation of the mechanoreceptors effecting the pain-gate mechanism or through stimulation of the descending inhibitory controls.

Mechanoreceptors within the joint capsule and spinal ligaments are stimulated by the tension created by spinal manipulation. This inhibits the small-diameter nociceptor afferent input to the ascending pathways at spinal cord level via the gating mechanism described above. The relief of pain achieved reduces the reflex muscle spasm and an increase in the range of movement occurs.

The periaqueductal grey (PAG) area of the brain, as a control centre for endogenous analgesia, is considered to play an important role in the control of pain. Two different forms of analgesia may be produced: an opioid form that seems to be associated with sympathetic inhibition and takes a period of time to develop and a non-opioid form that is associated with sympathetic excitation that has a more rapid onset. Spinal manipulation has an immediate effect, producing pain relief within seconds or minutes due to the non-opioid form, associated with sympathetic excitation that is related to mechanical nociception. Over a period of about 20–45 min the analgesia changes to the opioid form associated with sympathetic inhibition. Spinal manipulation provides an appropriate stimulus to activate the descending pain inhibitory systems from the PAG to the spinal cord (Wright 1995).

It must not be forgotten that spinal manipulation can also relieve pain through the placebo effect of skilful handling and care. Indeed, Ernst (2000) offers the opinion that 'the success of manipulation is largely due to a placebo effect'. Further discussion on this topic is outside the scope of this book except to acknowledge the role of the placebo effect as one of the myriad of factors that can affect treatment outcomes. It is not possible to quantify this effect, although many trials try to eliminate its effect by establishing controls.

Principles of application of spinal and sacroiliac joint manipulation

Certain principles need to be considered in order to apply the technique effectively.

A short- or long-lever arm is used and a torque or twisting force is usually applied, taking up the slack in the surrounding connective tissue to induce a passive movement at one or more spinal joints (Hadler et al 1987). The minimal amplitude, high velocity thrust is of great importance since tissues loaded quickly behave more stiffly and have a higher ultimate strength (see Ch. 2). Thus, as the spinal manipulative technique is applied, the force needed to affect the target tissue does not cause damage to the surrounding structures (Threlkeld 1992), i.e. the weak link in the chain effect.

Manipulative reduction is more likely to succeed if the joint space is increased. Therefore an element of distraction is usually included. Spinal manipulation, in particular, requires skilful handling that takes time and practice to acquire. The hands must be continuously sensitive to the end-feel of the joints and any abnormal end-feel, e.g. bony resistance or muscle spasm, should alert the manipulator to abandon the procedure.

Successful manipulation requires accurate clinical diagnosis and the choice of the right patient with knowledge of the effects, contraindications and limits of the technique. Thought, care and expert skill are essentials, together with an explanation to the patient of the diagnosis, treatment and possible complications, in order to gain informed consent. Safety is essential and the precautions necessary will be discussed in the appropriate chapters.

Peripheral manipulation

Manipulative rupture of shortened scar tissue may be appropriate in peripheral lesions. The aim of the technique is to manipulatively rupture unwanted adhesions, producing permanent elongation and restoring full painless function. The short toe-phase of the adhesions ensures that the slack is taken up more rapidly than in the surrounding normal tissue and the minimal amplitude, high velocity thrust causes macrofailure, or rupture, of the adhesions while the normal tissue remains intact. It is important that the elongation achieved should be maintained by the patient. In orthopaedic medicine, manipulative rupture of unwanted adhesions is applied in two situations:

Manipulative rupture of unwanted adhesions between a ligament and bone

Peripheral manipulation is applied to a chronic ligamentous sprain of two ligaments in the lower limb, the medial collateral ligament at the knee and the lateral collateral ligament at the ankle. Unwanted adhesions may have developed between the ligament and the underlying bone that disrupt the normal functional movement of the joint and on examination a non-capsular pattern of pain and limitation will be found. The ligament is prepared by deep transverse frictions to achieve an analgesic effect and the manipulation follows immediately.

Effective manipulation should achieve instant results and vigorous exercise is required to maintain the lengthening achieved. Rehabilitation must address all components contributing to the dysfunction.

To rupture adherent scar tissue at the teno-osseous junction of the common extensor tendon (tennis elbow)

A special manipulation (Mills' manipulation) is applied at the teno-osseous junction of the common extensor tendon as a treatment for tennis elbow (Ch. 6). The manipulation aims to elongate adhesions interfering with the mobility of the tendon at its insertion and within the adjacent tissues. The tendon is first prepared by deep transverse frictions, followed by the manipulation. The elongation gained must be maintained through exercise.

TRACTION

The terms *traction* and *distraction* have the same meaning in describing a force applied to produce separation of joint surfaces and widening of the joint space. There is a convention that traction is applied to spinal joints and distraction to peripheral joints, but this is not a hard and fast rule.

This section considers the theory underpinning the traction and distraction techniques used in orthopaedic medicine. Emphasis will be placed on the use of traction as a treatment for back and neck pain. Many other treatment modalities employ distraction in the treatment of peripheral joint lesions and the aims and effects will be described briefly here.

The general indications for traction and distraction will be mentioned, but these, together with the contraindications for treatment, will be discussed in greater detail in the following chapters.

The aims of traction were originally devised from Cyriax's hypotheses of the effects on the spinal joints. They have been developed subsequently to encompass the peripheral joints, where appropriate, and may be stated as follows and as listed in the box.

To relieve pain

Pain relief through the use of traction is gained by relieving pressure. Traction reduces the compression force, muscles relax and the pressure on the joint and pain-sensitive structures is reduced.

To create space

The application of distraction/traction creates a degree of space within the joint, allowing a displaced bulge or fragment, a loose body or a displaced carpal bone room to move.

To produce negative pressure within a joint

Creating space within the joint creates a suction effect that helps to move a displaced intra-articular fragment.

To tighten the ligaments around a joint

Tightening up of the ligaments around the joint produces a centripetal force. A disc displacement will tend to be pushed towards the centre as the traction is applied.

To reduce a peripheral loose body

Distraction is the main element of the manoeuvre, with a Grade A mobilization applied during traction. The aim is to move the displaced fragment to another area of the joint where it does not block joint movement.

DISCUSSION ON THE AIMS AND EFFECTS OF TRACTION

To provide some support for the aims, the following paragraphs set out to review the evidence for the effects and effectiveness of traction, particularly as a treatment for back and neck pain.

'Traction is generally considered to be an empirical treatment', stated Colachis & Strohm (1965) and, in spite of several well organized trials to demonstrate the contrary, this statement unfortunately continues to be true.

In these days of evidence-based practice, demands have been made for traction, as an expensive, time-consuming modality, to be stopped as a treatment until evidence for its effectiveness has been produced. Mathews & Hickling's presentation of their paper (1975) was criticized for not honestly stating that no evidence had been found and an editorial in the *British Medical Journal* ('Trial by traction', BMJ 1976) urgently called for thorough research into traction to avoid further waste of resources.

Swezey (1983) represented the views of the many who use traction when he acknowledged that 'there is a consensus among thoughtful clinicians that traction is useful, and until further study argues to the contrary, it deserves a place in our therapeutic armamentarium'. Sharing that view, Saunders (1998) set out to evaluate the reviews that were considered for the *Clinical Guidelines for the Management of Low Back Pain* (Waddell et al 1996) that concluded that 'traction does not appear to be effective for low back pain with radiculopathy'. Saunders provides an interesting discussion which addresses the methodological weaknesses of the studies selected for the review, suggesting that the randomized controlled trial on this single modality, aiming for statistical significance, is clinically inappropriate and that a multimodal approach to treatment, including the use of specific and general exercise programmes, is likely to be more realistic in the clinical setting. He compares the trials in the reviews to a separate series of articles which, while they may not have achieved statistical significance, have suggested that traction may be effective for a specific population.

Van der Heijden et al (1995), in one of the reviews considered by Waddell et al, acknowledge that the studies they included 'do not allow clear conclusions due to methodological flaws in their design and conduct'. Van der Heijden et al (1995) also designed a pilot study to compare the effect of high-dose continuous lumbar traction and low-dose continuous lumbar traction on the magnitude and rate of recovery for patients with low back pain. They tentatively concluded that traction seemed to be more effective than sham traction in the short term but acknowledged that the small numbers involved prevented the achievement of statistical significance. Following evaluation of the pilot study, it was extended by Beurskens et al (1997) to include a total of 151 subjects. Beurskens et al were meticulous in their methodology, including patient selection, but nonetheless the study failed to demonstrate a significant difference between the two groups.

A literature search conducted by van Tulder & Koes (2002) for *Clinical Evidence Concise*, the self-acclaimed 'international source of the best available evidence for effective health care', concluded that randomized control trials found conflicting evidence and no support for the effects of traction for both acute and chronic low back pain. The question of patient selection and the parameters of the studies reviewed are left unstated, however, and Saunders (1998) warns that we should avoid making judgements about traction based on reports drawn from reviews without critically reviewing the articles ourselves. There was no mention in the same issue of *Clinical Evidence Concise* for the effects of traction on cervical pain.

Traction has been documented as a treatment for back pain at least since the time of Hippocrates (Hume Kendall 1955). Cyriax himself developed his first traction bed in 1949 and collaborated with his physiotherapists on how it could be used to relieve the symptoms produced by nuclear disc protrusion. His belief was that pain of gradual onset, usually associated with leg pain, was due to nerve root compression from herniated nuclear material through a tear in the annulus, i.e. a disc protrusion (see Ch. 13).

Cyriax's hypothesis was that effective traction could produce a suction effect within the disc to draw the nuclear material centrally and away from the nerve root. At the same time a mechanical 'push' would be given to the herniated material by tightening the ligaments spanning the bulge – the posterior longitudinal ligament in particular. Andersson et al, cited in Lee & Evans (2001), studied intradiscal pressure and showed Cyriax's hypothesis of a suction effect to be unfounded. However, Cyriax had claimed that in order to achieve these effects traction would need to produce separation of the intervertebral and zygapophyseal joints between the vertebrae accompanied by tensioning of the intervertebral ligaments, and there is considerable evidence that this separation occurs.

To demonstrate the separation of the vertebrae, Cyriax (1982) compared two X-rays of the cervical spine taken before and after the application of 'fairly' strong manual traction for several seconds. He measured an increase of 2.5 mm at each of the joints between the fourth cervical and first thoracic vertebrae. His maximum manual traction had previously (in an experiment in 1955) been estimated to be 140 kg, but his use of the term 'fairly' implies something less than that. Similarly, before and after X-rays of the lumbar spine were superimposed upon each other after 50 kg of traction had been applied for 10 min, and a widening of the disc space was observed.

Judovitch (1952) took a series of X-rays as progressive poundages were applied to the cervical spine of seven patients. He observed that with 45 lb (20.5 kg) of static, vertical traction there was separation of the interbody joints of C2–C7 and a small widening of the zygapophyseal joints. A similar serial study was performed by Colachis & Strohm (1966), but using 30 lb (14 kg) of intermittent cervical traction at a 24° angle of pull. In all 10 subjects the mean separation of the vertebrae increased proportionally, both anteriorly and posteriorly, to a maximum at 25 min.

On the assumption that increased disc space with traction would be manifest in an increase in height, Worden & Humphrey (1964) applied sustained traction of up to 132 lb (60 kg) to normal fit males. The traction was divided between the head and thorax and pelvis and ankles for 1 h on each of several consecutive days. They demonstrated an average increase in height of 8 mm.

They continued to observe two subjects and noted that they lost their increased height at a rate of 4 mm per h. In the Colachis & Strohm study mentioned above, no increase in posterior separation remained at 20 min after the cessation of traction but the residual anterior separation was statistically significant (Colachis & Strohm 1966).

Mathews (1968) used epidurography, involving the injection of radiopaque contrast medium into the epidural space for subsequent radiological investigation, and applied 120 lb (55 kg) of lumbar traction to three patients, two with suspected disc protrusions and one control. In one patient the bulge of the protrusion began to decrease in depth from 4 min and was further decreased at 20 min, with partial recurrence on release.

Evidence was provided for Cyriax's proposed suction effect on observing a second patient where not only was there a reduction in the depth of the multiple protrusions, but also contrast medium appeared to have been drawn into the disc spaces, implying the production of negative pressure within the disc.

The apparent suction effect may be a sequel to the reduction of load on the disc when traction is applied. Nachemson (1980), with the use of a miniature intradiscal pressure transducer, measured the approximate load on the L3 disc in a 70 kg individual, in different postures and exercises. Minimal load of 30 kg was recorded on the disc with the subject in supine lying and this was reduced to 10 kg on the application of 30 kg of traction.

This finding provided foundation for Cyriax's suggestion that the same effect on a disc prolapse could be achieved in a short time with sustained traction as that brought about by weeks or months of bed rest. Bed rest had disadvantages in terms of expense, if prolonged hospitalization was involved, as well as incapacitating the patient. Lumbar traction, on the other hand, would allow the patient to continue with daily activities and commitments.

Lee & Evans (2001) have examined loads in the lumbar spine during traction therapy and propose that traction does not simply produce axial distraction of the spine. They suggest that traction also produces a flexion moment leading to an increase in the posterior height of the discs and a flattening of the lumbar lordosis. This effect is enhanced by the use of the Fowler's position (hips and knees flexed to 90°) and may have clinical significance in tightening the posterior annulus and the overlying posterior longitudinal ligament, theoretically stimulating mechanoreceptors and reducing a confined disc prolapse towards the relief of pain.

Lumbar flexion has been demonstrated to increase the size of the intervertebral foramina (Punjabi et al cited in Lee & Evans 2001) and this would tend to support the use of traction as a treatment tool to enlarge a pathologically narrowed foramen, i.e. with symptoms of spinal stenosis.

Since the ambulant position subjects the disc to compressive forces (Nachemson 1980), certain considerations need to be applied to prevent the loss of the benefits of traction between treatments. Cyriax (1982) claimed that traction needs to be:

- As strong as possible
- Applied for as long as is both practicable and tolerable
- Applied daily, or at least five times a week
- Applied continuously

When Cyriax proposed that the physiological and biomechanical effects of static traction were more effective at reducing a nuclear protrusion, the debate of continuous (static) versus intermittent traction had little evidence to support either side.

Wyke, referred to in Cyriax (1982), observed that motor activity in the sacrospinalis muscles increased as the distracting force was increased, until the mechanoreceptors in the tendons were stimulated, producing an inhibitory effect after which the stress was allowed to fall on the spinal joints. Cyriax claimed that electromyographic (EMG) silence in the sacrospinalis was not achieved until 3 min into the application of traction. For this reason he proposed that intermittent traction would not be as suitable to produce nuclear movement, since repeated pulls of shorter duration would continually elicit the stretch reflex, producing muscular contraction and preventing joint distraction.

Cyriax's argument for wanting to avoid muscular contraction is supported by the study of Goldie & Reichmann (1977) to examine the influence of traction on the cervical spine. They observed that the force of muscle contraction in the cervical spine could overcome a traction force in excess of 30 kg (66 lb).

However, Hood & Chrisman (1968) used EMG recordings of lumbar sacrospinalis activity to compare the effect of static and intermittent traction and found no difference. Moreover, Klaber Moffett et al (1990) investigated the effects of sustained cervical traction on neck musculature using EMG recordings. They applied 6–12 lb (3–5 kg) of traction for 20 min in the recumbent position, but found that relaxation was not induced.

Support for sustained, as opposed to intermittent, traction may lie in the hydrostatic behaviour of the disc (Nachemson 1980). Sustained traction would be expected to be more effective in producing creep in the tissues gradually to reduce the herniation by the combined effect of both suction from within the disc and the 'push' produced by the tightening of the tissues spanning the joint.

Onel et al (1989) performed computed tomographic investigation of 30 patients diagnosed as having disc prolapse to observe the effect of traction on lumbar disc herniations. While establishing that 45 kg of traction was effective in reducing disc herniations, it was also apparent that intervertebral joint and zygapophyseal joint space was increased, with associated stretching of all anatomical structures of the spine. Grieve (1981) had already acknowledged the much wider range of application of traction, irrespective of the disc. The effect of traction on other tissues would suggest that it should be seen as a useful and adaptable method of mobilization of the motion segment, or segments, as a whole. This being so, intermittent traction would also have a place in mobilizing stiffness in the motion segments, relieving pain through the stimulation of the mechanoreceptors and by increasing circulation, as well as by reducing the compressive effects.

INDICATIONS FOR SPINAL TRACTION

Cyriax (1982) identified factors from the patient's history, together with certain symptoms and signs, which he believed were characteristic of a nuclear disc protrusion. Treatment with sustained traction was therefore indicated to reduce the protrusion.

He stated that with a nuclear protrusion, the pain is usually of gradual onset, with no recollection of the mode or time of onset. There is usually little central pain, but referred pain is usually present in the arm or leg. The pattern of spinal movement is non-capsular and the movements provoke the limb pain.

Cyriax ascribed the pathology to posterolateral movement of the protrusion, compressing the dural nerve root sleeve and producing unilateral pain. Smyth & Wright (1958) had also proposed this mechanism but when, in the light of investigation, opinion moved away from the notion of a 'jelly-like' nucleus, thus refuting the possibility of a nuclear ooze, Cyriax's hypothesis was largely rejected. The empirical findings nonetheless remained that traction could afford relief with that particular onset and pattern of pain.

Mathews & Hickling (1975) suggested that traction should be applied to a defined syndrome rather than a specific condition. This would appear to be a more satisfactory premise against which clinicians from the myriad of musculoskeletal backgrounds can apply the basic principles, while the debate on pathology continues as fresh evidence emerges.

Apart from the application of mechanical traction, in the cervical spine most of the mobilization and manipulation techniques are performed under manual traction. In the rotational techniques in the lumbar spine, a degree of distraction is applied to the joints with the Grade C manipulation.

Clinical tip

When applying the techniques of traction or distraction to the cervical spine or peripheral joints, the following principles should be employed:

- Body weight should be used.
- The application of body weight should be achieved by leaning out with straight arms.
- The distraction/traction should be sustained for a moment or two to become established before proceeding with the manoeuvre.

INDICATIONS FOR TRACTION AT PERIPHERAL JOINTS

Stiff osteoarthritic joints respond well to distraction, as do joints demonstrating the capsular pattern following adaptive changes in response to traumatic arthritis. The distraction is applied to increase mobility, using longitudinal or lateral distraction techniques, which may produce separation of joint surfaces and assist mobilization by stretching the joint capsule and capsular ligaments.

It may be applied manually as a treatment in itself or in conjunction with mobilization and manipulation techniques.

Where signs and symptoms indicate the presence of a loose body in a joint, or a carpal bone needs to be relocated, distraction before Grade A mobilization is applied. The distraction of joint surfaces allows space for movement of the fragment, assisted by the accompanying suction effect which distraction tends to produce.

ORTHOPAEDIC MEDICINE INJECTION TECHNIQUES

The interested reader is referred to *Musculoskeletal Injection Skills* (Kesson et al 2003), in which injections are covered in more detail.

In orthopaedic medicine, injection techniques are often an alternative treatment to transverse frictions and mobilization techniques. Whereas transverse frictions and mobilization appear to be most efficacious when used together or with other physiotherapy modalities, injection techniques tend to stand alone, notwithstanding the attention to biomechanical or causative factors that should always be applied.

The drugs administered often have effects for some time after the application of treatment and they must be given time to achieve these beneficial effects. In many instances the orthopaedic medicine clinician has a choice of treatment, either injection or transverse frictions and mobilization (e.g. tendinopathy). In some cases an injection is more appropriate (e.g. bursitis), and in others, transverse frictions may be more appropriate (e.g. musculotendinous lesions). Injections tend to be more cost-effective when compared to manual therapy (e.g. capsulitis). The need for collaboration between the patient, physician and physiotherapist is emphasized to ascertain the best mode of treatment for the patient.

CORTICOSTEROID INJECTIONS

> **Uses in orthopaedic medicine**
> - Chronic tendinopathy and tenosynovitis
> - Acute and chronic bursitis
> - Inflammatory arthritis and acute episodes of degenerative osteoathrosis
> - Epidural, via sacral hiatus
> - Nerve entrapment syndromes
> - Some ligament sprains

Corticosteroids have a potent anti-inflammatory effect, much more dramatic than the anti-inflammatory effect of non-steroidal anti-inflammatory drugs (NSAIDs), and are therefore used therapeutically to achieve this effect in orthopaedic medicine. They are applied intraarticularly or intralesionally for chronic inflammatory lesions. The intense anti-inflammatory effect is beneficial in some acute lesions (e.g. acute bursitis, rheumatoid arthritis) but is unwanted in other conditions (e.g. acute muscle belly lesion and acute ligamentous lesions) because of its detrimental effects on collagen production.

As well as its anti-inflammatory effect, corticosteroids have other potent effects, including immunosuppression and a delay in the normal physiological process of healing. These effects cannot be separated from the beneficial effects of corticosteroids. Much of the reported unwanted effects of corticosteroids involve systemic, high dose applications of the drugs for long periods of time.

A locally applied injection of corticosteroid in orthopaedic medicine aims to achieve a rapid and intense local anti-inflammatory effect. The local effect will depend on the dose applied, the relative potency of the corticosteroid and its solubility, which determines the length of time it stays in the tissues. In orthopaedic medicine the aim is to give the smallest dose that will achieve the desired effects. Intra-articular injections are most appropriate if there is an inflammatory component, therefore they are indicated whenever a joint capsule is inflamed, e.g. in rheumatoid arthritis, traumatic arthritis and acute episodes of osteoarthrosis. Intralesional injections are applied to chronic tendinopathy, tenosynovitis, bursitis and some ligamentous sprains.

The use of corticosteroids would seem to affect all stages of the inflammatory process, the initial acute phase of heat, redness, swelling and pain, as well as the proliferative phases of repair and remodelling.

Corticosteroids also produce a potent immunosuppressive effect, which is why it is so important to pay attention to aseptic technique.

In this text the corticosteroid referred to is *triamcinolone acetonide*. Two different concentrations of triamcinolone acetonide, Adcortyl (10 mg/ml) and Kenalog (40 mg/ml), provide versatility for different applications. Other drugs and information are available on current data sheets.

Corticosteroid injection technique

The appropriate dose (corticosteroid alone, or mixed with local anaesthetic) will be determined by the size of the joint or lesion to be injected and the previous response to injection, if any.

TRIAMCINOLONE ACETONIDE

- Adcortyl 10 mg/ml for large-volume injections
- Kenalog 40 mg/ml for small-volume injections (Fig. 4.6)

Accurate needle placement is essential. This depends on clinical diagnosis. Knowledge of anatomy will allow accurate location of the lesion and avoid unnecessary complications. Points worth considering are:

- The tissue in which the lesion lies
- How deep the lesion lies
- The extent of the lesion
- The position of the patient to make the site of the lesion accessible
- The direction in which the needle should be inserted
- The length of needle and the size of syringe required

Figure 4.6   Containers of drugs in common use for musculoskeletal injections.

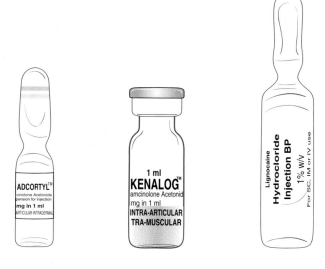

Unwanted side–effects of corticosteroid therapy

Most of the unpleasant side-effects of corticosteroid therapy relate to large, long-term doses of the drugs taken systemically. It is rare to produce systemic side-effects from a single local corticosteroid injection, but it can happen.

Post-injection flare is a self-limiting side-effect occurring 6–12 hours after injection once the local anaesthetic effect has subsided. Symptoms usually resolve in 72 hours, but may mimic infection, which should be suspected if symptoms do not settle in the expected time.

Local soft tissue atrophy and pigment changes. These may occur with inaccurate needle placement and/or leakage of fluid, particularly of long-acting corticosteroids, into subcutaneous tissue, and have been documented to promote fat necrosis, dermal atrophy, senile purpura, depigmentation and subcutaneous atrophy (Ponec et al 1977, Marks et al 1983, Grillet & Dequeker 1990). These subcutaneous changes may be reversible, although the patient may be left with long-lasting evidence of injection.

Connective tissue weakening is believed to occur due to a loss in tensile strength of the collagen tissue, possibly leading to tendon rupture in particular. The balance of collagen synthesis is altered to produce degradation of fibres and new immature scar tissue is laid down. Appropriate mobilization is required at the right time to encourage alignment of fibres and increased tensile strength. The corticosteroid will affect the normal tissue as well as the damaged tissue. During its time of action, corticosteroid potentially causes a weakening of collagen fibres, damaged and normal, and this should be recognized as a potential hazard. The patient is instructed to rest from aggravating activities while normal, pain-free function is encouraged, to provide mechanical stimulus for the new fibres. Since triamcinolone acetonide is absorbed within approximately a 2-week period, it would seem appropriate to advise the patient to rest for up to 2 weeks if practical.

Steroid arthropathy, a Charcot-type arthropathy, has been reported in association with corticosteroid injections; however, more recent reports have refuted this (Grillet & Dequeker 1990, Cameron 1995). It has been considered that the deterioration in the cartilage and joint may be more likely to be due to the underlying inflammatory or degenerative condition rather than the treatment with corticosteroids. It is appropriate to instruct the patient to rest following intra-articular injection. Cameron (1995) reviewed the evidence on steroid arthropathy and found that the greatest risk of its development is from prolonged, high-dose oral steroids in the presence of associated underlying disease. There is a general consensus that repeated corticosteroid injections into weight-bearing joints should be limited to a maximum of two, or perhaps three, per year because of the risk of steroid arthropathy. However, Raynauld et al (2003) conducted a randomized, double blind, placebo-controlled trial to determine the efficacy of long-term intra-articular corticosteroid injection (40 mg triamcinolone acetonide every 3 months) in osteoarthritis of the knee. The 1- and 2-year follow-up showed no difference in the loss of joint space over time between the corticosteroid injection group and the saline injected group. There was a trend in the corticosteroid group to show greater symptomatic relief with pain and stiffness significantly improved. The authors concluded that there was no significant deleterious effect on the anatomical joint structure in either group, indicating that repeated intra-articular injections are safe.

Iatrogenic (clinician induced) septic arthritis is a rare but avoidable side-effect. The 'no touch' technique described below is advised.

Systemic effects include: hyperglycaemia in a diabetic patient; facial flushing in the first 2–3 days and lasting a day or two; menstrual disturbance, including postmenopausal bleeding.

LOCAL ANAESTHETIC

> **Uses of local anaesthetic in orthopaedic medicine**
> - Used together with corticosteroids for diagnostic purposes and therapeutic pain relief for the patient.
> - To treat chronic bursitis.
> - As part of an epidural injection via the sacral hiatus.

The earliest local anaesthetic, cocaine, first used in 1860, was used as a local anaesthetic for surgery. A synthetic substitute, procaine, was developed in 1905 and many other compounds have since been produced.

Local anaesthetics work by penetrating the nerve sheath and axon membrane. They tend to block conduction more readily in small diameter, myelinated and unmyelinated nerve fibres. Nociceptive and sympathetic impulses are therefore blocked more readily (Rang et al 2003).

This pain-relieving effect of local anaesthetic is utilized in orthopaedic medicine for its therapeutic and diagnostic effects. Given together with corticosteroid, local anaesthetic allows immediate reassessment of the patient to confirm diagnosis and to ensure that the lesion has been completely infiltrated. It gives the patient initial pain relief and may reduce the effects of post-injection flare from corticosteroid injection.

In this text, lidocaine (lignocaine) hydrochloride will be used. It has a rapid rate of onset and moderate duration. It may be used as 0.5%, 1% or 2% solution and the maximum dose is 200 mg (given by infiltration to a fit adult of average weight, it would be unsafe to give this dose intravenously).

Unwanted side–effects of local anaesthetic

It is important to recognize the maximum dose of local anaesthetic in order to avoid the unwanted side-effects (Rang et al 2003) and patients should always be questioned about sensitivity to previous injections.

Central nervous system effects may initially be due to stimulation and may include feelings of inebriation and light-headedness, restlessness and tremor, confusion progressing to extreme agitation. Further increase in drug levels leads to depression of the central nervous system which may present as sedation, twitching, convulsion or respiratory depression which is potentially life-threatening.

Cardiovascular effects may present as a combination of myocardial depression and vasodilatation producing sudden hypotension which may be life-threatening. Myocardial depression occurs as a result of inhibition of sodium current in cardiac muscle. Vasodilatation is due to the local anaesthetic effect on the smooth muscle of the arterioles and sympathetic inhibition.

Allergic reactions are commonly an allergic dermatitis due to hypersensitivity, and, rarely, anaphylaxis, which is life-threatening.

'NO-TOUCH' TECHNIQUE

A 'no-touch' technique is essential to minimize the risk of infection. Avoid injecting in the presence of infection because the corticosteroid also has an immunosuppressive effect – further details can be found in *Musculoskeletal Injection Skills* (Kesson et al 2003):

- Explain the procedure to the patient
- Position the patient with the lesion accessible and mark the injection site (pen, thumb nail)
- Ensure that the injection site is medicolegally clean using an appropriate antiseptic (e.g. chlorhexidine in spirit)
- Wash and dry hands, preferably using surgical scrub
- Draw up the appropriate dosage of corticosteroid and local anaesthetic using disposable syringes and needles. Single-dose containers should be used wherever possible and discarded after use
- Change the needle, discarding the one used for drawing up the dose
- Give the injection without touching the needle or the injection site
- Withdraw the needle and apply the appropriate dressing
- Issue the patient with instructions to rest from aggravating factors and avoid painful movements for up to 2 weeks

NEEDLE SIZE (Fig. 4.7)

Figure 4.7   Needles in common use for musculoskeletal injections.

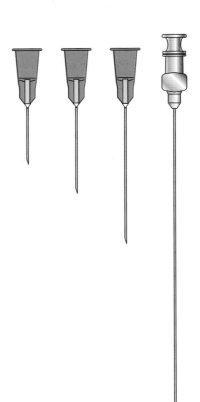

SYRINGES (Fig. 4.8)

Figure 4.8 Syringes in common use for musculoskeletal injections.

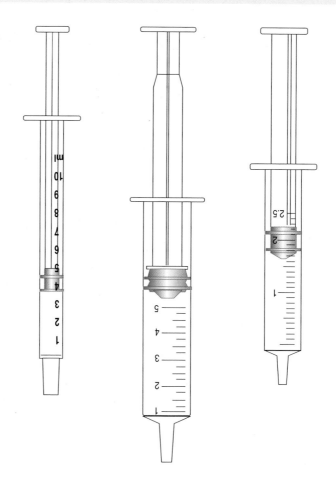

Two techniques are generally used to deliver the injection. A *bolus technique* is used for joint spaces and bursae, where no resistance is felt on pressing the plunger. A *peppering technique* is used for tendons and ligaments where a series of small droplets is delivered throughout the substance of the structure to cover the extent and depth of the lesion.

Lack of response to corticosteroid injection may require a review of the diagnosis and the technique. It is fairly common to have a relapse or recurrence of symptoms in soft tissue lesions. This is particularly likely if the patient returns to the overuse activity too soon or the cause of the problem is not properly investigated and remedied.

NON-STEROIDAL ANTI-INFLAMMATORY DRUGS

These are some of the most widely used drugs for musculoskeletal lesions as well as the symptoms of headaches, flu, colds and other minor aches and pains. However, nearly all NSAIDs have side-effects, the most notorious being gastrointestinal problems, which caution against their long-term use. NSAIDs seem to have their action within the injured tissue itself.

NSAIDs produce the following three main effects:

- *Anti-inflammatory*: they modify the inflammatory reaction by reducing vasodilatation, oedema and permeability of the postcapillary venules
- *Analgesic*: they reduce pain by inhibiting prostaglandin formation. They are therefore most effective in treating the chemical pain produced by inflammation in which the prostaglandins sensitize the nociceptors. They have little effect in mechanical pain, which is why they are not particularly effective in treating the acute pain assciated with recent disc protrusion
- *Antipyretic*: they reduce a raised temperature, but have no effect on the normal body temperature

NSAIDs commonly prescribed include ibuprofen, naproxen, indomethacin, piroxicam, diclofenac and aspirin.

In acute inflammatory musculoskeletal lesions (e.g. acute muscle belly lesions, acute ligament sprains and acute tenosynovitis) it is probably better to allow the first 3–5 days of the inflammatory phase to pass before using anti-inflammatory drugs such as the corticosteroids (Boruta et al 1990). If the condition is very painful, NSAIDs may be administered, or other analgesics such as paracetamol, together with the physical treatments of controlled and precise mobilization coupled with protection, relative rest, ice, compression and elevation (PRICE). In chronic inflammatory states, however, the use of corticosteroid injection is strongly indicated and most beneficial, but the patient should be instructed to rest following injection.

EPIDURAL INJECTIONS

Uses of epidural injections in orthopaedic medicine
- Hyperacute pain.
- Radicular pain.
- Chronic back or leg pain, with or without neurological deficit.
- Trial treatment for pain relief prior to consideration for surgery.

The use of epidural injections may be appropriate in the management of lumbar pain, with or without sciatica (see Ch. 13). The orthopaedic medicine approach is injection via the caudal route with the aim of bathing the dura mater and sensitized nerve roots in anaesthetic to relieve pain. Bush & Hillier (1991) discuss three possible mechanisms of pain relief, citing Bhatia & Parikh and Gupta et al, who join Cyriax (1984) in the suggestion that the introduction of the fluid local anaesthetic into the epidural space is enough in itself to influence the relationship between the disc and nerve root. Bush & Hillier (1991) also cite Wall & Melzak in describing how, in spite of its short action, the local anaesthetic may nonetheless break a pain cycle. Corticosteroid is usually added to the solution, however, with the logic of reducing both the swelling and inflammation at the disc–nerve root interface as an additional benefit of the large volume injection (Bush & Hillier 1991).

It should be stressed that, although epidural injection via the caudal route can be performed as an outpatient procedure, the injection should only be carried out by an experienced medical practitioner who has undergone appropriate training.

The injection typically involves the introduction of 40–80 mg triamcinolone acetonide in 20–30 ml of 0.5% procaine hydrochloride introduced via the sacral hiatus, using a no-touch technique.

SCLEROSANT THERAPY (PROLOTHERAPY)

The aim of sclerosant therapy is to increase ligament or tendon mass and ligament–bone or tendon–bone strength. Experiments have shown a statistically significant increase in collagen fibril diameters (Liu et al 1983), suggesting that sclerosing solution has an influence on connective tissue at the insertion sites.

P2G

- Phenol 2% w/v
- Dextrose 25% w/v
- Glycerol 30% w/v

Other sclerosant solutions include hypertonic dextrose and sodium morrhuate.

P2G causes an intense inflammatory reaction at the site of injection. The intention in producing such an intense inflammatory reaction is to stimulate the formation of scar tissue. The immature scar tissue laid down is encouraged to contract and shorten by avoiding movement and stress during the repair and remodelling phases. The intense reaction causes considerable pain, but it would not be rational to use anti-inflammatory medication following sclerosant therapy.

Uses of sclerosant therapy in orthopaedic medicine
- Recurrent or chronic episodes of low back pain, with or without leg pain.
- Recurrent sacroiliac joint subluxation.
- Other conditions associated with ligamentous laxity, e.g. subluxing capitate bone.

Unwanted side–effect of sclerosant therapy

Strong phenol penetrates the nerve endings producing a local anaesthetic effect (Goodman & Gilman 1970) which is permanent. It is not known whether the very low concentrations used in sclerosant injections has any effect other than antiseptic.

SUMMARY OF PRINCIPLES OF ORTHOPAEDIC MEDICINE TREATMENT APPLIED TO SOFT TISSUE LESIONS

The following table is not intended as a recipe, but acts as a guide to the integration of the principles of orthopaedic medicine into clinical practice.

Acute muscle belly lesions	■ PRICE ■ Gentle transverse frictions in a shortened position, six sweeps after analgesic effect ■ Grade A mobilization ■ Progressing to an increased depth of transverse frictions and Grade A+ mobilization until the full range of movement is restored ■ Ideally treat daily, or as often as possible, in the early phase
Chronic muscle belly lesions	■ Deep transverse frictions in shortened position, 10 min after analgesic effect ■ Grade A+ mobilization ■ No resisted exercise or Grade B mobilization (i.e. stretching) until pain-free on testing through the application of selective tension (when stretching is only indicated if the structure is judged to be restricting range)
Musculotendinous lesions (usually chronic)	■ Deep transverse frictions in accessible position, 10 min after analgesic effect ■ Grade A+ mobilization ■ Corticosteroid injection is not contraindicated, but the above regimen is generally thought to be more effective
Acute tenosynovitis	■ PRICE ■ Gentle transverse frictions, six sweeps after analgesic effect ■ Grade A mobilization
Chronic tenosynovitis	■ Corticosteroid injection, bolus technique between tendon and sheath ■ Relative rest (Grade A mobilization) *OR* ■ Deep transverse frictions, tendon on a stretch ■ Grade A mobilization
Chronic tendinopathy, teno-osseous junction	■ Corticosteroid injection, peppering technique at the bone–tendon interface ■ Relative rest (Grade A mobilization) *OR* ■ Deep transverse frictions, 10 min after analgesic effect ■ Grade A mobilization ■ Mills' manipulation, special technique for tennis elbow
Stage I capsulitis	■ Corticosteroid injection, bolus technique ■ Relative rest (Grade A mobilization), progressing to increased mobilization once pain settles *OR* ■ Grade B mobilization
Stage II capsulitis	■ Corticosteroid injection, bolus technique ■ Relative rest (Grade A mobilization), progressing to increased mobilization once pain settles *OR* ■ Grade A mobilization, distraction techniques
Stage III capsulitis	■ Grade B mobilization

Acute bursitis	■ Corticosteroid injection, peppering or bolus technique ■ Relative rest (Grade A mobilization)
Chronic bursitis	■ Corticosteroid injection, large volume local anaesthetic, low dose, ideally bolus technique ■ Relative rest (Grade A mobilization)
Acute ligament lesion	■ PRICE ■ Gentle transverse frictions, six sweeps after analgesic effect ■ Grade A mobilization ■ Progressing to an increased depth of transverse frictions and Grade A+ mobilization until the full range of movement is restored ■ Ideally treat daily, or as often as possible, in the early phase
Chronic ligament lesion	■ Deep transverse frictions, 10 min after analgesic effect ■ Grade A+ mobilization ■ Manipulation applied to chronic medial collateral ligament sprain of the knee and lateral ligament sprain of the ankle following the application of sufficient deep transverse frictions to achieve analgesic effect *OR* ■ Corticosteroid injection ■ Relative rest (Grade A mobilization)
Ligamentous laxity	■ Sclerosant therapy (prolotherapy) ■ Relative rest
Loose body	■ Grade A mobilization applied under strong manual traction
Subluxed carpal/tarsal bone	■ Grade A mobilization applied under strong manual traction
Acute cervical lesion	■ 'Bridging' mobilization technique ■ Grade A mobilization
Subacute/chronic cervical lesion	■ Mobilization under manual traction, progressing to manipulation if necessary (NB: vertebrobasilar artery test should be conducted before manipulation)
Acute lumbar lesion	■ 'Pretzel' mobilization technique ■ Grade A mobilization ■ Caudal epidural injection
Subacute/chronic lumbar lesion	■ Mobilization techniques ■ Manipulation ■ Traction ■ Caudal epidural injection
Sacroiliac joint lesion	■ Mobilization techniques ■ Manipulation ■ Exercise

References

Abenhaim L, Bergeron A M 1992 Twenty years of randomized trials of manipulative therapy for back pain: a review. Clinical and Investigative Medicine 15:527–535

Adams M A, Hutton W C 1981 The relevance of torsion to the mechanical derangement of the lumbar spine. Spine 6:241–248

Adams M, Bogduk N, Burton K et al 2002 The biomechanics of back pain. Churchill Livingstone, Edinburgh

Akeson W 1990 The response of ligaments to stress modulation and overview of the ligament healing response. In: Daniel D et al (eds) Knee ligaments: structure, function, injury and repair. Lippincott, Williams & Wilkins, Philadelphia, p 315–327

Akeson W, Amiel D, La Violette D 1967 The connective tissue response to immobility: a study of chondroitin-4 and 6-sulfate and dermatan sulfate changes in periarticular connective tissue of control and immobilised knees of dogs. Clinical Orthopaedics 51:183–197

Akeson W, Woo S L-Y, Amiel D et al 1973 The connective tissue response to immobility: biochemical changes in periarticular connective tissue of the immobilised rabbit's knee. Clinical Orthopaedics 93:356–362

Akeson W, Amiel D, Woo S L-Y 1980 Immobility effects on synovial joints, the pathomechanics of joint contracture. Biorheology 17:95–110

Akeson W, Amiel D, Abel M F et al 1986 Effects of immobilization on joints. Clinical Orthopaedics and Related Research 219:28–37

Amiel D, Woo S L-Y, Harwood F L, Akeson W H 1982 The effects of immobilization on collagen turnover in connective tissue: a biochemical-biomedical correlation. Acta Orthopaedica Scandinavica 53:325–332

Amis A A 1985 Biomechanics of ligaments. In: Jenkins D H R (ed) Ligament injuries and their treatment. Chapman and Hall, London p 3–28

Arem A J, Madden J W 1976 Effects of stress on healing wounds, 1: intermittent noncyclical tension. Journal of Surgical Research 20:93–102

Assendelft W J J, Morton S C, Yu E I et al 2003 Spinal manipulative therapy for low back pain: a meta-analysis of effectiveness relative to other therapies. Annals of Internal Medicine 138(11):871–881

Barker M E 1994 Spinal manipulation: a general practice study. Journal of Orthopaedic Medicine 16:42–44

BMJ 1976 Trial by traction [editorial]. British Medical Journal 1(6000):2–3

Bogduk, N 1997 Clinical anatomy of the lumbar spine and sacrum, 3rd edn. Churchill Livingstone, Edinburgh

Boruta P M, Bishop J O, Braly W G et al 1990 Acute lateral ankle ligament injuries: a literature review. Foot and Ankle 11:107–113

Bowsher D 1994 Modulation of nociceptive input. In: Wells P E, Frampton V, Bowsher D (eds) Pain management by physiotherapy, 2nd edn. Butterworth Heinemann, Oxford, p 30–31

Brandy W D, Irion J M 1994 The effect of time on static stretch on the flexibility of the hamstring muscles. Physical Therapy 74(9):845–852

Brandy W D, Irion J M, Briggler M 1997 The effect of time and frequency of static stretching on the flexibility of the hamstring muscles. Physical therapy 77(10):1090–1096

Braverman D, Schulman R 1999 Massage techniques in rehabilitation medicine. Physical Medicine and rehabilitation Clinics of North America 10(3):631–649

Brodeur R 1995 The audible release associated with joint manipulation. Journal of Manipulative and Physiological Therapeutics 18(3):155–164

Brosseau L, Casimiro L, Milne S et al 2002 Deep transverse friction massage for treating tendinopathy (Cochrane review). The Cochrane Library 2 Online. Available: htt://www.athensams.net June 2002

Buerskens S A J, de Vet H C, Köke A J et al 1997 Efficacy of traction for nonspecific low back pain: 12-week and 6-month results of a randomized clinical trial. Spine 22(23):2756–2762

Burke-Evans E, Eggers G W N, Butler J K et al 1960 Experimental immobilization and remobilization of rat knee joints. Journal of Bone and Joint Surgery 42A:737–758

Bush K, Hillier S 1991 A controlled study of caudal epidural injections of triamcinolone plus procaine for the management of intractable sciatica. Spine 16(5):572–575

Bush K, Cowan N, Katz D E et al 1992 The natural history of sciatica associated with disc pathology. Spine 17:1205–1212

Cameron G 1995 Steroid arthropathy: myth or reality? A review of the evidence. Journal of Orthopaedic Medicine 17:51–55

Carreck A 1994 The effect of massage on pain perception threshold. Manipulative Physiotherapist 26:10–16

Chamberlain G J 1982 Cyriax's friction massage: a review. Journal of Orthopaedic and Sports Physical Therapy 4:16–22

Chambers Dictionary 1998 Chambers Harrap, Edinburgh

Chartered Society of Physiotherapy 1998 Guidelines for the management of soft issue injury with PRICE during the first 72 hours. Association of Chartered Physiotherapists in Sports Medicine

Cherkin D C, Sherman K J, Deyo R A et al 2003 A review of the evidence for the effectiveness, safety and cost of acupuncture, massage therapy and spinal manipulation for back pain. Annals of Internal Medicine 138(11):898–907

Colachis S C, Strohm B R 1965 A study of tractive forces and angle of pull on vertebral interspaces in the cervical spine. Archives of Physical Medicine and Rheumatology 46:820–830

Colachis S C, Strohm B R 1966 Effect of duration of intermittent cervical traction on vertebral separation. Archives of Physical Medicine and Rehabilitation 47:353–359

Colloca C J, Keller T S 2001 Electromyographic reflex responses to mechanical force, manually assisted spinal manipulative therapy. Spine 26(10):1117–1124

Committee on Safety of Medicines 1995 Tendon damage associated with quinolone antibiotics. HMSO, London

Conway P J W, Herzog W, Zhang Y et al 1993 Forces required to cause cavitation during spinal manipulation of the thoracic spine. Clinical Biomechanics 8:210–214

Cook J L, Khan K M, Maffulli N, Purdam C 2000 Overuse tendinosis, not tendinopathy, part 2: applying the new approach to patellar tendinopathy. Physician and Sports Medicine 28(6):31–41

Cramer G D, Tuck N R Jr, Knudsen T et al 2000 Effects of side-posture adjusting on the lumbar zygapophyseal joints as evaluated by magnetic resonance imaging: a before and after study with randomization. Journal of Manipulative and Physiological Therapeutics 23(6):380–394

Cyriax J 1982 Textbook of orthopaedic medicine, 8th edn. Baillière Tindall, London, vol 1

Cyriax J 1984 Textbook of orthopaedic medicine, 11th edn. Baillière Tindall, London, vol 2

Cyriax J H, Cyriax P J 1983 Illustrated manual of orthopaedic medicine. Butterworth, London

Davidson C, Ganion L, Gehlsen G et al 1997 Rat tendon morphologic and functional changes resulting from soft tissue mobilisation. Medicine and Science in Sports and Exercise 29(3):313–319

de Bruijn R 1984 Deep transverse friction: its analgesic effect. International Journal of Sports Medicine 5:35–36

Dolan P, Adams M A 2001 Recent advances in lumbar spinal mechanics and their significance for modelling. Clinical Biomechanics 16(Suppl. 1):S8–S16

Drechsler W, Knarr J, Snyder-Mackler L 1997 A comparison of two treatment regimes for lateral epicondylitis: a randomised trial of clinical interventions. Journal of Sport Rehabilitation 6: 226–234

Enneking W F, Horowitz M 1972 The intra-articular effects of immobilization of the human knee. Journal of Bone and Joint Surgery 54:973–985

Ernst E 2000 Does spinal manipulation have specific treatment effects? Family Practice 17(6):554–556

Evans P 1980 The healing process at cellular level: a review. Physiotherapy 66:256–259

Farfan H F, Cossette J W, Robertson G H et al (1970) The effects of torsion on the lumbar intervertebral joints: the role of torsion in the production of disc degeneration. Journal of Bone and Joint Surgery [American] 52:468–497

Evans D 2002 Mechanisms and effects of spinal high velocity, low amplitude thrust manipulation: previous theories. Journal of Manipulative and Physiological Therapeutics 25(4):251–262

Gal J M, Herzog W, Kawchuk G N et al 1995 Forces and relative vertebral movements during SMT to unembalmed post-rigor human cadavers: peculiarities associated with joint cavitation. Journal of Manipulative and Physiological Therapeutics 18(1):4–9

Gehlsen G, Ganion L, Helfst R 1998 Fibroblastic responses to variation in soft tissue mobilization pressure. Medicine and Science in Sports and Exercise 31(4):531–535

Gibbons P, Collins A 2001 Comparison of high velocity low amplitude manipulation with cavitation verses [sic] non-cavitation: effect upon atlanto-axial rotation asymmetry in asymptomatic subjects. Journal of Orthopaedic Medicine 23(1):2–8

Gibbons P, Tehan P 2001 Patient positioning and spinal locking for lumbar spine rotation manipulation. Manual Therapy 6(3):130–138

Goats G C 1994 Massage – the scientific basis of an ancient art, part 1: the techniques. British Journal of Sports Medicine 28:149–152

Goldie I F, Reichmann S 1977 The biomechanical influence of traction on the cervical spine. Scandinavian Journal of Rehabilitation Medicine 9:31–34

Goodman L S, Gilman A 1970 The pharmacological basis of Therapeutics, 4th edn. Macmillan, New York

Gregory M A, Deane M N, Mars M 2003 Ultrastructural changes in untraumatised rabbit skeletal muscle treated with deep transverse friction. Physiotherapy 89(7):408–416

Grieve G P 1981 Common vertebral joint problems. Churchill Livingstone, Edinburgh

Grillet B, Dequeker J 1990 Intra-articular steroid injection: a risk benefit assessment. Drug Safety 5:205–211

Hadler N M, Curtis P, Gillings D B et al 1987 A benefit of spinal manipulation as adjunctive therapy for acute low back pain: a stratified controlled trial. Spine 12:703–706

Hardy M A 1989 The biology of scar formation. Physical Therapy 69:1014–1023

Hardy M, Woodall W 1998 Therapeutic effects of heat, cold and stretch on connective tissue. Journal of Hand Therapy 11(2):148–156

Harvey E, Burton A K, Moffett J K et al 2003 Spinal manipulation for low-back pain: a treatment package agreed by the UK chiropractic, osteopathy and physiotherapy professional associations. Manual Therapy 8(1):46–51

Hemmings B, Smith M, Graydon J, Dyson R 2000 Effects of massage on physiological restoration, perceived recovery and repeated sports performance. Sports Medicine 34:109–115

Herzog W, Conway P J, Kawchuk G N et al 1993 Forces exerted during spinal manipulative therapy. Spine 18:1206–1212

Herzog W, Scheele D, Conway P J 1999 Electromyographic responses of back and limb muscles associated with spinal manipulative therapy. Spine 24(2):146–152

Hood L B, Chrisman D 1968 Intermittent pelvic traction in the treatment of the ruptured intervertebral disk. Physical Therapy 48:21–30

Hsieh C-Y J, Adams A H, Tobis J et al 2002 Effectiveness of four conservative treatments for subacute low back pain; a randomized clinical trial. Spine 27(11):1142–1148

Huebscher R 1998 An overview of massage, part 1: history, types of massage, credentialing and literature. Nurse Practitioner Forum 9(4):197–199

Hume Kendall P 1955 A history of lumbar traction. Physiotherapy 41:177–179

Hunter G 1994 Specific soft tissue mobilization in the treatment of soft tissue lesions. Physiotherapy 80:15–21

Ingham B 1981 Transverse friction massage for the relief of tennis elbow. Physician and Sports Medicine 9:116

Iwatsuki H, Ikuta Y, Shinoda K 2001 Deep friction massage on the masticatory muscles in stroke patients increases biting force. Journal of Physical Therapy Science 13(1):17–20

Järvinen M J, Lehto M U K 1993 The effects of early mobilization and immobilization on the healing process following muscle injuries. Sports Medicine 15:78–89

Judovitch B 1952 Herniated cervical disc. American Journal of Surgery 84:646–656

Katavitch L 1998 Differential effects of spinal manipulative therapy on acute and chronic muscle spasm: a proposal for mechanisms and efficacy. Manual Therapy 3(3):132–139

Keller T S, Colloca C J 2000 Mechanical force spinal manipulation increases trunk muscle strength assessed by electromyography: a comparative clinical trial. Journal of Manipulative and Physiological Therapeutics 23(9):585–595

Kelly E 1997 The effects of deep transverse frictional massage to the gastrocnemius muscle. Journal of Orthopaedic Medicine 19:3–9

Kesson M, Atkins E, Davies I 2003 Musculoskeletal injection skills. Butterworth Heinemann, Oxford

Khan K M, Cook J L 2000 Overuse tendon injuries: where does the pain come from? Sports Medicine and Arthroscopic Review 8:17–31

Klaber Moffett J A, Hughes G I, Griffiths P 1990 An investigation of the effects of cervical traction, part 2: the effects on the neck musculature. Clinical Rehabilitation 4:287–290

Koes B W, Bouter L M, Geert J M G et al 1995 Methodological quality of randomized clinical trials on treatment efficacy in low back pain. Spine 20(2):228–235

Koes B W, Assendelft W J J, Geert J M G et al 1996 Spinal manipulation for low back pain: an updated systematic review of randomized clinical trials. Spine 21(24):2860–2873

Krismer M, Haid C, Rabl W 1996 The contribution of anulus fibers to torque resistance. Spine 21: 2551–2557

LaBan M M, Taylor R S 1992 Manipulation: an objective analysis of the literature. Orthopaedic Clinics of North America 23:451–459

Lamb D W 1994 A review of manual therapy for spinal pain. In: Boyling J, Palastanga N (eds) Grieve's Modern manual therapy, 2nd edn. Churchill Livingstone, Edinburgh

Lee R Y W, Evans J H 2001 Loads in the lumbar spine during traction therapy. Australian Journal of Physiotherapy 47:102–108

Lee M, Steven G P, Crosbie J et al 1996 Towards a theory of lumbar mobilisation – the relationship between applied manual force and movements of the spine. Manual Therapy 1(2):67–75

Lehman G J, Vernon H, McGill S M 2001 Effects of a mechanical pain stimulus on erector spinae activity before and after a spinal manipulation in patients with back pain: a preliminary investigation. Journal of Manipulative and Physiological Therapeutics 24(6):402–406

Lehto M, Duance V C, Restall D 1985 Collagen and fibronectin in a healing skeletal muscle injury. Journal of Bone and Joint Surgery 67B:820–828

Levangie P K, Norkin C C 2001 Joint structure and function: a comprehensive analysis. F A Davis, Philadelphia

Liu Y K, Tipton C M, Matthes R D et al 1983 An in situ study of the influence of a sclerosing solution in rabbit medial collateral ligaments and its junction strength. Connective Tissue Research 11:95–102

Loitz B J, Zernicke R F, Vailas A C et al 1988 Effects of short-term immobilization versus continuous passive motion on the biomechanical and biochemical properties of the rabbit tendon. Clinical Orthopaedics and Related Research 244:265–271

Low J, Reed A 1994 Electrotherapy explained: principles and practice. Butterworth Heinemann, Oxford

McGregor A, Wragg P, Gedroyc W M W 2001 Can interventional MRI provide an insight into the mechanics of a posterior-anterior mobilisation? Clinical Biomechanics 16:926–929

Marks J G, Cano C, Leitzel K et al 1983 Inhibition of wound healing by topical steroids. Journal of Dermatologic Surgery and Oncology 9:819–821

Mathews J A 1968 Dynamic discography: a study of lumbar traction. Annals of Physical Medicine 9:275–279

Mathews J A, Hickling J 1975 Lumbar traction: a double-blind controlled study for sciatica. Rheumatology and Rehabilitation 14:222–225

Melzack R, Wall P D 1988 The challenge of pain, 2nd edn. Penguin, Harmondsworth.

Mixter W J, Barr J S 1934 Rupture of the intervertebral disc with involvement of the spinal canal. New England Journal of Medicine 211:210–215

Nachemson A 1980 Lumbar intradiscal pressure. In: Jayson M I V (ed) The lumbar spine and back pain, 2nd edn. Pitman, London, p 341–358

Noren R, Trafimow J, Andersson G B J et al 1991 The role of facet joint tropism and facet angle in disc degeneration. Spine 16:530–532

Norris C M 1998 Sports injuries: diagnosis and management for physiotherapists, 2nd edn. Butterworth Heinemann, Oxford

Noyes F 1977 Functional properties of knee ligaments and alterations induced by immobilization. Clinical Orthopaedics and Related Research 123:210–242

O'Donaghue C 1994 Manipulation trials. In: Boyling J, Palastanga N (eds) Grieve's Modern manual therapy, 2nd edn. Churchill Livingstone, Edinburgh, p 661–672

Onel D, Tuzlaci M, Sari H et al 1989 Computed tomographic investigation of the effect of traction on lumbar disc herniations. Spine 14:82–90

Peacock E E 1966 Some biochemical and biophysical aspects of joint stiffness. Annals of Surgery 164:1–12

Pellecchia G L, Hamel H, Behnke P 1994 Treatment of infrapatellar tendinopathy: a combination of modalities and transverse friction massage versus iontophoresis. Journal of Sports Rehabilitation 3:135–145

Ponec M, de Haas C, Bachra, B N et al 1977 Effects of glucocorticosteroids on primary human skin fibroblasts. Archives for Dermatological Research 259(2):117–123

Priestley G C 1978 Effects of corticosteroids on the growth and metabolism of fibroblasts cultured from human skin. British Journal of Dermatology 99:253–261

Rang H P, Dale M M, Ritter J M et al 2003 Pharmacology, 5th edn. Churchill Livingstone, Edinburgh

Raynauld et al 2003

Roland M, Waddell G, Klaber Moffett J et al 1996 The back book. Stationery Office, Norwich

Salter R B 1989 The biologic concept of continuous passive motion of synovial joints. Clinical Orthopaedics and Related Research 242:12–25

Sandoz, R 1976 Some physical mechanisms and effects of spinal adjustments. Annals Swiss Chiropractic Association 6:91–141

Saunders H D 1998 The controversy over traction for neck and low back pain. Physiotherapy 84(6):285–288

Saunders S 2000 Orthopaedic medicine course manual. Saunders, London

Schwellnus M P, Mackintosh L, Mee J 1992 Deep transverse frictions in the treatment of iliotibial band friction syndrome in athletes: a clinical trial. Physiotherapy 78:564–568

Shekelle P G 1994 Spine update: spinal manipulation. Spine 19:858–861

Solinger A B 1996 Oscillations of the vertebrae in spinal manipulative therapy. Journal of Manipulative and Physiological Therapeutics 19(4):238–243

Smyth M J, Wright V 1958 Sciatica and the intervertebral disc. Journal of Bone and Joint Surgery 40A:1401

Stratford P W, Levy D R, Gauldie S et al 1989 The evaluation of phonophoresis and friction massage as treatments for extensor carpi radialis tendonitis: a randomised controlled trial. Physiotherapy Canada 41:93–99

Swezey R L 1983 The modern thrust of manipulation and traction therapy. Seminars in Arthritis and Rheumatism 12:322–331

Takai S, Woo S L-Y, Horibe S et al 1991 The effects of frequency and duration of controlled passive mobilization on tendon healing. Journal of Orthopaedic Research 9:705–713

Taylor J R, Twomey L T 1986 Age changes in lumbar zygapophyseal joints: observations on structure and function. Spine 11:739–745

Threlkeld A J 1992 The effects of manual therapy on connective tissue. Physical Therapy 72:893–902

Tipton C M, Vailas A C, Matthes R D 1986 Experimental studies on the influences of physical activity on ligaments, tendons and joints: a brief review. Acta Medica Scandinavica 711(Suppl.):157–168

Twomey L 1992 A rationale for the treatment of back pain and joint pain by manual therapy. Physical Therapy 72(12):885–892

Van der Heijden G J M G, Beurskens A J H M, Dirx M J M et al 1995a Efficacy of lumbar traction. Physiotherapy 81(1):29–35

Van der Heijden G J M G, Buerskens A J H M, Koes B W et al 1995a The efficacy of traction for back and neck pain: a systematic, blinded review of randomized clinical trial methods. Physical Therapy 75:93–104

Van Tulder M, Koes B 2002 Review – Low back pain and sciatica. In: Clinical evidence concise. BMJ Publishing, London

Van Tulder M W, Koes B W, Bouter L M 1997 Conservative treatment of acute and chronic nonspecific low back pain: a systematic review of randomized controlled trials of the most common interventions. Spine 22(18):2128–2156

Vasseljen O 1992 Low level laser versus traditional physiotherapy in the treatment of tennis elbow. Physiotherapy 78:329–334

Verhaar J A N, Walenkamp, G H I M, van Mameren H et al 1996 Local corticosteroid injection versus Cyriax-type physiotherapy for tennis elbow. Journal of Bone and Joint Surgery 78B:128–132

Vernon H 2000 Qualitative review of studies of manipulation-induced hypoalgesia. Journal of Manipulative and Physiological Therapeutics 23(2):134–138

Vicenzino B, Wright A 2002 In: Strong J, Unruh A M, Wright A et al (eds) Pain: a textbook for therapists. Churchill Livingstone, Edinburgh

Videman T 1986 Connective tissue and immobilization: key factors in musculoskeletal degeneration? Clinical Orthopaedics 221:26–32

Waddell G, Feder G, McIntosh A et al 1996 Low back pain evidence review. Royal College of General Practitioners, London

Warren C G, Lehmann J F, Koblanski J N 1971 Elongation of the rat tail tendon: effect of load and temperature. Physical Medicine and Rehabilitation 52:465–474

Weiner I J, Peacock E E 1971 Biologic principles affecting repair of flexor tendons. Advances in Surgery 5:145–188

Wells P 1994 Manipulative procedures. In: Wells P E, Frampton V, Bowsher D (eds) Pain management by physiotherapy, 2nd edn. Butterworth Heinemann, Oxford, p 187–212

Winter B 1968 Transverse frictions. South African Journal of Physiotherapy 24:5–7

Woo S L-Y 1982 Mechanical properties of tendons and ligaments, II: the relationship of immobilization and exercise on tissue remodelling. Biorheology 19:385–408

Woo S L-Y, Matthews J, Akeson W et al 1975 Connective tissue response to immobility: correlative study of the biomechanical and biochemical measurements of normal and immobilised rabbit knees. Arthritis and Rheumatism 18:257–264

Woo S L-Y, Wang C W, Newton P O et al 1990 The response of ligaments to stress deprivation and stress enhancement. In: Daniel D et al (eds) Knee ligaments: structure, function, injury and repair. Lippincott, Williams & Wilkins, Philadelphia, p 337–349

Woodman R M, Pare L 1982 Evaluation and treatment of soft tissue lesions of the ankle and forefoot using the Cyriax approach. Physical Therapy 62:1144–1147

Worden R E, Humphrey T L 1964 Effect of spinal traction on the length of the body. Archives of Physical Medicine and Rehabilitation 44:318–320

Wright A 1995 Hypoalgesia post-manipulative therapy: a review of a potential neurophysiological mechanism. Manual Therapy 1:11–16

Wyke B 1967 The neurology of joints. Annals of the Royal College of Surgeons England 41(1):25–50

Wyke B 1979 The neurology of the cervical spine joints. Physiotherapy 65:72–76

Wyke B 1980 The neurology of back pain. In: Jayson M (ed) The lumbar spine and back pain, 2nd edn. Pitman, London

Zusman M 1994 What does manipulation do? The need for basic research. In: Boyling J D, Palastanga N (eds) Grieve's Modern manual therapy, 2nd edn. Churchill Livingstone, Edinburgh, p 651–672

SECTION 2

Practice of orthopaedic medicine

SECTION CONTENTS

INTRODUCTION TO SECTION 2

Section 2 adopts a regional approach, encompassing the shoulder, elbow, wrist and hand, cervical spine, thoracic spine, hip, knee, ankle and foot, lumbar spine and sacroiliac joint. Anatomy, assessment, lesions and treatment techniques are discussed in turn for each region.

Throughout this book, anatomy is presented on a 'need to know' basis, being confined to what is clinically relevant in the context of orthopaedic medicine. It is not intended that, through its presentation here, anatomy can be learned afresh, but rather that it should act as a reminder of the subject taught so stringently at undergraduate level. It may also stimulate the reader to return to specialized anatomy texts to explore each region in greater detail in the pursuit of increased accuracy, particularly in peripheral joint lesions, and enhanced clinical effectiveness.

This book is not intended to be a cookbook whose recipes must be followed rigidly in the application of the treatment techniques presented. In the sections on treatment indications and application, the words 'may' and 'might' will often be encountered. They are not intended to imply a wishy-washy attitude to practice, but rather to acknowledge the existence of options and to underline the fact that final decisions should rest with professionals, on the basis of judgement.

It has been our experience in teaching orthopaedic medicine that students gain confidence and competence more rapidly if they can at first be guided step by step through the techniques with feedback on their performance. Though unable to provide feedback, this book aims to enable students to check treatment techniques in the unsupervised clinical situation, and reflective self-evaluation is encouraged to help to develop the skills from there.

Chapter 5

The shoulder

SUMMARY

The shoulder can be a minefield of misdiagnosis with lesions grouped under the broader, non-specific headings of 'rotator cuff syndrome', 'impingement' or 'frozen shoulder'. Diagnosis can be difficult if lesions coexist. It is not uncommon to find a tendinopathy or bursitis in conjunction with a secondary arthritis. Reference of pain from the cervical region may mimic that from the shoulder requiring assessment of both joints to be sure of the origin of the symptoms. Shoulder pain may also be due to pathology in the chest and visceral stuctures making thorough examination essential.

Knowledge of anatomy and the use of selective tension aid the incrimination of the causative structure. Palpation then identifies the specific site of the lesion to which effective treatment can be applied. The orthopaedic medicine treatment techniques discussed below should be integrated into clinical practice alongside techniques drawn from other modalities; the importance of addressing the cause as well as the symptoms cannot be stressed enough.

This chapter outlines the relevant anatomy of the shoulder region with guidelines for palpation. The assessment procedure follows, incorporating the pertinent elements of the subjective and objective examination towards the identification of shoulder lesions. The lesions are discussed and treatments are suggested, based on the principles of theory and practice.

ANATOMY

INERT STRUCTURES

In the shoulder region, simultaneous coordinated movements occur at four articulations between the scapula, clavicle, humerus and sternum: the glenohumeral joint, acromioclavicular joint, sternoclavicular joint and scapulothoracic joint. The glenohumeral joint (shoulder joint) is the most mobile joint in the body and is the first link in a mechanical chain of levers that allows the arm to be positioned in space. Movement at the spinal joints increases the range of movement available to the glenohumeral joint (Nordin & Frankel 2001).

The large, flat *scapula* is suspended by its muscles against the posterolateral thoracic wall and overlies the second to seventh ribs in the neutral position. It is attached to the strut-like clavicle by the acromioclavicular joint and together they position, steady and brace the shoulder laterally, so that the arm can clear the trunk. The clavicle transmits the weight of the upper limb to the axial skeleton via the coracoclavicular and costoclavicular ligaments, and the glenohumeral joint provides the upper limb with its wide range of movement.

The inferior junction of the medial and lateral borders of the scapula forms the *inferior angle*, which lies over the seventh rib and is crossed by latissimus dorsi. The lateral border provides the origins of teres major below and teres minor above. The medial border is long, providing attachment for the levator scapulae and the rhomboid muscles; it joins the short superior border at the *superior angle*. The *suprascapular notch* lies at the junction of the superior border with the coracoid process. This notch is converted by the *superior transverse scapular ligament* into a foramen for the passage of the suprascapular nerve. The suprascapular vessels pass above it.

The dorsal surface of the scapula is divided by the spine of the scapula into fossae above and below. The smaller upper *supraspinous fossa* gives origin to the supraspinatus muscle and the lower, larger *infraspinous fossa* gives origin to infraspinatus. The two fossae communicate laterally at the *spinoglenoid notch* through which runs the suprascapular nerve. The costal surface shows a slight hollowing for the origin of subscapularis and its medial border is roughened for the insertion of serratus anterior.

The lateral angle of the scapula is broadened to form the pear-shaped *glenoid fossa* that articulates with the head of the humerus at the glenohumeral joint. A roughened *supraglenoid tubercle* gives origin to the long head of biceps and a roughened *infraglenoid tubercle* gives origin to the long head of triceps.

The *spine of the scapula* is subcutaneous and having arisen from the upper dorsal surface of the scapula it widens laterally, projecting forwards to form the distinctive *acromion process*. When the acromion is viewed laterally it may be observed to be flat, slightly curved or to have an anterior hook-like process. The last two may predispose to rotator cuff pathology since they reduce the vertical dimensions of the subacromial space (Flatow et al 1994, Pratt 1994, Hulstyn & Fadale 1995).

The lower border of the crest of the spine of the scapula is continuous with the lateral border of the acromion and forms a useful palpable bony landmark, the *posterior angle of the acromion*. The anteromedial border of the acromion shows an oval facet for articulation with the clavicle at the acromioclavicular joint.

Just above the glenoid fossa, the prominent hook-like *coracoid process* springs up and forwards to lie below the outer clavicle. With the arm in the anatomical position, the coracoid points directly forwards to form a prominent palpable bony landmark.

The *clavicle* is subcutaneous, running horizontally between the acromion process of the scapula and the manubrium sterni, with which it articulates. On its lateral aspect is a small oval facet that articulates with the acromion at the acromioclavicular joint.

Inferiorly and laterally is a rounded conoid tubercle from which a roughened trapezoid line runs forwards and laterally. Both give attachment to the separate parts of the coracoclavicular ligament, which firmly fastens the clavicle to the scapula via the coracoid process.

The upper part of the humerus expands to bear a head and the greater and lesser tuberosities. The *head of the humerus* is approximately hemispherical and provides an articulating surface that is much greater than its scapular counterpart, the glenoid fossa. Surrounding the head of the humerus is a slight constriction that represents the *anatomical neck* and separates the head from the two tuberosities. The head of the humerus joins the shaft at the *surgical neck*, so called because it is the common site of fracture of the humerus.

The *greater tuberosity* is large and quadrilateral and is the most lateral palpable bony landmark at the shoulder. Projecting laterally beyond the acromion, it is covered by the deltoid muscle and is continuous with the shaft of the humerus below. Three articular facets *sit* on its superior and posterior surface for the attachment of supraspinatus, infraspinatus and teres minor. Supraspinatus inserts into the highest or superior facet, infraspinatus into the middle and teres minor into the lower or inferior facet. In reality these tendons are not separate, but together with subscapularis, they interdigitate at their insertions to form a fibrous thickening of the capsule, the rotator cuff. The sharp medial edge of the greater tuberosity forms the lateral lip of the *bicipital groove (intertubercular sulcus)* which receives the insertion of pectoralis major.

The *lesser tuberosity* is a bony projection that lies below and lateral to the coracoid process. It receives the insertion of subscapularis on its medial aspect and its sharp lateral edge forms the medial lip of the bicipital groove which receives the insertion of teres major.

The *sternoclavicular joint* is a synovial joint between the medial end of the clavicle and a notch on the superolateral aspect of the manubrium sterni. A fibrocartilaginous disc is positioned between the joint surfaces. It is an important joint since it is the point of attachment of the upper limb to the axial skeleton.

The *acromioclavicular joint* is a synovial plane joint with its articular surfaces covered with fibrocartilage. A wedge-shaped fibrocartilaginous disc drops down into the joint from the superior aspect of the joint capsule, producing a partial division of the joint. The articular facet on the lateral aspect of the clavicle is directed inferolaterally and the corresponding facet on the medial border of the acromion is directed superomedially, producing a tendency for the clavicle to override the acromion. The plane of the joint tends to be variable, but may run slightly obliquely, sloping medially from superior to inferior. The joint is surrounded by a fibrous capsule that is thickened superiorly and inferiorly by the parallel fibres of the capsular ligaments running between the two bones (Fig. 5.1). The stability of the acromioclavicular joint is provided by the strong accessory coracoclavicular ligament.

The clavicle acts as a strut or brace and allows the scapula to rotate and glide forwards and backwards. The movements at the acromioclavicular joint are passive, in the same way as the sacroiliac joint. The small amounts of movement available make it impossible to determine a capsular pattern, although as a synovial joint it can be affected by arthritis.

Figure 5.1   Acromioclavicular joint, showing intra-articular disc and ligaments. From Anatomy and Human Movement by N Palastanga D Field and R Soames. Reprinted by permission of Elsevier Ltd.

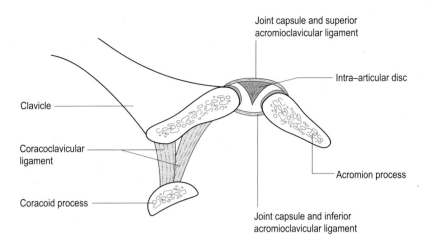

The *coracoclavicular ligament* is separate from the acromioclavicular joint, but in strongly binding the scapula to the clavicle via the coracoid process it provides a stabilizing component to the joint. The ligament has two parts, the trapezoid and conoid ligaments, which are separate anatomically and functionally. The more horizontal trapezoid ligament acts as a hinge for scapular motion, while the more vertical conoid ligament acts as a longitudinal axis for scapular rotation. Together, the ligaments prevent medial displacement of the acromion under the clavicle.

The *glenohumeral joint* is a synovial ball-and-socket joint between the head of the humerus and the glenoid fossa of the scapula, deepened by the fibrocartilaginous glenoid labrum (Fig. 5.2). The two articular surfaces are incongruent, with the relatively large head of the humerus providing a surface area three to four times that of the glenoid fossa (Hulstyn & Fadale 1995). The enormous range of movement is therefore at the expense of joint stability. With no inherent bony stability available, stability is dependent primarily upon the static effects of the capsuloligamentous structures and the dynamic effects of the surrounding muscles. The limited joint volume and a negative intra-articular pressure provide a form of static stability. The action of muscle forces, mainly the rotator cuff, produces compression of the head of the humerus into the glenoid labrum, providing important dynamic stability and steering the joint surfaces during movement (Speer 1995).

The *joint capsule*, lined with synovium, is thin and spacious, with a large volume of normally between 15 and 30 ml (Cailliet 1991, Halder & An 2000). It attaches to the edge of the glenoid medially and surrounds the anatomical neck of the humerus laterally, except for its inferomedial part that descends to attach to the shaft of the humerus, approximately 1 cm below the articular margin. The inferomedial portion forms a loose axillary pouch or fold and consists of randomly organized collagen fibres (Hulstyn & Fadale 1995). Although this arrangement facilitates movement, this part of the capsule is relatively weak as it is not supported by muscles and therefore is often subject to strain.

Figure 5.2   Cross-section of glenohumeral joint showing internal structure. From Anatomy and Human Movement by N Palastanga D Field and R Soames. Reprinted by permission of Elsevier Ltd.

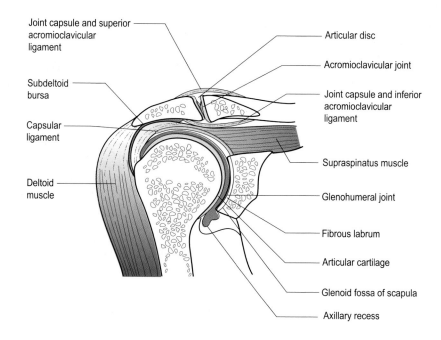

Figure 5.3   External aspect of glenohumeral joint showing axillary pouch and capsular ligaments.

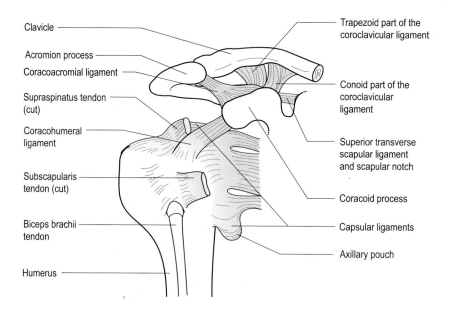

The capsular fibres are mainly horizontal and are reinforced anteriorly by three capsular ligaments, the *superior, middle and inferior glenohumeral ligaments*, which are only evident on the interior aspect of the capsule (Fig. 5.3). The three bands together form a Z-shape reinforcement to the anterior capsule (Kapandji 1982). The inferior glenohumeral ligament complex plays a major stabilizing role in supporting the humeral head in a hammock or broad sling, particularly during abduction (Hulstyn & Fadale 1995, Speer 1995). All three bands of the glenohumeral ligaments are taut in lateral rotation and abduction stresses the middle and inferior bands. This may be significant in the development of the capsular pattern of the shoulder joint.

The rotator cuff muscles (supraspinatus, infraspinatus, teres minor and subscapularis) act as extensible ligaments to support the capsule, assisted by the long heads of triceps and biceps. Much of the capsule is less than 1 mm thick, but it is thickened to between 1 and 2 mm near its humeral attachment where it receives the rotator cuff tendon fibres (Hulstyn & Fadale 1995). The rotator interval is a fibrous gap between the supraspinatus and subscapularis tendons and is therefore part of the rotator cuff. It is composed of fibres from supraspinatus and subscapularis together with the coracohumeral ligament, the superior glenohumeral ligament and parts of the capsule. The key structure of the interval was determined to be the coracohumeral ligament, which attaches between the dorsolateral aspect of the base of the coracoid and the greater, and to some extent the lesser, tuberosities. It would seem to be important for inferior stability of the glenohumeral joint and in limiting lateral rotation (Jost et al 2000), possibly contributing to the capsular pattern if the interval becomes reduced.

The wide range of movement available at the glenohumeral joint consists of flexion, extension, abduction, adduction, medial and lateral rotation that all combine to allow circumduction. The range of elevation may be up to 180° and may occur through flexion in the sagittal plane, or abduction through the coronal plane. The most functional movement is abduction in the plane of the scapula, known as *scaption*. This is not a fixed plane but occurs 30–40° anterior to the coronal plane of the humerus (Frame 1991). It places deltoid and supraspinatus in an optimal position to elevate the arm (Nordin & Frankel 2001). Abduction is accompanied by lateral rotation in the coronal plane which allows the greater tuberosity to clear the acromion; scaption does not involve this element of concomitant lateral rotation (Frame 1991).

Active elevation consists of abduction from 0–60° occurring at the glenohumeral joint, 60–120° occurring at the scapulothoracic joint and 120–180° occurring at the glenohumeral and scapulothoracic joints together with side flexion of the trunk to the opposite side (Kapandji 1982). Approximately 90° of passive glenohumeral abduction is achieved with the inferior angle of the scapula fixed. The range of lateral rotation is 80–90° and medial rotation 100–110°, with full range only achieved by taking the arm behind the back.

Rolling and translational (gliding) movements also occur and the glenohumeral joint surfaces can be separated by distraction. Muscle forces acting on the joint stabilize it and produce a combination of shearing and compression forces, maintaining the humeral head in the glenoid fossa.

The nerve supply to the glenohumeral joint is mainly from the C5 segment.

Cameron (1995) looked at the shoulder as a weight-bearing joint. Although this joint is traditionally considered to be non-weight-bearing in character, he applied simple physical principles showing this not to be the case. With the weight of the adult arm estimated to be approximately 5 kg, forces equivalent to three times body weight are transmitted through the shoulder during simple daily activities.

The *coracoacromial ligament* is an accessory ligament of the shoulder joint, forming an osseoligamentous arch over the superior aspect of the shoulder joint and the subacromial bursa. It is triangular in shape and approximately 1 cm wide. Its apex attaches to the anterior aspect of the acromion and its base to the lateral aspect of the coracoid process. The coracoacromial arch is separated from the underlying tendons by the subacromial bursa. The coracoacromial ligament is unusual in that it attaches to two parts of the same bone, probably functioning as a buffer, it provides stability for the head of the humerus against upwards displacement and protects it from direct vertical trauma (Petersilge et al 1997).

Numerous small bursae are associated with the shoulder joint. An anterior *subscapular bursa* lies between the tendon of subscapularis and the anterior capsule, consistently communicating with the joint. The synovial lining of the joint extends to form a sheath around the long head of biceps in the bicipital groove. A bursa, which communicates with the joint, may be present between the tendon of infraspinatus and the posterior capsule.

The *subacromial bursa (synonymous with subdeltoid bursa)* is independent of the shoulder joint and normally does not communicate with it. It was described by Codman in 1934 as the largest and most complicated bursa in the body forming a secondary scapulohumeral joint (Beals et al 1998). It therefore has a special role in the biomechanics of the shoulder joint and is frequently a cause of pain. It is a smooth synovial sac containing variable thin bands or plicae and is surrounded by fatty areolar tissue (Hulstyn & Fadale 1995). Beals et al (1998) identified by cadaver studies that only the anterior half of the under surface of the acromion is contained within the subacromial bursal cavity, which may have implications for injection of the subacromial bursa, particularly if a posterior approach is used. Its deep layer lies over the rotator cuff tendons and the head of the humerus (Cooper et al 1993). Medially it extends under the acromion to the acromioclavicular joint line and laterally it caps the greater tuberosity, separating it from the overlying deltoid muscle.

The *subacromial space* is sometimes considered to be a joint (Kapandji 1982, Pratt 1994). This is not a true articulation but it is critical to shoulder movement. As supraspinatus pulls the greater tuberosity superiorly and medially, the walls of the subacromial bursa glide over one another allowing the head of the humerus to slide (Netter 1987). The subacromial space is approximately 7–14mm deep (Frame 1991) and is occupied by the subacromial bursa, the supraspinatus tendon, the superior part of the capsule of the shoulder joint and the tendon of the long head of biceps. The tightly packed structures move constantly in relation to one another and there is the potential for friction and degeneration. Inflammation, degeneration, the shape of the acromion or degeneration of the acromioclavicular joint can all contribute to a reduction of the vertical proportions or stenosis of the subacromial space. Impingement of a painful structure in the space may produce a painful arc between 60 and 120° of abduction.

CONTRACTILE STRUCTURES

Four short muscles (supraspinatus, infraspinatus, teres minor and subscapularis) pass from the scapula to the head of the humerus and these are known as the rotator cuff. The rotator cuff muscles are particularly important to the function of the shoulder, working together as extensible ligaments to provide dynamic stability, maintaining and centralizing the head of the humerus in the glenoid fossa. Shoulder movement, particularly elevation, is governed by force couples that involve the interaction of deltoid and the rotator cuff muscles (Nordin & Frankel 2001). The rotator cuff muscles maintain the joint's apposition, preventing excessive superior translatory movement that would lead to instability.

As the rotator cuff tendons insert into the head of the humerus they blend with the capsule of the joint forming a thickened common tendinous cuff. Fibres from subscapularis and infraspinatus interdigitate with those of supraspinatus in their deep layer, facilitating the distribution of forces directly or indirectly over a wider area (Clark & Harryman 1992). The tendon of the long head of biceps exits the capsule through a reinforced foramen at the junction of the insertions of supraspinatus and subscapularis onto the humerus (Hulstyn & Fadale 1995). These tendons are frequently a source of pain through degeneration and overuse.

Supraspinatus (suprascapular nerve C4–C6) takes origin from the medial two-thirds of the suprascapular fossa. The fibres, which are bipennate, converge to pass under the acromion, blending with the capsule of the shoulder joint and adjacent tendon fibres of subscapularis and infraspinatus, inserting mainly into the upper of the three facets on the greater tuberosity. As the tendon passes to its insertion it appears to be reinforced by the coracohumeral ligament that runs parallel and is firmly adherent to it (Clark & Harryman 1992). Supraspinatus produces abduction of the glenohumeral joint but its exact role in the mechanism of shoulder movement is controversial.

Supraspinatus, together with the other rotator cuff muscles, stabilizes the head of the humerus, providing horizontal compression and reducing vertical displacement. It is considered to be responsible for initiating abduction by holding the head of the humerus down on the glenoid, before deltoid takes over at approximately 20°, to provide the force for abduction (Palastanga et al 2002, Pratt 1994). However, both supraspinatus and deltoid have been shown to be active throughout the range of abduction with an early rise in tension in supraspinatus fixing the humeral head, and enabling deltoid to work at a better mechanical advantage (Cailliet 1991, Frame 1991). It may be that deltoid and supraspinatus can initiate and complete a full range of abduction independently.

Infraspinatus (suprascapular nerve C4–C6) is a thick triangular muscle that takes origin from the medial two-thirds of the infraspinous fossa. Its fibres converge to form a broad, thick tendon, passing over the posterior joint capsule, with which it blends, and inserting into the middle of the three facets on the greater tuberosity of the humerus, some of its fibres interdigitating with the adjacent supraspinatus. Together with teres minor, with which it is sometimes fused, infraspinatus produces lateral rotation of the glenohumeral joint during elevation.

Teres minor (axillary nerve C5–C6) takes origin from the upper two-thirds of the lateral border of the scapula, above the origin of teres major. It inserts into the lowest of the three facets on the posterior aspect of the greater tuberosity blending with the posterior capsule as it passes over it. It functions with infraspinatus to produce lateral rotation of the glenohumeral joint.

Subscapularis (upper and lower subscapular nerve C5–C6) takes origin from the medial two-thirds of the subscapular fossa on the costal surface of the scapula, and inserts by a broad, thin, membranous tendon into the lesser tuberosity of the humerus. It reinforces the anterior capsule, from which it is partially separated by a bursa which communicates with the joint. It functions to produce medial rotation of the glenohumeral joint. Fibres from subscapularis and supraspinatus blend together to contribute to the rotator interval (see above).

Trapezius (spinal accessory nerve, XI and ventral rami of C3–C4) is a large, flat triangular muscle forming a trapezium with its opposite number. It has a long line of attachment from the superior nuchal line, external occipital protruberance, ligamentum nuchae and the spinous processes and intervening supraspinous ligament from C7 to T12. The upper fibres descend to the posterior border of the lateral third of the clavicle, the middle fibres pass horizontally to the medial border of the acromion and the lower fibres pass upwards to the crest of the spine of the scapula. In conjunction with other muscles, trapezius stabilizes the scapula for functional movement of the arm and the individual portions of the muscle assist other muscles in producing primary movement. The upper fibres of trapezius and levator scapulae suspend the scapula against the thoracic cage and are constantly active during ambulation (Paine & Voight 1993). Trapezius together with serratus anterior forms a force couple to rotate the scapula on the thoracic wall (Frame 1991).

Rhomboids, major and minor (rhomboid branch of the dorsal scapular nerve, C4–C5), form a line of attachment from the lower ligamentum nuchae and the spines of C7 to T5 and pass to the medial border of the scapula, to assist in its stabilization against the thoracic cage. The rhomboids are active in scapular retraction, which is essential for overhead throwing movements and swimming strokes, e.g. crawl (Paine & Voight 1993).

Levator scapulae (C3–C5) descends from the transverse processes of the atlas and axis to the medial upper scapular border. Together with the rhomboids it controls and positions the scapula.

Latissimus dorsi (thoracodorsal nerve C6–C8) has an extensive origin from the lumbar spine, thoracolumbar fascia and thorax. The fibres converge towards the humerus, attaching to the inferior angle of the scapula as they pass by. The tendinous fibres twist through an angle of

180° before inserting into the floor of the bicipital groove. At the shoulder latissimus dorsi extends, adducts and medially rotates the humerus.

Teres major (lower subscapular nerve, C6–C7) passes from the lower dorsal aspect of the scapula near the inferior angle to insert into the medial lip of the bicipital groove. It functions together with latissimus dorsi to adduct and medially rotate the humerus and together they form the posterior fold of the axilla. In conjunction with pectoralis major, teres major stabilizes the shoulder joint.

Deltoid (axillary nerve C5–C6) gives the shoulder its rounded contour. The muscle has three sets of fibres which all converge to insert into the deltoid tubercle in the middle of the lateral aspect of the shaft of the upper humerus. The anterior fibres attach to the anterior border of the lateral third of the clavicle and assist flexion and medial rotation. The middle fibres attach to the acromion, assisting abduction, and the posterior fibres attach to the lower lip of the crest of the spine of the scapula assisting extension and lateral rotation. The direction of the muscle fibres is almost vertical and the muscle's basic action is to elevate the head of the humerus up into the overhanging coracoacromial arch (Cailliet 1991). Overall, deltoid is a powerful abductor of the glenohumeral joint but its function is dependent on supraspinatus and the other rotator cuff muscles.

Pectoralis major (lateral and medial pectoral nerves, clavicular part C5–C6: sternocostal part C7–C8, T1) is a thick triangular muscle, originating as two separate parts from the anterior chest wall to insert into the lateral lip of the bicipital groove. As the fibres cross to the arm they twist to form the anterior axillary fold. The two parts of the muscle are both powerful adductors and medial rotators of the humerus; the clavicular part produces flexion. Together with latissimus dorsi, pectoralis major acts in climbing activities and is involved in pushing and throwing.

Pectoralis minor (both pectoral nerves, C6–C8) passes from the upper ribs to the coracoid process. In conjunction with other muscles that anchor the scapula, pectoralis minor protracts, depresses, rotates and tilts the scapula.

Serratus anterior (long thoracic nerve C5–C7, descending on its external surface) has an extensive origin from the side of the thorax, passing round the thoracic cage to insert into the medial border of the costal surface of the scapula. It is responsible for stabilizing the scapula during elevation and protraction of the scapula in the functional activities of reaching and pushing. Loss of its nerve supply leads to winging of the scapula.

Movement of the scapula on the thoracic cage occurs at the scapulothoracic joint between two fascial planes, the most superficial of which lies between subscapularis and serratus anterior (Kapandji 1982, Pratt 1994). The surrounding muscles stabilize this joint and dynamically position the glenoid fossa to facilitate efficient glenohumeral movement (Paine & Voight 1993).

Coracobrachialis (musculocutaneous nerve C5–C7) originates from the tip of the coracoid process, where it forms a conjoint tendon with the short head of the biceps, and inserts into the medial aspect of the middle of the shaft of the humerus. It adducts the humerus, its position being analogous to the adductor group of muscles at the hip.

Biceps brachii (musculocutaneous nerve C5–C6) has a short head arising from the tip of the coracoid process and a long head originating within the capsule of the glenohumeral joint from the supraglenoid tubercle and adjacent glenoid labrum. The intracapsular part of the tendon is surrounded by a double sheath, an extension of the synovial lining of the glenohumeral joint (Williams 1998). The long head passes through the subacromial space and exits the joint behind the transverse humeral ligament, emerging between the insertions of supraspinatus and subscapularis. It continues on into the bicipital groove together with its synovial sheath. The two muscle bellies fuse to insert into the tuberosity of the radius via the biceps tendon. Biceps has its main effect at the elbow where it is a powerful supinator and elbow flexor. The long head exerts a stabilizing effect on the superior aspect of the shoulder joint, which may be important if the shoulder becomes less stable (Itoi et al 1994). Its passage laterally, then turning a 90° angle into the bicipital groove, assists forward flexion of the shoulder (Cailliet 1991).

Triceps (radial nerve C6–C8) originates by three heads. The long head arises from the infraglenoid tubercle of the scapula and the glenoid labrum, where it exerts a stabilizing effect on the shoulder joint. It also assists adduction and extension movements of the humerus from the flexed position. The lateral head originates from the humerus above and lateral to the spiral groove, and the medial head from the posterior humerus below the spiral groove. The three heads come together to insert into the olecranon process. The main action of the triceps is to extend the elbow.

GUIDE TO SURFACE MARKING AND PALPATION

POSTERIOR ASPECT
(Fig. 5.4)

Palpate the *inferior angle of the scapula* which, in most people, can be grasped between a finger and thumb. Abducting the arm may make the inferior angle easier to locate as it advances around the chest wall.

Figure 5.4   Posterior aspect of the shoulder.

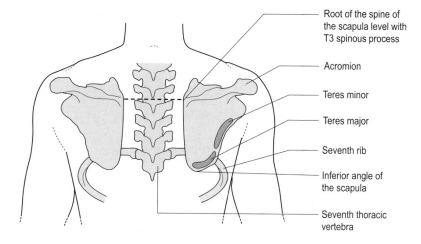

- Root of the spine of the scapula level with T3 spinous process
- Acromion
- Teres minor
- Teres major
- Seventh rib
- Inferior angle of the scapula
- Seventh thoracic vertebra

Palpate along the medial and lateral borders of the scapula. The lower medial border is subcutaneous and more readily palpable, lying parallel to and approximately three fingers' width from the spinous processes. Visualize the position of *latissimus dorsi* as it crosses the inferior angle, and track the *teres major and minor* muscles that take origin from the lateral border of the scapula. Teres major originates below teres minor.

The *crest of the spine of the scapula* may be visible and is readily palpable. Feel it sloping medially down to meet the medial border of the scapula at the level of the spinous process of T3.

Palpate the lateral end of the spine of the scapula and follow the lower border round until it joins the lateral border of the acromion. A sharp 90° angle is formed here, the *posterior angle of the acromion*, which is a useful bony landmark.

Palpate the flat upper surface of the *acromion* which is subcutaneous and forms the summit of the shoulder, lying just lateral to the acromioclavicular joint. Palpate the anterior edge of the acromion with an index finger and the posterior angle with a thumb, to appreciate its width.

LATERAL ASPECT

Palpate the lateral edge of the acromion. Note its depth and visualize the position of the subacromial bursa beneath it. Follow the anterior and posterior portions of the *deltoid muscle* down on to its insertion into the deltoid tubercle.

ANTERIOR ASPECT
(Fig. 5.5)

Palpate the *clavicle*; it is usually visible and palpable throughout its length in most people. Start at the medial end and follow the anterior

Figure 5.5   Anterior aspect of the shoulder.

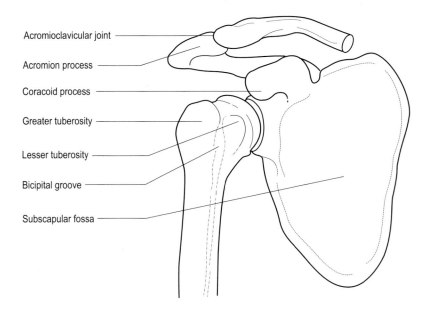

Acromioclavicular joint

Acromion process

Coracoid process

Greater tuberosity

Lesser tuberosity

Bicipital groove

Subscapular fossa

curve as it lies over the first rib, then the reverse curve that produces a hollow at the lateral end of the clavicle. Below this hollow, between deltoid and pectoralis major, lies the infraclavicular fossa.

Palpate the *acromioclavicular joint* line that lies approximately 1–2 cm, or a thumb's width, medial to the lateral border of the acromion. The clavicular end of the joint may project a little higher than the acromion since it overrides it slightly, and this may produce a slight step down between the clavicle and acromion. The joint line should be palpable from above. Apply a downwards pressure on the lateral end of the clavicle and ask the model (or patient) to flex and extend the shoulder to feel movement at the joint.

Below the junction of the lateral third and the medial two-thirds of the clavicle, in the lateral infraclavicular fossa, feel the prominent *coracoid process* which forms an anterior projection when the arm is resting at the side. This is covered by the anterior deltoid and deep palpation – which may be uncomfortable – is necessary. With a finger on the coracoid process, abduct the arm and the coracoid should move out from under your palpating finger.

Moving slightly downwards and laterally from the coracoid process, palpate the *lesser tuberosity* of the humerus. Immediately lateral to it is the *bicipital groove* and further laterally still, the *greater tuberosity* should be palpable.

Place the arm in the anatomical position and feel the greater tuberosity lying laterally and the lesser tuberosity lying anteriorly on either side of the bicipital groove. Relax the arm, allowing it to fall into the more functional position with some medial rotation, and feel the greater tuberosity lying more anteriorly and the lesser tuberosity medially.

The *greater tuberosity* can be easily located as it lies in line with and above the lateral epicondyle of the humerus. It can be grasped with the thumb, index and middle fingers placed on its anterior, superior and posterior surfaces. Note its width. The greater tuberosity is slightly wider from anterior to posterior than the acromion process. Try to visualize its three facets for the insertions of supraspinatus, infraspinatus and teres minor.

PALPATION OF THE INSERTIONS OF THE ROTATOR CUFF TENDONS

To palpate *supraspinatus*, the greater tuberosity must be brought forwards from under the acromion to expose its superior facet. Position the patient sitting up at an angle of about 45° against the couch. Medially rotate and extend the arm to position it behind the back (Fig. 5.6). Palpate for the anterior edge of the acromion and locate the greater tuberosity. The tendon of supraspinatus is running directly forwards between the two bony points, roughly in line with the position of a shoulder strap (remember that you have turned the greater tuberosity to lie more anteriorly). The tendon of insertion is approximately one finger's width.

To palpate *infraspinatus*, the greater tuberosity must be brought backwards from under the acromion to expose its middle facet. Position the patient in prone lying with the weight supported on the forearms. Ensure that the elbow is placed directly below the shoulder and laterally

Figure 5.6   Position of arm for palpation of the supraspinatus tendon.

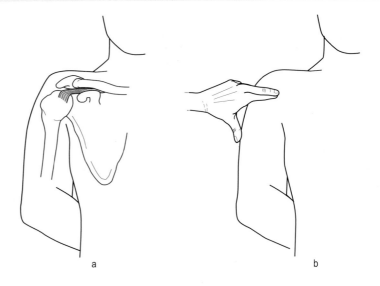

a

b

rotate and adduct the shoulder (Fig. 5.7). Palpate for the posterior angle of the acromion and locate the greater tuberosity. The tendon of infraspinatus runs parallel to the spine of the scapula to insert into the greater tuberosity, immediately below the posterior angle of the acromion. The tendon of insertion is approximately two fingers wide. Together with the insertion of *teres minor* the tendon is three fingers wide.

Figure 5.7   Position of arm for palpation of the infraspinatus tendon.

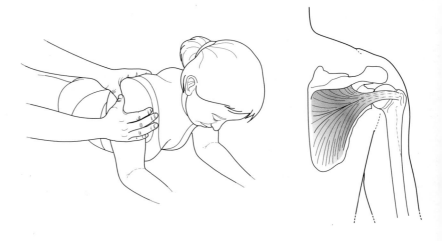

Figure 5.8   Position of arm for palpation of the subscapularis tendon.

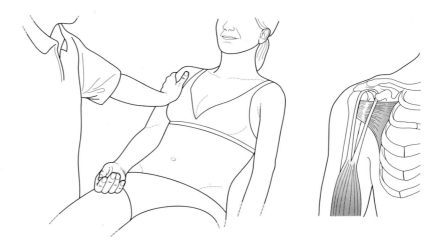

To locate *subscapularis*, position the arm with the humerus in the anatomical position. Either palpate the coracoid process and move laterally and slightly downwards, or identify the bicipital groove and move directly medially to find the sharp lateral lip of the lesser tuberosity (Fig. 5.8). Follow round onto the medial aspect of the lesser tuberosity to locate the insertion of subscapularis. The tendon itself cannot be felt and the underlying bone is tender to palpation. The tendon is approximately three fingers wide.

COMMENTARY ON THE EXAMINATION

The history at the shoulder is important, although it probably will not reveal a conclusive diagnosis. Cyriax (1982) considered the shoulder to be an 'honest' joint but most clues are related to the anatomy at the shoulder and are revealed in the objective examination rather than in the patient's account. Lesions may be complicated and due to a contribution of several factors. For instance, pain tends to cause immobility and it is not uncommon to find a secondary capsulitis accompanying bursitis or tendinopathy.

OBSERVATION

A general observation of the patient's *face, posture and gait* will alert the examiner to abnormalities and serious illness. Acute subacromial bursitis produces a constant acute pain that disturbs sleep and the patient looks tired.

The acute shoulder is usually held in a position of comfort, i.e. medially rotated with the elbow flexed and supported. An alteration in the rhythmical arm swing may be obvious. The head of the humerus is so positioned in the glenoid that functional movements tend to occur in diagonal patterns and this should be evident in the arm swing during gait activity.

Due to the many anatomical components that make up the shoulder region and the interrelationship between the function of each group, lesions can be subtly complicated. Multiple lesions can exist and instability can produce secondary problems at the shoulder. In focusing on the differential diagnosis of specific lesions, orthopaedic medicine looks at common lesions at the shoulder. For more detailed coverage of shoulder instability and its relationship to shoulder lesions the reader is referred to the other texts that cover this subject.

HISTORY (SUBJECTIVE EXAMINATION)

The *age, occupation, sports, hobbies and lifestyle* of the patient may give clues to diagnosis. The younger patient engaged in physical work or active in sport may have a minor instability problem or a labral tear related to overuse, producing secondary impingement. The middle-aged patient may present with overuse rotator cuff lesions, impingement or chronic bursitis. In the older age group, degenerative rotator cuff lesions or tears with secondary or idiopathic capsulitis may occur. Overuse injuries are a common cause of pain felt at the shoulder and the lifestyle of the patient can be directly responsible for the condition. Knowledge of lifestyle is useful to advise the patient on preventing recurrence.

Shoulder injuries are common in throwing sports, swimming and all overhead activities. Tennis strokes involve rotation, abduction and elevation, leading to repetitive and stressful use of the arm in the overhead position, possibly causing impingement and instability (McCann & Bigliani 1994). It is relevant to know which is the dominant arm.

Throwing has several different mechanisms, for example the straight-arm throw of the javelin, the centrifugally induced velocity of hammer throwing, the explosive push of putting the shot or the spinning pull of the discus thrower. A 'dead arm' syndrome may be produced during the acceleration phase of throwing, when the arm becomes useless and drops down by the side. It may be associated with pins and needles and takes several minutes to recover. It is considered to be due to momentary subluxation of the glenohumeral joint associated with compression of the brachial plexus (Copeland 1993, Clarnette & Miniaci 1998).

The *site* of the pain does not reliably indicate the site of the lesion. The shoulder joint and its surrounding capsule, ligaments and muscles are mainly derived from the C5 segment. Lesions of any of these structures will cause the pain to be referred into the C5 dermatome which extends into the anterolateral aspect of the arm and forearm as far as the base of the thumb. The most common point of referral for these structures is to the area over the insertion of deltoid. Rotator cuff pathology usually produces anterolateral shoulder pain (Clarnette & Miniaci 1998). The more irritable the lesion, the further the referral of pain into the C5 dermatome, such that the *spread* of pain will give an indication of the severity of the lesion. As a deep joint lying proximally in its dermatome, the glenohumeral joint has the potential to refer pain over a considerable distance. The cervical spine may produce pain in the shoulder area or refer pain into the C5 dermatome, therefore it will need to be excluded as a source of symptoms.

The acromioclavicular joint and surrounding ligaments produce an accurate localization of pain over the joint. This is because, in contrast to the glenohumeral joint, the acromioclavicular joint is a superficial joint giving little reference.

The *symptoms and behaviour* need to be considered. The shoulder area is a point of referral of pain from other deep structures. The cervical spine in particular can refer pain to the area and visceral problems may mimic musculoskeletal lesions. The diaphragm is a C4 structure and will produce pain felt at the point of the shoulder if affected by adjacent conditions such as pleurisy.

The *onset* of the pain may be sudden or gradual. If the onset was sudden it is important to know if there was any related trauma, with the possibility of fracture. A fall on the outstretched hand may initiate a traumatic shoulder joint capsulitis or, less commonly, chronic subacromial bursitis, tendon strain or acromioclavicular joint sprain.

Acromioclavicular lesions are usually associated with a traumatic onset.

An acute subacromial bursitis has a characteristic sudden onset with no apparent cause.

The common shoulder lesions of overuse tendinopathy, bursitis or capsulitis, present most typically with a gradual onset of pain due to overuse factors. A capsulitis may be precipitated by trauma, but this is often minor and the patient cannot recall the incident. Stiffness and loss of functional movement are usually indicative of capsulitis. Tendinopathy may be provoked by overstretching or contraction against strong resistance. The *duration* of the symptoms gives an indication of the stage the lesion has reached in the inflammatory cycle.

Non-specific shoulder pain may be associated with nerve entrapment, which would be confirmed by signs of objective weakness but with no pain on shoulder movements (Biundo & Harris 1993, Schulte & Warner 1995).

The *behaviour* of the pain is relevant to diagnosis with the common lesions producing typical musculoskeletal pain on movement which is eased by rest. The patient should be asked if the pain is constant or only present on movement, giving an indication of the irritability of the lesion. Chronic overuse tendinopathy or bursitis often produces a dull ache rather than a pain, although twinges of pain may be experienced if impingement occurs during movement. An acute subacromial bursitis produces severe pain that is constant and often unrelenting, disturbing sleep. A capsulitis shows an increasing worsening pain, referring further and further into the C5 dermatome. The inflammatory nature of the pain may be obvious in complaints of pain and stiffness on waking. 'Catching' pain may be described on activities such as reaching for a seat belt or into the back of the car, or placing an arm in a coat sleeve, and may indicate impingement of structures under the coracoacromial arch.

Three questions
- Does the pain spread below the elbow? (site and spread)
- Can you lie on that side at night? (symptoms)
- Is the pain constant? (behaviour)

The behaviour can also help to assess the severity and irritability of the lesion as well as distinguish it from a lesion that is referring pain into the shoulder area. If the patient is unable to lie on that side because the increase in pain disturbs sleep, the lesion is irritable. It may indicate a chronic subacromial bursitis, rotator cuff lesion or more commonly an irritable capsulitis. Sleeping postures may cause stress in structures, inducing microtrauma or impingement.

A loss of functional activity such as being unable to do up a bra or reach into the back pocket will indicate limitation of movement. There may be evidence of shoulder instability or labral tears in patients complaining of 'clicking', 'snapping' or feeling as if the shoulder is 'coming out'. Crepitus or grating sounds may indicate degenerative changes.

To distinguish the lesion from one of cervical or thoracic origin the patient should be questioned about the presence of paraesthesia, and whether pain is increased on a cough, sneeze or deep breath. Heaviness, tiredness, puffiness, sweating or altered temperature may indicate associated or referred autonomic symptoms.

Assessment of *other joint involvement* will indicate generalized arthritis, possibly rheumatoid. It is also interesting to note if the patient has had previous shoulder problems since both 'frozen shoulder' (adhesive capsulitis) and acute subacromial bursitis often affect the other shoulder some years after the first incidence. In frozen shoulder the patient may complain of cervical involvement and there may be associated trigger points over the posterior aspect of the shoulder (Grubbs 1993). This may be due to compensatory overuse of other muscles and holding the shoulder in a position of ease, or may be indicative of abnormal neural mobility.

The *past medical history* will alert the examiner to serious illness and operations encountered by the patient. The patient should be specifically asked about a history of diabetes since there is an association between diabetes mellitus and the development of a frozen shoulder (Owens-Burkhart 1991, Clarnette & Miniaci 1998). The examiner should be on the alert for possible contraindications to treatment. An indication of the patient's current state of health is necessary and the patient should be asked about recent unexplained weight loss. Tumours involving the shoulder area are rare but a history of primary tumour should raise the suspicion of metastatic disease as a possible diagnosis (Clarnette & Miniaci 1998).

Medications currently being taken by the patient are determined to eliminate possible contraindications to treatment. The amount of analgesia required by the patient gives an indication of the severity of the lesion.

From the history, the possible diagnoses are noted. If the eventual diagnosis is one of capsulitis, three special questions relating to the spread of pain and provocation factors asked during the history (see marginal box and above) will give an indication of the severity of the lesion and act as a guide to treatment.

INSPECTION

The patient should undress to enable the area to be inspected in a good light.

A general inspection will determine any *bony deformity*. Look at the position of the cervical spine and take an overall view of the spinal curvatures in general. The general posture of the patient can be important and any observations of asymmetry are recorded if they are relevant to the presenting condition. It has been postulated that abnormal cervical and thoracic posture, particularly an increased thoracic kyphosis, alters the resting position of the scapula and may be related to shoulder pain caused by overuse (Greenfield et al 1995).

The attitude of the shoulder should be noted. Is one higher than the other or excessively medially rotated? In a frozen shoulder, one shoulder may be held higher than the other due to pain, with the scapula elevated and retracted. The position of the scapulae should be noted. Are they more or less symmetrical, lying approximately three fingers from the midline, or are they excessively retracted or protracted? There may be evidence of winging of the scapula but this is usually more obvious on movement.

Lumps, scars, bony prominences and bruising should be observed. A prominent bump at the end of the clavicle may signify an old fracture or dislocation of the acromioclavicular joint.

Colour changes and swelling are unusual findings at the shoulder unless associated with direct trauma. *Muscle wasting* is suspected if the spine of the scapula is prominent, due to neuritis or rotator cuff rupture. In chronic rotator cuff tendinopathy and/or degenerative tears, wasting of supraspinatus and infraspinatus may be obvious. The 'pop-eye' deformity of a rupture of the long head of the biceps is usually obvious, but the patient does not particularly complain of pain. In deltoid atrophy, squaring of the shoulder occurs as deltoid is no longer rounded out over the humeral head and may be indicative of anterior dislocation (Clarnette & Miniaci 1998).

STATE AT REST

Before any movements are performed, the state at rest is established to provide a baseline for subsequent comparison.

The suggested sequence for an objective examination of the shoulder will now be given, followed by a commentary including the reasoning in performing the movements and the significance of the possible findings.

The examination of the shoulder should first exclude possible cervical lesions, therefore six active cervical movements are performed and if a pattern of signs emerges implicating the cervical spine, then a full assessment of this region must be conducted.

Three elevation tests are conducted for the glenohumeral joint. Since the shoulder is considered to be an 'emotional' area, active elevation indicates the patient's willingness to move the joint. The range of movement and level of pain should then be consistent with other findings as the objective examination proceeds.

Passive elevation is added to assess pain, range of movement and end-feel. The normal end-feel of passive elevation is elastic. Any limitation of passive elevation suggests that the capsular pattern exists at the glenohumeral joint and this will be confirmed when the passive glenohumeral movements are assessed individually.

EXAMINATION BY SELECTIVE TENSION (OBJECTIVE EXAMINATION)

Eliminate the Cervical Spine

- Active cervical extension (Fig. 5.9a)
- Active right cervical rotation (Fig. 5.9b)
- Active left cervical rotation (Fig. 5.9c)
- Active right cervical side flexion (Fig. 5.9d)
- Active left cervical side flexion (Fig. 5.9e)
- Active cervical flexion (Fig. 5.9f)

Shoulder Elevation Tests

- Active elevation through flexion (Fig. 5.10)
- Passive elevation (Fig. 5.11)
- Active elevation through abduction for a painful arc (Figs 5.12 and Fig. 5.13)

Passive Glenohumeral Movements

- Passive lateral rotation (Fig. 5.14)
- Passive abduction (Fig. 5.15)
- Passive medial rotation (Fig. 5.16)

Resisted Tests

- Resisted shoulder abduction (Fig. 5.17)
- Resisted shoulder adduction (Fig. 5.18)
- Resisted shoulder lateral rotation (Fig. 5.19)
- Resisted shoulder medial rotation (Fig. 5.20)
- Resisted elbow flexion (Fig. 5.21)
- Resisted elbow extension (Fig. 5.22)

Accessory Test for Acromioclavicular Joint or Lower Fibres of Subscapularis

- Passive shoulder flexion and adduction (scarf test) (Fig. 5.23)

Palpation

- Once a diagnosis has been made, the structure at fault is palpated for the exact site of the lesion

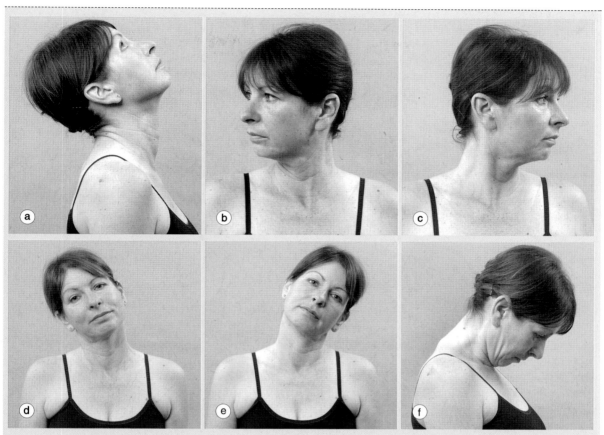

Figure 5.9   Six active movements of the cervical spine: (a) extension; (b, c) rotations; (d, e) side flexions; (f) flexion.

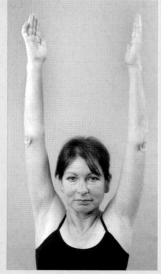

Figure 5.10   Active shoulder elevation.

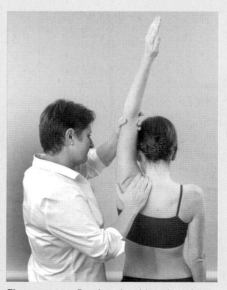

Figure 5.11   Passive shoulder elevation.

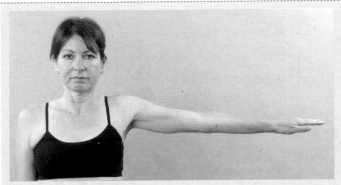

Figure 5.12   Active elevation through abduction, looking for a painful arc.

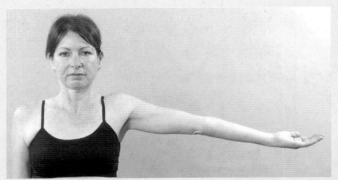

Figure 5.13   Varying arm position to explore for a painful arc.

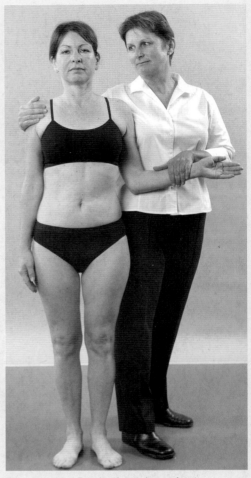

Figure 5.14   Passive lateral rotation.

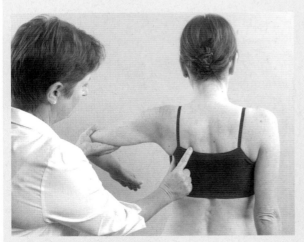

Figure 5.15   Passive abduction.

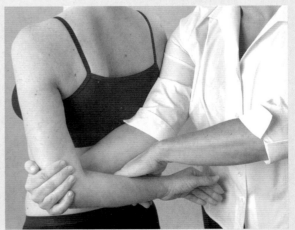

Figure 5.16   Passive medial rotation.

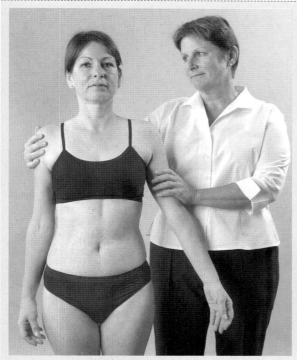

Figure 5.17   Resisted abduction.

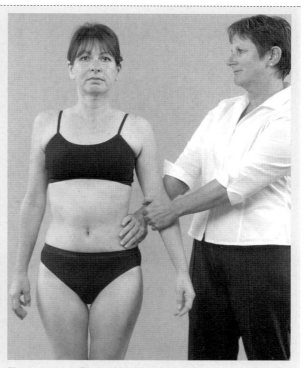

Figure 5.18   Resisted adduction.

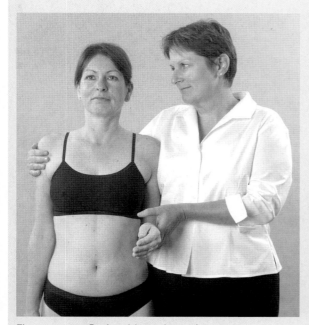

Figure 5.19   Resisted lateral rotation.

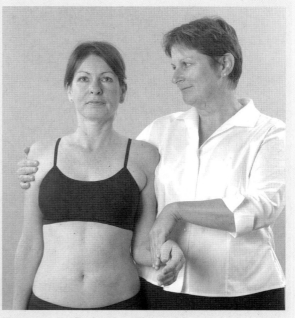

Figure 5.20   Resisted medial rotation.

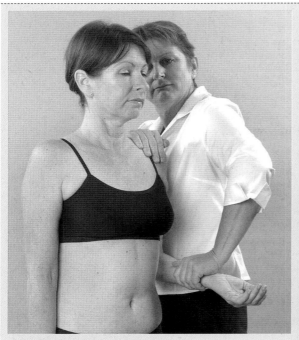

Figure 5.21   Resisted elbow flexion.

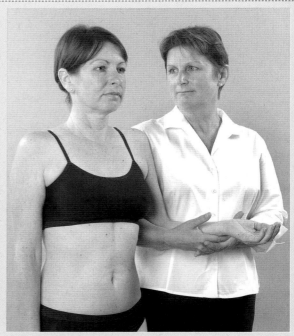

Figure 5.22   Resisted elbow extension.

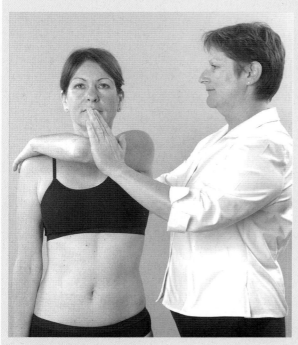

Figure 5.23   The scarf test.

Active elevation through abduction is conducted in the coronal plane to assess for the presence of a painful arc. This involves abduction to 90° followed by lateral rotation, to enable the greater tuberosity to clear the coracoacromial arch. The test performed in this way is usually consistent with the patient's account of symptoms. However, functionally, the arm is more commonly lifted through scaption (see p. 000).

A painful arc is a localizing sign and indicates impingement of a painful structure in the subacromial space – which structure will only be revealed by completing the full examination procedure. An arc is more easily elicited on active movement as contraction of the muscle groups tends to raise the humeral head and reduce the space; it is generally found between 60 and 120° of abduction.

Be prepared to explore for a painful arc, especially in the light of findings later in the examination, remembering that a diagnosis is not made until the full examination has been completed. The position may be modified to place the rotator cuff tendons into a more vulnerable position for compression against the coracoacromial arch.

Elevation of the humerus through abduction in the coronal plane favours compression of the distal end of the supraspinatus tendon. Abduction with lateral rotation, palm up, brings the upper part of subscapularis to face upwards to be compressed against the arch, while abduction with medial rotation brings infraspinatus forwards and increases the possibility of its compression. Forward elevation in the sagittal plane combined with lateral rotation, palm up, compresses the tendon of the long head of the biceps (Burns & Whipple 1993).

The passive glenohumeral movements are conducted looking for pain, range of movement and end-feel. Since variation in movement between individuals is probable, movements should always be compared with the other side. However, variation between sides may exist, for example in tennis players or fast bowlers, who may have a greater range of one rotation, at the expense of the other, on the dominant side. Passive lateral and medial rotation have a normal elastic end-feel; passive abduction is assessed for range of movement only, since it is not possible to appreciate the end-feel. Assessment of the passive glenohumeral movements may confirm the presence of the capsular pattern, indicating arthritis.

As movements become limited in the capsular pattern they develop an abnormally 'hard' end-feel. The capsular pattern results in overall limitation of passive elevation. Limitation or pain at the end of range of lateral rotation only may be a sign of early capsulitis.

It may not be possible to fully assess the range of medial rotation in severe capsulitis since the accompanying limitation of abduction prevents the arm from being placed behind the patient's back. As a guide for subsequent comparison, measure the range of movement against certain landmarks that can be reached by the hand, e.g. pocket, buttock, waist, inferior angle of scapula.

Subacromial bursitis provides a typical example of a non-capsular pattern of movement at the shoulder. While the acromioclavicular joint does not demonstrate its own capsular pattern, it produces a non-capsular pattern of movement at the glenohumeral joint.

Capsular pattern at the glenohumeral joint
- Most limitation of lateral rotation.
- Less limitation of abduction.
- Least limitation of medial rotation.

The resisted tests are conducted looking for pain and reduced power which will indicate a muscle lesion or possible neurological involvement. The resisted tests performed in the upright position apply a degree of upwards shearing and compression to the glenohumeral joint in stabilizing the head of the humerus. For this reason the resisted tests may be accessory signs in subacromial bursitis, or show involvement of the joint. To confirm diagnosis, the resisted tests may be repeated in lying, with some joint distraction, where the effect of compression and shear on the joint is reduced (Figs 5.24 and 5.25).

Figure 5.24   Resisted shoulder abduction with distraction.

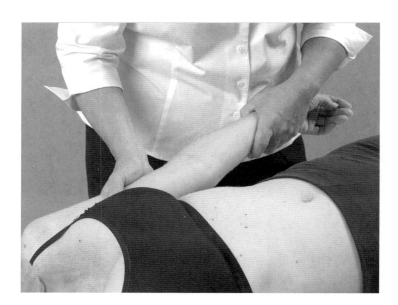

Figure 5.25   Resisted elbow extension with distraction.

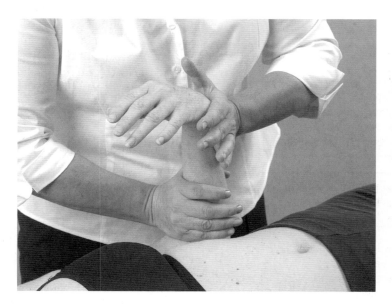

Resisted abduction tests mainly supraspinatus; resisted adduction tests latissimus dorsi and pectoralis major; resisted lateral rotation tests mainly infraspinatus and teres minor; resisted medial rotation tests mainly subscapularis; resisted elbow flexion tests biceps; and resisted elbow extension tests triceps. The anatomical interdigitation of the tendinous insertions of the rotator cuff tendons means that the resisted tests described may not definitively implicate one tendon; subsequent palpation of the structures implicated will identify the site of the lesion.

Painful weakness on resisted testing may indicate partial rupture, but it may be difficult to decide whether a test is producing real or apparent weakness since the patient is limited by pain from making a maximal effort (Pellecchia et al 1996).

In athletes it may be difficult to produce positive findings, especially on resisted testing, as the symptoms may only be provoked during the athletic or sporting activity itself. It may be necessary for the patient to provoke the pain before the examination is carried out.

An accessory test, the 'scarf' test (as in putting a scarf over the opposite shoulder), may be performed to localize the lesion. This compresses the acromioclavicular joint or impinges the lower fibres of the subscapularis tendon against the coracoid process. It may also be positive as part of the 'muddle' of signs of a chronic subacromial bursitis.

Palpation is conducted for the site of the lesion, but only along the structure determined to be at fault since the shoulder is notorious for tender trigger points.

Through this scheme, a working diagnosis is established on which to base a treatment programme, with constant monitoring and reassessment. This approach is just one possible way of assessing the shoulder. Pellecchia et al (1996) looked at the intertester reliability of the Cyriax evaluation and showed it to be highly reliable in the assessment of patients with shoulder pain, facilitating the identification of diagnostic categories for subjects with shoulder pain.

However, the approach does not investigate hypermobility at the shoulder with consequent instability, and the reader is recommended to employ provocative instability tests as appropriate. In addition, specific impingement tests and tests for labral tears can be employed as necessary. The examination of neural structures can also be incorporated into the procedure.

CAPSULAR LESIONS

Capsular pattern at the glenohumeral joint
- Most limitation of lateral rotation.
- Less limitation of abduction.
- Least limitation of medial rotation.

The movements limited in the capsular pattern have a characteristic 'hard' end-feel, although this is less marked in the early stage, and any restriction of the glenohumeral range is usually consistent with an overall loss of shoulder elevation. The presence of the capsular pattern at the shoulder indicates arthritis. Commonly this is idiopathic, primary arthritis or traumatic or secondary arthritis. This is synonymous with frozen shoulder or adhesive capsulitis, as discussed below. Less commonly, the shoulder can be affected by degenerative osteoarthrosis, rheumatoid arthritis or any of the spondyloarthropathies.

'FROZEN SHOULDER' (ADHESIVE CAPSULITIS)

The term *frozen shoulder* is commonly used by the general public to describe any stiff or painful shoulder, but it is an overused term, much criticized, since it appears to avoid a more specific diagnosis. It is, however, an easy term to use and describes the signs and symptoms indicating involvement of the capsule of the shoulder joint, which is the key factor.

The natural history of the condition is that it follows a pattern of increasing signs and symptoms (freezing), followed by a plateau stage (frozen) before a slow, spontaneous recovery of partial or complete function (thawing). Recovery tends to occur within 1—3 years (Wadsworth 1986). A short painful period is associated with a short recovery period and a longer painful period with a longer period of recovery (Owens-Burkhart 1991).

Several authors have reviewed the history of the frozen shoulder (Wadsworth 1986, Owens-Burkhart 1991, Anton 1993). It was first described by Duplay in 1872 and Codman was responsible for using the term 'frozen shoulder' in 1934, but used it in association with rotator cuff tendinopathy. Neviaser introduced the concept of 'adhesive capsulitis' in 1945 because of the appearance of the thickened, adherent capsule that could be peeled from the bone like sticky plaster.

The cause of the condition is unknown. It is probably multifactorial, including a period of immobilization due to pain, and may include local periarticular inflammatory and degenerative changes. Association with other lesions has been reported, including cervical spine disorders, dysfunction of neural structures, thoracic spine immobility, thoracic surgery, trauma, neurological disease, reflex sympathetic dystrophy, cardiovascular disease, stroke, systemic disease, in particular diabetes mellitus, and the presence of immunological factors, e.g. human leukocyte antigen (HLA)-B27 (Jeracitano et al 1992, Anton 1993, Grubbs 1993, Stam 1994).

Pathology of frozen shoulder

In a review of the literature, various authors observed and reported the following changes seen at arthrography, arthroscopy and surgery (Wadsworth 1986, Owens-Burkhart 1991, Wiley 1991, Uhthoff & Sarkar 1992, Anton 1993, Grubbs 1993, Uitvlugt et al 1993, Stam 1994, Bunker & Anthony 1995, Bunker et al 2000, Smith et al 2001):

- Volumes of less than 10 ml, compared with the normal intra-articular volume, and a failure to fill the subscapularis bursa or biceps tendon sheath
- Inflammatory changes, adhesion formation, erythematous fibrinous pannus over the synovium and loss of the redundant axillary fold
- Fibrosis, not inflammation, with changes similar to those seen in Dupuytren's disease of the hand
- Retraction of the capsule away from the greater tuberosity, thickening of the coracohumeral ligament and subscapularis tendon and a loss of the normal interval between the glenoid and humeral head

Involvement of the joint capsule seems to be a common feature to all cases studied, but the above list shows that debate still continues over the nature of that involvement.

Frozen shoulder consists of a spontaneous onset of gradually increasing shoulder pain, referring to the deltoid region, and forearm if severe, with an increasing limitation of movement. Lundberg (1969) divided the syndrome into primary or secondary types:

- Primary frozen shoulder is idiopathic
- Secondary frozen shoulder occurs follows a precipitating cause

Causes of secondary frozen shoulder may include trauma or any condition which causes immobilization of the shoulder, e.g. neurological conditions, fracture and pain associated with bursitis or tendinopathy, thyroid disease, cardiac disease, thoracic surgery, pulmonary disease, diabetes mellitus, postmenopausal hormonal changes, or psychological factors such as depression, apathy and emotional stress (Owens-Burkhart 1991, Stam 1994, Siegel et al 1999).

The steroid-sensitive arthritis and traumatic arthritis described by Cyriax (1982) fit into the primary and secondary groups, respectively.

Primary frozen shoulder

Cyriax (1982) called this condition 'steroid-sensitive arthritis' or 'monoarticular rheumatoid arthritis'. The condition seems particularly resistant to physical treatment, but responds well to corticosteroid injection.

The patient's condition follows a typical pattern:

- The patient is usually between 40 and 70 years old
- Women are affected slightly more frequently than men
- There is no reason for the onset
- The condition progresses slowly to spontaneous recovery over 2–3 years
- Recurrence of the condition in the other shoulder within 2–5 years is common (Cyriax 1982)

Secondary frozen shoulder

This type of arthritis most frequently occurs secondary to trauma but the condition can be secondary to a number of conditions, some of which are listed above. A painful shoulder may be kept relatively immobile by involuntary muscle spasm, contributing to pain and stiffness, but the close proximity of other anatomical structures may also be relevant. The subacromial bursa, rotator cuff tendons and the long head of the biceps are all closely related to the capsule of the shoulder joint and it may be possible for changes in these structures to have a secondary effect on the capsule.

If precipitated by trauma, the incident may be minor and the initial pain usually settles. Therefore the patient may have difficulty recalling a traumatic incident or associating it with the onset of the pain. As a guideline, the condition can be classified into three stages, each of which gives an indication of the irritability of the lesion and a suggested programme of treatment. The three special questions taken from the history (see below) and the assessment of the degree of capsular pattern, together with the end-feel of the passive movements, provide reliable diagnostic criteria.

Stage 1

After the precipitating incident, the initial pain settles. Approximately 1 week later, pain develops and gradually increases. The pain is felt over the area of deltoid, but as inflammation increases, the pain is referred further into the C5 dermatome. The extent of reference of pain indicates the degree of severity of the condition. This stage develops over several weeks and pain is the key feature, not the limited movement.

Since the shoulder joint has a wide range of movement, the early developing capsular pattern may not affect function and the patient may be oblivious to the loss of movement at this stage. Diagnosis in this early stage is not easy but it becomes conclusive once the capsular pattern of limited movement occurs. If treated early enough, it may be possible to abort the progressive cycle of the condition. Unfortunately, as pain is the main feature of this stage and not loss of function, patients may not seek help for the condition early enough.

The examination of the patient provides a set of signs and symptoms that classifies the patient as a stage 1 capsulitis and indicates a possible line of treatment.

From the history the three special questions reveal that:

- The pain is usually above the elbow
- The pain is not usually constant
- The patient can usually sleep on that side at night

The objective examination shows that:

- A minor capsular pattern exists (this may involve lateral rotation only)
- The end-feel of passive movements remains relatively elastic, but is harder than the normal end-feel

The history and examination indicate a relatively non-irritable joint capsule that may respond to corticosteroid injection or Grade B mobilization. Of course, any mobilizing technique can be applied to such a joint and the treatment programme for each individual patient is formulated based on the therapist's experience. Orthopaedic medicine treatment techniques will be described below.

Stage 2   Pain and loss of function are now the key features of the condition. The capsular pattern has developed to affect abduction and medial rotation adversely, and, subjectively, the latter is the most inconvenient functional movement for the patient to lose. As the pain gradually peaks and spreads, the patient notices an inability to reach into a back pocket, for example, or do up a bra. The limitation of lateral rotation is apparent in that the patient is unable to comb the hair.

From the history the three special questions reveal that:

- The pain usually spreads beyond the elbow
- The pain is usually constant
- The patient usually cannot sleep on that side at night

The objective examination shows that:

- A full capsular pattern is present
- The characteristic 'hard' end-feel of arthritis exists due to involuntary muscle spasm and capsular contracture

The history and examination reveal an irritable joint capsule. The presence of the capsular pattern is marked and the accessory glenohumeral movements will also be lost. Adhesion formation in the axillary fold, tightness in the anterior capsular ligaments, shortening of subscapularis and contracture of the rotator interval combine to limit lateral rotation and abduction significantly, producing the capsular pattern. At this stage corticosteroid injection may be used to treat the pain and/or relatively gentle pain-free mobilization may be applied to restore accessory range. The orthopaedic medicine treatment techniques will be described below.

Stage 3   If the patient progresses through the complete cycle of the condition, this represents the stage of recovery. The pain is settling and receding and full functional movement is returning. However, the end result of the condition may leave the patient with a degree of pain and some limited movement, especially lateral rotation and full elevation. Shaffer et al (1992), in a long-term follow-up (average 7 years) of idiopathic frozen shoulder treated non-operatively, showed 50% of patients to have residual mild pain or stiffness of the shoulder, or both. Limitation of lateral rotation was present when restriction of movement was a feature.

Stage 3 shows similar signs and symptoms to stage 1 and the same treatment may be applied together with rehabilitation, including strengthening and stretching exercises, towards full function.

TREATMENT TECHNIQUES FOR FROZEN SHOULDER

There is no standard agreed treatment for frozen shoulder. Various approaches have been advocated, including analgesic drugs, corticosteroid injections, mobilization techniques and exercises of various forms, manipulation under anaesthetic, brisement (forcible breaking of adhesions) or distension arthrography, arthroscopic distension and surgical release of adhesions (Hsu & Chan 1991, Hulstyn & Weiss 1993, Sharma et al 1993, Ogilvie-Harris et al 1995). The aim of treatment in each of these measures, as in the use of orthopaedic medicine techniques, is to relieve pain and restore function.

For primary frozen shoulder, i.e. steroid-sensitive arthritis, Cyriax (1982) suggested a course of intra-articular injections of corticosteroids to treat the pain. These are given over increasing intervals and, with the relief of pain, a gradual increase in movement occurs with recovery to full function.

For secondary frozen shoulder, i.e. traumatic arthritis, the clinician has a choice of treatment dependent upon the stage of irritability and the techniques available. Those recommended in orthopaedic medicine will be described, but the reader is urged not to be limited to this choice, but to draw on experience of other mobilization techniques that can be incorporated to provide an individual treatment programme for each patient.

Injection of the glenohumeral joint (Cyriax & Cyriax 1983, Cyriax, 1984)

Suggested needle size: 21G × 1½ in (0.8 × 40 mm) or 2 in (0.8 × 50 mm) green needle

Dose: 20–30 mg triamcinolone acetonide in a total volume of 3–4 ml

Position the patient either comfortably in prone lying or sitting in a chair (Fig. 5.26). Place the affected arm to rest in medial rotation across the abdomen with the elbow flexed.

Stand behind the patient and place your thumb on the posterior angle of the acromion and your index or middle finger on the coracoid process. Insert the needle 1 cm below your thumb placed on the acromion and direct it forwards towards the index finger placed on the coracoid process (Fig. 5.27). Once the needle rests against the articular surface, deliver the injection as a bolus, withdrawing slightly if there is resistance.

Figure 5.26 Injection of the glenohumeral joint, sitting.

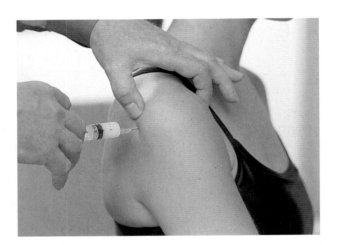

Figure 5.27 Injection of the glenohumeral joint, showing direction of approach and needle position.

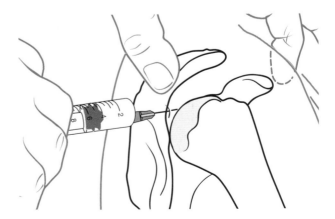

An explanation of the condition and prognosis is important. The principle is to give another injection if the pain begins to peak, which usually occurs at increasing intervals. Generally not more than three or four injections are given in total. The patient is instructed to apply relative rest for up to 2 weeks and then to begin pain-free mobilization. Injections of corticosteroid are efficacious in treating frozen shoulder providing the patients selected fulfill the diagnostic criteria based on Cyriax, described above in stages 1, 2 and 3 of the condition (Cameron 1995).

Jacobs et al (1991) looked at the effect of administrating intra-articular steroids with distension for the management of the early frozen shoulder. Fifty patients with frozen shoulder were divided into three treatment groups: a distension group only, a steroid group only and a steroid and distension group. A total of three injections were offered at 6-week intervals using the posterior approach described above. All patients were provided with an information sheet explaining capsulitis and a home exercise programme.

All patients entered into the study showed improvement during treatment, with a decreased need for analgesia and improvement in pain symptoms. A significantly increased rate of improvement in the range of passive abduction and forward flexion occurred in the two groups treated with intra-articular corticosteroid, indicating a positive role for the use of corticosteroids in the early frozen shoulder.

Grade B mobilization (Saunders 2000)

Grade B mobilization (see Ch. 4) is applied to the non-irritable joint only. The aim is to relieve pain and increase the range of movement. Heat may be used to assist the technique. The condition, prognosis and treatment are explained carefully to the patient since the recovery time may be prolonged over many months, or even years, and the patient must be encouraged to continue the stretching techniques at home, eventually taking over treatment, with the therapist remaining in a supervisory role for as long as necessary.

Position the patient comfortably in lying with the arm in as much elevation as possible (Fig. 5.28). Place a hand on the sternum or scapula to stabilize the thorax and the other hand over the patient's raised elbow to apply a stretch into elevation. The principles of Grade B mobilization are applied (see Ch. 4) and the arm is returned under some distraction for comfort (Fig. 5.29).

This technique is fairly aggressive and will cause a certain amount of post-treatment soreness. The pain may be aggravated for 2–4 hours and this should be explained to the patient. An increase in mobility is often reported before the reduction of pain but both are indications for continued treatment.

Figure 5.28 Grade B mobilization of the glenohumeral joint.

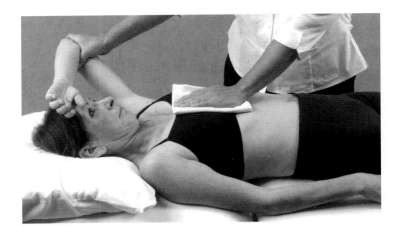

Figure 5.29 Returning the arm from the elevated position, with distraction for comfort.

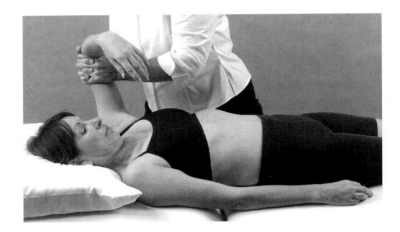

Distraction techniques

These are a form of Grade A mobilization since they occur within the pain-free range of movement. The aim is to restore the accessory range of movement to the joint. The techniques can be applied together with Grade B mobilization in the non-irritable joint or alone in the more irritable joint. Once accessory range returns in the irritable joint and the end-feel of the limited movements regains some elasticity, the joint is deemed to be non-irritable and techniques can be progressed, adding Grade B mobilization.

Lateral distraction (Cyriax & Cyriax 1983, Cyriax 1984)

Position the patient comfortably in supine lying close to the edge of the couch, which is raised to approximately hip height. Place a pillow under and around the arm to support it in the loose packed position of adduction and some medial rotation. Place a hand into the axilla to apply the lateral distraction while simultaneously applying counterpressure to the patient's elbow, resting against your hip (Fig. 5.30). The distraction is held for as long as possible and repeated often.

Figure 5.30   Lateral distraction.

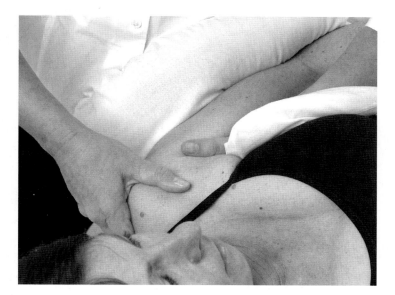

Caudal distraction

Position the patient as above. Hook your forearm into the crook of the patient's flexed elbow (Fig. 5.31). Apply sustained and repeated caudal distractions.

A 'seat belt' can be used to aid the distraction techniques, but the reader is referred to courses and texts on 'seat belt therapy' for the description of its use. Other mobilizing techniques can also be incorporated into this regime.

Figure 5.31   Caudal distraction.

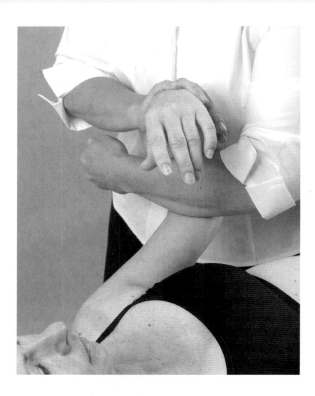

NON-CAPSULAR LESIONS

CHRONIC SUBACROMIAL BURSITIS (SYNONYMOUS WITH SUBDELTOID BURSITIS)

Chronic subacromial bursitis may be a relatively common cause of pain at the shoulder. However, it can present a challenge to diagnosis because of the muddled picture presented on examination. The bursa's intimate relationship with the capsule, the rotator cuff tendons and the biceps tendon makes it difficult to diagnose definitively and treatment response can help to confirm or refute diagnosis.

Furthermore, lesions can coexist, and a primary lesion can indirectly affect the structures closely related to it. In reviewing the anatomy it will be seen that the inner synovial aspect of the bursa is also the outer aspect of the rotator cuff, the supraspinatus tendon in particular. Therefore, they cannot be separated and a lesion of one may affect the other.

Prolonged inflammation can cause adhesion formation between the layers of the bursa and may produce a secondary frozen shoulder. In an unwell patient subacromial abscess or infective bursitis may be suspected (Ward & Eckardt 1993).

Chronic subacromial bursitis has a gradual onset of pain due to the microtrauma of overuse. Together with rotator cuff lesions, chronic bursitis is a common cause of pain in athletes using the arm in the overhead position, e.g. racket sports, throwing activities of all kinds, swimming, etc. Occasionally it can be directly caused by a fall on the outstretched hand or may be due to the congenital shape of the acromion process reducing the vertical height of the subacromial space and producing impingement. Altered joint mechanics, posture, incorrect or overtraining and muscle imbalances which affect the steering mechanism of the rotator cuff tendons are all factors which may contribute to chronic bursitis at the shoulder.

The patient complains of a low-grade ache over the insertion of deltoid and may not be able to sleep on that side at night. On examination there is a non-capsular pattern of movement, often with pain felt at the end of range of passive elevation. A painful arc may be present and various resisted tests may also produce the pain. The room in the subacromial space is minimal and impingement under the coracoacromial arch may inflame the bursa, producing a painful arc on movement.

The application of resisted tests produces some compression of the glenohumeral joint and subacromial space. This produces a characteristic muddle of signs associated with a bursitis. The pain may be on the application of resistance, on the release of resistance or may produce several positive signs, e.g. pain on resisted abduction, lateral rotation and elbow extension. The resisted tests may not be consistent and on reassessment of the patient a completely different set of resisted tests may be present.

Treatment, ideally, consists of an injection of a large volume of low-dose local anaesthetic together with an appropriate amount of corticosteroid.

Injection of chronic subacromial bursitis

Suggested needle size: 21G × 1½ in (0.8 × 40 mm) green needle
Dose: 20 mg triamcinolone acetonide in a total volume of 7 ml

---

Position the patient comfortably in sitting with the arm hanging by the side. Locate the lateral border of the acromion and insert the needle just below, at an oblique angle upwards with respect to the acromion (Fig. 5.32). According to Beals et al (1998), the bursa lies under the

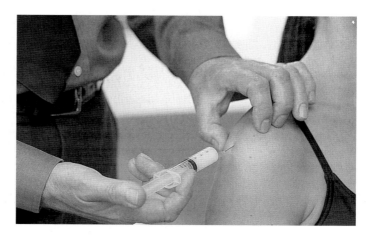

Figure 5.32 Injection of the subacromial bursa.

Figure 5.33   Injection of the subacromial bursa showing direction of approach and needle position.

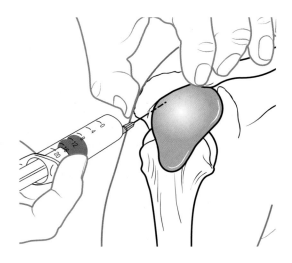

anterior half of the acromion, so accurate needle placement is important. Insert the needle and deliver the injection as a bolus, having detected the area, or areas, of less resistance (Fig. 5.33). The synovial folds and adhesions within the bursa may present a resistance to the injection and it may be necessary to deliver the injection by a series of withdrawals and reinsertions. The patient is advised to maintain a period of relative rest for approximately 2 weeks following injection.

As mentioned above, it may be difficult to distinguish chronic subacromial bursitis from chronic rotator cuff tendinopathy and injection into the subacromial space may be an appropriate choice of treatment when such a dilemma occurs.

Attention should be paid to the mechanism by which the bursa becomes involved, as described above. An explanation is given to the patient together with restoration of balanced forces, aiming to ensure normal shoulder movement and to avoid excessive superior translation.

ACUTE SUBACROMIAL BURSITIS

The existence of this condition as described by Cyriax 1983 and Cyriax & Cyriax 1993 is controversial and it may be the same as, or a similar to, a condition described by others as acute calcific tendinitis. The calcific deposit in the rotator cuff, usually supraspinatus, increases in size and ruptures into the subacromial bursa (Berg 1997). This provides a plausible explanation for the acute onset and intensity of the pain in the relatively short acute phase and its subsequent resolution over 7–10 days into the subacute phase, with the condition usually resolving in approximately 6 weeks. MRI scanning would confirm the presence of calcific deposits and/or inflammation in the subacromial space or overlying rotator cuff.

Acute subacromial bursitis is a completely separate entity from chronic subacromial bursitis, described above. It has a typical presentation of a rapid onset of pain for no apparent reason. The pain is felt in the shoulder area; it rapidly increases in severity and within hours the pain is referred into the whole C5 dermatome. The patient may look tired and unwell as the condition is very painful and disturbs sleep. Since the bursa is an extra-articular structure, it is not protected by involuntary muscle spasm. Voluntary muscle spasm is responsible for the patient holding the arm in an antalgic position and in the attempt to sleep, the patient loses the protective voluntary muscle spasm, waking with severe pain. Severe twinges of pain are experienced on attempted active movement, especially abduction, which compresses the painful bursa in the subacromial space.

On examination, a non-capsular pattern of limited movement is present. Voluntary muscle spasm is responsible for producing an empty end-feel on examination, where the examiner is aware that much more range is available but the patient will not tolerate further movement. Usually full lateral rotation can be coaxed, especially with a little distraction applied to the joint, but the range of abduction is severely limited by pain, indicating a non-capsular pattern. Swelling and tenderness may be present along the lateral border of the acromion.

The condition is self-limiting and is usually very much better within 7–10 days, clearing completely within 6 weeks, but prone to recurrence (Cyriax 1982). Treatment does not alter the course of the condition but should take the form of pain-relieving modalities and an explanation to the patient. The application of transcutaneous nerve stimulation and oral administration of analgesics are appropriate. Advice should also be given on sleeping position, suggesting that the arm should be well-supported by pillows, bandaged to the side or supported inside a tight-fitting tee shirt to maintain comfort when the protective muscle spasm is lost. A collar-and-cuff sling provides less support but may be used if the patient is unable to tolerate the compression of the previous suggestions.

An injection of corticosteroid is usually helpful, although it may increase the pain initially as the bursa is already swollen and very painful. The technique is the same as for chronic subacromial bursitis, but less volume is used.

Injection of acute subacromial bursitis

Suggested needle size: 21G × $1\frac{1}{2}$ in (0.8 × 40 mm) green needle
Dose: 20 mg triamcinolone acetonide in a total volume of 3 ml

---

ACROMIOCLAVICULAR JOINT

The pain from the acromioclavicular joint is characteristically felt in the epaulette region of the shoulder. The onset may be precipitated by trauma – either a fall on the outstretched hand or a direct blow such as a heavy fall against the wall while playing squash, in a rugby tackle or at touchdown.

On examination, a non-capsular pattern of glenohumeral movement is present with pain felt at extremes of passive elevation, lateral and medial rotation; the acromioclavicular joint itself does not display a capsular pattern as such. The diagnosis is confirmed by a positive scarf test reproducing the pain by compressing and shearing the joint.

Degenerative osteoarthrosis affects the acromioclavicular joint, especially in those who have been extremely active in sport (Stenlund 1993). Overuse can provoke a traumatic arthritis of the degenerate joint. The degenerative changes cause narrowing and osteophyte formation, which can have a secondary effect on the structures in the subacromial space.

Allman classified injuries of the acromioclavicular joint into three categories (Cailliet 1991, Hartley 1995):

- *Type I* injury is sprain or partial tearing of the capsuloligamentous fibres with local pain and tenderness and no joint instability.
- *Type II* injury involves tearing of capsuloligamentous fibres and minor subluxation, but as the coracoclavicular ligament remains intact, there is no instability.
- *Type III* injury is dislocation of the acromioclavicular joint with disruption of the capsule and the coracoclavicular ligament. Treatment for type III injury is usually surgery.

Orthopaedic medicine treatment may be useful in type I and II lesions. Corticosteroid injection of the joint may be curative or, if the superior aspect of the capsular ligament is involved, it may be treated with transverse frictions.

Injection of the acromioclavicular joint (Cyriax & Cyriax 1983, Cyriax, 1984)

Suggested needle size: 23G × 1 in (0.6 × 25 mm) blue needle or 25G × $\frac{5}{8}$ in (0.5 × 16 mm) orange needle
Dose: 10 mg triamcinolone acetonide in a total volume of 0.5 ml

---

Position the patient comfortably in sitting or half-lying and palpate the superior aspect of the joint line (Fig. 5.34). There is considerable variation in the size, shape and direction of the joint surfaces and if the joint is narrowed by degenerative changes it may be difficult to enter. The needle may have to be angled obliquely inferomedially and the presence of the articular disc may make entry difficult. Insert the needle into the joint and deliver the injection as a bolus, or pepper the superior ligament if needle entry proves to be difficult (Fig. 5.35). The patient is advised to maintain a period of relative rest for approximately 2 weeks following injection.

Figure 5.34 Injection of the acromioclavicular joint.

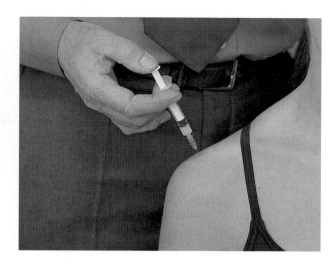

Figure 5. 35 Injection of the acromioclavicular joint showing direction of approach and needle position.

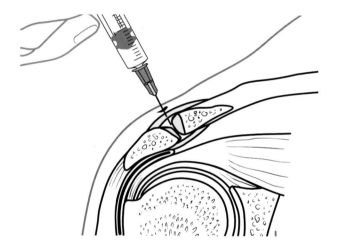

Transverse frictions to the superior acromioclavicular capsular ligament (Cyriax & Cyriax 1983, Cyriax, 1984)

Stand behind the seated patient and palpate the joint line. Using an index finger reinforced by a middle finger, thumb-down on the scapula for counterpressure, direct the pressure down on to the tender ligament and impart the transverse frictions in an anteroposterior direction. The grade of application will depend on the irritability of the lesion (Fig. 5.36).

Other mobilization techniques can be incorporated into the treatment regime for acromioclavicular strain and management may include strapping or taping the joint, particularly if the injury is type II.

Figure 5.36   Transverse frictions to the acromioclavicular joint.

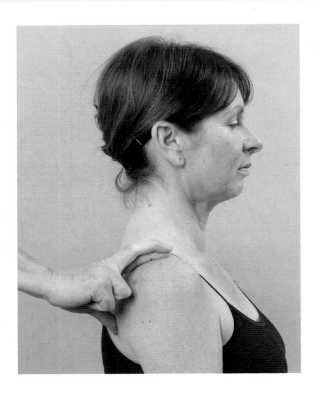

CONTRACTILE LESIONS

The more common contractile lesions at the shoulder involve the rotator cuff tendons, particularly supraspinatus. Rotator cuff lesions can vary from simple tendinopathy to degeneration and partial or complete thickness tears. The lesion may be secondary to subacromial impingement and may also involve the subacromial bursa and tendon of the long head of the biceps, which all lie in very close proximity. Tendinopathy may lead to secondary capsulitis through abnormal movement patterns due to pain.

Tendinopathy occurs from the cumulative effects of microtrauma which has a gradual onset, usually due to overuse. Single traumatic incidents may produce tendinopathy but this is unusual, and the effect of trauma in this case is more likely to cause tearing of an already degenerate tendon. Pain is localized to the deltoid area and, although the patient may be aware of a vague ache, the pain is considerably increased by use and movements such as reaching, pushing and pulling, in particular those activities associated with using the hands above shoulder level.

On examination, pain is reproduced on the appropriate resisted test and there may be localizing signs of a painful arc and/or positive scarf test. Resisted abduction may implicate supraspinatus, resisted lateral rotation may implicate infraspinatus and teres minor and resisted medial rotation may implicate subscapularis. However, as discussed above, the tendons interdigitate and insert to form a tendinous cuff, therefore it may not be possible to make a definitive diagnosis. Two or more resisted tests may be positive and subsequent palpation will determine the site of the lesion. Passive movements should be of full range with a normal end-feel, but occasionally the opposite passive movement or end-range passive elevation reproduces the pain by stretching or compressing the tendinous insertion respectively. A further complication may be a secondary capsulitis, in which case a capsular pattern will be superimposed on the non-capsular pattern described above.

Early onset of tendinopathy may respond to conservative treatment and corticosteroid injection or transverse frictions may be successful. However, tendinopathy involves focal degenerative changes within the tendon leading to partial or full thickness tears; further complications may include involvement of the nearby subacromial bursa or biceps tendon, or involve subtle instability or lesions of the glenoid labrum.

'Impingement syndrome' is a generic term for rotator cuff lesions encompassing all stages of tendon disease. Impingement may be due to subacromial space stenosis, inflammation and/or fibrosis of the contents of the space. Anatomical anomalies, particularly type III hook-shaped acromions or congenital subacromial stenosis, may predispose to impingement syndrome (Farley et al 1994, Frieman et al 1994, Burkhart 1995).

Microtrauma of the cuff tendons may interfere with their stabilizing function, allowing the humeral head to ride higher in the glenoid and further reducing the subacromial space. Impingement may be associated with shoulder instability, degenerative changes in the acromioclavicular joint, osteophyte formation, degenerative spur formation under the acromion and thickening of the coracoacromial ligament.

The rotator cuff, especially supraspinatus, maintains the subacromial space by depressing the head of the humerus to prevent superior translation during abduction and elevation movements. Repetitive use, fatigue or overload results in cumulative microtrauma, and the cuff muscles are unable to resist this superior translation, leading to subtle instability (Copeland 1993).

Patients under 35 years, particularly athletes using the arm in the overhead position (e.g. swimming, tennis, squash, javelin, golf), in which large ranges of movement, forces, acceleration and repetitive movements are involved, may present with signs of impingement. This may be secondary to minor instability, possibly involving labral tears (Copeland 1993, Jobe & Pink 1993, 1994). Subtle or subclinical subluxation reduces the maximum congruency of the glenoid and it appears that the supraspinatus and infraspinatus tendons are pinched in the posterosuperior labrum. The combination of instability, impingement and rotator cuff lesions should be considered in the younger athlete and the management directed at improving movement patterns to correct the instability (Iannotti 1994).

In patients over 35 years, changes occur in the subacromial space which are related to degeneration and the ageing process. Fatigue and degeneration of fibres may produce muscle imbalances which lead to altered neuromuscular control and abnormal movement patterns. The humeral head is no longer effectively depressed and superior translation occurs, compromising the subacromial space (Copeland 1993, Wilk & Arrigo 1993, Greenfield et al 1995).

The impingement syndrome involves inflammation and oedema in the subacromial bursa in the first instance, and secondary thickening and fibrosis is followed by partial or full tears of the rotator cuff. The tears are usually longitudinal and on the undersurface of the tendons, which may be relatively avascular compared with the bursal surface (Cailliet 1991, Uhthoff & Sarkar 1992, Copeland 1993, Fukuda et al 1994, McCann & Bigliani 1994). Early tendon lesions may involve intrasubstance tears and calcific deposits can occur within the substance of the tendon (Meister & Andrews 1993).

Neer (1983) was responsible for classifying the impingement syndrome into three progressive stages and provided additional evidence that impingement occurs against the anterior edge and undersurface of the anterior third of the acromion and the coracoacromial ligament; sometimes the acromioclavicular joint is involved but not the lateral edge of the acromion:

- *Stage I* impingement involves oedema and haemorrhage, characteristically seen in younger patients. Conservative treatment at this stage usually has good results and can reverse the condition
- *Stage II* follows repeated episodes of mechanical inflammation and the subacromial bursa may become thickened and fibrotic. This stage occurs in older patients and the shoulder functions well for light use but becomes symptomatic after overuse, particularly in the overhead position. Neer recommends conservative management, with surgery only considered if the condition fails to respond to treatment after an 18-month period
- *Stage III* involves incomplete or complete tears of the rotator cuff, biceps lesions and bone alteration of the anterior acromion and greater tuberosity. These are found almost exclusively in the over-40 age group, with tears of supraspinatus occurring in a ratio of 7:1 over biceps. Stage III lesions are referred for surgical opinion. Neer also states that in his experience, 95% of tears of the cuff are initiated by impingement wear rather than circulatory impairment or trauma, although trauma may enlarge an existing tear

Dalton (1994) reported that an area of hypovascularity in supraspinatus, 1 cm from its insertion, has been both proposed and disputed. A critical zone of vascular ischaemia has been proposed, existing between the supraspinatus tendon and the coracohumeral ligament, where degeneration and tears usually occur (Cailliet 1991). The critical zone is said to vary from being ischaemic when the vascular anastomosis is constricted, to hyperaemic when it is allowed to flow freely. The vessels are elongated when the arm is hanging by the side and compressed when the rotator cuff tendons contract to produce movement, both potentially causing relative ischaemia. Hyperaemia is said to occur only when the arm is passively supported at rest.

Clark & Harryman (1992), however, studied cadaver shoulders aged between 17 and 70 years and found no avascular area in supraspinatus. The blood vessels in the deeper tendon layers were found to be small compared with those in the superficial layers. There was no associated evidence of degeneration and the authors concluded that the blood supply was adequate for the metabolic needs of the tissue.

The aim of treatment for rotator cuff tendinopathy is to relieve pain and to restore full functional movement to the shoulder, the resisted tests often proving weak and painful. This weakness may be due to tears or muscle inhibition due to pain. The cause of the lesion should be determined and factors such as instability and muscle imbalance should be addressed, with the rehabilitation of movement patterns to ensure restoration of the dynamic stabilizing function of the rotator cuff. Excessive superior and anterior translation should be prevented, to avoid the long-term complications of impingement which may eventually lead to surgery.

SUPRASPINATUS TENDINOPATHY

A lesion in supraspinatus produces pain on resisted abduction. Weakness may also be present and it is difficult to be certain whether this is due to muscle inhibition because of the pain, or partial or full thickness tears of the tendon. A painful arc or pain at the end of range of passive elevation localizes the lesion to the distal end of the tendon, usually at the teno-osseous junction. If pain is produced on resisted abduction only, without this localizing sign, the lesion is probably at the musculotendinous junction. Either way, palpation will confirm the exact site of the lesion.

Currently the whole question of tendinopathy is under debate with inflammation disputed as a component of the problem and degeneration of the tendon proposed as the cause. This leads to questions being asked of the prognosis for the patient. An inflammatory problem is expected to resolve with treatment in up to approximately 3 weeks; a degenerative problem will take much longer (see discussion in Ch. 4). Furthermore, if the pathology of rotator cuff tendinopathy is degenerative, more questions are raised, such as why corticosteroid injection relieves pain. At the time of going to press this debate is current and the reader is advised to keep abreast of the research and to make judgements about treatment programmes in line with the best available evidence.

The following treatment techniques of injection and transverse frictions may be successful, but they do not stand alone and should be incorporated into a holistic treatment programme in which all components of the patient's problem are addressed, including eliminating the possible cause. Injection of the individual tendons may be appropriate, as discussed below, but there is growing controversy on whether this could contribute to degenerative change, leading to tendon rupture, although the current evidence does not support this. Controversy also surrounds the inflammatory model of tendinitis and therefore the appropriateness of anti-inflammatory treatments such as corticosteroid injection. Khan & Cook (2000) acknowledge that clinical experience and some studies show that corticosteroid injection produces short-term relief of pain in these lesions although the mechanisms for this pain relief are currently not known. A generic injection into the subacromial bursa may be more appropriate, particularly if impingement of the degenerate tendons produces inflammation in the subacromial space. It is up to clinicians to make that judgement based on current best practice and having also ascertained the views of their local orthopaedic consultants.

Injection of the teno–osseous junction of supraspinatus (Cyriax & Cyriax 1983, Cyriax 1984)

Suggested needle size: 25G $\times \frac{5}{8}$ in (0.5 × 16 mm) orange needle or 23G × 1 in (0.6 × 25 mm) blue needle
Dose: 10 mg triamcinolone acetonide in a total volume of 1 ml

Position the patient in sitting at an angle of 45°, medially rotating the shoulder and placing the arm behind the back to expose the tendon insertion (Fig. 5.37). Insert the needle perpendicular to the teno-osseous junction and deliver the injection using a peppering technique (Fig. 5.38). The patient is advised to maintain a period of relative rest for approximately 2 weeks following injection.

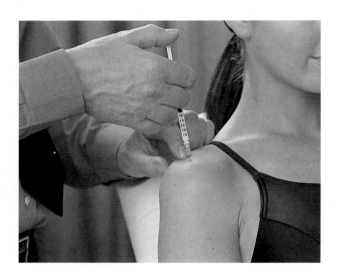

Figure 5.37   Injection of the supraspinatus tendon.

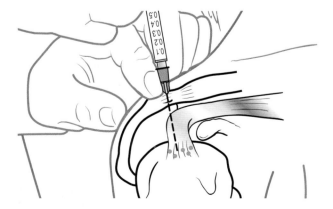

Figure 5.38   Injection of the supraspinatus tendon showing direction of approach and needle position.

Transverse frictions to supraspinatus (Cyriax & Cyriax 1983, Cyriax 1984)

Teno-osseous junction

Position the patient as above. Stand at the side of the patient and identify the area of tenderness. Place an index finger, reinforced by the middle finger onto the tendon and direct the pressure down onto the insertion (Fig. 5.39). Deliver the frictions transversely across the fibres, keeping the index finger parallel to the anterior edge of the acromion process. The supraspinatus tendon is approximately one finger wide (1 cm). Maintain the technique for 10 min after the analgesic effect has been achieved. Relative rest is advised where functional movements may continue, but no overuse or stretching until pain-free on resisted testing.

Musculotendinous junction of supraspinatus

Position the patient in sitting with the painful shoulder abducted to 90° and supported comfortably on the couch. Stand on the opposite side of the patient but facing forwards with your arm straight across and behind the patient's shoulders. Locate the musculotendinous junction in the 'V' created by the clavicle and the acromion process (Fig. 5.40). Using the middle finger reinforced by the index finger, direct the pressure down onto the tendon and deliver the transverse frictions by rotating the forearm for 10 min after the analgesic effect has been achieved. Relative rest is advised where functional movements may continue, but no overuse or stretching until pain-free on resisted testing.

Figure 5.39 Transverse frictions to the supraspinatus tendon, teno-osseous site.

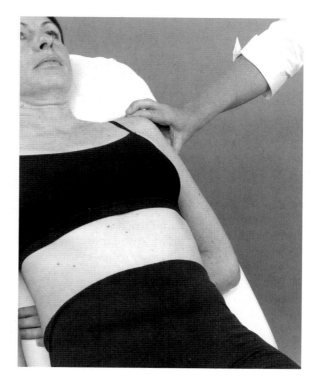

Figure 5.40 Transverse frictions to the supraspinatus tendon, musculotendinous junction.

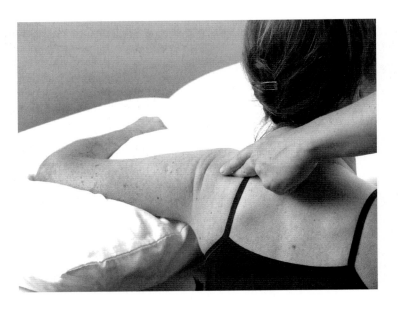

INFRASPINATUS TENDINOPATHY (+/– TERES MINOR)

A lesion in infraspinatus and teres minor produces pain on resisted lateral rotation. A painful arc and pain at the end of range of passive elevation indicate that the lesion lies at the distal end of the tendon, usually at the teno-osseous junction. If no arc is present the lesion is often a little further proximally in the body of the tendon. Palpation will confirm the exact site of the lesion.

> **Injection of the teno-osseous junction of infraspinatus** (Cyriax & Cyriax 1983, Cyriax 1984)
>
> Suggested needle size: 23G × 1 in (0.6 × 25 mm) or 23G × 1¼ in (0.6 × 30 mm) blue needle or 21G × 1½ in (0.8 × 40 mm) green needle
> Dose: 10 mg triamcinolone acetonide in a total volume of 1 ml

Position the patient in prone lying propped up on the elbows. Laterally rotate and adduct the affected arm to expose the greater tuberosity. Locate the area of tenderness over the greater tuberosity, which now lies approximately two fingers width below to the posterior angle of the acromion (Fig. 5.41). Insert the needle and deliver the injection by a peppering technique to the whole extent of the lesion, which may be up to 2–3 cm wide (Fig. 5.42). The patient is advised to maintain a period of relative rest for approximately 2 weeks following injection. The above position may be impossible or uncomfortable for the patient to maintain. An adapted position is described below for the transverse frictions.

Figure 5.41   Injection of the infraspinatus tendon.

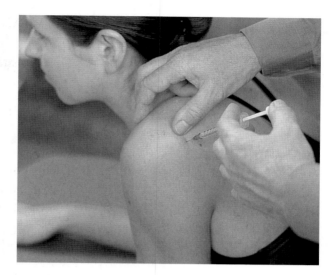

Figure 5.42   Injection of the supraspinatus tendon showing direction of approach and needle position.

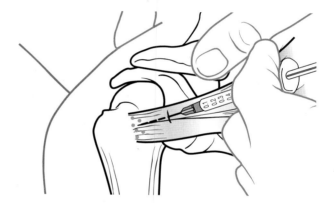

Transverse frictions to infraspinatus (Cyriax & Cyriax 1983, Cyriax 1984)

Position the patient as above, (Fig. 5.43) or, alternatively, place the patient in side lying and recreate the position described above, i.e. shoulder and elbow flexed to 90°, shoulder laterally rotated and adducted. Locate the area of tenderness and place a thumb on the area parallel to the direction of the tendon fibres; reinforce this with the other thumb (Fig. 5.44).

Standing back to apply body weight, press down onto the tendon and deliver a transverse sweep across the fibres, aiming to touch the posterior angle of the acromion with each stroke. The infraspinatus is two fingers (2 cm) wide; if teres minor is involved, the sweep should cover a width of three fingers (3 cm). Ten minutes' friction is delivered after achieving the analgesic effect. Relative rest is advised where functional movements may continue, but no overuse or stretching until pain-free on resisted testing.

Figure 5.43 Transverse frictions to the infraspinatus tendon.

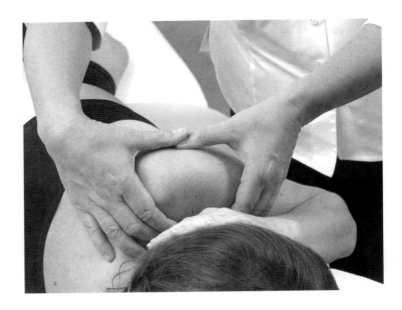

Figure 5.44 Alternative position for transverse friction massage of the infraspinatus tendon.

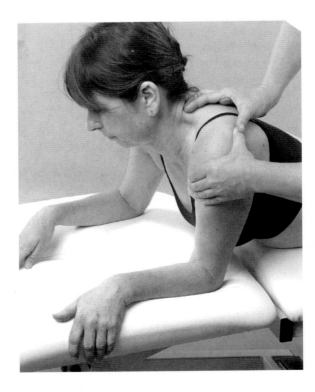

If the lesion lies in the body of the tendon, the technique for transverse frictions is the same, but applied a little more proximally at the site of the lesion, identified by palpation.

SUBSCAPULARIS TENDINOPATHY

A lesion in subscapularis produces pain on resisted medial rotation. A painful arc indicates a lesion in the upper fibres; a positive scarf test indicates a lesion in the lower fibres. Palpation will confirm the exact site of the lesion, which may cover a large area of tendon, i.e. approximately three fingers (3 cm) wide.

> **Injection of subscapularis** (Cyriax & Cyriax, 1983, Cyriax 1984)
>
> Suggested needle size: 23G × 1 in (0.6 × 25 mm) or 23G × 1¼ in (0.6 × 30 mm) blue needle
> Dose: 10 mg triamcinolone acetonide in a total volume of 1 ml

Position the patient in sitting with the arm supported to allow the humerus to rest in the anatomical position (Fig. 5.45). Locate the lesser tuberosity and deliver the injection by peppering technique to the full width of the lesion at the insertion onto the lesser tuberosity (Fig. 5.46).

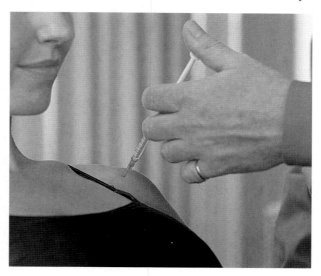

Figure 5.45   Injection of the subscapularis tendon.

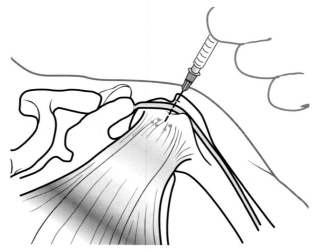

Figure 5.46   Injection of the subscapularis tendon showing direction of approach and needle position.

The patient is advised to maintain a period of relative rest for approximately 2 weeks following injection.

Transverse frictions to subscapularis (Cyriax & Cyriax 1983, Cyriax 1984)

Position the patient as above and locate the area of tenderness (upper fibres, lower fibres or both) on the medial aspect of the lesser tuberosity (Fig. 5.47). Place the thumb perpendicular to the direction of the fibres, parallel to the shaft of the humerus and directed laterally; deliver the transverse frictions in a superoinferior direction transversely across the fibres. The subscapularis tendon is approximately three fingers wide (3 cm). If the full width of the tendon is affected it may be necessary to divide the area into two sites for treatment as it is difficult to friction across the entire structure and a blister may be raised. Ten minutes' transverse frictions are delivered after the analgesic effect is achieved. Relative rest is advised where functional movements may continue, but no overuse or stretching until pain-free on resisted testing. The therapist's position can be varied to give better access to the tendon (Fig. 5.48).

Figure 5.47   Transverse frictions to the subscapularis tendon.

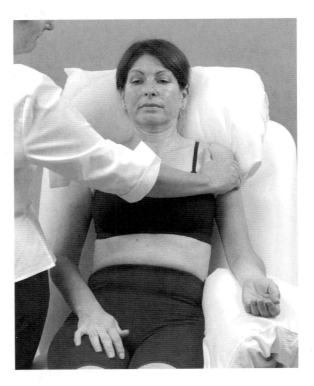

Figure 5.48   (a, b) Alternative
positions for transverse
frictions to the subscapularis
tendon.

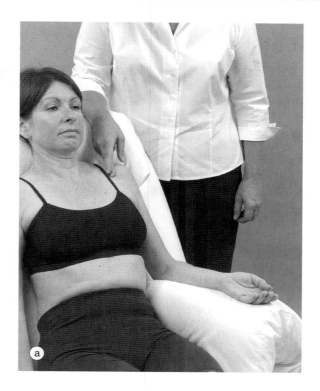

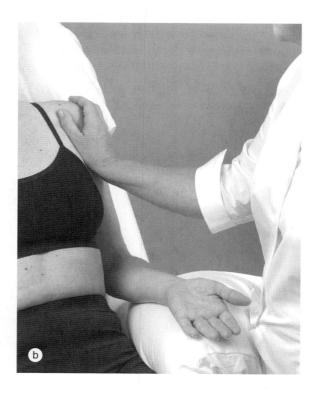

TENDINOPATHY OF THE LONG HEAD OF THE BICEPS

In its position in the subacromial space, the tendon of the long head of biceps may be involved in an impingement syndrome. It will produce pain felt at the shoulder on resisted elbow flexion. With the former lesion, a painful arc is usually present on forwards flexion of the shoulder with a straight arm and the palm uppermost.

Injection of the long head of the biceps in the bicipital groove

Suggested needle size: 23G × 1 in (0.6 × 25 mm) or 23G × 1$\frac{1}{4}$ in (0.6 × 30 mm) blue needle
Dose: 10 mg triamcinolone acetonide in a total volume of 1 ml

---

Position the patient in sitting with the arm supported so that the humerus rests in the anatomical position (Fig. 5.49). Locate the bicipital groove and slide the needle in parallel to the groove (Fig. 5.50). Deliver the injection by a bolus technique alongside the tendon. The patient is advised to maintain a period of relative rest for approximately 2 weeks following injection.

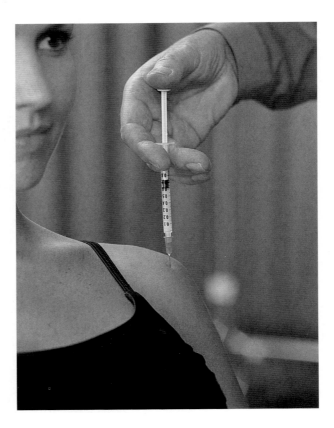

Figure 5.49   Injection of the long head of biceps tendon

Clarnette R G, Miniaci A 1998 Clinical examination of the shoulder. Medicine and Science in Sports and Exercise 30(4Suppl.):S1–6

Cooper D E, O'Brien S J, Warren R F 1993 Supporting layers of the glenohumeral joint: an anatomic study. Clinical Orthopaedics and Related Research 289:144–155

Copeland S 1993 Throwing injuries of the shoulder. British Journal of Sports Medicine 27:221–227

Cyriax J 1982 Textbook of orthopaedic medicine, 8th edn. Baillière Tindall, London, vol 1

Cyriax 1983?

Cyriax J 1984 Textbook of orthopaedic medicine, 11th edn. Baillière Tindall, London, vol 2

Cyriax J, Cyriax P 1983 Illustrated manual of orthopaedic medicine. Butterworths, London

Cyriax & Cyriax 1993?

Dalton S E 1994 The conservative management of rotator cuff disorders. British Journal of Rheumatology 33:663–667

Farley T E, Neumann C H, Steinbach L S et al 1994 The coracoacromial arch – MR evaluation and correlation with rotator cuff pathology. Skeletal Radiology 23:641–645

Flatow E L, Soslowsky L J, Ticker J B et al 1994 Excursion of the rotator cuff under the acromion. American Journal of Sports Medicine 22:779–788

Frame M K 1991 Anatomy and biomechanics of the shoulder. In: Donatelli R A (ed) Clinics in physical therapy, physical therapy of the shoulder. Churchill Livingstone, Edinburgh, p 1–18

Frieman B G, Albert T J, Fenlin J M 1994 Rotator cuff disease – a review of diagnosis, pathophysiology and current trends in treatment. Archives of Physical Medicine and Rehabilitation 75:604–609

Fukuda H, Hamada K, Nakajima T et al 1994 Pathology and pathogenesis of the intratendinous tearing of the rotator cuff viewed from en bloc histologic sections. Clinical Orthopaedics and Related Research 304:60–67

Greenfield B, Catlin P A, Coats P W et al 1995 Posture in patients with shoulder overuse injuries in healthy individuals. Journal of Orthopaedic and Sports Physical Therapy 21:287–295

Grubbs N 1993 Frozen shoulder syndrome – a review of the literature. Journal of Orthopaedic and Sports Physical Therapy 18:479–487

Halder A M, An K-N 2000 Anatomy and biomechanics of the shoulder. Orthopaedic Clinics of North America 31(2):159–176

Hartley A 1995 Practical joint assessment, upper quadrant, 2nd edn. Mosby, London

Hollingworth G R, Ellis R, Hattersley T S 1983 Comparison of injection techniques for shoulder pain – results of a double blind, randomized study. British Medical Journal 287:1339–1341

Hsu S Y C, Chan K M 1991 Arthroscopic distension in the management of frozen shoulder. International Orthopaedics 15:79–83

Hulstyn M J, Fadale P D 1995 Arthroscopic anatomy of the shoulder. Orthopaedic Clinics of North America 26:597–612

Hulstyn M J, Weiss A 1993 Adhesive capsulitis of the shoulder. Orthopaedic Review 22:425–433

Iannotti J P 1994 Evaluation of the painful shoulder. Journal of Hand Therapy 7:77–83

Itoi E, Newman S R, Kuechle D K et al 1994 Dynamic anterior stabilizers of the shoulder with the arm in abduction. Journal of Bone and Joint Surgery 76B:834–836

Jacobs L G H, Barton M A J, Wallace W A et al 1991 Intra-articular distension and steroids in the management of capsulitis of the shoulder. British Medical Journal 302:1498–1501

Jeracitano D, Cooper R, Lyon L J et al 1992 Abnormal temperature control suggesting sympathetic dysfunction in the shoulder skin of patients with frozen shoulder. British Journal of Rheumatology 31:539–542

Jobe F W, Pink M 1993 Classification and treatment of shoulder dysfunction in the overhead athlete. Journal of Orthopaedic and Sports Physical Therapy 18:427–432

Jobe F W, Pink M 1994 The athlete's shoulder. Journal of Hand Therapy 7:107–110

Jost B, Koch P, Gerber C 2000 Anatomy and functional aspects of the rotator interval. Journal of Shoulder and Elbow Surgery 9(4):336–341

Kapandji I A 1982 The physiology of the joints, upper limb, 5th edn. Churchill Livingstone, Edinburgh

Khan K M, Cook J L 2000 Overuse tendon injuries: where does the pain come from? Sports Medicine and Arthroscopic Review 8:17–31

Lundberg B J 1969 The frozen shoulder. Acta Orthopaedica Scandinavica. Supplementum 119:1–59

McCann P D, Bigliani L U 1994 Shoulder pain in tennis players. Sports Medicine 17:53–64

Meister K, Andrews J R 1993 Classification and treatment of rotator cuff injuries in the overhead athlete. Journal of Orthopaedic and Sports Physical Therapy 18:413–421

Neer C S 1983 Impingement lesions. Clinical Orthopaedics and Related Research 173:70–77

Netter F H 1987 Musculoskeletal system part I. Ciba Collection of Medical Illustrations, vol 8. Ciba-Giegy, New Jersey

Nordin M, Frankel V H 2001 Basic biomechanics of the musculoskeletal system, 3rd edn. Lippincott, Williams & Wilkins, Philadelphia

Ogilvie-Harris D J, Biggs D J, Fistsialos D P et al 1995 The resistant frozen shoulder: manipulation versus arthroscopic release. Clinical Orthopaedics and Related Research 319:238–248

Owens-Burkhart H 1991 Management of frozen shoulder. In: Donatelli R A (ed) Clinics in physical therapy, physical therapy of the shoulder. Churchill Livingstone, Edinburgh, p 91–116

Paine R M, Voight M 1993 The role of the scapula. Journal of Orthopaedic and Sports Physical Therapy 18:386–391

Palastanga N, Field D, Soames R 2002 Anatomy and human movement, 4th edn. Butterworth Heinemann, Oxford

Pellecchia G L, Paolino J, Connell J 1996 Intertester reliability of the Cyriax evaluation in assessing patients with shoulder pain. Journal of Orthopaedic and Sports Physical Therapy 23:34–38

Petersilge C A, Witte D H, Sewell B O et al 1997 Normal regional anatomy of the shoulder. MRI Clinics of North America 5(4):667–680

Pratt N E 1994 Anatomy and biomechanics of the shoulder. Journal of Hand Therapy 7:65–76

Schulte K R, Warner J J P 1995 Uncommon causes of shoulder pain in the athlete. Orthopaedic Clinics of North America 26:505–528

Shaffer B, Tibone J E, Kerlan R K 1992 Frozen shoulder – a long term follow-up. Journal of Bone and Hand Surgery 74A:738–746

Sharma R K, Bajekal R A, Bhan S 1993 Frozen shoulder syndrome. International Orthopaedics 17:275–278

Siegel L B, Cohen N J, Gall E P 1999 Adhesive capsulitis: a sticky issue. American Academy of Family Physician 59(1):1843–1852

Smith S P, Devaraj V S, Bunker T D 2001 The association between frozen shoulder and Dupuytren's disease. Journal of Shoulder and Elbow Surgery 10(2):149–151

Speer K P 1995 Anatomy and pathomechanics of shoulder instability. Clinics in Sports Medicine 14:751–760

Stam H W 1994 Frozen shoulder – a review of current concepts. Physiotherapy 80:588–598

Stenlund B 1993 Shoulder tendinitis and osteoarthrosis of the acromioclavicular joint and their relation to sports. British Journal of Sports Medicine 27:125–130

Uhthoff K J, Sarkar K 1992 Periarticular soft tissue conditions causing pain in the shoulder. Current Opinion in Rheumatology 4:241–246

Uitvlugt G, Detrisac D A, Johnson L J et al 1993 Arthroscopic observations before and after manipulation of frozen shoulder. Journal of Arthroscopic and Related Surgery 9:181–185

Wadsworth C T 1986 Frozen shoulder. Physical Therapy 66:1878–1883

Ward W G, Eckardt J J 1993 Subacromial/subdeltoid bursa abscesses, an overlooked diagnosis. Clinical Orthopaedics and Related Research 288:189–194

Wiley A M 1991 Arthroscopic appearance of frozen shoulder. Journal of Arthroscopic and Related Surgery 7:138–143

Wilk K E, Arrigo C 1993 Current concepts in the rehabilitation of the athletic shoulder. Journal of Orthopaedic and Sports Physical Therapy 18:365–378

Williams P L 1998 Gray's Anatomy: the anatomical basis of medicine and surgery, 38th edn. Churchill Livingstone, Edinburgh

Chapter 6

The elbow

SUMMARY

Tennis elbow is the most commonly encountered elbow problem in clinical practice and probably presents the greatest challenge. This chapter suggests an approach to its management, as well as addressing other common and more unusual lesions.

To aid diagnosis and accurate treatment, the chapter begins by outlining the relevant anatomy and provides guidelines for palpation. A commentary on the history and objective sequence follows, leading to discussion of the lesions which may be encountered, with suggestions for their effective treatment and management.

ANATOMY

INERT STRUCTURES

Together with the shoulder, the elbow functions to position the hand in space. Anatomically the elbow consists of two articulations, the elbow joint proper and the superior radioulnar joint, both contained within the same joint capsule.

The *elbow joint* proper is a synovial hinge joint between the distal end of the humerus, comprising the capitulum and trochlea, and the proximal ends of the radius and ulna. The articular capsule surrounds the articular margins, originating anteriorly around the coronoid and radial fossae of the humerus and inserting into the annular ligament and anterior border of the coronoid of the ulna. Posteriorly it attaches to the olecranon fossa of the humerus and the olecranon of the ulna.

In common with other synovial hinge joints, the relatively weak articular capsule is reinforced by strong collateral ligaments. The medial collateral ligament fans out from the medial epicondyle, where it is closely related to the common flexor tendon and primarily resists valgus stresses. The lateral collateral ligament is a strong triangular band fanning out from the lateral epicondyle, where it underlies and shares a close anatomical relationship with the common extensor tendon. It runs onto blend with the annular ligament below. The radial collateral ligament stabilizes the radial head, preventing varus stresses, and the annular ligament stabilizes the superior radioulnar joint. The elbow joint has two axes of motion and thus a greater inherent stability than the shoulder (Miyasaka 1999).

The *capitulum* is roughly hemispherical in shape and articulates with the radial head. The *trochlea* is pulley- or spool-shaped and extends from the anterior aspect of the distal end of the humerus to the olecranon fossa posteriorly. Its prominent medial ridge provides a valgus tilt which contributes to the carrying angle of the elbow joint. It articulates with the trochlear notch of the ulna.

On the distal, anterior surface of the humerus sit the radial and coronoid fossae, accommodating the rims of the radial head and coronoid process of ulna in full flexion. The olecranon fossa of the humerus accepts the olecranon process of the ulna in full extension. The proximal end of the radius consists of a head, neck and tuberosity. The radial head is cup-shaped superiorly for articulation with the capitulum. The periphery of the head is an articulating surface for the superior radioulnar joint, articulating with the inner surface of the annular ligament. The *radial tuberosity* gives insertion to the biceps tendon.

At the proximal end of the ulna is the massive, hook-shaped *olecranon process*. Anteriorly, the coronoid process arises with the radial notch on its medial side for articulation with the radius at the superior radioulnar joint. The elbow joint itself permits flexion and extension coupled with a small amount of adjunct rotation (Williams 1998). About 160° of passive flexion exists as the bones become almost parallel and the radial and coronoid fossae allow for extra functional movement by accommodating the flexor muscle bulk. The normal end-feel of elbow flexion is soft due to approximation of the flexor muscles. Passive extension is achieved by locking the olecranon into the olecranon fossa; it corresponds to a 180° angle and has a hard end-feel due to bone contact.

The elbow joint receives a nerve supply from the musculocutaneous, median and radial nerves anteriorly, and the ulnar and radial nerves posteriorly (C5–C8).

The *superior (proximal) radioulnar joint* is a uniaxial pivot joint permitting the movements of pronation and supination. These movements occur between the circumference of the radial head in the fibro-osseous ring created by the annular ligament and the radial notch of the ulna. The annular ligament is covered internally by a thin layer of articular cartilage.

Movement occurring at the superior and inferior radioulnar joints is rotation of the radius around the ulna to produce pronation and supination. The range of passive pronation is approximately 85° and passive supination 90°, normally with an elastic end-feel.

The *carrying angle (cubitus valgus)* is evident in the anatomical position. The medial end of the distal humerus projects more distally and anteriorly than the lateral, pushing the ulna laterally to produce this valgus angle. It is approximately 10–15° in men and 20–25° in women (Palastanga et al 2002). Miyasaka (1999) cites several references suggesting that the carrying angle in women is 13–16° and noting that one large study demonstrated no difference in the carrying angle between men and women.

The *cubital fossa* is situated on the anterior aspect of the elbow. Its proximal border is an imaginary line drawn between the two epicondyles of the humerus; its lateral border is brachioradialis and its medial border is pronator teres. On the floor of the fossa lies supinator and biceps and the roof is formed by the overlying skin and fascia. The contents of the cubital fossa, from lateral to medial, are the tendon of the biceps in the centre, the brachial artery and the median nerve.

CONTRACTILE STRUCTURES

Biceps brachii (musculocutaneous nerve C5–C6) has two heads of origin. The muscle ends in a stout tendon which attaches deeply to the posterior aspect of the radial tuberosity. As the tendon passes to its insertion it twists so that its anterior surface comes to rest laterally. The tendon is separated from the anterior aspect of the radial tuberosity by the subtendinous bicipital bursa. The bicipital aponeurosis arises anteromedially from the distal end of the tendon and sweeps medially to blend with the antebrachial fascia. Biceps is a powerful elbow flexor. Its secondary action, due to its insertion on the medial aspect of the radius, is to assist supinator in supination of the forearm, particularly with the elbow joint in 90° of flexion; it has no supinating action in the extended elbow.

Brachialis (musculocutaneous nerve C5–C6) takes origin from the anterior aspect of the lower half of the shaft of the humerus and inserts into the coronoid process of the ulna. As it crosses the elbow joint some of its deep fibres insert into the capsule of the elbow joint. Its action is to flex the elbow in either pronation or supination.

Brachioradialis (radial nerve C5–C7) passes from a long attachment on the upper two-thirds of the lateral supracondylar ridge of the humerus to the distal end of the radius just above the styloid. It flexes the elbow, being most effective in the mid-pronation–supination position.

Triceps (radial nerve C6–C8) has three heads of origin above the elbow, with its tendon inserting into the olecranon process. It is the main elbow extensor and is involved in pushing and thrusting activities as well as raising body weight on semiflexed elbows, as in getting up from a chair.

Pronator teres (median nerve C6–C7) has two heads of origin: a humeral head from just above the medial epicondyle, the coronoid process and from the common flexor tendon, and an ulnar head from the medial side of the coronoid process. It passes down and laterally to insert into a roughened area along the lateral aspect of the shaft of the radius. Its main action is to pronate the forearm, especially against resistance.

Pronator quadratus (median nerve C8, T1) binds the lower parts of the radius and ulna and is the principal pronator of the forearm.

Supinator (posterior interosseous nerve C5–C6) has its proximal attachment from the supinator crest of the ulna, lateral epicondyle of the humerus and the radial collateral and annular ligaments. It wraps round the elbow obliquely, laterally and distally, to insert into the proximal third of the radius, and supinates the forearm, bringing the palm of the hand to face upwards, whatever the degree of flexion at the elbow.

Extensor carpi radialis longus (radial nerve C6–C7) takes its main origin from the lower third of the lateral supracondylar ridge, in part deep to the origin of brachioradialis, and some origin from the common extensor tendon. It passes to the radial side of the base of the second metacarpal.

Extensor carpi radialis brevis (posterior interosseous nerve C7–C8) takes its main origin from the lateral epicondyle via the common extensor tendon, in part deep to extensor carpi radialis longus, and inserts into the radial side of the base of the third metacarpal. It is very commonly involved in tennis elbow.

Extensor carpi radialis longus and brevis extend the wrist and produce radial deviation. They work synergistically with the finger flexor tendons by holding the wrist in extension, allowing the finger flexors to form an effective grip (Palastanga et al 2002).

Other muscles which share the origin from the common extensor tendon with extensor carpi radialis brevis and are also responsible for wrist extension are extensor digitorum, extensor digiti minimi and extensor carpi ulnaris (which also produces ulnar deviation). All of these muscles are supplied by the posterior interosseous nerve (C7–C8).

Flexor carpi radialis (median nerve C6–C7) arises from the medial epicondyle via the common flexor tendon and becomes tendinous above the wrist, before passing through its own lateral compartment under the flexor retinaculum. It inserts into the bases of the second and third metacarpals.

Palmaris longus (median nerve C7–C8), often absent, arises from the medial epicondyle via the common flexor tendon and passes over, not under, the flexor retinaculum to attach to this and the palmar aponeurosis.

Flexor digitorum superficialis (median nerve C7–C8, T1) lies in a slightly deeper plane than the above flexor muscles and has a humeral head from the medial epicondyle via the common flexor tendon and a small radial head. It divides to pass under the flexor retinaculum before entering the fingers to attach to the middle phalanx of each.

Flexor carpi ulnaris (ulnar nerve C7–C8) has two heads of origin: a small humeral head from the medial epicondyle via the common flexor origin and an ulnar head from the ulna. It passes over the retinaculum into pisiform.

GUIDE TO SURFACE MARKING AND PALPATION

LATERAL ASPECT
(Fig. 6.1)

Palpate the *lateral supracondylar ridge*, which is a subcutaneous sharp ridge, giving part origin to extensor carpi radialis longus and brachioradialis.

The lateral supracondylar ridge terminates in the *lateral epicondyle*, a small bony projection which you will palpate more easily if the elbow is flexed.

Visualize the small facet on the anterolateral aspect of the lateral epicondyle which gives origin to the *common extensor tendon* of the superficial wrist extensor muscles. This facet is approximately the size of the patient's little finger nail.

Palpate the *head of the radius* on the lateral side of the extended forearm; it is located in a posterior depression just distal to the lateral epicondyle. Confirm the correct position by rotating the forearm to feel the radial head move under your finger.

Move proximally a short distance to palpate the *radiohumeral joint line*, just above the radial head. Here the gap between the head of the radius and the capitulum of the humerus should be obvious; flex your

Figure 6.1   Lateral aspect of the elbow in flexion.

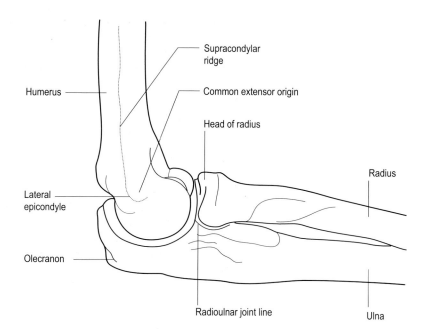

elbow and feel the joint open, providing the most accessible point for an intra-articular injection. Flexion past 45° tightens the joint capsule, making the joint line less obvious. Identify *brachioradialis*, the most superficial forearm muscle on the lateral side of the forearm, by flexing the elbow against resistance in the mid-pronation–supination position.

MEDIAL ASPECT (Fig. 6.2)

Palpate the *medial supracondylar ridge* which ends in the rounded knob of the *medial epicondyle*. Identify the medial epicondyle, which is subcutaneous and most easily felt with the elbow in extension. Palpate the anterior aspect of the medial epicondyle, which provides the attachment for the *common flexor tendon* of the superficial wrist flexor muscles.

Figure 6.2   Medial aspect of the elbow in extension.

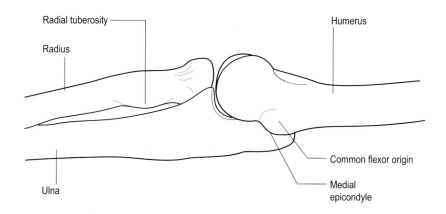

Visualize the position of the superficial wrist flexor muscles by placing the thenar eminence of one hand onto the opposite medial epicondyle, and spread the digits down the forearm to represent the following tendons (Fig. 6.3):

- *Thumb*: pronator teres
- *Index*: flexor carpi radialis
- *Middle*: palmaris longus
- *Ring*: flexor digitorum superficialis (deeper than the others and not so obvious)
- *Little*: flexor carpi ulnaris.

ANTERIOR ASPECT

It is not possible to palpate the joint line of the elbow anteriorly because of the position of the flexor muscles, but it can be visualized approximately 1 cm below the elbow flexor crease that connects the medial and lateral epicondyles (Miyasaka 1999, Palastanga et al 2002).

Figure 6.3 The position of the muscles arising from the common flexor origin.

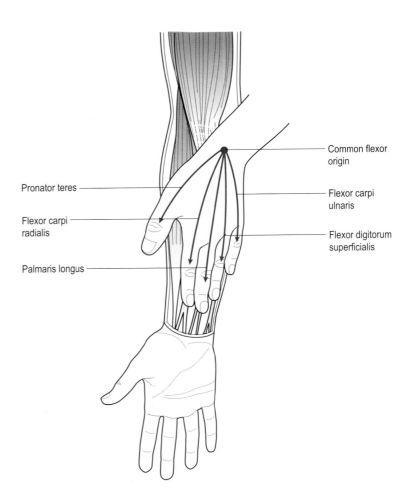

Common flexor origin

Pronator teres

Flexor carpi radialis

Palmaris longus

Flexor carpi ulnaris

Flexor digitorum superficialis

Locate the tuberosity of the radius by flexing the elbow to make the tendon of the biceps more obvious. Follow the tendon down to its insertion onto the radial tuberosity. The tendon of the biceps will be easily palpable as it passes deep into the cubital fossa, but the tuberosity may not feel distinct to the palpating finger, although it is tender to deep palpation.

Place the arm in the anatomical position of elbow extension and supination and note the obvious valgus angle, known as the *carrying angle*. It should be symmetrical bilaterally.

POSTERIOR ASPECT

Palpate the proximal surface of the *olecranon process*, the point of the elbow, which is subcutaneous and most easily palpated when the elbow is flexed. The olecranon gives insertion to triceps and a subcutaneous bursa, the olecranon bursa, lies under the loose skin at the back of the elbow.

COMMENTARY ON THE EXAMINATION

OBSERVATION

Before proceeding with the history, a general observation of the patient's *face, posture and gait* will alert the examiner to abnormalities and serious illness. The acute elbow is usually held in a position of flexion and a degree of supination, with medial rotation at the shoulder and the patient nursing the arm in a position of comfort.

Lesions commonly found at the elbow are due to overuse when abnormalities of posture are not usually observed.

HISTORY (SUBJECTIVE EXAMINATION)

The *age, occupation, sports, hobbies and lifestyle* of the patient may give an indication of the nature of the onset and cause of the injury, and will alert the examiner to possible postural or overuse problems. It may also give an indication of whether the source of the problem is in the cervical spine.

Age may be relevant, as certain conditions affect particular age groups, for example conditions such as 'pulled elbow' (a subluxation of the small radial head in the relatively immature annular ligament), which affects children in the 1–4 years age group. Degenerative osteoarthrosis generally affects the elderly, while rheumatoid arthritis may involve the elbow at any age. Loose bodies can occur in adolescents, associated with osteochondritis dissecans, or in the middle-aged/elderly group, associated with degenerative changes in the articular cartilage. The overuse lesions of tennis and golfer's elbow tend to be a problem of middle age as the ageing process causes the tendinous material to become less extensible and more prone to injury.

The elbow joint and surrounding structures are situated within the C5–C7 and T1 dermatomes. However, the *site* of pain is usually well-localized, indicating a less severe, superficial lesion. A *spread* of pain would indicate a more irritable lesion and possibly referral of pain from a deeper more proximal structure.

The patient may report local tenderness with an olecranon bursitis or, more commonly, with a tennis or golfer's elbow, which may produce a diffuse reference of pain into the forearm, as well as point tenderness over either the lateral or medial epicondyle, respectively.

The *onset* of the symptoms may be sudden, due to trauma, or gradual, due to overuse or arthritis. If the onset is traumatic in nature the mechanism of injury should be deduced. Acute injuries include dislocations and fractures of the radial head, olecranon and distal humerus (Safran 1995).

Hyperextension injuries may cause a capsulitis, or a fall on the outstretched hand may cause fracture (e.g. supracondylar, distal radius or ulna) and/or dislocation. Possible neurovascular complications, secondary to trauma, should be kept in mind.

A sudden onset of pain associated with locking of the elbow could indicate a loose body.

The duration of the symptoms may be long-standing. The commonest lesions at the elbow are due to chronic overuse and result in the enthesiopathies tennis elbow (lateral epicondylar tendinopathy) and golfer's elbow (medial epicondylar tendinopathy). The common tendons of the forearm flexors and extensors are susceptible to excessive use because they function across two joints. The causative factors may be intrinsic overload, from the force of muscle contraction; extrinsic overload, through excessive joint torque forces stressing the connective tissue, stretching and eventually disrupting it; or a combination of intrinsic and extrinsic forces (Safran 1995).

These overuse injuries are often associated with the middle-aged racquet sports player or individuals participating in throwing activities. Throwing motions may produce a valgus stress on the medial elbow and compressive forces at the lateral elbow. Such repetitive actions may result in microtrauma to the joint or surrounding tissues (Nicola 1992).

Climber's elbow affects brachialis, as climbing involves the use of the semi-flexed pronated forearm (Safran 1995). Overuse may cause friction between the radial tuberosity and the biceps tendon, resulting in inflammation of the biceps subtendinous bursa, or an overuse lesion in the tendon itself.

The duration of symptoms indicates the stage of the lesion in the inflammatory process. The common presentation of tennis or golfer's elbow is pain of weeks' or even months' duration, while the less common loose body has recurrent episodes of twinging, often resolving spontaneously. Arthritis is characterized by recurrent episodes of exacerbation of symptoms.

The *symptoms and behaviour* need to be considered. The behaviour of the pain indicates the nature of the lesion: mechanical lesions are eased by rest and aggravated by repeated movements, particularly those involved in the mechanism of the lesion. For example, tennis elbow gives an increase of pain on gripping activities – simple things such as lifting a cup or pulling up bedclothes. Patients often report that knocking the lateral aspect of the elbow can give excruciating pain and it is very tender to touch. Other symptoms described by the patient could include twinges of pain with locking of the elbow, usually just short of full extension, which would indicate a possible loose body. A twinge of pain in the forearm on gripping is also associated with a tennis elbow, causing the patient to drop the object and giving an apparent feeling of muscle weakness.

Paraesthesia may be indicative of nerve involvement and the exact location of these symptoms should be ascertained. Paraesthesia may be referred distally from the cervical spine, but as the ulnar nerve lies in an exposed location behind the medial epicondyle, it is occasionally subject to direct trauma.

Both the posterior interosseous nerve (passing between the two heads of supinator) and the median nerve (passing between the two heads of pronator teres) are susceptible to muscular compression. This may complicate the clinical presentation of either tennis or golfer's elbow and may be a reason for a poor response to treatment.

An indication of *past medical history, other joint involvement* and *medications* will establish whether contraindications to treatment exist, or that the lesion is part of an ongoing inflammatory arthritis.

INSPECTION

An inspection is conducted in standing with the upper limb resting in the anatomical position, if this can be achieved. Assess the overall posture from above down, looking for any *bony deformity*, noting the position of the head, the lordosis in the cervical spine, the position of both shoulders and the scapulae. Assess the carrying angle in the anatomical position, comparing it with the other side for symmetry.

Inspect for *colour changes*, including contusions and abrasions which are associated with direct trauma. These may be located at the point of the elbow or over either epicondyle. Bruising over the biceps or triceps muscles can occur in contact sports where a direct blow is possible. Abrasions may be a site of entry for bacteria, with septic olecranon bursitis being a possible result of such infection.

Muscle wasting may be evident in the forearm if a patient has a long or recurrent history of tennis elbow. Other muscle wasting would be unusual and would probably be a neurological sign associated with cervical pathology.

Swelling is usually associated with trauma. It may be diffuse, engulfing the elbow area, in which case the elbow will be fixed in the position of ease, to accommodate the swelling with minimal pain. The dimples seen at the back of a flexed elbow are obliterated if swelling is present, as here the capsule is lax and usually accommodates excess fluid.

Immediate swelling indicates bleeding and possibly a haemarthrosis. Swelling developing 6–24 h after trauma indicates synovial irritation and capsular involvement. Local swellings are associated with direct trauma. A localized soft, boggy, fluctuating swelling may be seen over the point of the elbow and is indicative of an olecranon bursitis. Occasionally patients complain of swelling over the lateral epicondyle in tennis elbow, but this is not always evident clinically.

PALPATION

Since the elbow is a peripheral joint, the joint is palpated for signs of activity. *Heat* indicates an active inflammation (Fig. 6.4), as does *synovial thickening* which is most easily palpable over the radial head in the more chronic state (Fig. 6.5). *Swelling* is usually most apparent in the dimples at the back of the elbow and may be palpated in that area. Other swellings such as nodules or associated with olecranon bursitis can also be palpated to assess whether they are hard or soft.

Figure 6.4   Palpation for heat.

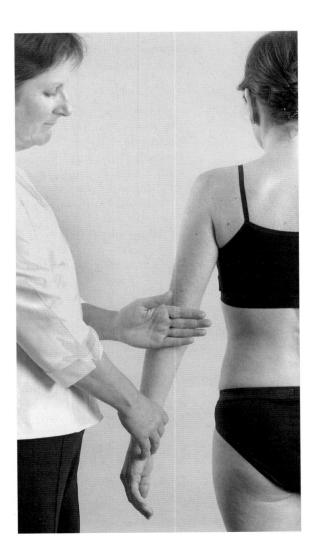

Figure 6.5   Palpation for synovial thickening.

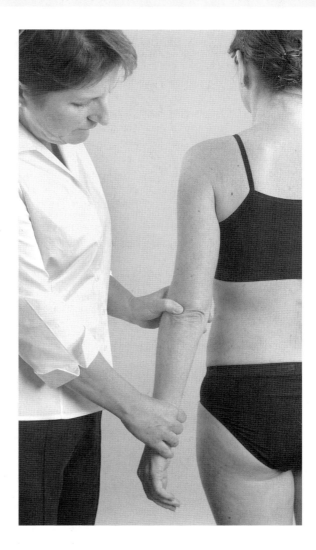

STATE AT REST   Before any movements are performed, the state at rest is established to provide a baseline for subsequent comparison.

The suggested sequence for the objective examination will now be given, followed by a commentary including the reasoning in performing the movements and the significance of the possible findings.

Elbow and Superior Radioulnar Joints

■ Passive elbow flexion (Fig. 6.6)
■ Passive elbow extension (Fig. 6.7)
■ Passive pronation of the superior radioulnar joint (Fig. 6.8)
■ Passive supination of the superior radioulnar joint (Fig. 6.9)
■ Resisted elbow flexion (Fig. 6.10)
■ Resisted elbow extension (Fig. 6.11)
■ Resisted pronation (Fig. 6.12 a,b,c)
■ Resisted supination (Fig. 6.12 a,b,c)

Pain Provocation Tests for Tennis and Golfer's Elbow

■ Resisted wrist extension for tennis elbow (Fig. 6.13 and 6.15a)
■ Resisted wrist flexion for golfer's elbow (Fig. 6.14 and 6.15b)

Palpation

■ Once a diagnosis has been made, the structure at fault is palpated for the exact site of the lesion

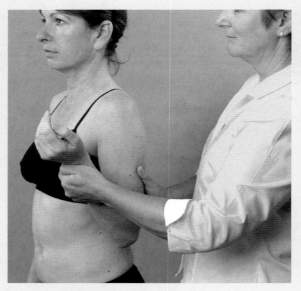

Figure 6.6   Passive elbow flexion.

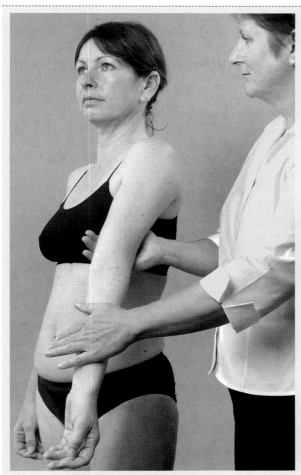

Figure 6.7   Passive elbow extension.

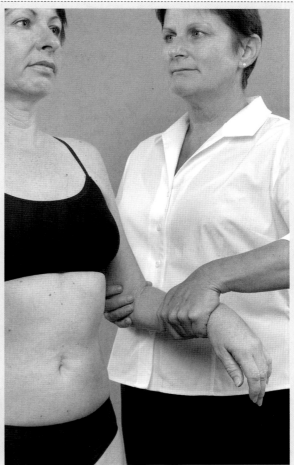

Figure 6.8   Passive pronation.

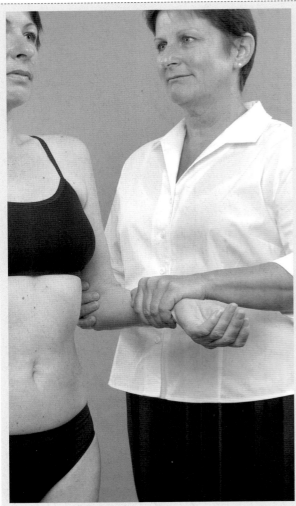

Figure 6.9   Passive supination.

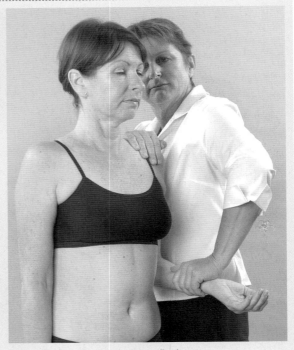

Figure 6.10   Resisted elbow flexion.

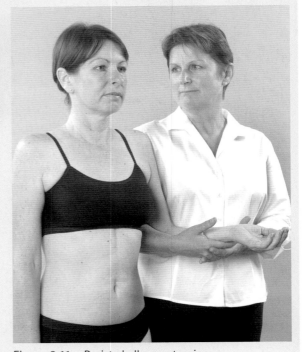

Figure 6.11   Resisted elbow extension.

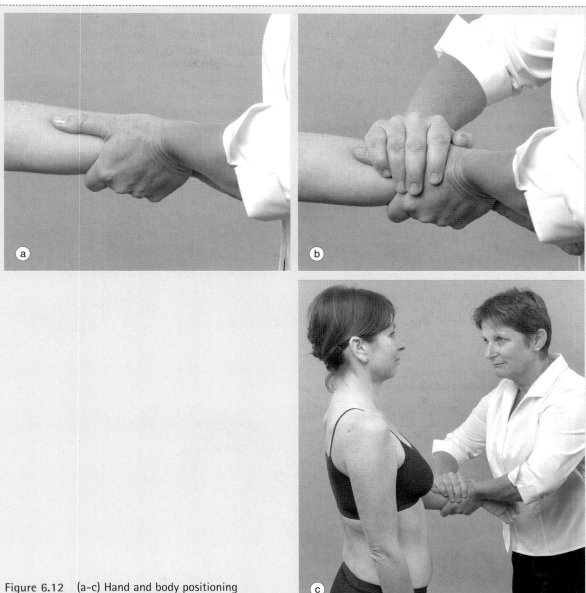

Figure 6.12   (a–c) Hand and body positioning
for resisted pronation and supination.

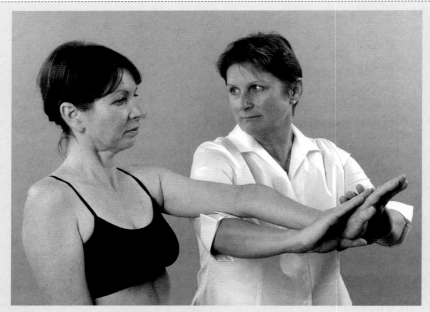

Figure 6.13   Resisted wrist extension.

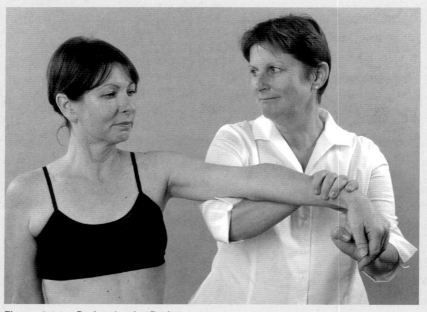

Figure 6.14   Resisted wrist flexion.

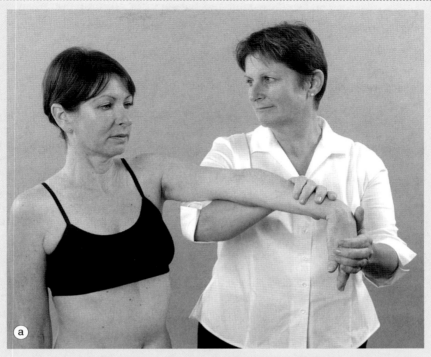

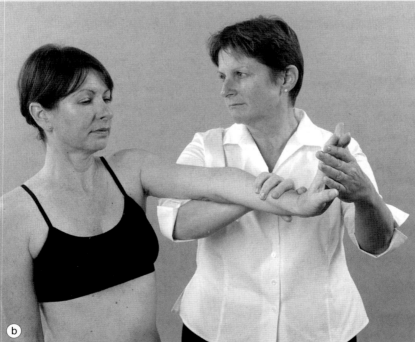

Figure 6.15   Examples of further provocative tests: (a) resisted wrist extension from the flexed position; (b) resisted wrist flexion from the extended position.

The elbow joint and the superior radioulnar joint are assessed by four passive movements looking for pain, range and end-feel. In the normal patient passive flexion has a 'soft' end-feel and passive extension has a 'hard' end-feel. At the superior radioulnar joint, passive pronation and supination have an 'elastic' end-feel. The signs elicited will establish whether or not the capsular pattern exists.

A loose body in the elbow joint produces a non-capsular pattern of movement with either limitation of passive flexion, or extension, but not both. The limited movement has an abnormal 'springy' end-feel.

The resisted tests are conducted for the muscles around the elbow, looking for pain and power. Resisted elbow flexion tests biceps and resisted elbow extension tests triceps. Resisted pronation tests pronator quadratus and pronator teres, but since pronator teres takes origin from the common flexor tendon, this may be an accessory sign in golfer's elbow. Resisted supination tests biceps, since it is assessed with the elbow flexed, and supinator.

Two provocative resisted tests are conducted at the wrist to assess the common extensor and common flexor tendons for tendinopathy. Resisted wrist extension and resisted wrist flexion are assessed with the elbow joint fully extended. Since they are not required to stabilize the elbow in this close packed or locked position, they contract strongly to resist the wrist movements. To provoke pain, further provocative tests can be applied for tennis elbow, e.g. passive wrist flexion, resisted wrist extension from the flexed position, resisted radial deviation and resisted middle finger extension. For golfer's elbow resisted wrist flexion can be assessed from the extended position.

CAPSULAR LESIONS

Capsular pattern of the elbow joint
■ More limitation of flexion than extension.

The capsular pattern indicates the presence of arthritis in the joint which, at the elbow, is frequently rheumatoid arthritis. Degenerative osteoarthrosis is of itself symptom-free, but traumatic arthritis may be secondary to overuse or trauma of a restricted joint. Treatment of choice is a corticosteroid injection into the elbow joint.

Injection of the elbow joint

Suggested needle size: 25G × ⁵/₈ in (0.5 × 16 mm) orange needle
Dose: 20 mg triamcinolone acetonide in a total volume of 3 ml

Capsular pattern of the superior radioulnar joint
■ Pain at the end of range of both rotations.

Sit the patient with the elbow flexed to approximately 45° and the forearm pronated (Fig. 6.16). Locate the radiohumeral joint line on the posterolateral aspect of the elbow. Insert the needle between the head of the radius and the capitulum (Fig. 6.17). Once intra-articular, deliver the injection as a bolus. The patient is advised to maintain a period of relative rest for approximately 2 weeks following injection.

Figure 6.16 Injection of the elbow joint.

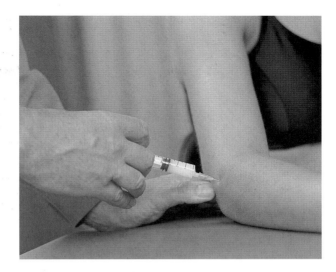

Figure 6.17 Injection of the elbow joint, showing direction of approach and needle position.

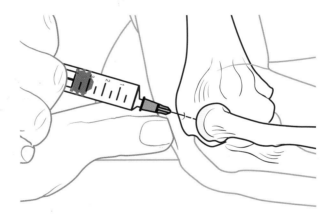

Traumatic arthritis can be treated with other physiotherapeutic modalities.

NON-CAPSULAR LESIONS

LOOSE BODY

Osteochondritis dissecans occurs in adolescents and can give rise to loose body formation, particularly with activities such as gymnastics, throwing and racket sports. Repeated compressive forces cause microtrauma between the radial head and capitulum and focal degeneration results in fragmentation and the formation of loose bodies (Ho 1995, Patten 1995). Surgical removal is advisable in this age group. Joji et al (2001) present a case report to demonstrate osteochondritis dissecans occurring in the medial aspect of the distal humerus of a 17-year-old baseball pitcher, which is deemed to be less common than osteochondritis with loose body formation found in the lateral aspect.

Loose bodies can also be encountered in the middle-aged or elderly group and may be associated with degenerative changes. Characteristically, the patient complains of a history of twinging pain, with the elbow giving way under pressure or locking, usually just short of full elbow extension. The history alone may be the only diagnostic evidence available since the loose body may spontaneously reduce. Sometimes diagnostic imaging may be necessary to identify and localize loose bodies before arthroscopic removal (Ho 1995).

On examination, a non-capsular pattern may exist with either a small degree of limitation of flexion or extension, but not both. The end-feel to the limited movement is abnormally springy.

The treatment of choice to reduce a loose body is strong traction together with Grade A mobilization, theoretically aiming to shift the loose body to another part of the joint and to restore full, pain-free movement.

There are two possible manoeuvres, both working towards elbow extension. The choice of starting manoeuvre is random and sometimes it may be necessary to try both and repeat the most successful, although sometimes one manoeuvre is sufficient. As with all mobilization techniques, the patient is reassessed after every manoeuvre and a decision made about the next, based on the outcome.

Mobilization for loose body in the elbow joint (Saunders 2000)

Towards extension and supination

Position the patient against the raised head of the couch, with the arm resting against a pillow. Use a butterfly grip with the thumbs placed on the flexor surface of the forearm, over the radius (Fig. 6.18). Face the direction of the supination movement and lift the leg farthest from the patient off the ground, leaning out to establish traction with straight arms. Step forwards, taking the elbow joint towards extension (not full range), while simultaneously rotating the forearm with several flicking movements towards supination (Fig. 6.19). The manoeuvre is easier to perform if you begin the rotation from a position of some pronation.

Figure 6.18   Hand position for mobilization for loose body in the elbow joint, towards extension and supination.

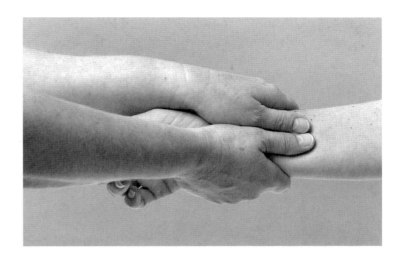

Figure 6.19   Body position for mobilization for loose body in the elbow joint, towards extension and supination: step forwards.

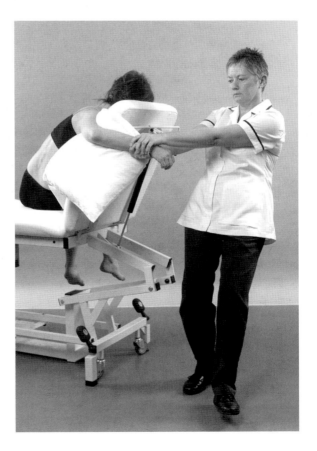

Towards extension and pronation

The patient's position is the same. Face the movement of pronation, placing the thumbs on the extensor surface of the forearm, over the radius (Fig. 6.20). Establish the traction as above and step backwards, simultaneously rotating the forearm with several flicking movements towards pronation (Fig. 6.21). The manoeuvre is easier to perform if you begin the rotation from a position of some supination.

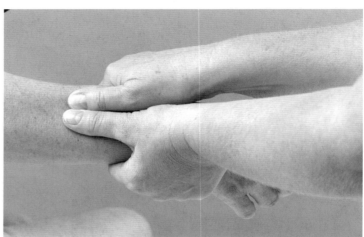

Figure 6.20   Hand position for mobilization for loose body in the elbow joint, towards extension and pronation.

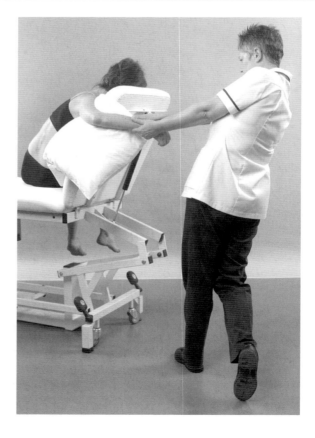

Figure 6.21   Body position for mobilization for loose body in the elbow joint, towards extension and pronation: step backwards.

The patient may need to be reviewed to assess the success of the treatment. Generally speaking, the manoeuvre is usually successful, but there are no guarantees that the condition will not recur. Excessive recurrences of the condition may need referral for surgery.

OLECRANON BURSITIS

Swelling and inflammation of the olecranon bursa can occur due to repeated pressure and friction, or to direct trauma of the bursa. The bursa is the most vulnerable structure to trauma on the posterior surface of the elbow and septic bursitis is not uncommon (Nicola 1992, Hoppmann 1993). The patient may present with an obvious swelling over the olecranon which is boggy and fluctuating. Provided sepsis is not present, conservative management includes aspiration, ice and non-steroidal anti-inflammatory drugs (Nicola 1992). Any physiotherapeutic modality may be applied and corticosteroid injection may be given in the absence of infection (for further information see Kesson et al 2003).

PULLED ELBOW

This condition usually presents to the general practitioner's surgery or the casualty department. Typically the child is aged between 1 and 4 years old and has a sudden onset of pain in the arm, followed by a reluctance to use the arm. The child is unhappy and holds the arm in elbow flexion and pronation. The arm is pain-free provided it is not moved.

There may be a history of the child stumbling or falling or it may occur if the child grabs the cot rails or other stationary object while falling. Frequently the child is accompanied by a guilty parent, if pulling a resistant toddler or lifting the child by the arms and swinging them in play was the cause.

The mechanism is thought to be a distal subluxation of the radial head through the annular ligament (Hardy 1978, Kohlhaas & Roeder 1995); however, X-rays taken before and after reduction show no evidence of displacement (Hardy 1978).

Reduction of a pulled elbow involves supporting the child's elbow with one hand, feeling the radial head and providing counterpressure to axial compression. Quickly pronate the forearm through a small range while maintaining axial compression until a click is felt. The reduction is confirmed by immediate use of the arm by the child, to the subsequent relief of the parent.

Adeniran & Merriam (1994) reported a case of 'pulled elbow' in a 21-year-old woman, as an exception to the usual age group of the condition. Spontaneous reduction occurred as the patient was positioned into supination for X-ray.

CONTRACTILE LESIONS

TENNIS ELBOW

Tennis elbow is the term commonly applied to a strain of the wrist extensor muscles at the site of their common origin from the anterolateral aspect at the lateral epicondyle of the humerus. In the past it has been commonly referred to as *lateral epicondylitis*, but the absence of inflammatory cells at the site of the lesion has led to this terminology being dropped. It is commonly a chronic lesion of more than 3 months' duration. *Tendinopathy* is a more appropriate description unless excision biopsy has been performed and the specific histopathological features of the specimen can be described, to be able to distinguish between tendinopathy and tendinosis (Khan & Cook 2000). It most commonly involves the extensor carpi radialis brevis tendon and is by far the most common lesion treated at the elbow, being five to eight times more common than golfer's elbow (Coonrad & Hooper 1973, Gellman 1992, Gabel 1999). The condition may be resistant to treatment and is prone to recurrence.

Tennis elbow was first described in 1898 by Runge as *writer's cramp* (Gellman 1992, Verhaar et al 1993). Of all diagnosed cases, 35–64% are associated with work-related activities, with tennis players representing 8% of the total diagnosed. Repetitive loading seems to be a factor, with low-load activities such as keyboarding possibly representing the majority of patients. Workplace stress contributes to psychosocial factors (Gabel 1999). Repetitive wrist movements and unaccustomed activities are often blamed. However, competitive tennis players are susceptible to tennis elbow, 50% of them experiencing at least one episode (Noteboom et al 1994). Altered biomechanics, particularly of the backhand stroke, predisposes tennis players to the condition (Schnatz & Steiner 1993).

The condition occurs in middle age with incidence of the condition peaking between the ages of 35 and 54 and with a duration of an average episode of between 6 months and 2 years (Assendelft et al 1996, Ernst 1992, Katarincic et al 1992). It affects the dominant arm most commonly, with epidemiological studies showing a prevalence of 1% in men and 4% in women (Verhaar et al 1993, Noteboom et al 1994).

The patient complains of a gradually increasing pain felt on the lateral aspect of the elbow and posterior aspect of the forearm, sometimes referred to the wrist and into the dorsum of the hand. The condition is so common that patients often make the diagnosis themselves. There is a constant ache which is aggravated by repeated gripping actions, together with rotation of the forearm. The gripping action is often related to occupational or sporting activities and rarely is tennis elbow related to direct trauma or a traumatic incident. The possibility of acute onset has been reported, however, in which case inflammatory changes might be present (Nirschl; Maffuli et al cited in Greenfield & Webster 2002).

Point tenderness is present over the lateral epicondyle and the patient will often experience excruciating pain when the elbow is knocked. An apparent muscle weakness may be reported, as pain is often accompanied by a severe twinge which causes the patient to drop relatively light objects (e.g. coffee cup). Pienimäki et al (2002) demonstrated similar subjective pain reports in tennis and golfer's elbow, but a greater reduction in grip strength associated with tennis elbow.

On examination there is usually a full range of pain-free movement at the elbow joint with pain on resisted wrist extension. Most authors seem to be in agreement that pain on resisted extension of the wrist and tenderness to palpation over the lateral epicondyle at the insertion of extensor carpi radialis brevis are pathognomic of the condition.

Greenfield & Webster (2002) conducted a survey of outpatient physiotherapists, seeking their opinion on current practice of tennis elbow, and identified 15 diagnostic tests with the above two tests being used most commonly. Passive wrist flexion stretches the common extensor tendon and other resisted tests which may be positive include resisted radial deviation and resisted extension of the middle digit, which preferentially stresses extensor carpi radialis brevis as it contracts synergistically, anchoring the third metacarpal to allow the digit to extend (Brukner & Khan 2002). A clinical observation of the authors suggests that apparent weakness on resisted wrist extension may be due to pain inhibition and this sign is a useful reassessment tool. Smidt et al (2002b) recommend the use of pain-free grip strength using a hand held dynamometer as a relatively easy test of functional disability in tennis elbow, showing it to have excellent reliability.

Mills' sign is sometimes used to confirm diagnosis. The forearm is fully pronated and the wrist joint flexed. While maintaining this position, passive elbow extension is performed and a positive sign is elicited if pain is reproduced at the lateral side of the elbow (Noteboom et al 1994, Sölveborn et al 1995).

Cervical spine examination and radial nerve tension testing were the most popular differential diagnostic tests in the study by Greenfield & Webster (2002). Since the above positioning for the Mills' test and the radial nerve tension test are similar, this may present a false positive result as symptoms would be provoked if neural tension and/or tendinopathy were present.

MECHANISM OF TENNIS ELBOW

The normal ageing process causes degenerative changes in collagen fibres and ground substance similar to the changes seen when tissues are immobilized (Akeson et al 1968). Degeneration and relative avascularity of the tendon make it susceptible to microtrauma through overuse activity.

The repeated gripping action may initially produce traction of the common extensor origin causing microtrauma and inflammation (Foley 1993). Microscopic and macroscopic tears occur at the common extensor origin, with the development of fibrous scar tissue and contracture. Eventually, degenerative foci and calcification can occur (Coonrad & Hooper 1973, Ernst 1992, Gellman 1992, Noteboom et al 1994).

Theoretically, initial inflammatory changes may produce a characteristic tendinopathy in an early acute lesion, but this is rarely seen clinically. Histologically, as the chronic condition develops, the degenerative features of tendinosis are thought to become paramount. This degenerative condition of the tendon is considered to be similar to the ongoing degenerative tendinosis seen in the Achilles tendon and rotator cuff tendons (Bennett 1994). With continued overuse, the degenerative changes lead to microscopic tearing and scar tissue development within the tendon. An area of vascular granulation tissue develops which contains many nociceptive nerve endings, possibly explaining why the lesion is so painful (Brukner & Khan 2002).

Chard et al (1994) conducted histological studies of normal and biopsy tendon specimens (rotator cuff tendinopathy and tennis elbow) to determine the mechanisms involved in tendon degeneration. The major mechanism of tennis elbow or rotator cuff was not inflammation, but a sequence of degenerative changes which increased with age, although chronic traction is believed to have an effect. The tendons studied were considered to have an area of relative avascularity which seemed to predispose them to degeneration.

The sequence of degeneration included changes in the blood vessel walls and fibroblasts and alteration in the gel to fibre ratio, with glycosaminoglycans replacing collagen fibres. This led to lack of maintenance of collagen turnover, loss of the wavy configuration of collagen fibres and transformation of the fibroblasts into chondrocyte-type cells, with subsequent cartilage formation, calcification and eventual bone formation. It would seem that as the degenerative process progresses the tendon fibroblasts undergo fibrocartilaginous change, ultimately to convert the tendon to bone. This theory is supported by Edelson et al (2001) who examined a large number of cadaver elbow specimens and found characteristic bone formation at the point of usual tenderness to palpation in the area that corresponded to the origin of extensor carpi radialis brevis. A C-shaped crescent of bone was identified along the posterior margin of the epicondyle, although it was also noted that the anatomical relationship of both the insertion of the tendon and the lateral collateral ligament complex at this point could not be distinguished.

Palpation determines the site of the lesion. Of the cases of tennis elbow encountered, 90% involve the teno-osseous junction of the common extensor tendon (Cyriax 1982). Stratford et al (1989) demonstrated only a 22.5% occurrence at this site, hypothesizing that patients with tenderness over the lateral epicondyle and recurrent cases have a poorer short-term prognosis. They suggest that Cyriax would have seen more resistant cases in consultant practice whereas their research was

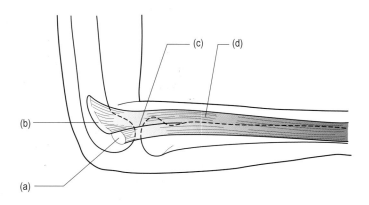

Figure 6.22   Four possible sites of tennis elbow: (a) teno-osseous junction (enthesis); (b) supracondylar ridge; (c) body of the common extensor tendon; (d) the muscle bellies.

conducted in primary care. If remaining with Cyriax's clinical estimate, however, the remaining 10% involve the body of the tendon, the extensor carpi radialis longus attachment on the supracondylar ridge or the muscle bellies (Fig. 6.22) (Cyriax 1982).

TREATMENT OF TENNIS ELBOW

Treatment of tennis elbow should always look to address the causative factors. A full explanation should be given so that the patient is responsible for modifying activities to give treatment, whatever the choice, the best possible opportunity. Lifting should be performed with a supination action rather than pronation (Gellman 1992), and various counterforce elbow or forearm supports are available to alter the stress on the common extensor origin or to rest the wrist to avoid strain. Patient and therapist can discuss the best choice for the individual patient.

With current knowledge that tendinopathy is more likely to be due to degenerative change than to inflammation, educating the patient in terms of prognosis becomes important. Many treatment options are available for the tendinopathies and several seem to have good pain relief in the short term. The patient needs to understand that a minimum of 3–6 months may be required to resolve their problem and that they have an important role to play in terms of activity modification (Gabel 1999).

Greenfield & Webster (2002) identified 24 different treatment modalities, demonstrating that physiotherapists use judgment, largely based on past experience, when choosing treatment for tennis elbow. Progressive stretch and strengthening were identified as popular treatments, with 67.5% of respondents using deep transverse frictions and 64.4% using Mills' manipulation (see below). Although not specified in the study, it is assumed that the regime of deep transverse frictions to prepare the tendon, followed by Mills' manipulation was used, as this is taught in the orthopaedic medicine approach.

Verhaar et al (1996), in a study of 106 subjects, demonstrated that in the short term, corticosteroid injection was more beneficial than deep transverse frictions and Mills' manipulation. Stratford et al (1989) failed to demonstrate statistical power in a study comparing deep transverse frictions with phonophoresis, and Vasseljen (1992) demonstrated that 'traditional physiotherapy' consisting of transverse frictions and ultrasound performed better under subjective, but not objective, testing when compared with laser treatment.

Drechsler et al (1997) compare two treatment regimes, a 'standard' treatment group exposed to several interventions including transverse frictions and a neural tension group exposed to mobilization of the radial nerve. The results showed no significant difference for any variable tested and the authors then attempted to validate the study through group analysis, incorporating further variables. While admitting that the study could have been confounded by these additions, they nevertheless concluded that neural and joint mobilizations together were superior to 'standard' treatment techniques.

Smidt et al (2003) evaluated current evidence of the effectiveness of physiotherapy for tennis elbow identifying 23 randomized controlled trials. Little evidence was found to either support or refute the use of physiotherapy. Lack of evidence was judged to be due to low statistical power, inadequate validity and insufficient reported data. There is a need to standardize outcome measures, to increase sample sizes and to include short, medium and long-term follow-up. A few valid studies were identified which suggested the potential effectiveness of some commonly used treatments. Ultrasound may be better than placebo in alleviating pain; ultrasound with transverse frictions may be more effective than laser; and stretching, muscle conditioning and occupational exercises may be better than ultrasound with transverse frictions.

From this discussion the authors acknowledge that the evidence to support the use of transverse frictions and Mills' manipulation is weak, but it should also be emphasized that these techniques have not been proven to be ineffective. It is interesting to note that the studies in general address inflammatory components rather than the degenerative features of tennis elbow.

Davidson et al (1997) and Gehlsen et al (1998) show some interesting support for the use of augmented soft tissue mobilizations in animal studies. Pressures, similar to those delivered by deep transverse frictions, are applied to promote the healing process in tendinopathy, which provides a stimulus for further investigation into transverse frictions. The controlled application of microtrauma through pressure is thought to promote fibroblastic activity leading to repair in the absence of inflammation (see Ch. 4).

Greenfield & Webster (2002) demonstrate the lack of consensus on the best practice for the treatment of tennis elbow, but with well over half of the respondents choosing transverse frictions and Mills' manipulation, positive clinical results can be assumed.

As mentioned above, Cyriax (1982) and Cyriax & Cyriax (1983) describe four possible sites of the lesion:

- Teno-osseous junction (enthesis) – *mainly extensor carpi radialis brevis*
- Supracondylar ridge – *origin of extensor carpi radialis longus*
- Body of the common extensor tendon
- The muscle bellies.

Tennis elbow at the teno-osseous junction

Cyriax (1982) and Cyriax & Cyriax (1983) describe this as the most common type of tennis elbow lesion, suggesting 90% occurrence at this site. As mentioned above, however, this may be an overestimation. Pain is localized to the common extensor tendon at the teno-osseous junction, mainly affecting the extensor carpi radialis brevis on the anterolateral aspect of the lateral epicondyle of the humerus. The facet for attachment of the common extensor tendon faces anteriorly and is approximately the size of the patient's little finger nail. The choice of treatment may be corticosteroid injection or Mills' manipulation.

The inflammatory model of chronic tendinopathy is under debate and the justification for corticosteroid injection is difficult in the absence of inflammation. Khan & Cook (2000) acknowledge that clinical experience and some studies show that corticosteroid injection produces short-term relief of pain in these lesions, although the mechanisms for this pain relief are currently not known. Corticosteroid injection for tennis elbow at the teno-osseous site is therefore still currently recommended. Once rendered pain-free, the patient, through normal movement, will encourage alignment of fibres and mobility of the scar. However, injection should not be considered to be a panacea and an entire management programme, including activity modification and supports or braces, should be adhered to (Gabel 1999).

Injection of tennis elbow, teno–osseous site

Suggested needle size: 25G × ⁵/₈ in (0.5 × 16 mm) orange needle
Dose: 10 mg triamcinolone acetonide in a total volume of 1 ml

---

Support the patient with the forearm resting on a pillow, the elbow flexed to approximately 90° and fully supinated (Fig. 6.23). Identify the area of tenderness over the teno-osseous junction of the common extensor tendon with the anterolateral aspect of the lateral epicondyle. Insert the needle from an anterior direction, perpendicular to the facet, and deliver the injection by a peppering technique (Fig. 6.24). The patient is advised to maintain a period of relative rest for approximately 2 weeks following injection.

Sölveborn et al (1995) conducted a study of 109 cases of tennis elbow treated with a single corticosteroid injection (10 mg triamcinolone) together with local anaesthetic. Bupivacaine (a long-acting local anaesthetic) was compared with lidocaine (lignocaine) (a short-acting local anaesthetic). An impressive improvement was reported 2 weeks after the injection, with the patients treated with bupivacaine showing a significantly better outcome. However, at 3 months the results in both groups showed deterioration and relapse, with patients seeking other treatments.

Figure 6.23   Injection of tennis elbow, teno–osseous site.

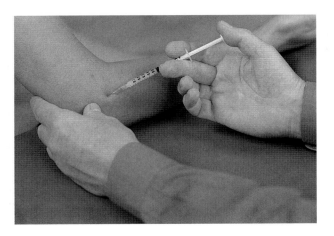

Figure. 6.24   Injection of tennis elbow, teno–osseous site, showing direction of approach and needle position.

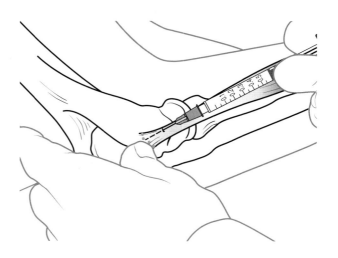

Verhaar et al (1996) conducted a prospective randomized trial of 106 patients with tennis elbow. They compared the effects of corticosteroid injections with Cyriax physiotherapy (i.e. deep transverse frictions followed by Mills' manipulation). Both groups showed significant improvement at 6 weeks, with the injection group demonstrating better results. However, at 1-year follow-up there was no significant difference between the groups, with 17 patients in the injection group and 14 patients in the physiotherapy group going onto eventual surgery. There were no adverse side-effects from either group. The authors reached the conclusion that, although corticosteroid injections alleviate pain in the short term, they do not address the cause of the condition. Since corticosteroid injection is more time-efficient than physiotherapy (three visits maximum for the injection group; 12 visits for the physiotherapy group), it was considered to be the more effective treatment in the short term. However, as mentioned above, the effect of corticosteroid injection on healing at different stages is uncertain.

Newcomer et al (2001) conducted a randomized controlled double blind trial on 39 subjects with symptoms present for less than 4 weeks. The experimental group received corticosteroid injection and rehabilitation, the control group sham injection and rehabilitation. The authors recorded that there was no significant change in the experimental group and that subjects improved over time with the rehabilitation programme. They concluded that injections were not justified in patients who had symptoms for less than 4 weeks and that rehabilitation should be the first line of treatment.

Smidt et al (2002a) showed short-term relief for corticosteroid injection, but physiotherapy consisting of ultrasound, deep transverse frictions and exercise was more effective in the long term, as was advice and pain medication from a family practitioner. However, there was no evidence of standardization of injection technique or of the way the physiotherapy programme was managed (Hart 2002).

Assendelft et al (1996), on reviewing the literature, determined that the existing evidence on effectiveness, optimal timing of injections, composition of injection fluid and adverse effects of injections is not conclusive, although they appear to be safe and effective in the short term (2–6 weeks). Three injections seem to be the recommended maximum in several reviews, with post-injection pain and subcutaneous atrophy being the adverse side-effects. Corticosteroid injections are relatively easy to administer and cheap, and specialist referral is not necessary.

An alternative treatment to corticosteroid injection is to aim to elongate the scar tissue by rupturing adhesions within the teno-osseous junction, thus making the area mobile and pain-free. This is achieved by a *Mills' manipulation*, which must be followed by stretching exercises to maintain the lengthening achieved. Before the Mills' manipulation can be performed, the teno-osseous junction is prepared by deep transverse frictions to produce an analgesic effect, in preparation for the manipulative technique.

G. Percival Mills described this technique for the treatment of tennis elbow in the *British Medical Journal* in 1928. On examining patients with tennis elbow, he found that on combined pronation and wrist and finger flexion, the elbow joint could not achieve full extension. He suggested that forcing the restricted movement (now known as Mills' manipulation) could be curative.

Mills' manipulation (cited in Cyriax & Cyriax 1983, Cyriax 1984)

The area should first be prepared by transverse frictions to produce an analgesic effect before applying the technique. Position the patient comfortably with the elbow fully supinated and in 90° of flexion, this exposes the tendon by allowing it to run directly forward from the anterior aspect of the epicondyle. Locate the anterolateral aspect of the lateral epicondyle and identify the area of tenderness (Fig. 6.25). Apply deep transverse frictions with the side of the thumb tip, applying the pressure in a posterior direction onto the teno-osseous junction (Fig. 6.26). Maintain this pressure while imparting deep transverse frictions in a direction towards your fingers, which should be positioned around the posteromedial side of the elbow for counterpressure.

The Mills' manipulation is performed immediately after the transverse frictions, providing the patient has a full range of passive elbow extension, demonstrated during the clinical examination process. If the patient does not have full passive elbow extension on examination, the manipulative thrust will affect the elbow joint, rather than the common extensor tendon, possibly causing a traumatic arthritis.

Position the patient on a chair with a back rest. Stand behind the patient:

Figure 6.25 Transverse frictions for tennis elbow, teno-osseous site.

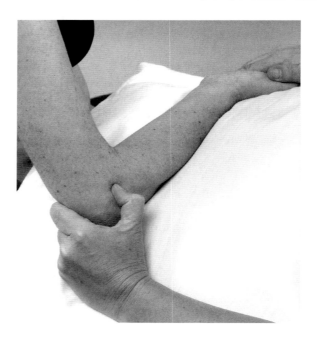

Figure 6.26 Transverse frictions for tennis elbow, teno-osseous site, showing site of anterolateral facet on the lateral epicondyle of the humerus, and the direction of application.

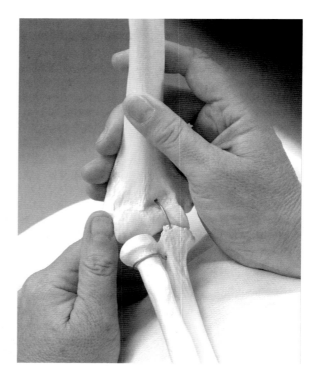

- Support the patient's arm under the crook of the elbow with the shoulder joint abducted to 90° and medially rotated. The forearm will automatically fall into pronation (Fig. 6.27).
- Place the thumb of your other hand in the web space between the patient's thumb and index finger and fully flex the patient's wrist and pronate the forearm (Fig. 6.28 a, b, c).
- Move the hand supporting the crook of the elbow onto the posterior surface of the elbow joint and, while maintaining full wrist flexion and pronation, extend the patient's elbow until you feel all the slack has been taken up in the tendon.
- Step sideways to stand behind the patient's head, taking care to prevent the patient from leaning away either forwards or sideways, which would reduce the tension on the tendon (Fig. 6.29).
- Apply a minimal amplitude, high velocity thrust (Grade C manipulation) by simultaneously side flexing your body away from your arms and pushing smartly downwards with the hand over the patient's elbow.

Figure 6.27   Mill's manipulation, starting position.

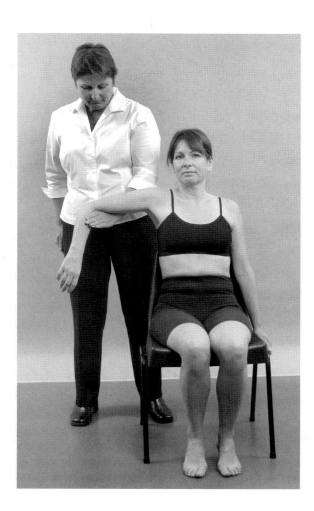

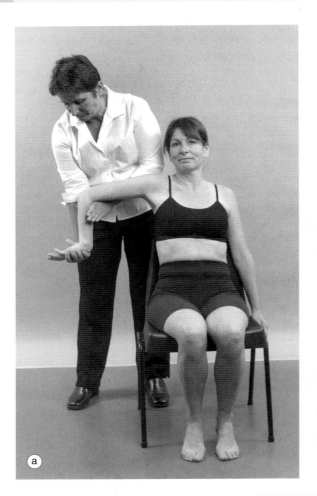

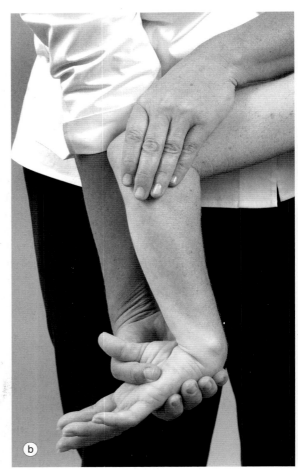

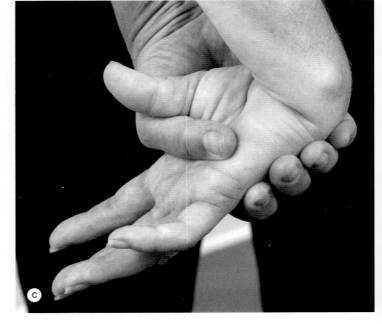

Figure 6.28   (a–c) The thumb placed in the palm, forearm pronated and wrist maintained in full flexion.

Figure 6.29   Positioning of hand on posterior aspect of extended elbow for application of the Grade C manipulation.

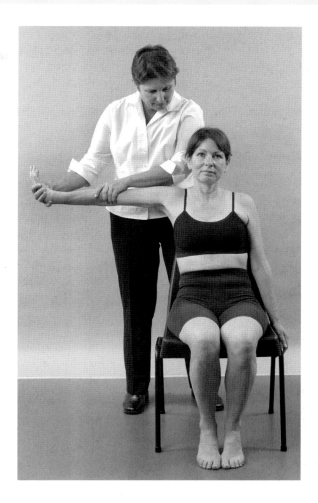

This manoeuvre is usually conducted once only at each treatment session since it is not a comfortable procedure for the patient and the effects of treatment often become fully apparent over the following few days. Between sessions the patient is instructed to continue stretching the tendon to maintain length and mobility.

THE RESISTANT TENNIS ELBOW

The short-term relief gained from either injection or physiotherapy is an indication that the causative factors and ideal treatment for tennis elbow still elude us. Injection or physiotherapy seem to work well for uncomplicated tennis elbow of recent onset. The chronic nature of the condition, however, means that most of us do not see patients until the condition is well-established. The disappointing results and recurrence of symptoms indicate that there may be one or more components involved in tennis elbow.

The gradual onset of tennis elbow means that problems can coexist within the elbow joint and surrounding neural structures. Pain may restrict the range of active movement and the relative immobilization may produce an associated capsular pattern in the elbow joint. Similarly, dysfunction at one site can cause dysfunction at others and adverse neural tension can be a primary cause or associated cause with tennis elbow (Yaxley & Jull 1993). A cervical lesion can refer pain into the forearm and mimic tennis elbow, or cervical syndromes can coexist with a lesion at the elbow.

Nerve entrapment at the elbow may be a complication (Noteboom et al 1994, Hartley 1995). The radial nerve divides into its terminal branches at the elbow and the posterior interosseous nerve passes between the deep and superficial head of supinator. The upper edge of the superficial head of supinator is a thickened fibrous band forming a firm arch known as the arcade of Frohse, which provides a possible site for nerve entrapment.

The musculotendinous, neural, neurological and articular components should be assessed in the resistant tennis elbow, although there is little evidence in the literature to confirm that addressing all possible components gives any better results. Some cases of tennis elbow come to surgery, involving tenotomy of the extensor tendons at the lateral epicondyle.

Transverse frictions to the origin of extensor carpi radialis longus from the supracondylar ridge (Cyriax & Cyriax 1983, Cyriax 1984)

Transverse frictions are the recommended treatment at this site. Position the patient with the elbow supported in 90° of flexion and the forearm in supination. Sit facing the patient and place the pad of your thumb against

Figure 6.30 Transverse frictions for tennis elbow, supracondylar ridge.

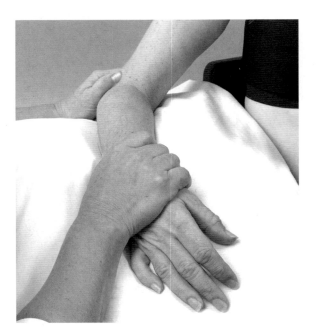

the lower third of the lateral supracondylar ridge (Fig. 6.30). Direct the pressure back against the ridge and impart the transverse frictions in a superoinferior direction. Relative rest is advised where functional movements may continue, but no overuse or stretching until pain-free on resisted testing.

Transverse frictions to the body of the common extensor tendon (Cyriax & Cyriax 1983, Cyriax 1984)

This variety of tennis elbow is less common. The area of tenderness is located in the region of the radial head. Injection of the tendon is controversial and treatment is preferably by transverse frictions.

Figure 6.31   Transverse frictions for tennis elbow, body of the tendon.

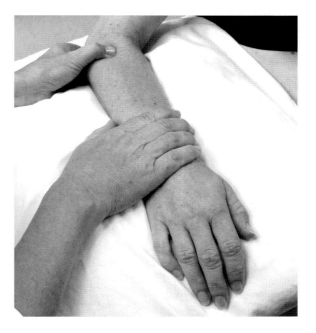

Position the patient with the elbow supported in 90° of flexion and the forearm supported in pronation (Fig. 6.31). Locate the body of the tendon over the radial head. Impart deep transverse frictions across the fibres for 10 min after some analgesia has taken effect. Relative rest is advised where functional movements may continue, but no overuse or stretching until pain-free on resisted testing.

Transverse frictions to the muscle bellies (Cyriax & Cyriax 1983, Cyriax 1984)

The lesion is in the bellies of the common extensor muscles lying deep to the brachioradialis. Treatment by transverse frictions is usually successful.

Figure 6.32   Transverse frictions for tennis elbow, muscle bellies.

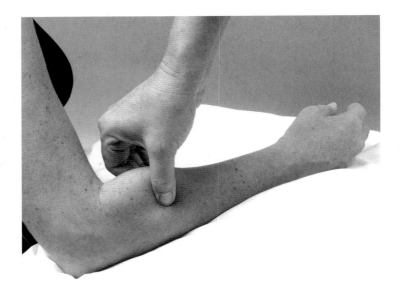

Position the patient with the forearm supported with the elbow flexed to 90° and the forearm in the mid-position (Fig. 6.32). Palpate for the site of the lesion deep to brachioradialis. Grasp the affected muscle fibres between a finger and thumb and impart the transverse frictions by a pinching pressure applied up and down in a superoinferior direction. Relative rest is advised where functional movements may continue, but no overuse or stretching until pain-free on resisted testing.

GOLFER'S ELBOW

Although not as common as tennis elbow, golfer's elbow has a similar presentation, aetiology, disease process and management.

The patient presents with a gradual onset of pain on the medial aspect of the arm. This may radiate distally, but in general it does not project as far as the pain seen in tennis elbow. The pain is aggravated by use and the elbow is often stiff after rest. Onset of symptoms may be associated with occupational overuse, sporting activities (e.g. tennis, bowling, archery) or hobbies (e.g. knitting, needlework) (Rayan 1992, Kurvers & Verhaar 1995). The motion of throwing may cause golfer's elbow as it produces a valgus stress at the elbow which has to be supported by the flexor muscles (Ho 1995). On examination, pain on resisted wrist flexion with the elbow extended reproduces the patient's pain.

The tendons involved in golfer's elbow control movement at two joints and are susceptible to overuse through overload. Stretching, valgus forces and intrinsic forces from muscle contraction all contribute to the condition (Safran 1995). In the degenerative process of golfer's elbow tendinosis is evident rather than the acute inflammatory changes of tendinopathy (Bennett 1994, Patten 1995).

Golfer's elbow, generally speaking, is a less complicated condition to treat than tennis elbow, but coexistent ulnar neuritis (cubital tunnel syndrome) may produce medial elbow pain with tenderness and paraesthesia in the distribution of the ulnar nerve (Kurvers & Verhaar 1995, O'Dwyer & Howie 1995). Some cases of golfer's elbow come to surgery, involving incision of the flexor tendons around the medial epicondyle, denervation of the epicondyle and transposition of the ulnar nerve.

There are two sites for the lesion: teno-osseous site and musculotendinous site.

TREATMENT OF GOLFER'S ELBOW

The common flexor tendon takes origin from the anterior aspect of the medial epicondyle. Palpation will identify the site of the lesion. Treatment may be by either corticosteroid injection or transverse frictions.

> **Injection of golfer's elbow, teno-osseous site** (Cyriax & Cyriax 1983, Cyriax 1984)
>
> Suggested needle size: 25G × ⁵/₈ in (0.5 × 16 mm) orange needle or 23G × 1 in (0.6 × 25 mm) blue needle
> Dose: 10 mg triamcinolone acetonide in a total volume of 1 ml

Teno-osseous site (enthesis)

Position the patient with the elbow supported in extension and fully supinated. Locate the anterior aspect of the medial epicondyle and identify the area of tenderness (Fig. 6.33). Insert the needle perpendicular to the facet and deliver the injection by a peppering technique (Fig. 6.34). Bear in mind the position of the ulnar nerve behind the medial epicondyle. The patient is advised to maintain a period of relative rest for approximately 2 weeks following injection.

Figure 6.33 Injection of golfer's elbow, teno-osseous site.

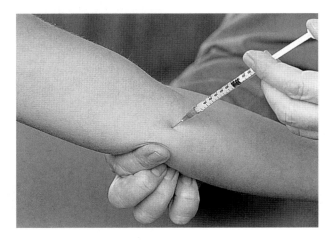

Figure 6.34   Injection of golfer's elbow, teno-osseous site showing direction of approach and needle position.

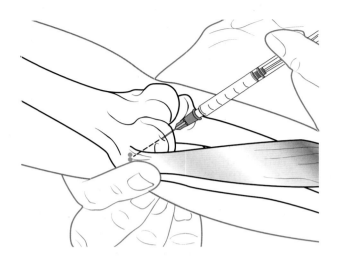

Figure 6.35   Transverse frictions for golfer's elbow, teno-osseous site.

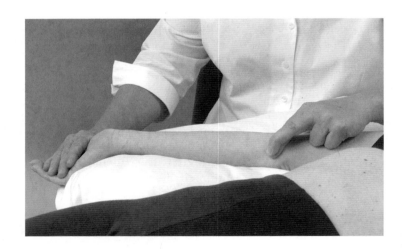

Figure 6.36   Transverse frictions for golfer's elbow, teno-osseous site, to give an indication of the direction of application.

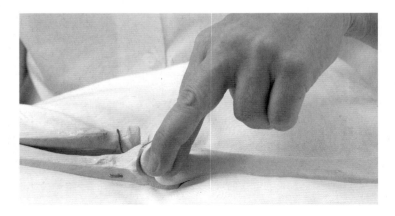

Transverse frictions for golfer's elbow, teno-osseous site (Cyriax & Cyriax 1983, Cyriax 1984)

Position the patient in supine lying with the elbow supported in extension and locate the area of tenderness on the anterior aspect of the medial epicondyle (Fig. 6.35). Using an index finger reinforced by the middle finger, and thumb for counterpressure, impart the transverse frictions by applying the pressure down onto the anterior aspect and sweeping transversely across the fibres (Fig. 6.36). Ten minutes' deep transverse frictions are delivered after the analgesic effect has been achieved. Relative rest is advised where functional movements may continue, but no overuse or stretching until pain-free on resisted testing.

Musculotendinous site

Transverse frictions for golfer's elbow, musculotendinous site

Transverse frictions are considered to be the most effective treatment here (Cyriax & Cyriax 1983, Cyriax 1984). Position yourself and the patient as above and, using the index finger, move 1 cm distally to palpate the musculotendinous junction at the inferior edge of the medial epicondyle (Fig. 6.37). Maintain the pressure against the bone and impart the frictions transversely across the fibres for 10 min after the analgesic effect has been achieved. Relative rest is advised where functional movements may continue, but no overuse or stretching until pain-free on resisted testing.

An alternative position may be used for the application of transverse frictions to both sites. The patient is seated on the treatment couch with the shoulder in lateral rotation, the elbow extended and the forearm fully supinated. The clinician stands alongside and facing the patient to support the elbow in extension. Using the other hand, transverse frictions can then be applied transversely across the fibres at each site (Figs. 6.38 and 6.39).

Figure 6.37   Transverse frictions for golfer's elbow, musculotendinous junction.

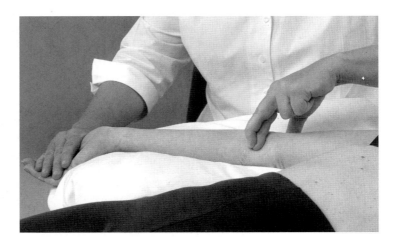

Figure 6.38   Transverse frictions for golfer's elbow, teno-osseous site. (Alternative position)

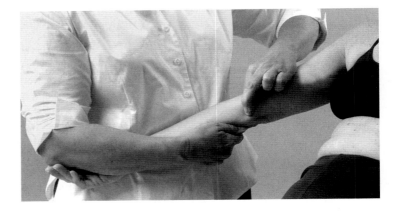

Figure 6.39   Transverse frictions for golfer's elbow, musculotendinous junction. (Alternative position)

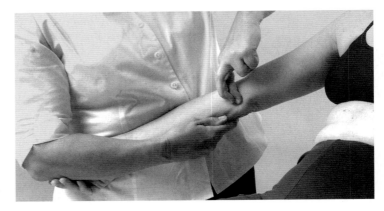

BICEPS

At the elbow, the lesion lies either in the muscle belly or at the insertion onto the radial tuberosity. The patient complains of pain at the elbow on resisted elbow flexion and resisted supination of the flexed elbow. Passive stretching into elbow extension can also cause pain.

Excessive friction may cause inflammation of the subtendinous biceps bursa and differential diagnosis from bicipital tendinopathy may be difficult. A muddled presentation of signs is found, confirming the diagnosis of bursitis. Pain may be reproduced on resisted elbow flexion, passive elbow extension and passive elbow pronation, as the bursa is squeezed against its insertion.

An injection of corticosteroid is the treatment of choice for the insertion of biceps, since the tendon of insertion lies deeply.

Injection of the insertion of biceps at the radial tuberosity (Cyriax & Cyriax 1983, Cyriax 1984)

Suggested needle size: 23G × 1 in (0.6 × 25 mm) blue needle
Dose: 10 mg triamcinolone acetonide in a total volume of 1 ml

Figure 6.40   Injection of biceps insertion at the radial tuberosity.

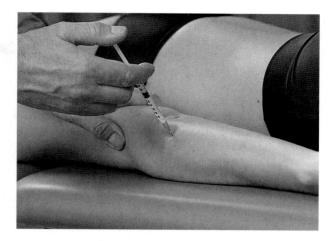

Figure 6.41   Injection of biceps insertion at the radial tuberosity, showing direction of approach and needle position.

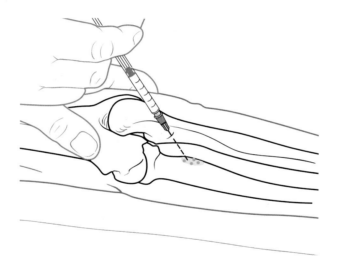

Position the patient in prone lying in the anatomical position. Without changing the position of the glenohumeral joint, carefully pronate the extended forearm keeping your thumb in contact with the radial head to confirm your position. Insert the needle between the radius and ulna approximately 2 cm distal to the radiohumeral joint line until the resistance of the tendon insertion is felt (Fig. 6.40). Deliver the injection by a peppering technique to the tendon and adjacent area if the bursa is also involved (Fig. 6.41) The patient is advised to maintain a period of relative rest for approximately 2 weeks following injection.

Figure 6.42   Transverse frictions to the insertion of biceps at the radial tuberosity

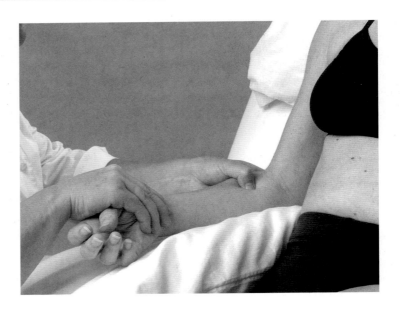

Transverse frictions to the insertion of biceps at the radial tuberosity (Cyriax & Cyriax 1983, Cyriax 1984)

Position the patient with the elbow joint flexed to 90° and supinated. With your thumb, locate the insertion of biceps at the radial tuberosity and apply pressure against it, deeply and laterally (Fig. 6.42) Wrap your fingers around the forearm to provide counterpressure. Deliver the transverse fictions by alternately rotating the patient's forearm between pronation and supination while maintaining the pressure against the radial tuberosity.

If the lesion lies in the muscle belly, the general principles of treatment can be applied (see Ch. 4).

TRICEPS

Distal rupture of the triceps tendon due to forced overload into extension is uncommon. A triceps muscle lesion is also rare, but would present with posterior elbow pain, increased by resisted elbow extension. The general principles of treatment can be applied.

References

Adeniran A, Merriam, W F 1994 Pulled elbow in an adult. Journal of Bone and Joint Surgery 76B:848–849

Akeson W H, Amiel D, La Violette D et al 1968 The connective tissue response to immobility: an accelerated ageing response. Experimental Gerontology 3:289–301

Assendelft W J J, Hay E M, Adshead R et al 1996 Corticosteroid injections for lateral epicondylitis: a systematic overview. British Journal of General Practice 46:209–216

Bennett J B 1994 Lateral and medial epicondylitis. Hand Clinics 10:157–163

Brukner P, Khan K 2002 Clinical sports medicine, 2nd edn., McGraw-Hill, Sydney

Chard M D, Cawston T E, Riley G P et al 1994 Rotator cuff degeneration and lateral epicondylitis: a comparative histological study. Annals of the Rheumatic Diseases 53:30–34

Cook J L, Khan K M, Purdam C R 2001 Conservative treatment of patellar tendinopathy. Physical Therapy in Sport 2:54–65

Coonrad R W, Hooper W R 1973 Tennis elbow: its course, natural history, conservative and surgical management. Journal of Bone and Joint Surgery 55A: 1177–1182

Cyriax J 1982 Textbook of orthopaedic medicine, 8th edn. Baillière Tindall, London, vol 1

Cyriax J 1984 Textbook of orthopaedic medicine, 11th edn. Baillière Tindall, London, vol 2

Cyriax J, Cyriax P 1983 Illustrated manual of orthopaedic medicine. Butterworths, London

Davidson C, Ganion L, Gehlsen G et al 1997 Rat tendon morphologic and functional changes resulting from soft tissue mobilisation. Medicine and Science in Sports and Exercise 29(3):313–319

Drechsler W, Knarr J, Snyder-Mackler L 1997 A comparison of two treatment regimes for lateral epicondylitis: a randomised trial of clinical interventions. Journal of Sport Rehabilitation 6:226–234

Edelson G, Kunos C A, Vigder F et al 2001 Bony changes at the lateral epicondyle of possible significance in tennis elbow syndrome. Journal of Shoulder and Elbow Surgery 10:158–164

Ernst E 1992 Conservative therapy for tennis elbow. British Journal of Clinical Practice 46:55–57

Foley A E 1993 Tennis elbow. American Family Physician 48:281–288

Gabel G T 1999 Acute and chronic tendinopathies at the elbow. Current Opinion in Rheumatology 11(2):138–143

Gehlsen G, Ganion L, Helfst R 1998 Fibroblast responses to variation in soft tissue mobilisation pressure. Medicine and Science in Sports and Exercise 31(4):531–535

Gellman H 1992 Tennis elbow lateral epicondylitis. Orthopedic Clinics of North America 23:75–82

Greenfield C, Webster V 2002 Chronic lateral epicondylitis: survey of current practice in the outpatient departments in Scotland. Physiotherapy 88 (10):578–594

Hardy R H 1978 Pulled elbow. Journal of the Royal College of General Practitioners 28:224–226

Hart L E 2002 Commentary on corticosteroid injections, physiotherapy or a wait-and-see policy for lateral epicondylitis. Clinical Journal of Sport Medicine 12(6):403–404

Hartley A 1995 Practical joint assessment, upper quadrant, 2nd edn. Mosby, London Ho C P 1995 Sports and occupational injuries of the elbow: MR imaging findings. American Journal of Roentgenology 164:1465–1471

Hoppmann R A 1993 Diagnosis and management of common tendinopathy and bursitis syndromes. Journal of the South Carolina Medical Association 89:531–535

Joji S, Murakami T, Murao, T 2001 Osteochondritis dissecans developing in the trochlea humeri: a case report. Journal of Shoulder and Elbow Surgery 10(3):295–297

Katarincic J A, Weiss A-P C, Akelman E 1992 Lateral epicondylitis tennis elbow: a review. Rhode Island Medicine 75:541–544

Kesson M, Atkins E, Davies I 2003 Musculoskeletal injection skills. Butterworth Heinemann, Oxford

Khan K M, Cook J L 2000 Overuse tendon injuries: where does the pain come from? Sports Medicine and Arthroscopic Review 8:17–31

Kohlhaas A R, Roeder J 1995 Tee shirt management of nursemaid's elbow. American Journal of Orthopedics 24:74

Kurvers H, Verhaar, J 1995 The results of operative treatment of medial epicondylitis. Journal of Bone and Joint Surgery 77A:1374–1379

Mills G P 1928 Treatment of tennis elbow. British Medical Journal 1:12–13

Miyasaka K C 1999 Anatomy of the elbow. Orthopaedic Clinics of North America 30(1):1–13

Newcomer K L, Laskowski E R, Idank D M et al 2001 Corticosteroid injection in early treatment of lateral epicondylitis. Clinical Journal of Sports Medicine 11(4):214–222

Nicola T L 1992 Elbow injuries in athletes. Primary Care 19:283–302

Noteboom T, Cruver R, Keller J et al 1994 Tennis elbow: a review. Journal of Orthopaedic and Sports Physical Therapy 19:357–366

O'Dwyer K J, Howie C R 1995 Medial epicondylitis of the elbow. International Orthopaedics 19:69–71

Palastanga N, Field D, Soames R 2002 Anatomy and human movement, 4th edn. Butterworth Heinemann, Oxford

Patten R M 1995 Overuse syndromes and injuries involving the elbow: MR imaging findings. American Journal of Roentgenology 164:1205–1211

Pienimäki T T, Siira P T, Vanharanta H 2002 Chronic medial and lateral epicondylitis: a comparison of pain, disability and function. Archives of Physical Medicine and Rehabilitation 83:317–321

Rayan G M 1992 Archery-related injuries of the hand, forearm and elbow. Southern Medical Journal 85:961–964

Safran M R 1995 Elbow injuries in the athlete. Clinical Orthopaedics and R Related Research 310:257–277

Saunders S 2000 Orthopaedic medicine course manual. Saunders, London

Schnatz P, Steiner C 1993 Tennis elbow: a biomechanical and therapeutic approach. Journal of the American Osteopathic Association 93:778–788

Smidt N, van der Windt D A, Assendelft W J 2002a Corticosteroid injections, physiotherapy or wait-and-see policy for lateral epicondylitis. Clinical Journal of Sport Medicine 12(6):403–404

Smidt N, van der Windt D A, Assendelft W J et al 2002b Interobserver reproducibility of the assessment of severity of complaints, grip strength and pressure pain threshold in patients with lateral epicondylitis. Archives of Physical Medicine and Rehabilitation 83:1145–1150

Smidt N, Assendelft W J, Arola H et al 2003 Effectiveness of physiotherapy for lateral epicondylitis: a systematic review. Annals of Medicine 35(1): 51–62

Sölveborn SA, Buch F, Mallmin H et al 1995 Cortisone injection with anaesthetic additives for radial epicondylalgia tennis elbow. Clinical Orthopaedics and Related Research 316:99–105

Stratford P W, Levy D R, Gauldie S et al 1989 The evaluation of phonophoresis and friction massage as treatments for extensor carpi radialis tendinopathy: a randomised controlled trial. Physiotherapy Canada 41(2):93–99

Vasseljen O 1992 Low level laser versus traditional physiotherapy in the treatment of tennis elbow. Physiotherapy 78:329–334

Verhaar J, Walenkamp G, Kester A et al 1993 Lateral extensor release for tennis elbow. Journal of Bone and Joint Surgery 75A:1034–1043

Verhaar J A N, Walenkamp, G H I M, van Mameren H et al 1996 Local corticosteroid injection versus Cyriax-type physiotherapy for tennis elbow. Journal of Bone and Joint Surgery 78B:128–132

Williams P L 1998 Gray's Anatomy: the anatomical basis of medicine and surgery, 38th edn. Churchill Livingstone, Edinburgh

Yaxley G A, Jull G A 1993 Adverse neural tension in the neural system: a preliminary study of tennis elbow. Australian Physiotherapy 39:15–22

Chapter 7

The wrist and hand

SUMMARY

Repetitive strain injury and work-related upper limb disorder have done much to focus the clinician on the differential diagnosis and causative factors of pain in the wrist and hand.

This chapter takes a pragmatic approach to the identification of specific lesions and suggests localized treatment, which may form a component of overall management. The detailed but relevant anatomy that forms a basis for accurate treatment is presented. Treatment for individual lesions is discussed, with emphasis on the application of principles to less commonly encountered lesions.

ANATOMY

INERT STRUCTURES

The *distal radioulnar joint* is a pivot joint between the head of the ulna and the ulnar notch of the radius. Mechanically linked to the superior radioulnar joint, it is responsible for the movements of pronation (85°) and supination (90°).

A *triangular fibrocartilaginous articular disc* closes the distal radioulnar joint inferiorly and is the main structure uniting the radius and ulna (Palastanga et al 2002). It lies in a horizontal plane, its apex attaching to the ulnar styloid and its base to the lower edge of the ulnar notch of the radius. The disc articulates with the lunate when the hand is in ulnar deviation. It adds to the stability of the joint and acts as an articular cushion for the ulnar side of the carpus, absorbing compression, traction and shearing forces but being prone to degenerative changes (Livengood 1992, Rettig 1994, Wright et al 1994, Steinberg & Plancher 1995).

The movements of pronation and supination rotate the radius around the ulna. Supination is stronger, hence the thread of nuts and screws which are tightened by supination in right-handed people.

There are two rows of carpal bones; on the palmar aspect, from the radial to the ulnar side they are:

scaphoid, lunate, triquetral, pisiform
trapezium, trapezoid, capitate, hamate.

The carpal bones all articulate with their neighbours, except pisiform, which is a separate bone situated on the front of the triquetral. The intercarpal joints are all supported by intercarpal ligaments.

The *wrist joint* proper is a biaxial, ellipsoid joint between the distal end of the radius and the articular disc, and the proximal row of carpal bones. However, the so-called wrist joint complex includes the *midcarpal joint* and has mobility as well as stability, which is important for the function of the hand. Movements are extension (passive, 85°), flexion (passive, 85°), ulnar deviation (passive, 45°) and radial deviation (passive, 15°). The close packed position of the wrist joint is full extension.

The joints are surrounded by a fibrous capsule, lined with synovial membrane and reinforced by collateral ligaments. Both collateral ligaments pass from the appropriate styloid process to the carpal bones on the medial and lateral side of the carpus. A fibrocartilaginous *meniscus* projects into the joint from the ulnar collateral ligament.

The *metacarpophalangeal joints* are ellipsoid; the *interphalangeal joints* are hinge joints. Both are supported by palmar and collateral ligaments and the extensor tendons and digital expansions support the dorsal surfaces of the joints. Flexor tendons are contained within fibrous sheaths which have thickened areas known as pulleys which may provide a restriction, producing 'trigger finger' (see below). At the wrist and in the hand, the tendons are contained within synovial sheaths (Williams 1998).

The *flexor retinaculum*, a strong fibrous band, creates a fibro-osseous passage, the *carpal tunnel*, through which pass the flexor tendons of the digits, the median nerve and vessels. The flexor retinaculum has four points of attachment: the pisiform and hook of hamate medially and the tuberosity of the scaphoid and ridge of trapezium laterally. Its attachment onto the trapezium splits to form a separate compartment for the tendon of flexor carpi radialis. The *median nerve* enters the carpal tunnel deep to palmaris longus. It shares its compartment of the carpal tunnel with nine tendons comprising the four tendons of flexor digitorum superficialis and the four tendons of flexor digitorum profundus and flexor pollicis longus. On leaving the carpal tunnel it supplies the thenar muscles before dividing into four or five digital branches.

The *trapeziofirst-metacarpal joint (first carpometacarpal joint)* is a saddle joint with a loose articular capsule and extensive joint surfaces giving it a wide range of movement. The first metacarpal has been rotated medially for the movement of opposition.

Flexion and extension occur in a plane parallel to the palm of the hand, while abduction and adduction occur in a plane at right angles to the palm of the hand (Fig.7.1 a, b, c, d)

The close packed position of the trapeziofirst-metacarpal joint is strong opposition, when great force is transmitted to the joint. The functionally opposed thumb is subjected to compressive stresses which make the joint vulnerable to degenerative osteoarthrosis.

The *radial artery* passes under abductor pollicis longus and extensor pollicis brevis, crossing the snuffbox obliquely towards the first dorsal interosseous muscle. Its position should be acknowledged so that it can be avoided when injecting the trapeziofirst-metacarpal joint.

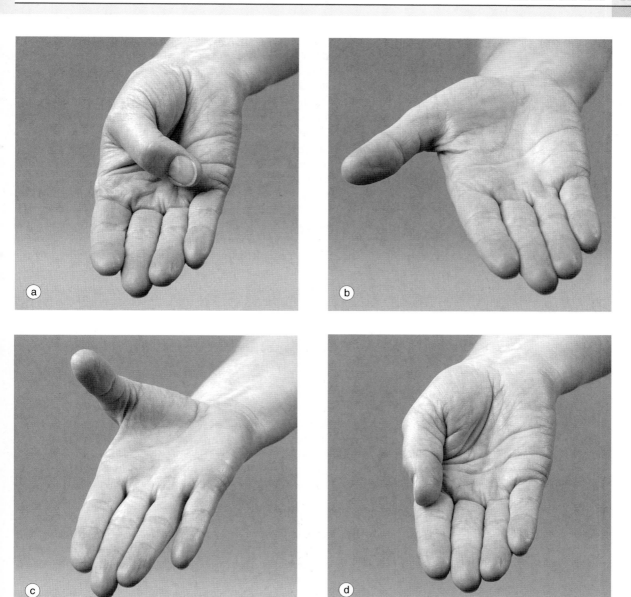

Figure 7.1   Movements of the
metacarpophalangeal joint
of the thumb a) flexion
b) extension c) abduction
d) adduction

CONTRACTILE STRUCTURES

Flexor carpi radialis (median nerve C6–C7) is the most lateral superficial flexor tendon. It passes through its own fibro-osseous compartment on the lateral side of the carpal tunnel, to insert into the base of the second and third metacarpals.

Palmaris longus (median nerve C7–C8) passes over, not under, the flexor retinaculum, to attach to the distal part of the flexor retinaculum and the palmar aponeurosis.

Flexor digitorum superficialis (median nerve C7–C8, T1) lies medial to palmaris longus, but is not as visible because it lies on a slightly deeper plane. In the carpal tunnel the four tendons are contained within the same synovial sheath, with tendons to the third and fourth fingers lying superficial to those to the second and fifth. The tendons divide to provide a passage for flexor digitorum profundus, before continuing onto insert either side of the middle phalanx.

Flexor carpi ulnaris (ulnar nerve C7–C8) is the most medial superficial flexor tendon and can be easily traced onto its insertion into pisiform. The tendon sends slips onwards as the pisohamate and pisofifth-metacarpal ligaments. The pisohamate ligament converts the space between pisiform and the hamate into a tunnel (tunnel of Guyon) for the passage of the ulnar vessels and nerves.

Flexor pollicis longus (median nerve C8, T1) passes through the lateral side of the carpal tunnel and inserts into the palmar aspect of the base of the distal phalanx of the thumb.

Flexor digitorum profundus (medial part supplied by the ulnar nerve; lateral part supplied by the median nerve C8, T1) divides into four tendons which lie deep to superficialis in the carpal tunnel. They pass through tunnels created by superficialis and attach to the distal phalanx of each finger.

The *lumbricals* are four small muscles which arise from the flexor digitorum profundus tendons and pass to the radial side of the dorsal digital expansions of each finger. With attachments that link flexor and extensor tendons, they function by flexing the metacarpophalangeal joints and extending the interphalangeal joints. The first two lumbricals are supplied by the median nerve, the third and fourth by the ulnar nerve, C8, T1.

Extensor carpi radialis longus (radial nerve C6–C7) and *extensor carpi radialis brevis* (posterior interosseous nerve C7–C8) pass deep to the tendons of abductor pollicis longus and extensor pollicis brevis, under the extensor retinaculum, to attach to the radial side of the base of the second and third metacarpals respectively.

Extensor digitorum (posterior interosseous nerve C7–C8) divides into four tendons which pass under the extensor retinaculum to insert into the dorsal digital expansions of the fingers.

Extensor digiti minimi (posterior interosseous nerve C7–C8) inserts into the dorsal digital expansion of the little finger.

Extensor carpi ulnaris (posterior interosseous nerve C7–C8) lies in a groove between the head of the ulna and the styloid process, under the extensor retinaculum. It attaches to the medial side of the base of the fifth metacarpal.

Abductor pollicis longus and *extensor pollicis brevis* (posterior interosseous nerve C7–C8) become tendinous and superficial in the lower forearm where they cross the tendons of extensor carpi radialis longus and brevis at the intersection point, a site of potential friction. They occupy the same synovial sheath in the first compartment of the extensor retinaculum and form the lateral border of the anatomical snuffbox. The abductor inserts into the base of the first metacarpal and the extensor into the base of the proximal phalanx. Because of its position, abductor pollicis longus has been considered both anatomically and functionally a radial deviator of the wrist (Elliott 1992a).

Extensor pollicis longus (posterior interosseous nerve C7–C8) deviates around the ulnar side of the dorsal tubercle of the radius, to pass to the base of the distal phalanx of the thumb. It forms the medial border of the anatomical snuffbox.

Extensor indicis (posterior interosseous nerve C7–C8) joins the ulnar side of the extensor digitorum tendon, passing to the index finger.

The *dorsal interossei* (ulnar nerve C8, T1) are four bipennate muscles arising from adjacent sides of the metacarpal bones and inserting into the dorsal digital expansion and base of the proximal phalanx of the appropriate finger. They are responsible for abducting the fingers from the midline of the middle finger.

The *palmar interossei* (ulnar nerve C8, T1) are four smaller muscles originating from the palmar aspect of the metacarpal bones and inserting into the dorsal digital expansions of the appropriate finger. They are responsible for adducting the fingers towards the middle finger.

GUIDE TO SURFACE MARKING AND PALPATION

PALMAR ASPECT
(Fig. 7.2)

Look for three creases (not distinct in everyone) on the palmar aspect of the lower forearm. The distal wrist crease joins pisiform and the tubercle of the scaphoid, the bones at the heel of the hand (Backhouse & Hutchings 1990), marking the proximal border of the flexor retinaculum.

Figure 7.2 Palmar aspect of the wrist showing position of the flexor retinaculum, its adjacent tendons and nerves.

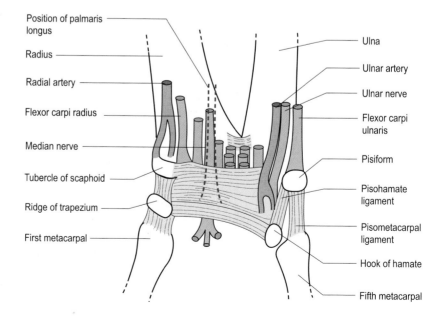

Position of palmaris longus
Radius
Radial artery
Flexor carpi radius
Median nerve
Tubercle of scaphoid
Ridge of trapezium
First metacarpal

Ulna
Ulnar artery
Ulnar nerve
Flexor carpi ulnaris
Pisiform
Pisohamate ligament
Pisometacarpal ligament
Hook of hamate
Fifth metacarpal

Figure 7.3   Bones of the hand. From Anatomy and Human Movement by N Palastanga D Field and R Soames. Reprinted by permission of Elsevier Ltd.

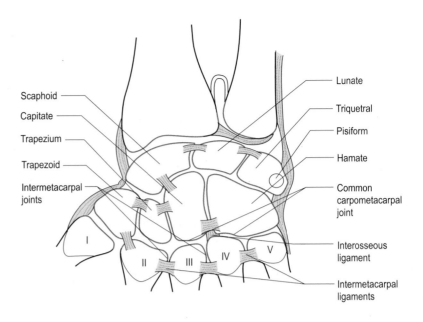

The middle crease joins the two styloid processes, marking the position of the wrist joint line, while the proximal crease (if present) marks the proximal extent of the flexor tendon sheaths.

Consider the position of the bones which make up the two rows of carpal bones (Fig. 7.3). From the radial to the ulnar side, an easy way to remember the order is:

simply learn the parts	scaphoid, lunate, triquetral, pisiform
that the carpus has	trapezium, trapezoid, capitate, hamate

Palpate the **radial and ulnar styloid processes** at the wrist; the radial styloid extends slightly more distally than the ulnar styloid.

Palpate **pisiform**, the pea-shaped sesamoid bone, which lies at the base of the hypothenar eminence, giving insertion to flexor carpi ulnaris.

Move a thumb approximately 1.5 cm distally and diagonally from pisiform, in the direction of the web between the thumb and index finger. Lying roughly in line with the ring finger is the **hook of hamate**. Palpate deeply and tenderness will confirm its presence.

Radially deviate the wrist to make the **tuberosity of the scaphoid** more prominent. It lies at the base of the thenar eminence, close to the tendon of flexor carpi radialis. Move a thumb from the tuberosity of the scaphoid, diagonally and distally approximately 1 cm, to lie in line with the index finger, and feel the **ridge of trapezium** through the bulk of the thenar eminence. It is best felt with the wrist joint in extension and is tender to deep palpation.

Joining the four points described above – pisiform, hook of hamate, tuberosity of scaphoid and ridge of trapezium – gives the position of the *flexor retinaculum*, which is approximately the size of the width of your thumb (Fig. 7.2).

Identify the superficial forearm flexor tendons as they cross the palmar aspect of the wrist from the radial to ulnar side. *Flexor carpi radialis* is the most lateral tendon. *Palmaris longus* passes over the flexor retinaculum and can be brought into prominence by opposing the thumb and little finger with the wrist flexed. *Flexor digitorum superficialis*, lying in a deeper plane, may not be readily palpable, but *flexor carpi ulnaris* can be followed down to its insertion onto the pisiform.

Palpate for the *radial pulse* on the palmar aspect of the lower radius lateral to flexor carpi radialis. The *ulnar pulse* can be palpated on the lower ulna, lateral to flexor carpi ulnaris.

Consider the position of the *median nerve* as it enters the carpal tunnel deep to palmaris longus. If palmaris longus is absent, oppose the thumb and little finger and the midline crease produced gives the position of the median nerve.

DORSAL ASPECT
(Fig. 7.4)

Pronate the forearm and the *head of the ulna* can be seen as a rounded elevation in the distal forearm. Palpate to the ulnar side of the head and feel the tendon of *extensor carpi ulnaris* in the groove between the head of the ulna and the *styloid process*.

Palpate the *inferior radioulnar joint* line, which lies approximately 1.5 cm laterally from the ulnar styloid. Confirm its presence by passively gliding the head of the ulna on the radius and feeling the joint line.

Figure 7.4   Dorsal aspect of the wrist.

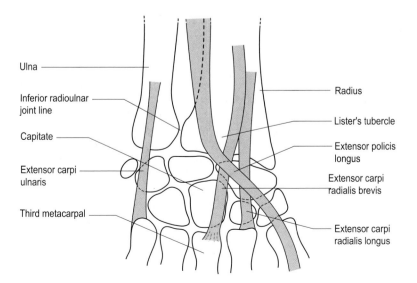

Ulna

Inferior radioulnar joint line

Capitate

Extensor carpi ulnaris

Third metacarpal

Radius

Lister's tubercle

Extensor policis longus

Extensor carpi radialis brevis

Extensor carpi radialis longus

On the lower end of the radius, palpate the *dorsal tubercle (of Lister)* lying roughly in line with the index finger. The tubercle is grooved on either side by the passing tendons. *Extensor carpi radialis longus and brevis* pass on its lateral side, while *extensor pollicis longus* passes on its medial side before taking a 45° turn laterally, where it can be traced to its insertion into the base of the distal phalanx of the thumb.

The *capitate* is the largest carpal bone and is roughly the size of the patient's thumb nail. It is wider dorsally and is roughly peg-shaped. It is situated in the centre of the carpus, articulating mainly with the third metacarpal distally, the trapezoid laterally, the hamate medially and the concavity formed by the scaphoid and lunate proximally (Steinberg & Plancher 1995, Williams 1998). To locate the position of the capitate, run your finger proximally down the shaft of the third metacarpal with the wrist in slight flexion and drop over the end into the shallow depression.

Place the wrist in flexion with the thumb relaxed to allow the tendon of extensor pollicis longus to fall out of the way and to expose the base of the metacarpals. Now palpate the insertions of *extensor carpi radialis longus and brevis* onto the radial side of the base of the second and third metacarpals respectively. The extensor carpi radialis brevis is probably the easier of the two to feel. Palpate the insertion of extensor carpi ulnaris onto the medial side of the base of the fifth metacarpal.

LATERAL ASPECT (Fig. 7.5)

Pronate the forearm and make a fist. The fleshy elevation seen at the distal end of the radius is formed by the musculotendinous junctions of *abductor pollicis longus and extensor pollicis brevis* as they wind around the lower radius, crossing over the tendons of extensor carpi radialis longus and brevis at the intersection point.

Locate the *anatomical snuffbox* (by extending the thumb) which is bordered by the tendons of abductor pollicis longus and extensor pollicis brevis laterally and by extensor pollicis longus medially. Palpate the *radial styloid* at the proximal end of the anatomical snuffbox and the trapeziofirst-metacarpal joint at the distal end.

Locate the tendons of abductor pollicis longus and extensor pollicis brevis; sometimes a V-shaped gap may be appreciated between the two.

Move the wrist into ulnar deviation and the scaphoid can be palpated distal to the radial styloid; it moves with the hand, whereas the radial styloid does not. The scaphoid can be grasped between your thumb posteriorly in the base of the snuffbox and your index finger anteriorly.

Move distally to palpate the trapezium lying between the scaphoid and the base of the first metacarpal.

Palpate the *trapeziofirst-metacarpal joint* line by running a thumb down the shaft of the first metacarpal into the anatomical snuffbox. Flex and extend the joint to check its location.

Palpate the *first dorsal interosseous* in the web between index finger and thumb; it can be made more prominent by resisting abduction of the index finger.

Figure 7.5   Tendons on the lateral aspect of the wrist.

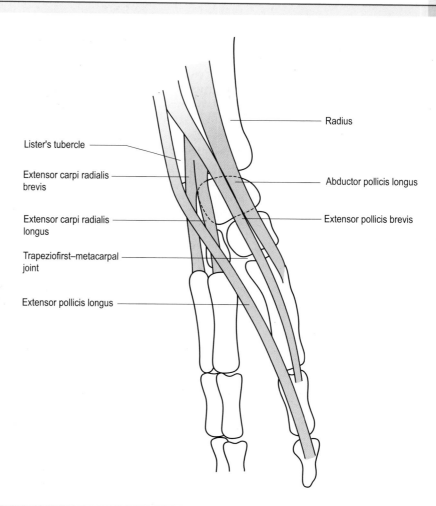

- Radius
- Lister's tubercle
- Extensor carpi radialis brevis
- Abductor pollicis longus
- Extensor carpi radialis longus
- Extensor pollicis brevis
- Trapeziofirst–metacarpal joint
- Extensor pollicis longus

COMMENTARY ON THE EXAMINATION

OBSERVATION

Before proceeding with the history, a general observation of the patient's *face, posture and gait* will alert the examiner to serious abnormalities or injuries. The painful hand may be held in an antalgic position, resting with the fingers parallel to each other and in a degree of flexion, the thumb in a neutral position. Possibly, the arm swing may be absent from the gait pattern and the hand held stiffly against the side. Difficulty with fine movement may be observed during undressing, indicating a problem with dexterity.

HISTORY (SUBJECTIVE EXAMINATION)

The *age, occupation, sports, hobbies and lifestyle* of the patient may give an indication of the cause and a possible diagnosis, since most problems in the lower forearm involve arthritis, trauma or overuse.

The *site* of pain is usually well-localized by the patient, with little *spread*, since these are peripheral joints and structures lying at the end of their respective dermatomes, with little scope for reference. The presence of paraesthesia or any apparent reference of pain may suggest a more proximal lesion, and all proximal joints must be examined, including the cervical spine. A fractured scaphoid gives localized pain and point tenderness in the anatomical snuffbox, while X-ray investigation may not show evidence of the fracture for several weeks (Livengood 1992).

The *onset* of the symptoms may be due to trauma, overuse or arthritis. If the onset is traumatic in nature, the possibility of fracture should be eliminated. Frequently, a direct injury involving a fall on the outstretched hand may cause fracture of the scaphoid or subluxation of the capitate or lunate bones, and may also cause a traumatic arthritis with soft tissue swelling and contusion. Indirect injury may also occur from a rotational force or maximal effort in racket sports (Rettig 1994).

Most injuries at the wrist and hand develop from repetitive overuse. Tendinopathy may result from frequent overstretching or unaccustomed activity. An overuse syndrome occurs when the level of repeated microtrauma exceeds the tissue's ability to adapt (Rettig 1994). Tensional overload or abnormal shear stresses can cause microtrauma at any point in the musculotendinous or ligamentous unit. The syndromes of carpal tunnel and de Quervain's (see below) may be associated with more proximal lesions, such as nerve entrapment or lesions of the cervical spine.

A hyperextension injury to the thumb is a relatively common sporting injury, producing a traumatic arthritis in either the trapeziofirst-metacarpal joint or the metacarpophalangeal joint. This may occur in skiing ('skier's thumb') or sports which involve ball-catching, e.g. volleyball, netball or goal-keeping in football.

Arthritis in the hand may be inflammatory, degenerative or traumatic. Rheumatoid arthritis is common in the smaller joints and therefore readily affects the joints of the wrist and hand where deformity is characteristic; it is usually bilaterally symmetrical. Any synovial space can be involved, including the tendon sheaths and bursae, as well as the joints. Juvenile chronic arthritis has less symmetrical joint involvement than adult rheumatoid arthritis.

Primary degenerative osteoarthrosis affects the trapeziofirst-metacarpal joints and the distal interphalangeal joints more readily. These joints are subjected to stress in the functional position and are used through all extremes of range, predisposing them to primary arthritis. Secondary degenerative osteoarthrosis can affect any joint.

The *duration* of symptoms indicates the stage of the lesion in the inflammatory process. Overuse syndromes have a gradual onset with symptoms present for many months. Rheumatoid arthritis and acute episodes of degenerative osteoarthrosis tend to have periods of remission and exacerbation while traumatic lesions may be of fairly short duration.

The *symptoms and behaviour* need to be considered. The behaviour of the pain indicates the nature of the lesion, with mechanical lesions eased by rest and aggravated by activity. Overuse lesions are worsened by repetition of the mechanism of trauma. The nature of the pain is also important: is it localized or vaguely diffuse, deep or superficial, sharp, burning, aching, constant or intermittent, getting worse or better, or staying the same?

The other symptoms described by the patient could include

paraesthesia. An accurate description of these associated symptoms is relevant to the source of pressure or nerve entrapment. The distribution of pins and needles and whether or not they possess edge and/or aspect helps to determine their origin. Stiffness of the hand may be relevant to arthritis or ligamentous lesions and it is therefore appropriate to know the daily pattern of the symptoms. Heat, coldness, sweating, dryness and other sensory changes may also be relevant, suggesting the vasomotor changes of Raynaud's disease or reflex sympathetic dystrophy.

An indication of *past medical history, other joint involvement and medications* will establish whether contraindications to treatment techniques exist.

INSPECTION

Fracture or dislocation commonly occurs with a fall on the outstretched hand and shows obvious *bony deformity* and *swelling*. Subluxation, e.g. of the capitate, may be seen as a bump on the dorsum of the hand with the wrist in flexion.

Deformities of the fingers are commonly associated with rheumatoid arthritis or may result from forced hyperextension injuries, as in wicket keepers, for example. If an extensor tendon is avulsed or torn from the distal phalanx, a mallet finger occurs with flexion of the distal interphalangeal joint. This can be associated with sporting injuries or may simply occur if the finger is forcibly caught, while making the bed, for example. A bony swelling of the distal interphalangeal joint is a characteristic deformity known as a Heberden's node, associated with primary degenerative osteoarthrosis.

Degenerative osteoarthrosis of the trapeziofirst-metacarpal joint produces a capsular pattern which may draw the thumb into a position of flexion and medial rotation with bony osteophytes obvious at the base of the thumb. Dupuytren's contracture is a deformity with contraction of the palmar fascia, causing flexion of principally the ring and little fingers. Clubbed fingers may be indicative of systemic disease.

Colour changes, which may indicate circulatory involvement, should be further investigated by palpating for the arterial pulses. The fingers, in particular, can give clues to serious underlying pathology and the colour and shape of the fingers and nails should be noted. Bruising may be apparent, resulting from direct trauma and may be associated with abrasions on the palm due to a fall on the outstretched hand.

Muscle wasting may be obvious in the flattening of the thenar muscles, producing the ape-like hand with the thumb moving back in line with the other fingers. This indicates involvement of the median nerve in the carpal tunnel or possibly cervical nerve root pressure. Similarly, the ulnar nerve or lower cervical nerve root compression involves the hypothenar eminence and if the intrinsic muscles are involved, a claw hand develops. Involvement of the radial nerve affects the wrist extensors and produces a dropped wrist.

Swelling indicates active inflammation and the wrist may be fixed in the mid-position due to the presence of a joint effusion. Contusions with swelling are due to direct trauma. Excessive friction of the skin causes callus and blister formation, e.g. rowing and gymnastics. Ganglia are mucus-filled cysts, which are commonly seen around the wrist, particularly on the dorsum of the hand. They are common between the second and fourth decades of life (Smith & Wernick 1994) and if symptomatic may be burst or require surgical excision. Rheumatoid nodules may be present.

PALPATION

Since these are peripheral joints, palpation for signs of activity is conducted. Temperature changes are assessed and **heat** indicates an active inflammation, while cold may indicate circulatory problems (Fig. 7.6). It may be appropriate to palpate the ulnar and/or radial pulse (Fig.7.7). **Synovial thickening** is usually palpated on the dorsum of the wrist (Fig. 7.8). **Swelling** is usually observed around the wrist where it may be fusiform, unilateral or bilateral. Other swellings, such as nodules or ganglia, can be palpated to assess whether they are hard or soft.

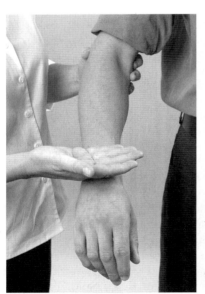

Figure 7.6   Palpation for heat.

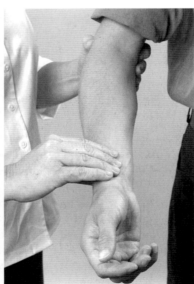

Figure 7.7   Palpation for radial pulse

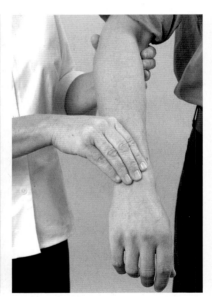

Figure 7.8   Palpation for synovial thickening.

STATE AT REST

Before any movements are performed, the state at rest is established to provide a baseline for subsequent comparison.

The suggested sequence for the objective examination will now be given, followed by a commentary including the reasoning in performing the movements and the significance of the possible findings.

Inferior Radioulnar Joint

- Passive pronation (Fig. 7.9)
- Passive supination (Fig. 7.10)

Wrist Joint

- Passive flexion (Fig. 7.11)
- Passive extension (Fig. 7.12)
- Passive ulnar deviation (Fig. 7.13)
- Passive radial deviation (Fig. 7.14)
- Resisted flexion (Fig. 7.15)
- Resisted extension (Fig. 7.16)
- Resisted ulnar deviation (Fig. 7.17)
- Resisted radial deviation (Fig. 7.18)

Trapeziofirst–Metacarpal Joint

- Passive extension and adduction (Fig. 7.19)
- Resisted flexion (Fig. 7.20)
- Resisted extension (Fig. 7.21)
- Resisted abduction (Fig. 7.22)
- Resisted adduction (Fig. 7.23)

Interossei

- Resisted finger abduction (Fig. 7.24) for the dorsal interossei
- Resisted finger adduction (Fig.7.25) for the palmar interossei

Palpation

- Once a diagnosis has been made, the structure at fault is palpated for the exact site of the lesion

Fingers:

- Passive and resisted testing of the fingers is not performed

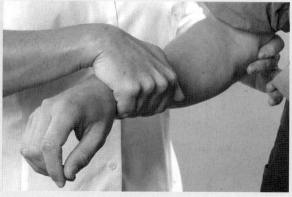

Figure 7.9   Passive pronation.

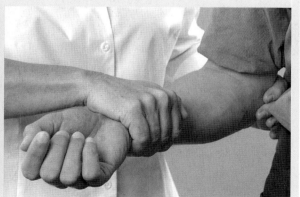

Figure 7.10   Passive supination.

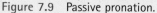

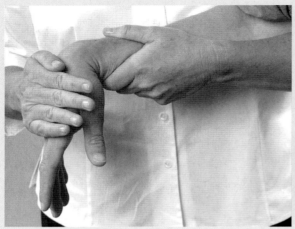

Figure 7.11   Passive flexion.

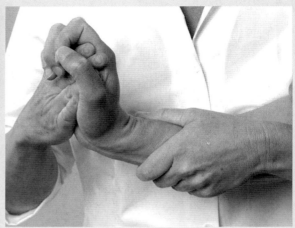

Figure 7.12   Passive extension.

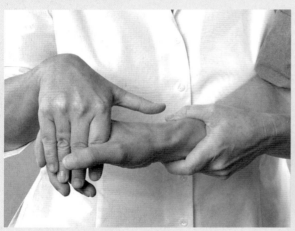

Figure 7.13   Passive ulnar deviation.

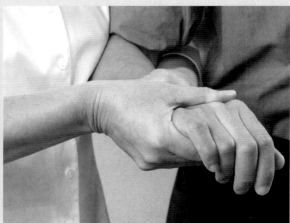

Figure 7.14   Passive radial deviation.

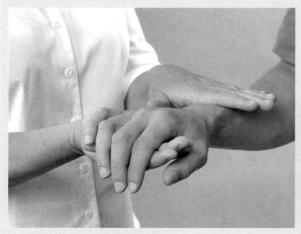

Figure 7.15   Resisted flexion.

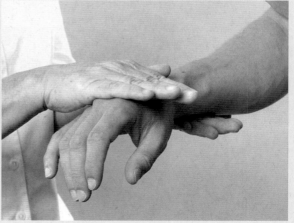

Figure 7.16   Resisted extension.

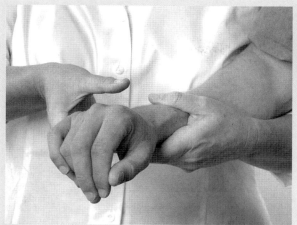

Figure 7.17   Resisted ulnar deviation.

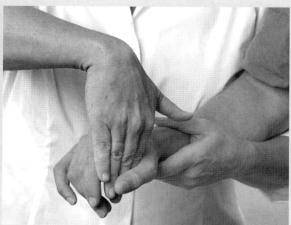

Figure 7.18   Resisted radial deviation.

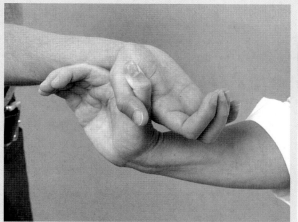

Figure 7.19   Passive extension and adduction of the thumb.

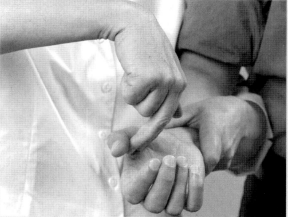

Figure 7.20   Resisted thumb flexion.

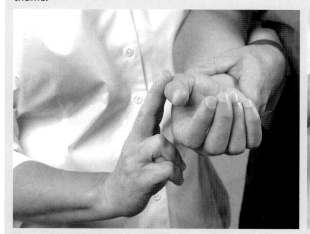

Figure 7.21   Resisted thumb extension.

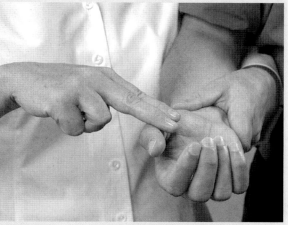

Figure 7.22   Resisted thumb abduction.

Figure 7.23   Resisted thumb adduction.

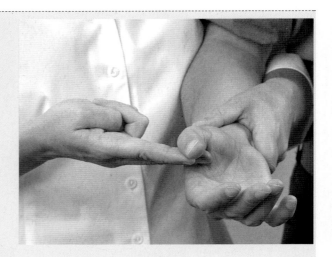

Figure 7.24   Resisted finger abduction for dorsal interossei.

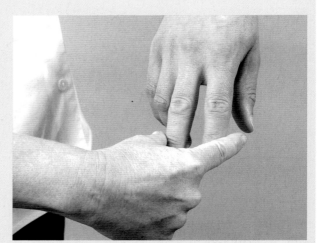

Figure 7.25   Resisted adduction for palmar interossei.

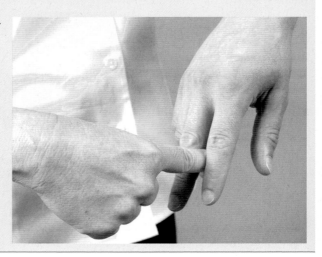

The inferior radioulnar joint gives pain felt at the wrist and is assessed using two passive movements, passive pronation and supination, looking for pain, range of movement, end-feel and the presence of the capsular pattern. Both rotations normally have an elastic end-feel.

The wrist joint is then assessed by four passive movements, looking for pain, range of movement and end-feel. Passive flexion normally has an elastic end-feel due to tissue tension and passive extension a hard end-feel, while both deviations normally display an elastic end-feel. The presence of the capsular pattern indicates the existence of arthritis; the non-capsular pattern may be due to a subluxed carpal bone, e.g. the capitate, or collateral ligament strain.

The contractile structures at the wrist are then assessed by resisted tests looking for pain and power. A positive finding requires palpation of the appropriate anatomical structure to establish the exact site of the lesion. The trapeziofirst-metacarpal joint is assessed by passive application of one combined movement, passive extension and adduction, which is always painful if the capsular pattern is present.

The contractile structures around the thumb are assessed by resisted tests looking for pain and power. Resisted flexion assesses flexor pollicis longus, resisted extension assesses extensor pollicis longus and brevis, resisted abduction assesses abductor pollicis longus and resisted adduction assesses adductor pollicis.

The interossei are assessed by two resisted tests looking for pain and power. Resisted finger abduction assesses the dorsal interossei and resisted finger adduction assesses the palmar interossei.

Passive and resisted movements of the fingers are not part of the routine examination, but included if necessary. Passive movements may establish the capsular patterns described below.

CAPSULAR LESIONS

The presence of the capsular pattern at the joints indicates arthritis. Rheumatoid arthritis more readily affects the smaller joints and is seen as symmetrical involvement of the joints in the wrist and hand with deformity characteristic of the condition. Primary degenerative osteoarthrosis affects the trapeziofirst-metacarpal and distal interphalangeal joints more readily. The thumb may be flexed towards the palm of the hand by the contracted anterior joint capsule and the distal interphalangeal joints of the fingers may show the characteristic Heberden's nodes. Trauma may produce traumatic arthritis and fracture of a carpal bone should be eliminated.

Arthritis in the wrist and hand responds to corticosteroid injection. An alternative treatment for the trapeziofirst-metacarpal joint is described.

INFERIOR (DISTAL) RADIOULNAR JOINT

The inferior radioulnar joint is most commonly affected by rheumatoid arthritis.

> **Injection of the inferior radioulnar joint** (Cyriax & Cyriax 1983, Cyriax 1984)
>
> Suggested needle size: 23G × 1 in (0.6 × 25 mm) blue needle
> Dose: 10 mg triamcinolone acetonide in a total volume of 1 ml

---

Capsular pattern of the inferior radioulnar joint
- Pain at end of range of both rotations.

Position the patient with the forearm supported in full pronation. Identify the inferior radioulnar joint line and insert the needle, which may need to be angled, into the joint (Fig. 7.26). Give the injection as a bolus once intracapsular (Fig. 7.27). The patient is advised to maintain a period of relative rest for approximately 2 weeks following injection.

Figure 7.26   Injection of the lower radio-ulnar joint.

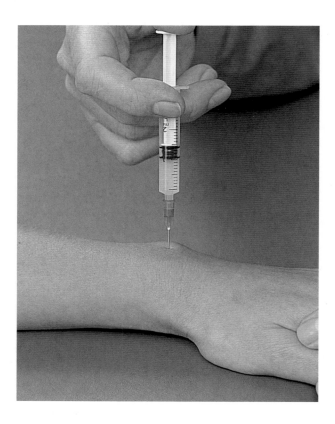

Figure 7.27   Injection of the lower radio-ulnar joint showing direction of approach and needle position.

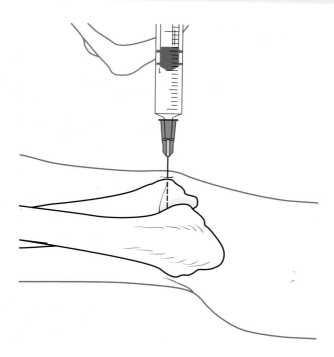

WRIST JOINT

The wrist joint is most commonly affected by rheumatoid arthritis and traumatic arthritis.

> **Injection of the wrist joint**
>
> Suggested needle size: 23G × 1 in (0.6 × 25 mm) blue needle
> Dose: 20 mg triamcinolone acetonide in a total volume of 3 ml

> **Capsular pattern of the wrist joint**
> - Equal limitation of flexion and extension.
> - Eventual fixation in the mid-position.

Position the patient with the wrist supported and the forearm in full pronation (Fig. 7.28). Locate a point of entry which may be at either side of the extensor carpi radialis brevis tendon.

Give the injection as a bolus once the needle is intracapsular (Fig. 7.29). Alternatively, in the rheumatoid wrist, or if degeneration is sufficient to prevent access to the joint, make two or three needle insertions and pepper the area of synovial thickening with a series of withdrawals and reinsertions. This technique is not comfortable for the patient. The patient is advised to maintain a period of relative rest for approximately 2 weeks following injection.

Figure 7.28   Injection of the wrist joint.

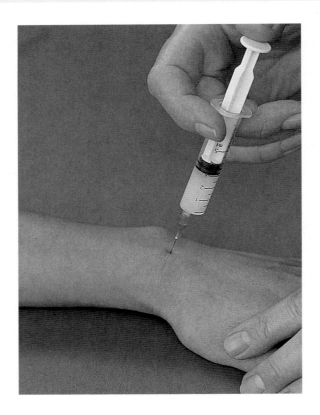

Figure 7.29   Injection of the wrist joint showing direction of approach and needle position.

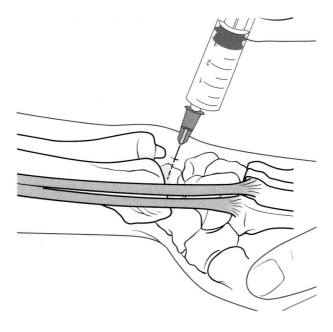

TRAPEZIOFIRST–METACARPAL JOINT

Capsular pattern of the trapeziofirst–metacarpal joint
- Most limitation of extension.

The patient complains of pain and tenderness at the base of the thumb and on using the thumb under compression, e.g. writing, gripping. It is a condition common in middle-aged women (Livengood 1992) and X-ray confirms the diagnosis. An axial compression test applies longitudinal pressure down the shaft of the first metacarpal to grind the articular surfaces together. If positive, it confirms the diagnosis of arthritis and differentiates the condition from de Quervain's tenosynovitis (see below).

Confirmation of the capsular limitation can be made by asking the patient to put the hands into the prayer position and spreading the thumbs, comparing the two sides.

Injection of the trapeziofirst–metacarpal joint (Cyriax & Cyriax 1983, Cyriax 1984)

Suggested needle size: 25G × ⁵/₈ in (0.5 × 16 mm) orange needle
Dose: 10 mg triamcinolone acetonide in a total volume of 0.5 ml

Position the patient with the hand resting comfortably. The patient can apply a degree of distraction to the affected thumb (Fig. 7.30). Identify the joint line by running your thumb down the first metacarpal into the anatomical snuffbox to locate the joint line. Insert the needle into the joint and give the injection as a bolus (Fig. 7.31). Alternatively, if the thenar eminence is flattened, identify the joint line anteriorly. In either case, osteophyte formation may make the injection difficult. The patient is advised to maintain a period of relative rest for approximately 2 weeks following injection.

Figure 7.30   Injection of the trapeziofirst-metacarpal joint.

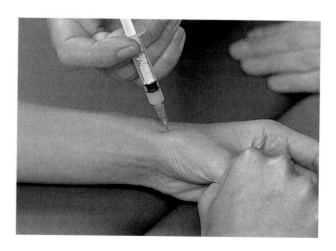

Figure 7.31   Injection of the trapeziofirst-metacarpal joint showing direction of approach and needle position.

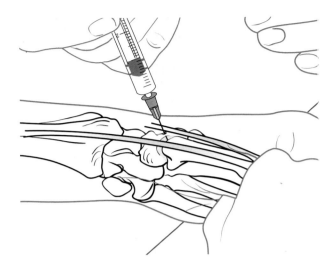

Transverse frictions to the anterior capsular ligament of the trapeziofirst-metacarpal joint (Cyriax & Cyriax 1983, Cyriax 1984)

Place the thumb comfortably into extension and adduction. Apply deep transverse frictions with the thumb or index finger reinforced by the middle finger (Fig. 7.32). Direct the friction down onto the anterior capsular ligament and apply the sweep transversely across the fibres. Maintain the technique for 10 min after achieving an analgesic effect. The principles for stretching capsular adhesions can be applied, e.g. Grade B mobilization, and distraction is a useful technique to apply to this joint.

Figure 7.32   Transverse frictions to the anterior capsular ligament of the trapeziofirst-metacarpal joint.

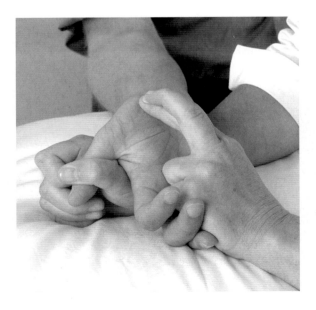

FINGER JOINTS

Injection of the finger joints

Suggested needle size: 25G × ⁵/₈ in (0.5 × 16 mm) orange needle
Dose: 5–10 mg triamcinolone acetonide in a total volume of 0.5–0.75 ml

Capsular pattern of the finger joints
- Slightly more limitation of flexion than extension.

Identify the affected joint. With knowledge of the position of the tendons and ligaments around it, find a point of convenient access, usually on the dorsal aspect avoiding the digital expansions (Figs 7.33 and 7.35). Angle the needle obliquely and, once intra-articular, give the injection as a bolus (Figs 7.34 and 7.36). The patient is advised to maintain a period of relative rest for approximately 2 weeks following injection.

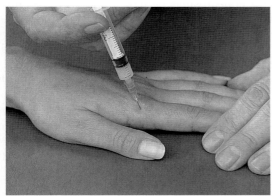

Figure 7.33   Injection of the metacarpophalangeal joint.

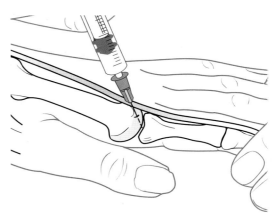

Figure 7.34   Injection of the metacarpophalangeal joint showing direction of approach and needle position.

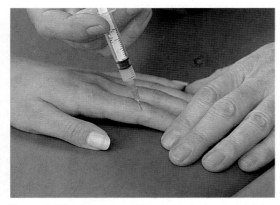

Figure 7.35   Injection of the interphalangeal joint.

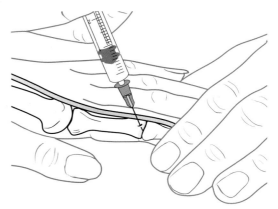

Figure 7.36   Injection of the interphalangeal joint showing direction of approach and needle position.

NON–CAPSULAR LESIONS

SUBLUXED CARPAL BONE

The capitate is particularly prone to dorsal subluxation or displacement because it is roughly peg-shaped, with its dorsal surface slightly wider than its palmar surface. The lunate sits between scaphoid and triquetral, and the lower end of the radius and the articular disc, and may displace anteriorly when the wrist is forced into extension (Norris 1998). Posterior displacements may also occur.

Either bone may displace, but commonly it is the capitate. The mechanism of injury involves a fall on the outstretched hand or repeated compression through the extended wrist, as occurs in gymnastics, for example, causing the capitate to displace dorsally. The patient may complain of pain and limited movement and may be concerned about the bump seen on the dorsum of the hand. Occasionally a subluxed capitate may have been present for a long duration when there is less chance of successful relocation.

On examination there is a non-capsular pattern. Passive extension is painful and limited by a bony block. Passive flexion can usually achieve full range, but the patient experiences pain at the end of range. A bony bump may be obvious on passive flexion, but this should not be confused with the base of the third metacarpal which is also prominent. Diagnosis is dependent upon the appropriate history and the presence of the non-capsular pattern.

The principle of treatment applied here is to relocate the carpal bone by a thrust applied to the capitate under strong traction. This is a mobilization technique performed under strong traction, not a manipulation at the end of range. The technique for the capitate mobilization will be explained below, but this can be adapted if another carpal bone is displaced.

Reduction of the capitate (Saunders 2000)

Locate the capitate by running a thumb down the shaft of the third metacarpal to its base and onto the adjacent displaced capitate (Fig. 7.37). Place one thumb, reinforced by the other, on top of the capitate (Fig. 7.38), and wrap your fingers comfortably around the patient's thenar and hypothenar eminences (Fig. 7.39).

Placing your little finger into the web between the patient's thumb and index finger will prevent you from flexing the patient's wrist during the technique.

Position the patient's proximal row of carpal bones level with the edge of the couch. Instruct an assistant to fix this proximal row of carpal bones with the web of the hand parallel to the edge of the couch and reinforced with the other hand, to give counterpressure (Fig. 7.40).

Place your feet directly under the patient's hand and lean back to apply strong traction (Fig. 7.41). Allow this traction to establish for a few seconds to separate the two rows of carpal bones. Apply a sharp thrust downwards on the capitate to assist its relocation.

Re-examine the patient to assess the results and repeat if necessary.

If pain persists after relocation, the ligaments surrounding the capitate may be treated with deep transverse frictions (Fig. 7.42 a,b).

Figure 7.37   Palpating for the
capitate bone at the base of
the third metacarpal.

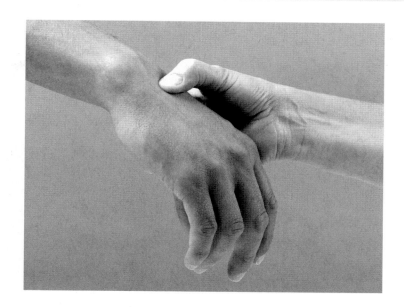

Figure 7.38   Thumb position
for the reduction of the
capitate.

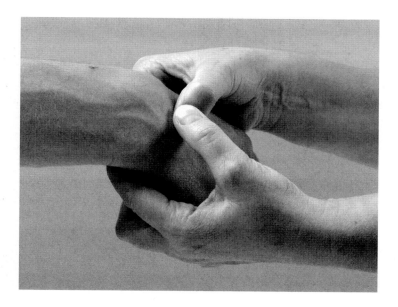

Figure 7.39   Finger position for the reduction of the capitate.

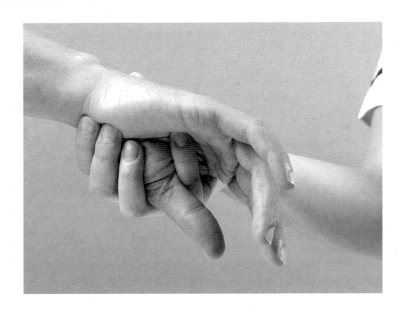

Figure 7.40   Assistant's hand position for the reduction of the capitate.

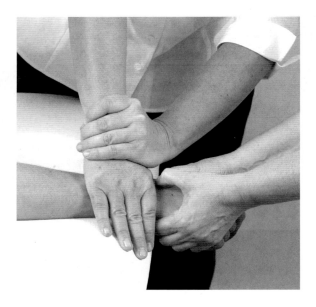

Figure 7.41   Body position for the reduction of the capitate.

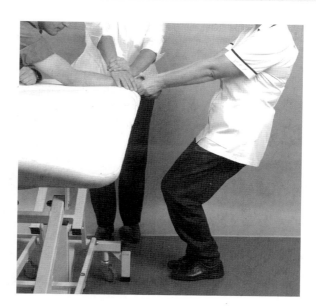

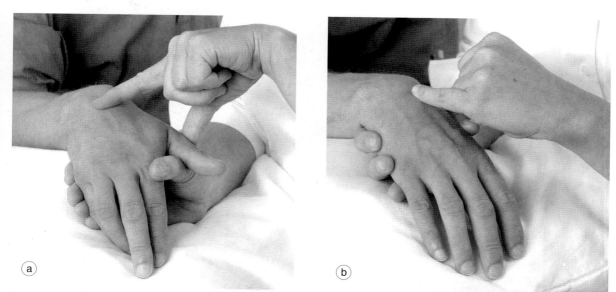

Figure 7.42   Transverse frictions to the capitate ligaments: (a) horizontal for vertical fibres and (b) vertically for horizontal fibres.

COLLATERAL LIGAMENTS AT THE WRIST JOINT

The collateral ligaments may be sprained by a traumatic overstretching of the joint in the appropriate direction to stress the ligament, or by repetitive microtrauma due to overuse. The patient complains of localized pain, and stretching the ligament by passive movement in the opposite direction reproduces this pain. The ligament is tender to palpation.

Radial collateral ligament sprain produces pain on passive ulnar deviation and a sprained ulnar collateral ligament produces pain on passive radial deviation. Either lesion may be treated by applying the principles of corticosteroid injection using a peppering technique, or by deep transverse frictions, having placed the hand in a suitable position to gain access to the ligament (Figs 7.43–7.48).

The patient is advised to maintain a period of relative rest for approximately 2 weeks following injection.

Injection of the collateral ligaments

Suggested needle size: 25G × ⁵/₈ in (0.5 × 16 mm) orange needle
Dose: 10 mg triamcinolone acetonide in a total volume of 0.5 ml

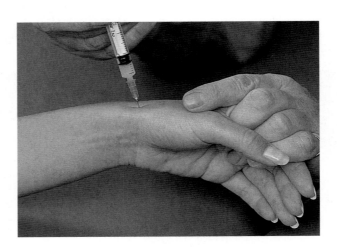

Figure 7.43   Injection of the radial collateral ligament.

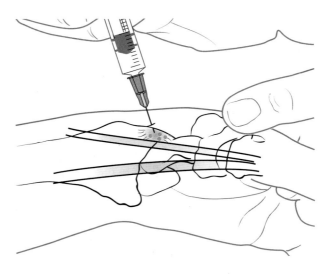

Figure 7.44   Injection of the radial collateral ligament showing direction of approach and needle position.

Figure 7.45   Injection of the ulnar collateral ligament.

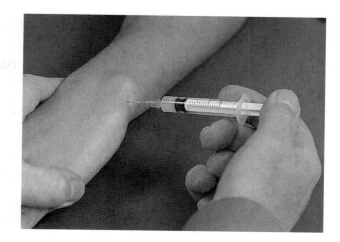

Figure 7.46   Injection of the ulnar collateral ligament showing direction of approach and needle position.

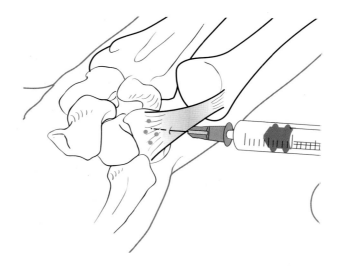

Figure 7.47   Transverse frictions to the radial collateral ligament.

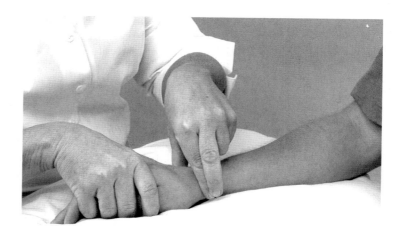

Figure 7.48   Transverse frictions to the ulnar collateral ligament.

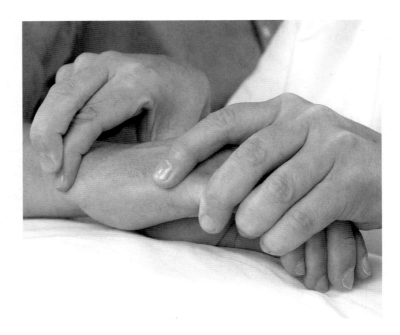

CARPAL TUNNEL SYNDROME

The mechanism of the lesion is uncertain, but involves some compression of the median nerve in the carpal tunnel. Mechanical and vascular factors are believed to be involved, with inflammation increasing the size of structures lying within the tunnel, causing swelling and compression, with scarring affecting the perineural vasculature (Anderson & Tichenor 1994). The muscles of the thenar eminence may be affected by denervation, abductor pollicis brevis in particular, causing the thumb to fall back into line with the other digits and flattening of the thenar eminence.

Anything which reduces the already tight space in the tunnel compresses the nerve. Intrinsic factors include inflammation and swelling of any structure within the tunnel, or reduction of the size of the tunnel itself: tenosynovitis, hypothyroidism, diabetes mellitus, pregnancy and obesity, rheumatoid arthritis and acromegaly (Kumar & Clark 2002). External factors include trauma, pressure, repetitive occupational or leisure activities, repeated gripping or squeezing, excessive vibration from heavy machinery, keyboard use, knitting, woodworking, using power tools, or racket sports. It occurs more commonly in women between the ages of 40 and 60 (Norris 1998).

The presenting symptoms and signs of carpal tunnel syndrome are variable. The patient usually complains of an aching, burning sensation, with tingling or numbness of the finger tips. Paraesthesia is experienced in the radial three and a half digits on the palmar surface. About 70% of patients experience numbness at night and 40% complain of pain radiating proximally into the lower forearm with simultaneous paraesthesia felt in the fingers (Smith & Wernick 1994). The symptoms may wake patients at night and they may gain relief by shaking or rubbing the hands (Cailliet 1990). Patients may complain of a loss of dexterity and sensitivity, with clumsiness of hand function.

On examination, flattening of the thenar eminence may be observed if median nerve compression has occurred. Objective sensory loss may be found in prolonged cases of compression with weakness of the thenar muscles, especially abductor pollicis brevis, if the motor branch is involved.

Tinel's sign and Phalen's test are usually used to confirm diagnosis, although it should be recognized that these tests are not perfect diagnostic indicators. False-negative and false-positive rates have been reported of between 25 and 50%. Nerve conduction studies show diminished nerve velocity across the wrist in 90% of patients who go onto have proven nerve compression at surgery (Smith & Wernick 1994).

Tinel's sign for median nerve compression in the carpal tunnel involves tapping the flexor retinaculum. It is positive if pins and needles are elicited in the radial three and a half digits (Hoppenfeld 1976, Hartley 1995).

Phalen's test applies compression to the median nerve in the carpal tunnel, achieved by maintaining maximum wrist flexion. The test is positive if pins and needles are reproduced. A normal hand would develop tingling if this position were maintained for 10 min or more; a patient with carpal tunnel syndrome will report the onset of pain, numbness and tingling within 1–2 min. If symptoms are not reproduced within 3 min the test may be considered to be negative (Hoppenfeld 1976, Cailliet 1990, Vargas Busquets 1994, Hartley 1995).

The 'link test' can be applied to assess muscle strength; the thumb and individual fingers are opposed in turn and the examiner attempts to break the link, which should be impossible if the patient possesses normal muscle power.

Examination of the cervical spine and neural tension testing should be conducted if there is any suspicion that the lesion lies more proximally.

Treatment of carpal tunnel syndrome

The causative factors should be discussed with the patient and attempts made to avoid repetitive actions. Symptomatic relief may be gained from a corticosteroid injection. The patient may be fitted with a wrist support splint to wear at night, to avoid flexion. If injection is unsuccessful or relief is short-term only, surgical release of the flexor retinaculum may be considered. Significant weakness of the thenar muscles will usually be an indication for surgery.

Injection of the carpal tunnel (Cyriax & Cyriax 1983, Cyriax 1984)

Suggested needle size: 23G × 1 in or 1 1/4 in (0.6 × 25/30 mm) blue needle
Dose: 20 mg triamcinolone acetonide

Position the patient with the wrist supported in extension. Choose a point of entry between the distal and middle wrist creases on the ulnar side of palmaris longus. If palmaris longus is absent, oppose the thumb

Figure 7.49   Injection of the carpal tunnel.

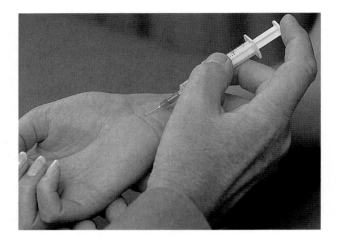

Figure 7.50   Injection of the carpal tunnel showing direction of approach and needle position.

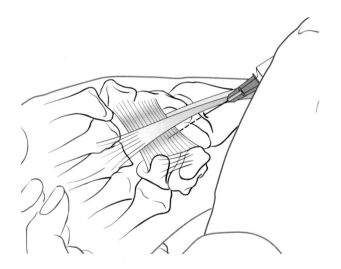

and little finger to produce a midline crease as a guide and keep to the ulnar side (Fig 7.49). Angle the needle parallel to and between the flexor tendons, until it is under the flexor retinaculum, and give the injection as a bolus within the tunnel (Fig. 7.50). Be careful to check that there is no paraesthesia before injecting to avoid injury to the median nerve. The patient is advised to maintain a period of relative rest for approximately 2 weeks following injection.

FIBROCARTILAGE TEARS AND MENISCAL LESIONS

A triangular fibrocartilaginous disc is related to the distal radioulnar joint inferiorly and a fibrocartilaginous meniscus projects into the wrist joint from the ulnar collateral ligament. These intra-articular structures are prone to degenerative changes, tears and occasionally displacement.

Trauma, such as a fall on the outstretched hand or repetitive joint over-loading, can cause degeneration and tears. Central or radial tears are the most common (Rettig 1994).

A mechanical lesion involving tear or displacement of any part of the intra-articular complex presents with pain and clicking felt on the ulnar side of the wrist. On examination the clicking may be appreciated by the examiner palpating the wrist while simultaneously pronating and supinating the forearm. Passive ulnar deviation may reproduce the pain, and point tenderness may be felt just distal to the ulnar styloid. To confirm diagnosis of a mechanical lesion of the intra-articular complex, the wrist is placed into extension and ulnar deviation and axial compression is applied to the ulnar side of the wrist while the wrist is passively circumducted.

Treatment may involve strong distraction to reduce possible displacement, or the patient may be referred for arthroscopy and excision.

TRIGGER FINGER OR THUMB

Trigger finger or thumb is a snapping phenomenon producing a painful catch as a flexor tendon is caught at a thickened pulley of the sheath during flexion and then released during forced extension (Smith & Wernick 1994, Murphy et al 1995). Palmar trauma or irritation can cause thickening of the tendon, sheath or annular pulley and a palpable nodule may exist. Some 35% of cases involve the flexor pollicis longus tendon and 50% involve the middle or ring finger flexor tendons (Smith & Wernick 1994). The condition may be secondary to systemic disease such as rheumatoid arthritis or diabetes mellitus.

Treatment by corticosteroid injection may be curative, restoring painless, smooth full range of movement to the digit (Murphy et al 1995).

Injection of trigger finger or thumb

Suggested needle size: 25G × 5/8 in (0.5 × 16 mm) orange needle
Dose: 10 mg triamcinolone acetonide in a total volume of 0.5 ml

Identify the area of thickening and deliver the injection by a peppering technique (Figs 7.51 and 7.52). The patient is advised to maintain a period of relative rest for approximately 2 weeks following injection.

Figure 7.51 Injection for trigger finger.

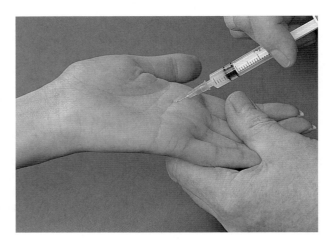

Figure 7.52 Injection for trigger finger showing direction of approach and needle position.

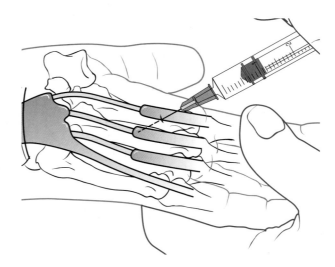

CONTRACTILE LESIONS

Tendinopathy at the teno-osseous junction of a tendon and tenosynovitis affecting the tendon in its sheath, as it runs under either the flexor or extensor retinacula, are common lesions found at the wrist and hand. Overuse is the most likely cause of the lesion, which may be a simple tendinopathy, tendinosis or tenosynovitis of a single unit, or part of an overall more complex syndrome known as repetitive strain injury or work-related upper limb disorder.

Tendinopathy at the teno-osseous junction can be treated by injection using a peppering technique or transverse frictions.

Tenosynovitis can be treated by transverse frictions applied with the tendon on a stretch to restore the gliding function of the tendon sheath, graded according to the irritability or severity of the lesion, or corticosteroid injection delivered between the tendon and its sheath. All sites are subjected to relative rest from overusing or aggravating factors following treatment.

Common contractile lesions will be discussed.

DE QUERVAIN'S TENOSYNOVITIS

This condition, originally described in 1895, is a commonly seen tenosynovitis involving the tendons of abductor pollicis longus and extensor pollicis brevis in the first extensor compartment at the wrist (Elliott 1992a, Livengood 1992, Rettig 1994, Klug 1995).

Uncomplicated inflammation of the shared synovial sheath is known as de Quervain's tenosynovitis. If the shared sheath is thickened due to scarring associated with chronic inflammation it becomes stenotic (Marini et al 1994); it is then known as de Quervain's stenosing tenosynovitis. Occasionally a ganglion is associated with the condition, especially if it is chronic (Tan et al 1994, Klug 1995).

Women are more commonly affected and the condition may be bilateral in up to 30% of patients (Klug 1995). Onset is occasionally due to direct trauma but more usually due to repetitive occupational or leisure activities. Shea et al (1991) reported a case of de Quervain's tenosynovitis associated with repeated gear-shifting in a mountain bike rider. Gout or rheumatoid arthritis may be associated conditions and Chen & Eng (1994) described a case of early tuberculous tenosynovitis mimicking de Quervain's tenosynovitis.

Pain is felt on the radial side of the wrist with point tenderness over the radial styloid. Pain is aggravated by movements into ulnar deviation, forced flexion/adduction of the thumb and wringing movements of the hand, especially into ulnar deviation. Crepitus may be audible during movements of the wrist.

On examination a local, thickened swelling may be obvious, especially to palpation (Anderson & Tichenor 1994), with the pain reproduced on resisted thumb abduction and extension. Passive movements of the thumb also reproduce the pain as the tendon is pushed or pulled through the thickened, inflamed sheath.

The axial grind test for arthritis of the trapeziofirst-metacarpal joint should be negative in de Quervain's tenosynovitis.

Finkelstein's test, placing the patient's thumb in the palm of the hand and positioning the hand into ulnar deviation produces excruciating pain over the radial styloid. If positive it is pathognomic of de Quervain's tenosynovitis (Shea et al 1991, Livengood 1992, Elliott 1992b, Rettig 1994).

The treatment of choice for de Quervain's stenosing tenosynovitis is a corticosteroid injection. Weiss et al (1994) compared the use of corticosteroid and lidocaine (lignocaine) to splinting alone and established better results in the injection group. If the symptoms are not completely cleared, the injection may be repeated.

Injection for de Quervain's tenosynovitis

Suggested needle size: 25G × ⁵/₈ in (0.5 × 16 mm) orange needle
Dose: 10 mg triamcinolone acetonide in a total volume of 1 ml

Position the patient in sitting, with the wrist supported, holding the thumb in a degree of flexion and the wrist in ulnar deviation and slight extension. Identify the tendons of abductor pollicis longus and extensor pollicis brevis and the V-shaped gap between them at the base of the first metacarpal. Insert the needle between and parallel to the two tendons (Fig. 7.53). Give the injection as a bolus into the shared sheath (Fig. 7.54). If the injection has been correctly placed a slight swelling will be seen around the tendons. The patient is advised to maintain a period of relative rest for approximately 2 weeks following injection.

Figure 7.53   Injection for de Quervain's tenosynovitis.

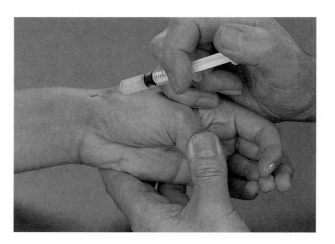

Figure 7.54   Injection for de Quervain's tenosynovitis showing direction of approach and needle position.

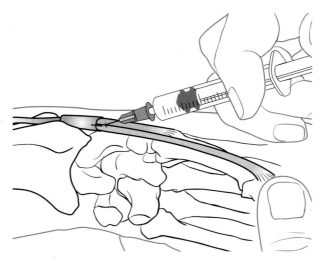

Transverse frictions for de Quervain's tenosynovitis

Alternatively, deep transverse frictions may be applied. Place the thumb into flexion and ulnar deviation at the wrist, to put the tendons on the stretch (Fig. 7.55). Direct the frictions down onto the tendons using two fingers side by side and sweep transversely across the fibres. Apply 10 min of deep transverse frictions after the analgesic effect is achieved. Relative rest is advised where functional movements may continue, but no overuse or stretching until pain-free on resisted testing. A splint to support the thumb in the resting position may be helpful.

Figure 7.55 Transverse frictions for de Quervain's tenosynovitis.

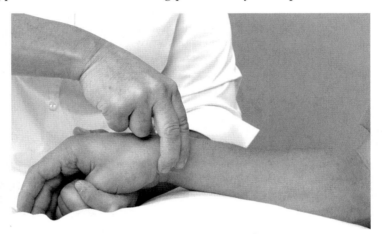

As de Quervain's tenosynovitis is a chronic lesion, it may form part of a syndrome involving occupational overuse and it may be necessary to include a full examination of the cervical spine and upper limb, including neural tension. All components of the condition should be treated appropriately.

INTERSECTION SYNDROME OR OARSMAN'S WRIST

The intersection point between two sets of tendons (abductor pollicis longus/extensor pollicis brevis and extensor carpi radialis longus/brevis) occurs at a point on the radius approximately 4 cm proximal to the wrist (Livengood 1992, Klug 1995). It is a point of potential friction between the structures as they exert tension in different directions. This could produce tenosynovitis of the tendons as they pass under the extensor retinaculum or, more commonly, inflammation of the musculotendinous junction in the lower forearm.

Cyriax (1982) referred to this as myosynovitis with crepitation of the muscle bellies, a condition which occasionally also affects the tibialis anterior muscle. Brukner & Khan (2002) attribute the condition to bursitis between the two sets of tendons. The condition is provoked by overuse and the patient presents with acute pain and the classical signs of inflammation, heat, redness, swelling and disturbed function. Crepitation is usually audible on movement, but objective testing is difficult due to restriction by pain.

Transverse frictions for intersection syndrome

Treatment begins immediately with protection, rest and ice to control pain and inflammation. Assuming the condition is due to tenosynovitis, gentle transverse frictions are given, ideally on a daily basis, and the patient usually recovers relatively quickly.

Position the patient comfortably on a pillow. Identify the area of tenderness, which is obvious on the lower radial aspect of the forearm. Place a thumb along the length of the painful tendons and by abduction and adduction of the thumb or pronation and supination of your forearm, impart the frictions transversely across the fibres (Fig. 7.56). Begin gently to achieve the analgesic effect, then follow this with approximately six good sweeps to produce movement. Relative rest is advised where functional movements may continue, but no overuse or stretching until pain-free on resisted testing. This condition is commonly provoked by overuse and the patient may need instruction in manual handling tasks and activity modification.

Figure 7.56   Transverse frictions for intersection syndrome.

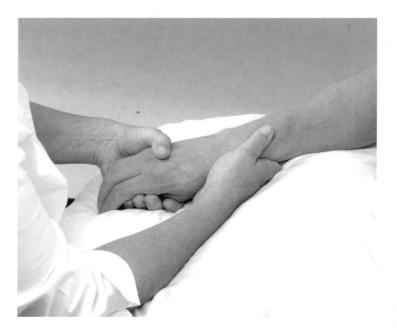

Injection of tendon lesions

Suggested needle size: 25G × ⁵/₈ in (0.5 × 16 mm) orange needle
Dose: 10 mg triamcinolone acetonide in a total volume of 1 ml
given as a bolus between the tendon and its sheath
given by peppering technique at the teno-osseous junction

Extensor carpi ulnaris tendinopathy

After de Quervain's, tenosynovitis of extensor carpi ulnaris is the next most common tenosynovitis at the wrist (Klug 1995). Tenosynovitis or tendinopathy at the teno-osseous junction is usually due to repetitive overuse, sometimes occurring in the non-dominant hand of the tennis player who uses a double-handed backhand when the take back involves an extreme position of ulnar deviation (Rettig 1994).

Direct trauma may cause subluxation of the tendon from the groove between the head of the ulna and the styloid process (Livengood 1992, Rettig 1994). The patient complains of pain and clicking on the ulnar side of the wrist. When the extended wrist is actively taken from radial to ulnar deviation, the subluxation of the tendon can be observed and this will help differentiate the condition from a triangular fibrocartilage or meniscal lesion.

Treatment applies the techniques of corticosteroid injection, either injecting between the tendon and sheath in tenosynovitis or peppering the insertion at the base of the fifth metacarpal (Figs 7.57 and 7.58). Alternatively, transverse frictions can be used, with the tendon on the stretch in tenosynovitis (Fig. 7.59) and against the insertion for the teno-osseous junction.

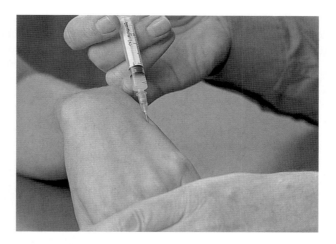

Figure 7.57   Injection for extensor carpi ulnaris at teno-osseous site.

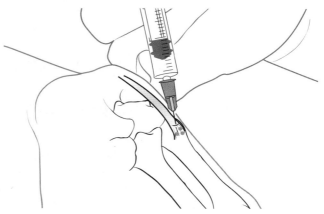

Figure 7.58   Injection for extensor carpi ulnaris at teno-osseous site showing direction of approach and needle position.

Figure 7.59   Transverse frictions for extensor carpi ulnaris tenosynovitis.

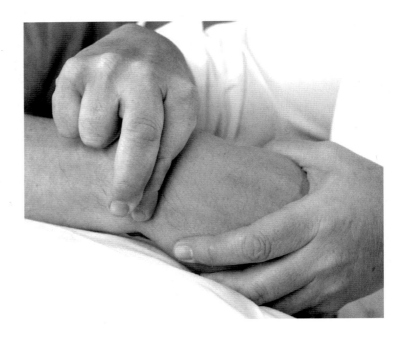

EXTENSOR CARPI RADIALIS LONGUS AND BREVIS TENDINOPATHY

The lesion is usually at the teno-osseous junction where it is due to repetitive overuse, or it may be associated with a bony metacarpal protuberance or boss (Rettig 1994, Bergman 1995). Pain is felt on resisted wrist extension and resisted radial deviation.

The principles of corticosteroid injection or transverse frictions are applied to treat the lesion. Position the patient with the wrist in flexion to expose the base of the metacarpals and to allow the long extensor tendon to the thumb to fall out of the way. Identify the site of the lesion by palpation at the radial side of either the base of the second or third metacarpals (Fig. 7.60). Deliver the corticosteroid injection by a peppering technique (Fig. 7.61), or direct the transverse frictions down on to the insertion and sweep transversely across the fibres (Fig. 7.62).

Figure 7.60   Injection for extensor carpi radialis longus or brevis tendons at teno-osseous site.

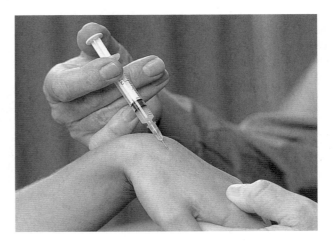

Figure 7.61 Injection for extensor carpi radialis longus or brevis tendons at teno-osseous site showing direction of approach and needle position.

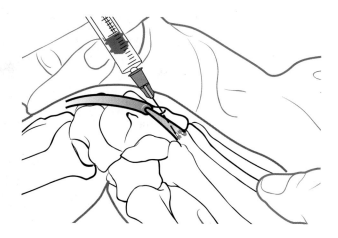

Figure 7.62 Transverse frictions to extensor carpi radialis longus or brevis tendons at teno-osseous site.

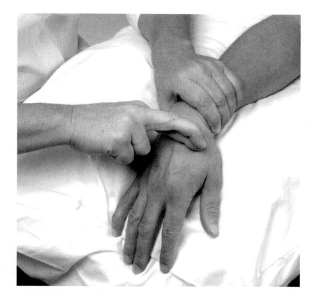

FLEXOR CARPI ULNARIS TENDINOPATHY

Insertional tendinopathy can occur proximal or distal to the teno-osseous junctions at the pisiform. Treatment consists of a corticosteroid injection delivered by a peppering technique into the lesion (Figs 7.63 and 7.64) or transverse frictions.

Remember the position of the ulnar nerve, lying just lateral to the tendon, so that you can avoid it if injecting.

If applying transverse frictions at the proximal site, direct your thumb down onto pisiform (Fig. 7.65). With the patient's little finger flexed, to relax the hypothenar eminence, apply transverse frictions to the distal site (Fig. 7.66). Sweep transversely across the fibres at either site.

Figure 7.63 Injection for flexor carpi ulnaris tendinopathy, proximal site.

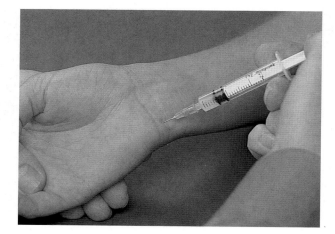

Figure 7.64 Injection for flexor carpi ulnaris tendinopathy, proximal site, showing direction of approach and needle position.

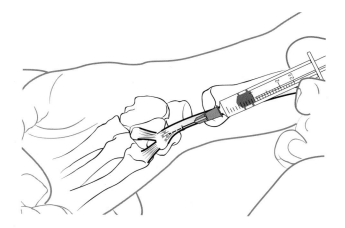

Figure 7.65 Transverse frictions to flexor carpi ulnaris tendinopathy, proximal site.

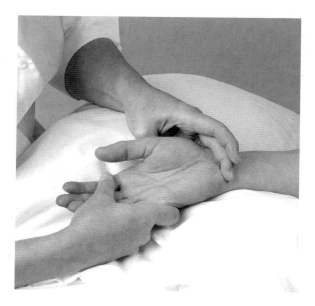

Figure 7.66 Transverse frictions to flexor carpi ulnaris tendinopathy, distal site.

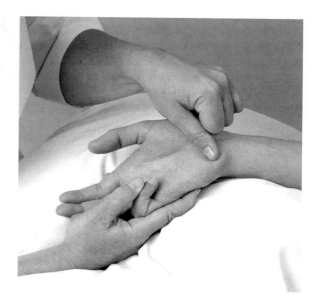

INTEROSSEOUS MUSCLE LESIONS

Strain of the dorsal interossei more commonly affects musicians and tennis players, for example. The patient presents with a vague pain at the metacarpophalangeal joint or between the metacarpals which is exacerbated by repeated gripping (Rettig 1994). Pain will be reproduced by resisted abduction of the appropriate finger.

The treatment of choice is transverse frictions. Palpation will determine the site, but it is often from the origin of the interosseous muscle on one metacarpal. Direct your pressure against the metacarpal and perform the sweep parallel to the shaft (Fig. 7.67).

Figure 7.67 Transverse frictions to the dorsal interossei.

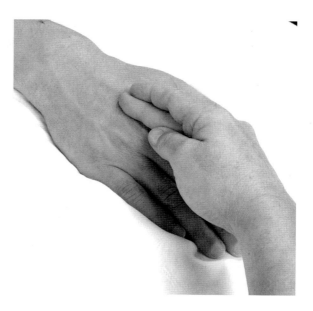

References

Anderson M, Tichenor C J 1994 A patient with de Quervain's tenosynovitis: a case study report using an Australian approach to manual therapy. Physical Therapy 74:314–326

Backhouse K M, Hutchings R T 1990 A colour atlas of surface anatomy – clinical and applied. Wolfe Medical, London

Bergman A G 1995 Synovial lesions of the hand and wrist. MRI Clinics of North America 3:265–279

Brukner P, Khan K 2002 Clinical sports medicine. McGraw Hill, Sydney

Cailliet R 1990 Soft tissue pain and disability, 2nd edn. F A Davis, Philadelphia

Chen W-S, Eng H-L 1994 Tuberculous tenosynovitis of the wrist mimicking de Quervain's disease. Journal of Rheumatology 21:763–765

Cyriax J 1982 Textbook of orthopaedic medicine, 8th edn. Baillière Tindall, London, vol 1

Cyriax J 1984 Textbook of orthopaedic medicine, 11th edn. Baillière Tindall, London, vol 2

Cyriax J, Cyriax P 1983 Illustrated manual of orthopaedic medicine. Butterworths, London

Elliott B G 1992a Abductor pollicis longus – a case of mistaken identity. Journal of Hand Surgery 17B:476–478

Elliott B G 1992b Finkelstein's test: a descriptive error that can produce a false positive. Journal of Hand Surgery 17B:481–482

Hartley A 1995 Practical joint assessment – lower quadrant, 2nd edn. Mosby, London

Hoppenfeld S 1976 Physical examination of the spine and extremities. Appleton Century Crofts, Connecticut

Kesson H, Atkins E, Davies I 2003 Musuloskeletal injection skills. Butterworth Heinemann, Oxford

Klug J D 1995 MR diagnosis of tenosynovitis about the wrist. MRI Clinics of North America 3:305–312

Kumar P, Clark, M 2002 Clinical medicine, 5th edn. Baillière Tindall, London

Livengood L 1992 Occupational soft tissue disorders of the hand and forearm. Wisconsin Medical Journal 91(10):583–584

Marini M, Boni S, Pingi A et al 1994 De Quervain's disease: diagnostic imaging. Chirurgia Degli Organi Di Movimento 79:219–223

Murphy D, Failla J M, Koniuch M P 1995 Steroid versus placebo injection for trigger finger. Journal of Hand Surgery 20A:628–631

Norris C M 1998 Sports injuries: diagnosis and management for physiotherapists, 2nd edn. Butterworth Heinemann, Oxford

Palastanga N, Field D, Soames R 2002 Anatomy and human movement, 4th edn. Butterworth Heinemann, Oxford

Rettig A 1994 Wrist problems in the tennis player. Medicine and Science in Sports and Exercise 26:1207–1212

Saunders S 2000 Orthopaedic medicine course manual. Saunders, London

Shea K G, Shumsky I B, Shea O F 1991 Shifting into wrist pain – de Quervain's disease and off-road mountain biking. Physician and Sports Medicine 19:59–63

Smith D L, Wernick R 1994 Common nonarticular syndromes in the elbow, wrist and hand. Postgraduate Medicine 95:173–188

Steinberg B D, Plancher K D 1995 Clinical anatomy of the wrist and elbow. Clinics in Sports Medicine 14:299–313

Tan M Y, Low C K, Tan S K 1994 De Quervain's tenosynovitis and ganglion over first dorsal extensor retinacular compartment. Annals Academy of Medicine 23:885–886

Vargas Busquets M A V 1994 Historical commentary: the wrist flexion test Phalen's sign. Journal of Hand Surgery 19:521

Weiss A P, Akelman E, Tabatabai M 1994 Treatment of de Quervain's disease. Journal of Hand Surgery 19A:595–598

Williams P L 1998 Gray's Anatomy: the anatomical basis of medicine and surgery, 38th edn. Churchill Livingstone, Edinburgh

Wright T W, del Charco M, Wheeler D 1994 Incidence of ligament lesions and associated degenerative changes in the elderly wrist. Journal of Hand Surgery 10A:313–318

Chapter **8**

The cervical spine

SUMMARY

Safety is of paramount importance in the application of manual techniques to the cervical spine. As a contribution to safety, this chapter begins with a summary of the key points of cervical anatomy, highlighting structures involved in the pre-treatment testing procedures and the treatment techniques themselves.

Differential diagnosis and the elements of clinical examination will be discussed. Patients with a mechanical lesion, and thus suitable for the treatments subsequently described, will be identified. The contraindications to treatment will be emphasized and guidelines for safe practice will be given, since both are of vital importance.

ANATOMY

The spinal column is a series of motion segments, each of which consists of an interbody joint and its two adjacent zygapophyseal joints. The resultant bony canal is protective, but while the structural arrangement of the lumbar spine as a whole is suited to weight-bearing, movement and stability, the cervical spine is designed principally for mobility.

The cervical spine is the most mobile area of the spine and its wide range and variety of movement are related to changes in the direction of vision, the positioning of the upper limbs and hands, and locomotion. It is also an area of potential danger as it gives bony protection to major blood vessels that supply the brain and the spinal cord (Taylor & Twomey 1994, Nordin & Frankel 2001).

Anatomically and functionally, the cervical spine can be divided into two segments. The *upper segment* consists of the atlas and the axis (C1 and C2). Its structure is designed for mobility, with approximately one-third of cervical flexion and extension and over half of axial rotation occurring at this level (Mercer & Bogduk 2001). The *lower segment* consists of the remaining cervical vertebrae (C3–C7), and contributes to overall mobility.

The *atlas* (C1) is composed of two lateral masses, supporting articular facets, and their joining anterior and posterior arches. The superior facets articulate with the head at the *atlanto-occipital joints* and their condylar shape facilitates nodding movements of the head (Netter 1987, Mercer & Bogduk 2001). The inferior facets articulate with the axis at the *atlantoaxial joints* where rotation is the principal movement. The *axis* (C2) has broad superior articular facets which support the lateral masses of the atlas and which are responsible for bearing the axial load of the head and atlas, transmitting the load to the rest of the cervical spine. The axis supports the *dens or odontoid process* on its superior surface, the dens providing a pivot around which the atlas rotates at the synovial median atlantoaxial joint (Mercer & Bogduk 2001). There is no intervertebral disc between the atlas and axis.

The internal ligaments of the upper cervical segment are particularly important to its stability (Fig. 8.1). The *tectorial membrane* is a superior extension of the posterior longitudinal ligament that covers the dens and its ligaments, acting as protection for the junction of the spinal cord and the medulla. The *transverse ligament* of the atlas is a strong horizontal band with extensions passing vertically and horizontally from its mid-point to form a ligamentous complex called the *cruciform ligament*. This, together with the *apical ligament* of the dens, is responsible for keeping the dens in close contact with the atlas. Any instability in the upper cervical segment, e.g. as occurs with rheumatoid arthritis, trauma or Down's syndrome, is an absolute contraindication to orthopaedic medicine techniques.

The lower cervical segment consists of typical cervical vertebrae C3–C6 and the atypical C7 which is known as the *vertebra prominens* because of its long spinous process. A typical cervical vertebra consists of a small, broad, weight-bearing *vertebral body* (Fig. 8.2), the superior surface of which is raised on each side, rather like a bucket seat, to form *unciform processes*. The unciform processes articulate with corresponding facets

Figure 8.1   Upper cervical internal ligaments. From Functional Anatomy of the Spine by Oliver J and Middleditch A. Reprinted by with permission of Harcourt Education Ltd.

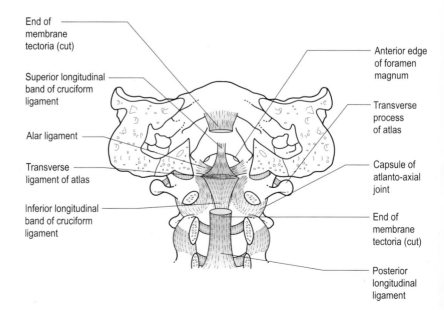

End of membrane tectoria (cut)

Superior longitudinal band of cruciform ligament

Alar ligament

Transverse ligament of atlas

Inferior longitudinal band of cruciform ligament

Anterior edge of foramen magnum

Transverse process of atlas

Capsule of atlanto-axial joint

End of membrane tectoria (cut)

Posterior longitudinal ligament

Figure 8.2 Typical cervical vertebra. From Anatomy and Human Movement by N Palastanga D Field and R Soames. Reprinted by permission of Elsevier Ltd.

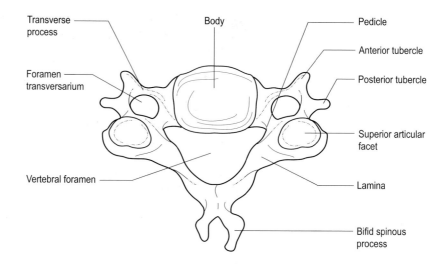

Transverse process

Body

Pedicle

Anterior tubercle

Foramen transversarium

Posterior tubercle

Superior articular facet

Vertebral foramen

Lamina

Bifid spinous process

on the vertebra above to form the **uncovertebral joints** or the **joints of Luschka**.

Posteriorly lie two short **pedicles** and two long, narrow **laminae** forming the vertebral arch which, together with the vertebral body, surround a large, triangular **vertebral canal**. The laminae come together to form a bifid **spinous process**. Superior and inferior **articular processes**, at the junction of the pedicles and laminae, articulate at the synovial **zygapophyseal joints** which form an articular pillar on either side of the spine.

Short, gutter-shaped **transverse processes** slope anterolaterally to transport the emerging nerve root. The **foramen transversarium**, a distinctive feature in the transverse processes on each side of the cervical vertebrae, houses the vertebral artery.

The ligaments of the lower cervical segment assist stability and allow mobility. The **anterior longitudinal ligament** protects the anterior aspect of the intervertebral joints and, with other anterior soft tissues, limits cervical extension. The **ligamentum nuchae** is a strong, fibroelastic sheet protecting the joints posteriorly and providing an intermuscular septum. The **ligamentum flavum** is a highly elastic ligament linking adjacent laminae. In the cervical spine it allows separation of the vertebrae during flexion and assists the neck's return to the upright posture. Its elastic properties also allow it to return to its original length, so preventing buckling into the spinal canal where it can sometimes compromise the spinal cord. The **posterior longitudinal ligament** passes from the axis to the sacrum and is at its broadest in the cervical spine where it covers the entire floor of the cervical vertebral canal, supporting the disc and possibly preventing its posterior displacement. It is taut in flexion and relaxed in extension. Mercer & Bogduk (1999) identify three distinct layers of the posterior longitudinal ligament. The deep layer, consisting of short fibres, spans each intervertebral joint and extends in an alar (wing-shaped) pattern as far as the posterior end of the base of the uncinate process, where it is believed to compensate for a deficient posterior annulus fibrosus.

THE JOINTS OF THE CERVICAL SPINE

The joints of the lower cervical segment consist of the interbody joint anteriorly and the two zygapophyseal joints posteriorly. The interbody joint is made up of the intervertebral joint and the uncovertebral joints. When stacked, the joints can be considered to form three pillars in a triangular formation, the vertebral bodies and uncinate processes forming the anterior column and the two articular pillars formed by the zygopophyseal joints arranged posteriorly (Mercer & Bogduk 1999).

The *intervertebral joint* is a symphysis formed between the relatively avascular intervertebral disc and the adjacent vertebral bodies. The disc contributes to mobility and, as it ages, assists the uncovertebral joints in providing translatory glide to the movements of flexion and extension (see below).

The *uncovertebral joints* (joints of Luschka) are formed between the unciform processes and corresponding facets on the vertebral body above (Fig. 8.3), though their existence has been challenged (Mercer & Bogduk 1999). They may be true synovial joints or adventitious fibrous joints which have developed through clefts or fissures in the lateral corners of the annulus fibrosis of the intervertebral disc originally described by Hurbert von Luschka in 1858 (Prescher 1998). These fissures are absent in young children and appear to develop in conjunction with the development of the unciform process. Once formed, the fissures in the annulus develop a pseudocapsule in which vascularized synovial folds have been seen. Prescher relates the development of these fissures and the uncovertebral 'joint' to the development of the cervical lordosis resulting in a change in configuration and the magnitude of the loads transmitted through the cervical spine. This results in strong shear forces

Figure 8.3 Uncovertebral joints. From Anatomy and Human Movement by N Palastanga D Field and R Soames. Reprinted by permission of Elsevier Ltd.

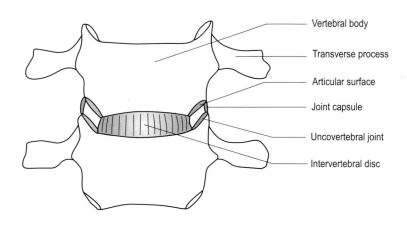

Vertebral body

Transverse process

Articular surface

Joint capsule

Uncovertebral joint

Intervertebral disc

being transmitted through the intervertebral disc, particularly during rotation and side flexion. C3–C5 are the most loaded segments and it is at these levels that the fissures in the disc first appear.

The uncovertebral joints also contribute to mobility by providing a translatory gliding component to flexion and extension as well as stabilizing the spine by limiting the amount of side flexion. The gliding component produces shear which extends horizontal fissuring of the disc medially from the uncovertebral joints. This, together with the degenerative process, may eventually produce a bipartite disc (Taylor & Twomey 1994).

The position of the uncovertebral joints gives bony protection to the nerve root from posterolateral disc displacement. As synovial 'joints', degenerative changes can have an effect on the uncovertebral joints. Osteophyte formation on the uncinate process occurs predominantly in the lower cervical segments. Posterior osteophytes can encroach on the intervertebral canal leading to compression of the emerging spinal nerve root, whereas anterior osteophytes may compress the vertebral artery.

The *zygapophyseal joints* are synovial plane joints with relatively lax fibrous capsules to facilitate movement. The articular facets are angled at approximately 45° to the vertical so that side flexion and rotation of the lower cervical spine occur as a coupled movement. This angle of inclination adds to the component of translatory glide during flexion and extension (Taylor & Twomey 1994).

A number of intra-articular structures have been described, particularly vascular synovial folds, similar to the alar folds of the knee, as well as fat pads and meniscoid structures. All are highly innervated and can be a potential source of pain (Oliver & Middleditch 1991, Taylor & Twomey 1994). As synovial joints the zygapophyseal joints are prone to degenerative changes and, being placed near the exiting nerve root, osteophyte formation may affect the size of the intervertebral foramen.

Orthopaedic medicine treatment is traditionally based on the discal model, but it should be remembered that any structure that receives a nerve supply can be a potential source of pain. Since the cervical spine is made up of individual motion segments, a lesion of one part of the segment will tend to influence the rest of that segment. Similarly, treatment directed to one part of a segment will affect the segment as a whole.

INTERVERTEBRAL DISCS

There are six cervical discs which facilitate and restrain movement as well as transmit load from one vertebral body to the next (Fig. 8.4). Cervical discs are approximately 5 mm thick (Palastanga et al 2002) and the thinnest of all the intervertebral discs. Each forms part of the anterior wall of the intervertebral foramen and is thicker anteriorly, contributing to the cervical lordosis. The intervertebral disc consists of an annulus fibrosus, nucleus pulposus, and transitional superior and inferior vertebral end-plates.

The difference in function between the lumbar and cervical spine and the traditionally accepted view that cervical discs are smaller versions of lumbar discs does not hold true. Mercer & Bogduk (1999) acknowledged

Figure 8.4 Cervical vertebrae, interbody joint and posterior elements. From Anatomy and Human Movement by N Palastanga D Field and R Soames. Reprinted by permission of Elsevier Ltd.

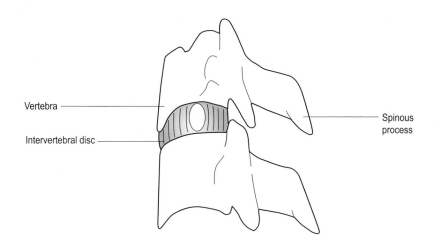

Vertebra

Intervertebral disc

Spinous process

this in their investigation of the form of the human adult intervertebral cervical disc and its ligaments. At birth the nucleus consists of no more than 25% of the entire disc and it undergoes rapid degeneration with age so that, by the age of 30, the nucleus is undistinguishable as such.

The structure of the *annulus fibrosus*, described by Mercer & Bogduk, is different anteriorly and posteriorly. The *anterolateral annulus* forms a crescent shape when viewed from above, thicker in the median plane and thinner laterally, tapering out to the unciform processes. It forms a dense, anterior interosseous ligament. The fibres arise from the superior surface of the lower vertebra, fanning out in an alar fashion laterally, but in the midline form a tightly interwoven pattern with fibres from opposite sides, not the true laminate structure as seen in the lumbar spine. A distance of 2–3 mm from the surface of the anterior annulus, collagen fibres have been found embedded with proteoglycans and forming a fibrocartilaginous mass which has a pearly appearance and the consistency of soap. On a deeper plane, the fibrocartilaginous mass becomes more homogeneous and less laminated, forming what the authors interpret as the nucleus of the disc. Clefts, presumably the uncovertebral 'joints', are seen to extend into the fibrocartilaginous core laterally at the uncovertebral region, partially into the core in younger patients but totally transecting the posterior two-thirds of the disc in older specimens. Covering the clefts in the uncovertebral region is thin periosteofascial tissue, the annular fibres being deficient here.

The *posterior annulus* demonstrates different features to the anterior annulus. It consists of a thin layer of one set of vertically orientated collagen fibres, not more than 1 mm thick, passing between adjacent vertebrae and extending out as far as the unciform process on each side where no oblique posterior annular fibres were found. Deep to this is the fibrocartilaginous core. It would appear that the deep layer of the posterior longitudinal ligament, with short fibres spanning each intervertebral joint, compensates for the lack of annular fibres in the posterior part of the disc, supporting the nucleus posteriorly. Posterolaterally the alar fibres of the posterior longitudinal ligament alone contain the nucleus and these may become torn or stretched by a bulging disc, or nuclear material may herniate under or through them.

The *vertebral end-plate* offers protection by preventing the disc from bulging into the vertebral body. It acts as a semipermeable membrane which, by diffusion, facilitates the exchange of nutrients between the vertebral body and the disc.

Cyriax (1982) stated that 'from a clinical point of view nuclear protrusions form only a small minority of cervical disc displacements'. He postulated that a true nuclear disc lesion occurs only in adolescents and young adults, presenting as an acute torticollis. His hypothesis would seem to be substantiated by Taylor & Twomey (1994) who suggested that early degeneration of the cervical nucleus makes nuclear protrusion in the cervical spine unlikely, unless precipitated by severe trauma. They regarded a central bar-like protrusion of the annulus to be more likely to occur in the cervical spine. This appears to be refuted by the work of Mercer & Bogduk (1999) described above, given the relatively deficient posterior cervical annulus identified. Perhaps, like lumbar discs, herniated cervical discs may consist of degenerate nuclear material. Posterolateral herniation of the disc could be possible through the weak supporting alar fibres of the posterior longitudinal ligament in the uncovertebral region. Indeed, one specimen from the Mercer & Bogduk study (1999) illustrates a disc bulge and a herniation, both below their respective alar fibres.

The position of the uncovertebral joints and the large vertebral canal in the cervical spine may both also exert a protective influence on disc movement. Degenerate cervical discs may prolapse directly posteriorly, encroaching on the dura through the posterior longitudinal ligament, rather than laterally at the uncovertebral region, to affect the dural nerve root sleeve and underlying nerve root in the intervertebral canal. Alternatively, discal material may be reflected posterolaterally in the vertebral canal by the stronger median part of the posterior longitudinal ligament to cause unilateral pressure on the dura.

The triangular vertebral canal is at its largest in the cervical spine and even though the cervical cord is enlarged in this region, there may be room for a prolapse to be accommodated. Posterolateral prolapse through the weaker alar portion in the uncovertebral region may encroach on the dural nerve root sleeve and underlying nerve root. However, it would seem that only a very large posterolateral prolapse would be able to compress the nerve root at the same level, unless there is canal stenosis caused by osteophyte formation, an infolding ligamentum flavum or congenital factors. Since the extent of pain referral is thought to be related to the amount of pressure on the dural nerve root sleeve (Mooney & Robertson 1976), brachial pain is not as commonly associated with cervical disc lesions as sciatica is with lumbar disc lesions. Dural pressure due to a cervical disc tends to produce central or unilateral scapular pain; the hypothetical reasons for this have been discussed above.

It is assumed that cervical discs are innervated in a similar way to lumbar discs, since no studies have refuted this as yet. At least the outer third and possibly the outer half of the annulus fibrosis receives a nerve supply from branches of a posterior longitudinal plexus, derived from the cervical sinuvertebral nerves, as well as from a similar plexus formed from cervical sympathetic trunks and the vertebral nerves, and from penetrating branches from the vertebral nerve (Bogduk 1994). Mendel et al (1992) found evidence of nerve fibres and mechanoreceptors in the posterolateral region of the annulus.

The cervical disc may produce either primary disc pain or pain due to the mechanical effect of secondary compression of pain-sensitive structures with associated chemical or ischaemic effects. The mechanism of pain produced by disc displacement is covered in greater detail in Chapter 13 since much of the investigative work on pain production has been performed in the lumbar region and no studies have been identified which relate to the cervical spine. If findings can be extrapolated to the cervical spine, disc material is thought to undergo a process of degradation which contributes to its herniation. The chemical mediators of inflammation may play a role in the pathophysiology of cervical radiculopathy which renders the nerve root pain-sensitive (Kang et al 1995).

CERVICAL SPINAL NERVES

There are eight cervical spinal nerves, each approximately 1 cm long, that, together with the dorsal root ganglion, occupy a large, funnel-shaped intervertebral foramen (Fig. 8.5). The *spinal nerve* is composed of one dorsal or posterior nerve root and one anterior or ventral nerve root, the ventral nerve root emerging more caudally from the dura mater (Tanaka et al 2000). The dorsal nerve root carries sensory fibres and the

Figure 8.5 Formation of a spinal nerve. From Functional Anatomy of the Spine by Oliver J and Middleditch A. Reprinted by with permission of Harcourt Education Ltd.

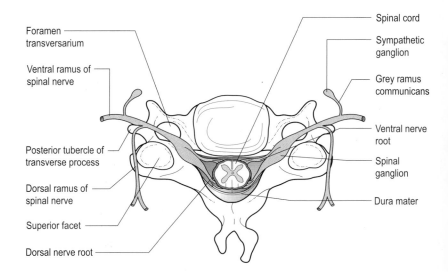

Labels:
- Foramen transversarium
- Ventral ramus of spinal nerve
- Posterior tubercle of transverse process
- Dorsal ramus of spinal nerve
- Superior facet
- Dorsal nerve root
- Spinal cord
- Sympathetic ganglion
- Grey ramus communicans
- Ventral nerve root
- Spinal ganglion
- Dura mater

Figure 8.6 Horizontal direction of emerging nerve roots. From Anatomy and Human Movement by N Palastanga D Field and R Soames. Reprinted by permission of Elsevier Ltd.

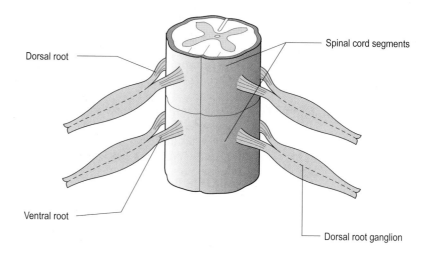

Dorsal root

Spinal cord segments

Ventral root

Dorsal root ganglion

ventral nerve root, motor fibres. The spinal nerve occupies one fourth to one third of the intervertebral foramen diameter and carries with it an investment of the dura mater, the dural nerve root sleeve. The **dural nerve root sleeve** is sensitive to pressure and produces pain in a segmental distribution. Cervical spinal nerves generally emerge horizontally and therefore the nerve roots are vulnerable to pressure only from the disc at that particular level, producing signs and symptoms in one segment only (Fig. 8.6). Indication of more than one nerve root involvement should be considered suspicious until proved otherwise.

However, Tanaka et al (2000), in a cadaver study, showed that the roots below C5 reached their intervertebral foramen with increasing obliquity making compression of more than one nerve root below this level possible. At the C7–T1 disc 78% of specimens showed that the C8 nerve roots did not have any contact with the disc at the entrance of the intervertebral foramen, which probably accounts for the low frequency of C8 radiculopathy. Nerve root compression was found to occur at the entrance of the intervertebral foramen and was determined to be due to herniated discs and osteophytes in the uncovertebral region anteriorly, and to the superior articular process, ligamentum flavum and periradicular fibrous tissue posteriorly (Tanaka et al 2000). Motor impairment, therefore, is suggestive of anterior compression from a disc prolapse or degenerative changes in the uncovertebral region, whereas sensory change is indicative of compression due to changes in the posterior structures. Of course a large disc prolapse or gross degenerative change, anteriorly or posteriorly, may compress both elements of the nerve root.

After it leaves the intervertebral foramen, the spinal nerve root immediately divides into **ventral and dorsal rami**. The **sinuvertebral nerve** is a mixed sensory and sympathetic nerve, receiving origin from the ventral ramus and the grey ramus communicans of the sympathetic system. The nerve returns through the intervertebral foramen and gives off ascending, descending and transverse branches to supply structures at, above and below the segment (Williams 1998, Oliver & Middleditch 1991, Palastanga et al 2002). The structures it supplies include the dura mater, posterior longitudinal ligament and the outer part of the annulus of the intervertebral disc (Bogduk 1994).

VERTEBRAL ARTERY

Anatomically the vertebral artery is divided into the following four sections, which include two right-angled bends where it is vulnerable to internal and external factors which tend to compromise blood flow (Fig. 8.7) (Williams 1998, Oliver & Middleditch 1991):

- Its origin from the subclavian artery
- Its passage through each foramen transversarium except C7. In this section it gives off spinal branches which supply the spinal cord and its sheaths via the intervertebral foramen
- The first right-angled bend, turning medially to pass behind the lateral mass of the atlas
- The second right-angled bend, to turn vertically to enter the foramen magnum to unite with the other vertebral artery to form the basilar artery, which passes onto contribute to the circle of Willis

Anatomical anomalies and variations exist and commonly one vertebral artery is narrower than its partner. Clinically it is important to recognize vertebrobasilar signs and symptoms since these contraindicate certain

Figure 8.7 Pathway of vertebrobasilar arteries. From Anatomy and Human Movement by N Palastanga D Field and R Soames. Reprinted by permission of Elsevier Ltd.

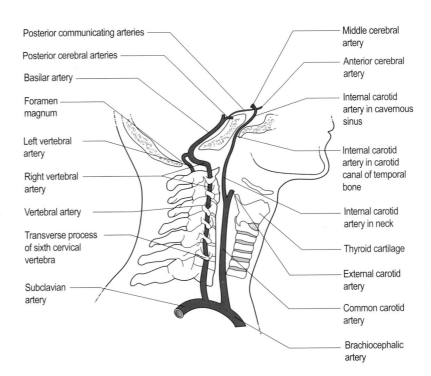

Posterior communicating arteries
Posterior cerebral arteries
Basilar artery
Foramen magnum
Left vertebral artery
Right vertebral artery
Vertebral artery
Transverse process of sixth cervical vertebra
Subclavian artery

Middle cerebral artery
Anterior cerebral artery
Internal carotid artery in cavernous sinus
Internal carotid artery in carotid canal of temporal bone
Internal carotid artery in neck
Thyroid cartilage
External carotid artery
Common carotid artery
Brachiocephalic artery

cervical manoeuvres. The artery is elastic, particularly in its first and third sections, which allow it to accommodate to movement. Degenerative changes in the artery itself, in the intervertebral canal, uncovertebral joints and zygapophyseal joints make it vulnerable to blockage as well as possibly distorting its pathway.

DIFFERENTIAL DIAGNOSIS AT THE CERVICAL SPINE

An understanding of the anatomy at the cervical spine, together with a detailed history and examination of the patient, will help with the selection of patients suitable for manual treatment and contribute to safe practice. The two areas of danger in this region are the vertebral arteries and the spinal cord and certain signs and symptoms will become evident on examination which would exclude some patients from manual treatment techniques (see below).

Similarly, there are non-mechanical causes of neck pain in which manual treatment techniques are either contraindicated or not appropriate. The following section will be divided into two parts. The first covers *mechanical lesions* attributed to the discal model, which present a set of signs and symptoms that help to establish diagnosis and to rationalize treatment programmes. The second covers the ***non-mechanical causes*** of neck pain and associated signs and symptoms. On the whole, these patients are not appropriate for treatment with manual orthopaedic medicine treatment techniques and require suitable referral.

As well as being a primary source of pain, the disc, through prolapse into the vertebral or intervertebral canal, can have a secondary effect on any pain-sensitive structure lying within. This effect can be mechanical through compression and distortion, chemical through the inflammatory process and ischaemic through the pressure of oedema. For further information on these theories, the reader is referred to Chapter 13. Although the differences in the anatomy and function of the cervical and lumbar spine must be acknowledged, no studies have been unearthed to reflect patterns of pain production specific to the cervical spine. For the time being, therefore these have been extrapolated from the lumbar model.

A central herniation of cervical disc material produces central and/or bilaterally referred symptoms. A unilateral herniation produces unilaterally referred symptoms. Reference of pain arising from compression of the central structures is characteristically multisegmental, i.e. over many segments (see Ch. 1). Involvement of the unilateral structures, dural nerve root sleeve and/or the nerve root produces segmentally referred signs and symptoms.

Since the disc degenerates early in the cervical spine, disc lesions tend to produce a pattern of symptoms which indicate a progression of the same condition. The symptoms are age-related with a pattern of increasing frequency and severity. Eventually the nerve root may become involved.

The anatomy of the zygapophyseal joint with its intra-articular structures makes it susceptible to possible mechanical derangement. Signs and symptoms of zygapophyseal joint derangement may mimic those of a disc lesion, and treatment of the intervertebral joint will also affect these joints. While acknowledging these possibilities, the approach in orthopaedic medicine is based on the discal model, since no other theory seems to fit as well with the clinical presentation of patients. However, some would consider that conclusive proof is still wanting.

Disc lesions in the cervical spine need to be reduced to prevent them contributing further to the degenerative process. A central prolapse in particular may cause osteophyte formation through ligamentous traction which may eventually threaten the spinal cord. Cyriax (1982) was emphatic in pointing out the danger of not reducing an early, minor cervical disc lesion for this reason as there comes a time when manipulation will not have an effect and a point at which it may be dangerous. Elderly patients with osteophytic cord compression often report the onset of paraesthesia associated with cervical extension and for that reason it would seem that particular attention should be paid to restoring cervical extension which would act as an indicator that reduction had been effected.

The cervical disc lesions produce a pattern of signs and symptoms and a set of clinical models has been established to aid diagnosis and establish treatment programmes. These are outlined later in this chapter. The models should be used as a general guide to the clinical diagnosis and treatment of cervical disc lesions. All show a non-capsular pattern on examination.

The following terminology will be used to describe disc lesions:

Disc protrusion

- Discal material passes into the weakened degenerate structure of the annulus, where it can produce primary disc pain since the outer annulus receives a nerve supply.

Disc prolapse

- Discal material passes through a ruptured annulus and/or posterior longitudinal ligament into the vertebral or intervertebral canal where it has a secondary effect on pain-sensitive structures: the posterior longitudinal ligament, dura mater, dural nerve root sleeve, nerve root and dorsal root ganglion. The sequela of this is sequestration of the disc.

Both forms of cervical disc lesion are suitable for orthopaedic medicine manual techniques, providing no contraindications exist.

OTHER CAUSES OF NECK PAIN, ARM PAIN AND ASSOCIATED SIGNS AND SYMPTOMS

Generally, this group of conditions does not respond to the manual techniques described in this chapter and indeed some may be absolute contraindications. There may, however, be some overlap, particularly with the degenerative conditions and the techniques may be attempted, provided contraindications have been eliminated.

Arthritis in any joint presents with the capsular pattern. Arthritis occurs in synovial joints in the cervical spine and involves the zygapophyseal and uncovertebral joints. In the cervical spine the

> **Capsular pattern of the cervical spine**
> - Equal limitation of side flexions.
> - Equal limitation of rotations.
> - Some limitation of extension.
> - Usually full flexion.

capsular pattern is demonstrated by the cervical spine as a whole. The limited movements have the 'hard' end-feel of arthritis. The pattern of symmetrical limitation of the side flexions and rotations is distinctive when compared with the asymmetrical pattern of limitation seen in disc lesions. The early degeneration of the cervical intervertebral disc occurs concurrently with degenerative changes within the other joints. The history will indicate the type of arthritis: degenerative osteoarthrosis, inflammatory or traumatic.

- *Degenerative osteoarthrosis* involves damage to hyaline cartilage and subchondral bone with sclerosis and osteophyte formation. Cervical movements become limited in the capsular pattern. Stiffening of the neck is particularly evident on rotation when the patient may, for example, have difficulty in reversing the car. Painful symptoms occur during acute exacerbations of the condition, precipitated by trauma or overuse.

  The upper cervical segments are particularly involved in the degenerative process, with marked loss of rotation. Degenerative changes in the neck are often referred to as cervical spondylosis. However, despite gross X-ray changes, there may be little in the way of symptoms.

  It is possible to have a disc lesion in an older degenerative neck, i.e. noncapsular pattern, superimposed onto a capsular pattern. The disc lesion can be treated with manual traction and the degenerative osteoarthrosis does not present a contraindication to treatment in itself. However, rotation under traction should be wisely avoided due to the close proximity of the degenerate zygopophyseal and uncovertebral joints to the course of the vertebral artery (see below).

  Degenerative changes in the uncovertebral joints lead to osteophyte formation which may encroach on the nerve root or adjacent vertebral arteries, causing problems through direct compression. Degenerative changes of the synovial joints may alter or distort the path of the vertebral artery, leading to symptoms of its compromise.

- *Matutinal headaches* may be due to ligamentous contracture around the upper two cervical joints, the atlanto-occipital and atlantoaxial joints. A condition called 'old man's matutinal headache' exists in which the patient, an elderly man, wakes every morning with a headache which usually eases after a few hours (Cyriax 1982). Mobilization techniques, particularly manual traction, may be appropriate for this condition.

- *Tinnitus and vertigo* may be associated symptoms of degenerative osteoarthrosis of the cervical spine. They can respond well to the techniques, but the vertebrobasilar system must be ruled out as a cause of the symptoms.

- *Osteophytic root palsy* produces a gradual onset of aching in the arm, usually with paraesthesia, as the osteophytes develop. The patient is usually elderly and will have objective neurological signs of weakness in the arm affecting one nerve root only. Since disc lesions presenting in this way are unusual in this age group, orthopaedic medicine techniques would be contraindicated.

- *Cervical myelopathy* may develop in association with degenerative changes in the cervical spine. Stenosis of the central canal occurs through osteophytic formation and hypertrophy and buckling of the ligamentum flavum develops. The osteophytes, a disc prolapse or a ligamentous fold may exert pressure on the spinal cord and a gradual onset of symptoms occurs with increasing disability. There may be pain, dysaesthesia of the hands consisting of numbness and tingling, clumsiness and weakness of the hands, weakness and evidence of spasticity of the lower limbs (Jenkins 1979, Connell & Wiesel 1992). The orthopaedic medicine treatment techniques described below would be contraindicated.

- *Zygapophyseal joints* could conceivably produce symptoms individually and in isolation to the other joints in the segment. As synovial joints they are prone to degenerative changes along with the other joints in the segment. Aprill et al (1989) suggested that distinct patterns of pain referral were associated with individual cervical zygapophyseal joints but others have refuted the existence of a facet syndrome (Schwarzer et al 1994).

- *Cervical or cervicogenic headache* describes a pain perceived to originate in the head, but whose source is in the cervical spine (Bogduk 1992). It consists of an aching or deep pain localized to the neck, suboccipital and frontal region, precipitated or aggravated by neck movements or sustained neck postures, especially flexion. There is limitation of passive neck movements, changes in muscle contour, texture or tone and abnormal tenderness of the neck muscles (Sjaastad 1992; Beeton & Jull 1994; Jull 1994a, 1994b; Nilsson 1995, Schoensee et al 1995). The upper three cervical segments are most commonly involved and associated symptoms may consist of nausea, visual disturbances, dizziness or lightheadedness (Jull 1994a, 1994b). There are many forms of headache and the overlapping symptoms make it difficult to isolate headache due to primary cervical dysfunction. Orthopaedic medicine treatment techniques can be considered as an option if diagnosis is due to cervical dysfunction.

- *Polymyalgia rheumatica* affects the middle and older age group, women more than men. It presents as pain and stiffness in the neck and shoulder girdle accompanied by fatigue, low-grade fever, depression and weight loss, and responds dramatically to small doses of oral corticosteroids (Hazelman 1995).

- *Giant cell arteritis or temporal arteritis* is a condition closely related to polymyalgia rheumatica. It is a vasculitis of unknown aetiology affecting the elderly. The patient presents with a severe temporal headache and scalp tenderness. The condition is treated urgently with high-dose steroids, to prevent blindness (Hazelman 1995).

- *Rheumatoid arthritis* is an inflammatory polyarthritis, affecting females more than males, with its onset usually between the ages of 40 and 50. It tends to follow a relapsing and remitting course. The synovial membrane becomes inflamed and thickened to become continuous with vascular tissue – a condition known as pannus. The pannus causes typical destructive changes of ligaments, cartilage and bone (Walker

1995). Rheumatoid arthritis can also involve extra-articular soft tissues, e.g. Achilles tendon, plantar fascia (Kumar & Clark 2002).

It is uncommon for rheumatoid arthritis to affect the cervical joints only, without its manifestation elsewhere, and it most commonly affects the smaller peripheral joints bilaterally. However, in patients with rheumatoid arthritis it may be silent in the cervical joints and there may be no clinical evidence of cervical spine involvement (Clark 1994).

The mechanism of the disease in the spinal joints is the same as that seen in peripheral joints, with ligament, cartilage and bone destruction. This loss of the supporting infrastructure of the spine, particularly of the upper cervical segment, is a potential hazard for significant neurological involvement of the brainstem and cervical spinal cord. Atlantoaxial subluxation is the most common manifestation, but cranial settling (vertical intrusion of the dens) and subaxial subluxation may also occur (Clark 1994, Zeidman & Ducker 1994, Mathews, 1995). Rheumatoid arthritis is therefore an absolute contraindication to orthopaedic medicine techniques.

- *Traumatic arthritis* is produced by significant trauma causing inflammation in the cervical synovial joints and therefore a capsular pattern. This may occur following a whiplash injury. Once the capsular pattern has settled, there may be evidence of an underlying disc lesion to which mobilization can be carefully applied, providing there is no damage to the vertebrobasilar system.

- *Whiplash* injury occurs when a car is struck from behind, often while the occupants of the involved car are unaware. A hyperextension injury followed by a hyperflexion injury occurs. During the hyperextension phase the anterior structures, the intervertebral discs, anterior longitudinal ligament and anterior muscles can be damaged or torn and the posterior structures compressed. During the hyperflexion phase the dens may impact against the atlas, and the atlanto-occipital joint, posterior ligaments and zygapophyseal joints can be involved (Bogduk 1986). Generally, a whiplash injury may produce some pain initially, but it is not until later that the ligaments stiffen and produce a secondary capsular pattern due to the trauma.

Significant bony or ligamentous damage causes immediate pain with a reluctance to move the neck. X-ray evidence of cervical instability is an absolute contraindication to orthopaedic medicine techniques. A history of recent whiplash injury has been identified as a possible risk factor of vascular accident (Kleynhans & Terrett 1985).

Taylor & Twomey (1993) conducted an autopsy study of neck sprains and showed clefts associated with vertebral end-plate lesions in trauma victims. These were distinct from the uncovertebral clefts and central fissures associated with degeneration of cervical discs. These so-called rim lesions involved the avascular cartilage end-plates and the outer annulus and, in further experiments, showed a poor response to healing. They may be responsible for the chronic pain often associated with whiplash injuries. Posterior disc herniation through a damaged annulus and haemarthrosis of the zygapophyseal joints were also observed in the trauma victims and this is clinically significant in treating the early whiplash. The acute sprain of the joints makes this an irritable lesion which requires pain relief and reduction of inflammation. Early mobilization – in line with the principles for acute lesions laid out in Chapter 4 – may be applied, providing gross bony injury and instability are not present.

Evidence exists to support early mobilization in whiplash-type injuries to avoid the chronic pain syndrome developing, with its associated psychosocial factors (Mealy et al 1986, McKinney 1989). In the hyperacute stage, gentle techniques are applied, including Grade A mobilization, providing there is no serious pathology. The patient is given the responsibility for management of the condition, and is instructed about posture and exercise, advice to avoid excessive reliance on a collar, appropriate pillow support and adequate analgesia.

Serious, non-mechanical conditions may present with signs and symptoms similar to those of a mechanical presentation. For this reason, careful examination is necessary to eliminate serious disease which would be contraindicated for orthopaedic medicine treatment. Patients may present with local symptoms which are rarely provoked by movement or posture. On examination it may be difficult to reproduce the symptoms. Other more generalized features may also be present, such as increasing and unrelenting pain, night pain, weight loss, general malaise, fever, raised erythrocyte sedimentation rate or other symptoms, e.g. cough.

- *Spinal infections* may include osteomyelitis or epidural abscess. The organism responsible may be *Staphylococcus aureus*, *Mycobacterium tuberculosis* or, rarely, *Brucella* (Kumar & Clark 2002).
- *Malignant disease* is usually extradural with bone metastases produced most commonly from primaries in the bronchus, breast, prostate, kidney or thyroid. There may be a history of a gradual onset of pain and stiffness, the pain tends to be unrelenting and night pain is usually a feature. The pain is not relieved by different postures. On examination active movements produce pain and limitation in all directions. The passive movements are prevented by the end-feel of a twang of muscle spasm and resisted movements are painful and possibly weak. All of these signs and symptoms are evidence of a gross lesion (Cyriax 1982). Neurological examination may reveal excessive muscle weakness involving several nerve roots, possibly bilaterally, in contrast to a disc lesion that tends to involve one nerve root only (Mathews 1995).
- *Primary tumours* (e.g. meningioma, neurofibroma, glioma) tend to present with a gradual onset of symptoms of cord compression and pain is not usually a major feature.
- *Pancoast's tumour* is carcinoma in the apex of the lung which may erode the ribs and involve the lower brachial plexus. There is severe pain in the shoulder and down the medial aspect of the arm, with evidence of T1 palsy. Cervical side flexion away from the painful side may be the only limited neck movement, with passive elevation of the shoulder on the symptomatic side also being painful (Cyriax 1982). Interruption of the sympathetic ganglia can produce Horner's

syndrome – constriction of the pupil and drooping of the eyelid on the side of the tumour (Kumar & Clark 2002).

- *Suprascapular, long thoracic and spinal accessory neuritis* usually present with pain in the scapula and upper arm of approximately 3 weeks' duration. On examination, the neck movements are full and do not reproduce the pain. There is weakness of the appropriate muscles supplied by the affected nerve. The cause may be unknown, or it may be due to trauma or follow a viral infection. Recovery is usually spontaneous over approximately 6 weeks.
- Suprascapular neuritis produces weakness of the supraspinatus and infraspinatus muscles
- Long thoracic neuritis produces weakness of the serratus anterior muscle and winging of the scapula
- Spinal accessory neuritis produces weakness of the sternocleidomastoid and trapezius muscles
- *Neuralgic amyotrophy* is an unusual cause of severe pain in the neck and scapular region with a bizarre pattern of muscle weakness in the infraspinatus, supraspinatus, deltoid, triceps and serratus anterior muscles. The cause of the condition is unknown, but it may follow viral infection or immunization and an allergic basis is postulated (Kumar & Clark 2002). It usually recovers spontaneously over several weeks or months, although recovery may be more prolonged in some cases.

  Thoracic outlet syndrome, reflex sympathetic dystrophy and work-related syndromes all present with upper limb signs and symptoms which are sometimes difficult to isolate into a simple diagnostic pattern, particularly if symptoms have been present for a long duration.
- *Thoracic outlet syndrome* is a term used for compression, entrapment and/or postural alterations affecting the brachial plexus and its accompanying neurovascular structures, although debate continues about its existence (Walsh 1994). Distal symptoms occur, usually due to compression of the lower trunk of the brachial plexus (C8, T1), but the upper and middle trunks can also be involved. The condition may be bilateral, with a burning, dull aching pain along the medial aspect of the forearm. Distal oedema may be associated with activity, sweating and heaviness, and circulatory changes may be seen in the hands. Paraesthesia occurs as the release phenomenon, coming on at night, some time after the pressure has been released.
- *Reflex sympathetic dystrophy* describes a complex disorder of the limbs with or without obvious nerve involvement. It consists of persistent peripheral burning pain and tenderness which is termed hyperaesthesia (an abnormal response to pain) or allodynia (pain in response to stimuli which are not normally noxious). Vasomotor and sensory changes consist of sweating, colour changes and trophic skin changes together with weakness, tremor, muscle spasm and contractures (Herrick 1995).

- *Work-related syndromes of the upper limb* are due to repetitive occupational overuse, producing musculoskeletal symptoms, once a certain threshold of activity is exceeded. Sometimes this may present as a simple tenosynovitis or tendinopathy but much more often it presents as a catalogue of symptoms which are non-specific. Diffuse aching, stiffness, muscle or joint tiredness are present with the chronic nature of the condition, perhaps leading to anxiety and depression (Bird 1995).

The preceding conditions are usually associated with factors that affect the mobility and circulation of the nervous system. Each component of each condition needs to be recognized and a suitable treatment programme established. Orthopaedic medicine techniques are not usually indicated unless specific lesions are diagnosed.

- *Fibromyalgia* presents, usually in women, as a complex of variable symptoms including widespread musculoskeletal pain of the neck, shoulders and upper limbs. Fatigue, headache, waking unrefreshed, subjective distal swelling, poor concentration, forgetfulness and weepiness have been described (Doherty 1995). Multiple hyperalgesic tender spots and non-restorative sleep are the main diagnostic features of fibromyalgia. There are several components to management: they include the use of relaxation techniques, exercise, hydrotherapy, physiotherapy, acupuncture, muscle relaxants and drugs to improve the quality of sleep. The condition is difficult to separate from endogenous depression and often responds to antidepressant medication (Huskisson 1995, Conference note).

- *Drop attacks* are episodes of weakness in the lower limbs, causing falling without loss of consciousness. They may be due to changes in tone in the lower limb originating in the brainstem, and appear to be related to transient ischaemic attacks (Kumar & Clark 2002). Any instability in the upper cervical segment – i.e. congenital ligamentous laxity of the atlanto-occipital joint, deformed odontoid process, cervical spondylosis or a spondylolisthesis – can produce drop attacks (Cyriax 1982, Hinton et al 1993). During the subjective examination the patient must be questioned about drop attacks and the result noted. Any history of drop attacks is an absolute contraindication to orthopaedic medicine treatment techniques.

  Subluxation of the atlantoaxial joint and hypermobility of the atlanto-occipital joint are associated with Down's syndrome and may occasionally lead to compression of the spinal cord. Clinicians involved in manipulation should be aware of this risk (Pueschel et al 1992, Department of Health 1995, Matsuda et al 1995).

- *Klippel–Feil syndrome* is associated with a limited range of cervical movement, short neck and low hairline. Patients usually have developmental abnormalities, including congenital fusion of cervical vertebrae, which may predispose them to the risk of neurological sequelae (Pizzutillo et al 1994).

- *Vertebrobasilar insufficiency* produces symptoms through a reduced blood flow in the vertebral arteries to the brain. Patients often relate their symptoms to particular head positions such as looking up (Toole & Tucker 1960). Anatomical anomalies are frequently seen in the vertebral arteries and their course through the cervical foramen transversarium. Often the two arteries vary considerably in diameter (Mitchell & McKay 1995) and extrinsic or intrinsic factors may decrease the lumen of the artery permanently or temporarily. Extrinsic factors include degenerative changes in the intervertebral, zygapophyseal and uncovertebral joints, with osteophyte formation, which may compress or alter the course of the artery. Intrinsic factors include arterial disease and thrombosis.

Wallenberg's syndrome or lateral medullary syndrome is probably the most recognized syndrome of brainstem infarction caused by vertebral artery pathology (Frumkin & Baloh 1990, Kumar & Clark 2002). The common site of injury to the vertebral artery following neck manipulation is at the level of the atlantoaxial joint. Injuries include intimal tearing, dissection or thrombus formation, intramural haematoma or vasospasm.

Dizziness and nausea are the main presenting symptoms of vertebrobasilar insufficiency. However, such symptoms are also associated with cervical dysfunction, therefore correct diagnosis is important. A full list of possible signs and symptoms of vertebrobasilar insufficiency is given with the description of the test later in this chapter.

COMMENTARY ON THE EXAMINATION

OBSERVATION

Before proceeding with the history, a general observation of the patient's *face, posture and gait* is made, noting the posture of the neck and the carriage of the head. Neck posture will give an immediate indication of the severity and possible irritability of the condition, e.g. a wry neck associated with acute pain in which the patient has developed an antalgic posture.

HISTORY (SUBJECTIVE EXAMINATION)

The history is particularly important at the spinal joints. Selection of patients for orthopaedic medicine treatment techniques relies on the discal model of diagnosis and certain aspects of the history will assist in this diagnosis as well as highlighting patients with contraindications to treatment.

The *age, occupation, sports, hobbies and lifestyle* of the patient may give an indication of the nature of onset and its relationship to habitual postural problems associated with a particular lifestyle.

The age of the patient is important, particularly at the cervical spine, since the type of cervical disc lesion is related to age. In the young patient, child or adolescent, neck pain may be associated with an acute torticollis, possibly a true nuclear disc lesion.

Disc lesions tend to occur in the middle-age group, with posterior or posterolateral herniation. Referred arm pain, due to a large posterolateral disc prolapse, usually occurs over the age of 35, through progressive prolapse. Arm pain presenting under the age of 35 may be indicative of serious pathology and this should be excluded. Degenerative changes in the intervertebral, uncovertebral and zygapophyseal joints occur in the older neck.

Occupation, sports, hobbies and lifestyle of the patient may contribute to the patient's signs and symptoms. Habitual postures can contribute to postural adjustment, altered biomechanics and muscle imbalance. Examples are provided by the head-forward posture of the visual display unit operator, the side-flexed posture of holding the telephone in the crook of the neck to leave the hands free, the flexed and rotated posture of the plumber or builder, or the head-extended posture allowing the arms to be used above the head in the painter or electrician. Athletes may assume certain postures related to their sport which may precipitate or contribute to their problem.

The *site and spread* of the symptoms give important clues to diagnosis in the cervical spine and highlight the importance of understanding the mechanisms of referred pain in a segmental or multisegmental pattern. Pain may be localized to the neck or occur in association with symptoms felt in the scapular area, chest, upper limb or head.

Nerve root compression in the cervical spine can only occur at the levels at which the nerve root can be compressed. In the mid and lower cervical regions the roots are under threat from the intervertebral discs, uncovertebral joints and zygapophyseal joints which form the boundaries of the intervertebral foramen. C1 and 2 nerve roots do not run in intervertebral foramina, therefore compression of these nerve roots is not the mechanism for upper cervical pain.

It is important to establish the nature of the *onset and duration* of the symptoms, not just of this current episode of pain, but of all previous episodes. Cervical disc lesions tend to be a progression of the same incident, and establishing a history of increasing and worsening episodes of pain assists diagnosis.

The onset may be sudden or gradual. It may be precipitated by a single incident, such as a whiplash injury due to a motor vehicle accident, or a sudden unguarded movement, such as missing a footing. If traumatic in onset, the exact mechanism should be established: was it hyperflexion, hyperextension or excessive rotation? If the condition developed gradually, is it associated with habitual postures, or a change in posture, such as sleeping in a different bed?

The patient with whiplash injury without serious bony complications presents with pain felt at the time of the trauma which settles. Twenty-four hours later, pain and stiffness develop due to the ligamentous involvement and muscular strain. The whiplash patient who has severe pain from the time of the trauma may have more serious underlying pathology, e.g. fracture and/or dislocation.

The duration of the symptoms helps to give a prognosis of the patient's condition as well as providing an indicator for serious pathology, being always on the alert for possible contraindications to treatment. Generally, the patient who presents with a short duration of symptoms responds better to treatment. Disc pathology tends to be self-limiting and generally symptoms will resolve spontaneously. With repeated episodes, however, this tends to take longer and longer. Nerve root compression may follow a mechanism of spontaneous recovery in 3 or 4 months, providing the patient loses the central symptoms.

Recurrent symptoms may indicate a cervical disc lesion or degenerative arthrosis which tends to present with periods of exacerbation of symptoms. Inflammatory arthritis may present a similar picture, but it has usually manifested itself in other joints before involving the cervical spine.

The *symptoms and behaviour* need to be considered. The behaviour of the pain will give an indication of the irritability of the condition. Make a note of the daily pattern of the pain. If it is easier first thing in the morning and worse as the day goes on, easing up again with rest, this could indicate a compression problem or a postural problem. If it is uncomfortable and stiff in the morning and painful on certain movements, this is indicative of an active arthritis. It may be due to an acute episode of degenerative osteoarthrosis, or inflammatory arthritis such as rheumatoid arthritis or ankylosing spondylitis. Pain not at all relieved by rest and with unrelenting night pain indicates serious pathology such as tumour.

Of what other symptoms does the patient complain? Pain on a cough, sneeze or straining, which cause an increase in the intrathecal pressure, may indicate disc compression or tumour. Paraesthesia may be related to nerve root compression. Sympathetic symptoms such as hot and cold feelings, heaviness, puffiness or circulatory symptoms may be related to nerve root compression or thoracic outlet syndrome, reflex sympathetic dystrophy or work-related upper limb disorder.

Other causes of neck pain and associated symptoms should be eliminated, such as thoracic outlet syndrome, which may produce similar symptoms to upper cervical syndromes. Symptoms may include facial pain, tinnitus, auditory and visual disturbances.

From the history, specific questions must be asked to eliminate vertebrobasilar artery problems and problems of instability in the upper cervical joints, which would contraindicate treatment. Explore any complaint of dizziness, nausea, faintness, tinnitus or visual problems. Ask specific questions about drop attacks, i.e. 'Do you ever fall to the ground without losing consciousness?' Establish the presence of pins and needles and numbness and note exactly where. Consider whether the distribution of these symptoms fits with segmental referral or is more a sympathetic feature. It may be pertinent to ask about headaches, fatigue and stress, or blurred or dull vision.

Other joint involvement will give an indication to previous problems which may or may not be related. Look for evidence of rheumatoid arthritis, usually in the smaller joints, remembering that the disease process may be quiet in the cervical spine. Ankylosing spondylitis usually starts in the sacroiliac joint(s) and lumbar spine or hips. Note the presence of generalized degenerative osteoarthrosis.

Ask about *past medical history* and consider any serious illness or operations. It is advisable to ask about previous trauma involving the neck: a history of whiplash is considered a risk factor in vascular accidents (Kleynhans & Terret 1985).

Check the *medications* currently taken by the patient, as anticoagulants and long-term systemic steroid use may present a contraindication to the treatment techniques. Ask about any pain-relieving drugs to give an indication of how much pain control is required by the patient and as antidepressants may also be prescribed for chronic pain they may give an indication of the patient's general pain profile.

INSPECTION

The patient should undress down to underwear to the waist, and be in a good light. A general inspection will reveal any **bony deformity**. The general spinal curvatures are appreciated, assessing for any increased or decreased cervical lordosis, tilt or rotation, abnormalities in the cervicothoracic junction and upper thoracic kyphosis, scoliosis, or the presence of an antalgic posture. Abnormal fatty tissue sometimes develops over C7, in association with postural deformity at the cervicothoracic junction and this is known as a dowager's hump. Similar fatty tissue can often be seen in rugby players in the front row of the scrum. The head carriage is also noted, looking for excessive protraction or retraction.

Colour changes and swelling would not be expected in the cervical spine unless associated with a history of direct trauma.

A neuritis would give the appropriate wasting of the muscles supplied by the nerve involved and the neck, shoulder and scapular area should be assessed for obvious **muscle wasting**. Some unusual nerve pathologies produce bizarre patterns of bilateral asymmetrical wasting, e.g. neuralgic amyotrophy. In disc pathology with nerve root compression, muscle wasting may not be obvious on inspection.

STATE AT REST

Before any movements are performed, the state at rest is established to provide a baseline for subsequent comparison.

The suggested sequence for the objective examination will now be given, followed by a commentary including the reasoning in performing the movements and the significance of the possible findings.

EXAMINATION BY
SELECTIVE TENSION
(OBJECTIVE
EXAMINATION)

Articular Signs

- Active cervical extension (Fig. 8.8)
- Active cervical right rotation (Fig. 8.9a)
- Active cervical left rotation (Fig. 8.9b)
- Active cervical right side flexion (Fig. 8.10a)
- Active cervical left side flexion (Fig. 8.10b)
- Active cervical flexion (Fig. 8.11)
- Passive cervical extension (Fig. 8.12)
- Passive cervical right rotation (Fig. 8.13a)
- Passive cervical left rotation (Fig. 8.13b)
- Passive cervical right side flexion (Fig. 8.14a)
- Passive cervical left side flexion (Fig. 8.14b)

Resisted Tests are not Part of the Routine Examination, but may be Applied here

- Resisted cervical extension (Fig. 8.15)
- Resisted cervical rotations (Fig. 8.16)
- Resisted cervical side flexions (Fig. 8.17)
- Resisted cervical flexion (Fig. 8.18)

Elimination of the Shoulder Joint

- Active shoulder elevation (Fig. 8.19)

Resisted tests for Objective Neurological Signs and Alternative Causes of Arm Pain; the Main Nerve Roots are Indicated in Bold

- Shoulder elevation, trapezius (Fig. 8.20): spinal accessory nerve XI C3, 4
- Shoulder abduction, supraspinatus (Fig. 8.21): C4, **5**, 6
- Shoulder adduction, latissimus dorsi, pectoralis major, teres major and minor (Fig. 8.22): C5, 6, **7**, **8**, T1
- Shoulder lateral rotation, infraspinatus (Fig. 8.23): C5, 6
- Shoulder medial rotation, subscapularis (Fig. 8.24), **C5, 6**
- Elbow flexion, biceps (Fig. 8.25): C5, **6**
- Elbow extension, triceps (Fig. 8.26): C6, **7**, 8
- Wrist extensors, (Fig. 8.27): C6, **7**, 8
- Wrist flexors, (Fig. 8.28): C6, **7**, **8**, T1
- Thumb adductors, adductor brevis (Fig. 8.29): **C8, T1**
- Finger adductors, palmar interossei (Fig. 8.30): **C8, T1**

Skin Sensation (Fig. 8.31)

- Thumb and index finger: C6
- Index, middle and ring fingers: C7
- Middle, ring and little fingers: C8

Reflexes

- Biceps (Fig. 8.32): C5, **6**
- Brachioradialis (Fig. 8.33): C5, **6**, **7**
- Triceps (Fig. 8.34): C6, **7**, **8**
- Plantar response (Fig. 8.35)

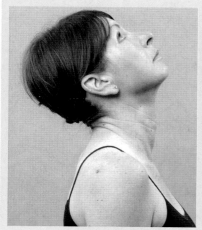 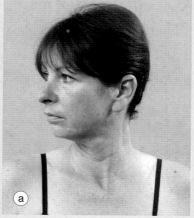 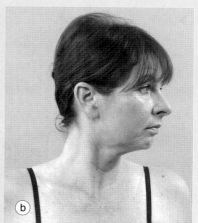

Figure 8.8   Active extension.   Figure 8.9   (a,b) Active rotations.

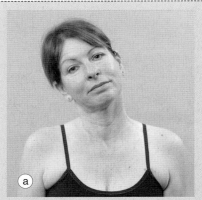

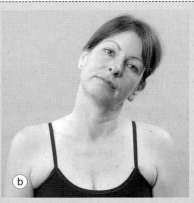

Figure 8.10 (a,b) Active side flexions.

Figure 8.11 Active flexion.

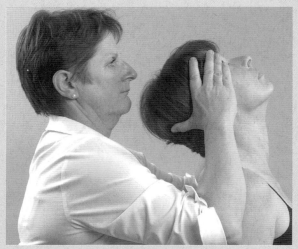

Figure 8.12 Passive extension.

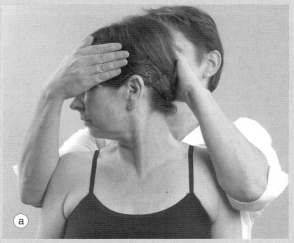

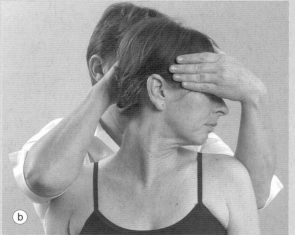

Figure 8.13 (a, b) Passive rotations.

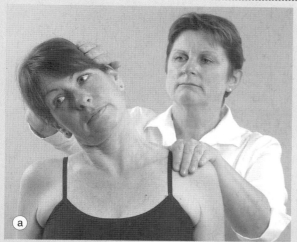

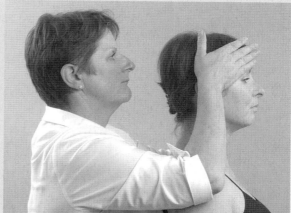

Figure 8.14 (a, b) Passive side flexions.

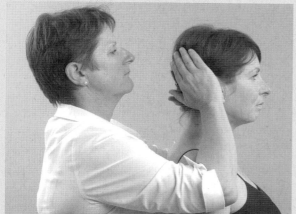

Figure 8.15 Resisted extension.

Figure 8.16 Resisted rotations.

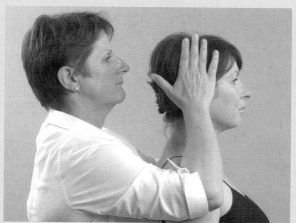

Figure 8.17 Resisted side flexions.

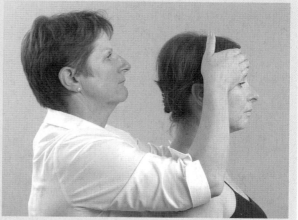

Figure 8.18 Resisted flexion.

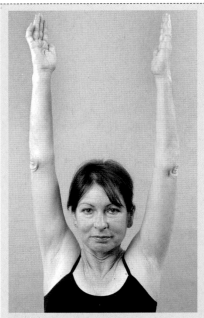

Figure 8.19   Active shoulder elevation to eliminate the shoulder as a cause of pain.

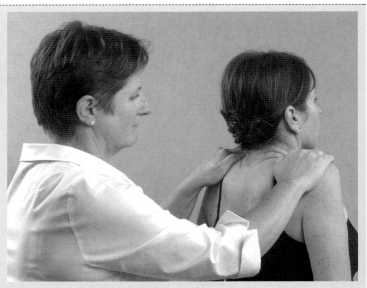

Figure 8.20   Resisted shoulder elevation.

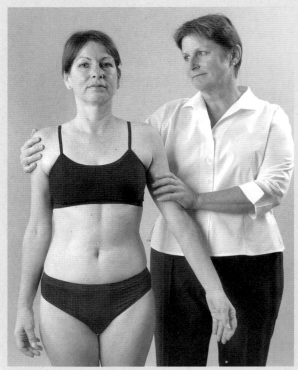

Figure 8.21   Resisted shoulder abduction.

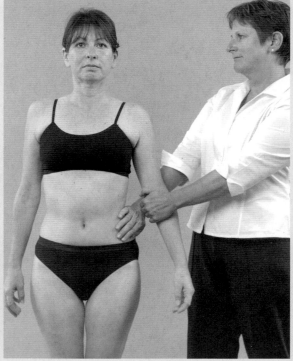

Figure 8.22   Resisted shoulder adduction.

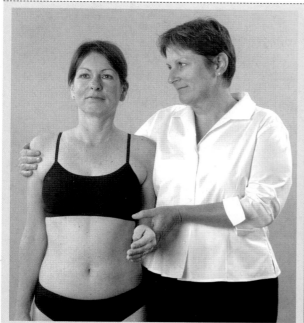

Figure 8.23   Resisted shoulder lateral rotation.

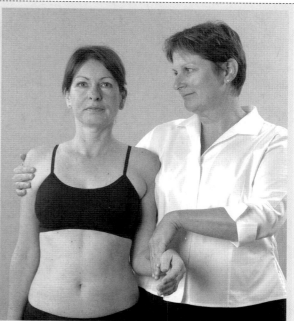

Figure 8.24   Resisted shoulder medial rotation.

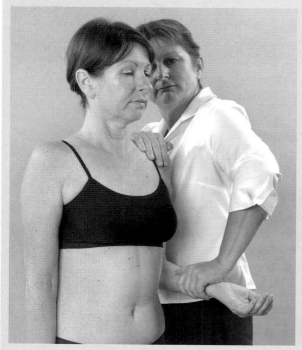

Figure 8.25   Resisted elbow flexion.

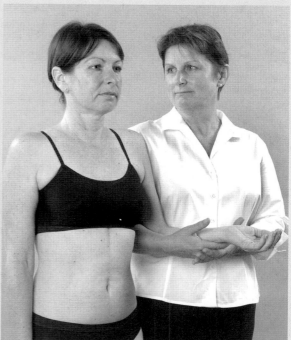

Figure 8.26   Resisted elbow extension

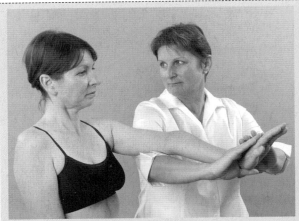

Figure 8.27   Resisted wrist extension.

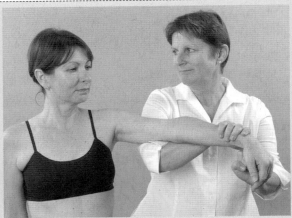

Figure 8.28   Resisted wrist flexion.

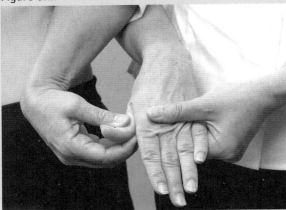

Figure 8.29   Resisted thumb adduction.

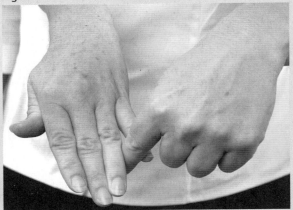

Figure 8.30   Resisted finger adduction.

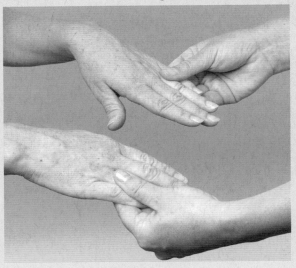

Figure 8.31   Checking skin sensation.

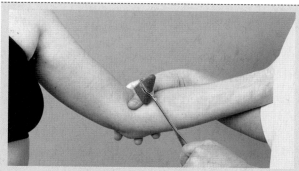

Figure 8.32   Biceps reflex.

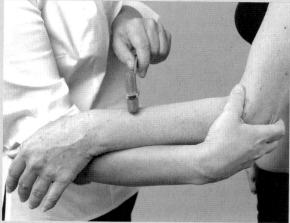

Figure 8.33   Brachioradialis reflex.

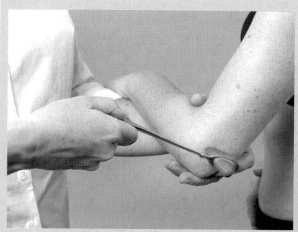

Figure 8.34   Triceps reflex

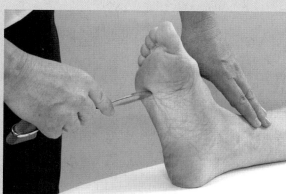

Figure 8.35   Plantar response.

The routine examination of the cervical spine includes active, passive and resisted movements. Since the spinal joints are considered to be a potential focus for 'emotional' symptoms, six active movements are conducted assessing willingness to move, range of movement and pain.

Capsular pattern of the cervical spine

- Equal limitation of side flexions.
- Equal limitation of rotations.
- Some limitation of extension.
- Usually full flexion.

The capsular or non-capsular pattern may also emerge from these active movements.

In a non-capsular pattern of the cervical spine, some movements are limited and/or painful and others are full and pain-free. The presence of a non-capsular pattern indicates a possible disc displacement. Normally movements at the cervical spine do not occur in isolation, but the examination procedure is conducted simply by assessing the individual movements. It should, however, be remembered that flexion and extension occur with a component of translatory glide, while side flexion and rotation occur as a coupled movement.

The passive movements are assessed to determine the true limitation of range of movement and the end-feel. The pattern of limited movements should be the same as that found on active movements, although the range may be slightly more. Normally passive extension has a hard end-feel, passive rotations an elastic end-feel and passive side flexions an elastic end-feel due to tissue tension. Passive flexion is not assessed because it would tend to aggravate the symptoms of disc lesion.

The resisted tests are not part of the routine examination at the cervical spine, but should be applied if there is a history of trauma, e.g. for a muscle lesion or suspected serious pathology such as fracture, metastases or illness behaviour. The resisted tests also assess the C1 and 2 nerve roots. Resisted flexion may produce pain in a disc lesion since it causes compression.

The shoulder joint complex is eliminated as a cause of pain by active elevation. If this is full range and pain-free, the shoulder can be eliminated from the examination.

Assessment for objective root signs is conducted by a series of resisted tests for the myotomes, looking for a pattern of muscle weakness which would indicate nerve root compression. Since it is also important to eliminate other causes of arm pain, the muscle groups are also assessed, looking for alternative causes of pain. This explains why the sequence appears to test the same nerve roots several times.

A quick check of skin sensation to light touch is made looking for differences. Paraesthesia commonly affects the distal end of the dermatomes and these are assessed, followed by the biceps, brachioradialis and triceps reflexes.

The plantar response is assessed by stroking up the lateral border of the sole of the foot and across the metatarsal heads. If the response is extensor, i.e. upgoing, it is indicative of an upper motor neuron lesion. The normal response is flexor.

The objective examination sequence provides a basic assessment framework to glean important information towards the selection of patients appropriate for the treatment techniques used in orthopaedic medicine. It also highlights possible contraindications and provides a guide for the specific treatments to be used.

Any other assessment procedures may be included throughout the sequence or explored separately afterwards, either to elicit extra information for the purposes of the application of other treatment modalities, or to confirm findings necessitating patient referral.

CERVICAL DISC LESIONS – A CLASSIFICATION SYSTEM OF THREE CLINICAL MODELS

In the past, treatment in orthopaedic medicine has been traditionally targeted at the disc, aiming to reduce displacement, relieve pain and restore movement. However, there is a lack of confidence in these traditional pathoanatomical diagnostic labels, since the cause of pain cannot be confidently localized to one specific structure. Consequently, several authors have established classifications to determine treatment programmes and to assist prognosis (McKenzie 1981, Riddle 1998, Laslett & van Wijmen 1999).

While not ideal, the presentation of signs and symptoms of cervical lesions has been classified here into clinical models adapted from Cyriax's original theories. These models are judgement based and contribute to the clinical decision-making process to rationalize appropriate treatment programmes, but are not intended to be restrictive. The reader is encouraged to be inventive, to draw on other experiences and to implement the approach into their existing knowledge when putting a treatment programme together for individual patients. The treatment techniques described are by no means a cure-all for every case of neck pain. However, uncomplicated lesions of recent onset may respond well to the mobilization and manipulative techniques of orthopaedic medicine. The key, as in the lumbar spine, is the selection of appropriate patients for treatment.

For the purposes of the following classification of lesions, a cervical lesion presents with the following features:

- An onset of neck pain which may be in a multisegmental or segmental distribution (see Ch. 1)
- A typical mechanical history that describes pain aggravated by activity and certain postures, such as sitting, and relieved by rest and postures such as lying
- Symptoms such as a cough or sneeze increasing the pain and possible paraesthesia in a segmental pattern
- No significant 'red' and 'yellow flags' present in the history
- Examination revealing a non-capsular pattern of movement
- No contraindications to treatment

CLINICAL MODEL 1: ACUTE TORTICOLLIS

Factors from the subjective examination

- Adolescent or young adult
- Mainly central, or short bilateral or unilateral neck pain
- Patient usually wakes with severe onset of pain, not attributable to any precipitating cause

Factors from the objective examination

- Antalgic posture
- Non-capsular pattern of painful movements
- *No* neurological signs

Treatment consists of reassurance to both the patient and parents and progressive positioning out of the deformity may expedite reduction. Pain-relieving modalities may be applied, e.g. analgesics, electrotherapy, massage and gentle mobilization. Gentle traction may be applied in the form of the 'bridging' technique and progressed to manual traction, depending on irritability. Traction is applied in line with the deformity if the neutral position cannot be assumed. The condition usually resolves spontaneously in 7–10 days.

This treatment procedure can be applied to any acute/irritable neck in the absence of contraindications, e.g. the acute whiplash patient or the patient who fits classification of Clinical Model 2, but who has adopted an antalgic 'wry' neck and is too irritable for the treatment regime suggested below.

CLINICAL MODEL 2

Factors from the subjective examination

- Central, or short bilateral or unilateral neck or scapular pain
- Gradual or sudden onset
- Patient may or may not recall the exact mode and time of onset

Factors from the objective examination

- Non-capsular pattern of painful and limited movements
- *No* neurological signs

Treatment of choice is to follow the cervical manual traction and mobilization routine described below, providing no contraindications to treatment exist.

CLINICAL MODEL 3: CERVICAL DISC LESION PRESENTING WITH REFERRED ARM SYMPTOMS

Factors from the subjective examination

- Patient usually over the age of 35
- Initial presentation of central or unilateral neck and/or scapular pain, followed by referred arm pain (the central pain ceasing or diminishing)
- Sudden or gradual onset
- Often part of a history of increasing, worsening episodes, therefore a progression of the above scenarios
- Patient may or may not recall the exact time and mode of onset
- Patient may complain of root symptoms, i.e. paraesthesia felt in a segmental pattern

Factors from the objective examination

- Non-capsular pattern of movements producing neck and/or arm symptoms
- Root signs may be present, i.e. muscle weakness, absent or reduced reflexes

The hypothesis is more readily rationalized here. Due to the nerve root involvement a large posterolateral prolapse of disc material has occurred, producing pain referred into the arm through compression of the dural nerve root sleeve or the nerve root itself. Pain, therefore, is segmental in distribution. If the nerve root is involved, there will be objective neurological signs. Since the nerve roots emerge horizontally in the cervical spine, only one nerve root should be involved in disc lesions. The quality of the pain helps to distinguish somatic and radicular pain (see Ch. 13).

Treatment is aimed at relieving pain. If neurological signs are present, manipulation is not strictly contraindicated provided the neurological signs are minimal and stable, i.e. non-progressive, and that no other contraindications exist. However, the more peripheral the signs and symptoms, the less likely it is to succeed, and other modalities, e.g. manual or sustained mechanical traction and mobilization, may be more effective in relieving symptoms. An epidural of corticosteroid and local anaesthetic may be indicated, but this is a specialist procedure usually conducted under ultrasonography. Since the natural history of disc herniation is one of recovery over time without the intervention of surgery, a mechanism of spontaneous recovery may occur (Saal et al 1996, Bush et al 1997).

TREATMENT OF CERVICAL DISC LESIONS

It is recommended that a course in orthopaedic medicine is attended before the treatment techniques below are applied in clinical practice (see Appendix).

Treatment of cervical disc lesions depends on the nature of the pain and classification of the symptoms (see above). If the pain is subacute and the symptoms not particularly irritable, a regime of mobilization can be commenced, progressing to manipulation if necessary. If the pain is acute and the symptoms highly irritable, a gentler approach to treatment is adopted. In chronic cervical conditions, a thorough examination may reveal several components to the diagnosis, adverse neural tension and muscle imbalance, for example, together with underlying psychological factors such as anxiety and depression. All components of the patient's condition must be addressed and the orthopaedic medicine approach and treatment techniques should form only part of the treatment programme. Their use is not intended to be exclusive.

In terms of likely response to manipulation, the ideal patient will fit into the pattern of signs and symptoms that indicate Clinical Model 2. In this model there will be a history of sudden or gradual onset of central, short bilateral or unilateral neck and/or scapular pain. On examination there is a non-capsular pattern of limited movement and no objective neurological signs. To be ideal in terms of likely effectiveness of treatment, the symptoms should be of recent onset and have minimum reference of pain. The more peripheral the symptoms, the less successful the techniques described tend to be.

Provided there are no contraindications to treatment, a regime of cervical mobilization is commenced. Treatment techniques are chosen based on a continuous assessment approach. After every technique the patient's comparable signs are reassessed.

Following each session of treatment, advice is given about neck care, general posture, sleeping postures and pillows. Maintenance exercises are given if they are appropriate and the patient is started on a self-help programme to prevent recurrence.

Mobilization and manipulation techniques in orthopaedic medicine usually produce immediate results. One, two or three sessions of treatment would be expected. If a patient is not responding to the approach, it is abandoned and other mobilization and treatment modalities attempted.

CONTRAINDICATIONS

As well as considering indications for treatment, it is essential to exclude patients with absolute contraindications. Although it is impossible to be absolutely definitive about all contraindications, – the so called 'red flags' to the cervical mobilization procedure discussed below – nothing can substitute for a rigorous assessment of the presenting signs and symptoms and an accurate diagnosis of a mechanical lesion.

Drop attacks are an absolute contraindication to the orthopaedic medicine cervical mobilization procedure, including manipulation, since these may be indicative of upper cervical instability or related to transient ischaemic attacks. Similarly, patients with a history of cerebrovascular accident, transient ischaemic attacks or other upper motor neuron lesion would be contraindicated and other treatment modalities should be considered if neck pain is a feature in these patients. Upper cervical spine instability is also associated with Down's syndrome patients and active cervical rheumatoid arthritic changes. Ligamentous laxity may be a feature of pregnancy, making pregnancy a relative contraindication to manipulation.

A gradual onset of increasing pain over 3 months may be indicative of inflammatory arthritis which may be a relative contraindication. Ankylosing spondylitis and other spondyloarthropathies, for example, may not affect the cervical spine, in which case the cervical mobilization regime discussed below would not be contraindicated and individual judgements would need to be made for each case. Rheumatoid arthritis, which usually affects the smaller joints symmetrically, may be progressing subclinically in the cervical spine, therefore the techniques discussed below would be contraindicated.

A subjective examination will screen a patient for symptoms of vertebrobasilar insufficiency and if present, the treatment regime discussed below would be absolutely contraindicated. However, dizziness, a major symptom of vertebrobasilar insufficiency, is more commonly a symptom of cervical dysfunction. Therefore accurate diagnosis is essential here in order to prevent a large group of patients being denied a very worthwhile treatment regime. The merits of the testing procedure for vertebrobasilar insufficiency will be discussed below and currently it is advisable to conduct a recognized test before applying manipulation. A positive vertebrobasilar test would be an absolute contraindication to manipulation. If the cause of dizziness cannot be ascertained, it would be wise to err on the side of caution.

Suspicious features indicative of non-mechanical lesions would be an absolute contraindication to the orthopedic medicine treatment regime. These symptoms should not be considered in isolation but in the general context of the whole examination procedure and may include unexplained weight loss, poor general health, pain unaffected by posture or activity, constant pain of which night pain is a feature and cord signs such as spastic gait and/or abnormal plantar response. The patient with a past history of primary tumour is not strictly contraindicated, but diagnosis of a mechanical lesion must be certain before proceeding with the treatment regime since the pain of bony metastases may mimic mechanical pain. Suspicious findings occur in Pancoast's tumour (a tumour in the apex of the lung) which may affect the lower trunks of the brachial plexus resulting in medial arm pain and T1 palsy. Objective examination may reveal provocation of pain by side flexion away from the painful side as the only positive cervical sign and this would be an unusual finding in a cervical disc lesion.

Symptoms of cervical disc lesions can generally be traced back to show a history of increasing and worsening episodes. Therefore cervical radiculopathy generally affects the over 35 age group. Of course, this can also occur in the younger age group, but diagnosis is again paramount, since this can be a suspicious feature associated with tumour. As in the lumbar spine, for the arm symptoms to be indicative of a mechanical lesion, the central symptoms are expected to subside considerably at the onset of arm pain. The nerve roots emerge horizontally, certainly in the upper cervical spine (see discussion in the anatomy section), therefore multiple nerve root involvement should be considered suspicious until the screening procedures in the subjective and objective examination confirm a mechanical diagnosis. Similarly double nerve root involvement is unusual, particularly as the vertebral canal in the cervical region is large and can more readily accommodate a disc prolapse than in the lumbar spine. Bilateral arm signs and symptoms would therefore be an unusual presentation of a mechanical lesion. If, during the application of manual traction, the patient experiences an onset of paraesthesia in a multisegmental distribution, i.e. both hands, then the procedure should be stopped. Cyriax (1993) suggested this phenomenon is due to adherent dura, presumably therefore having implications for the mobility of the spinal cord, and alternative treatment options should be explored.

Cord signs, which may be associated with cervical myelopathy, are an absolute contraindication to cervical manipulation. A central disc prolapse may encroach on the dura mater producing bilateral symptoms, therefore central techniques might be appropriate, but rotatory techniques under traction would not. The importance of reducing small uncomplicated disc lesions is important to prevent future degenerative changes threatening the spinal cord (Ombregt et al 2003).

The acute cervical lesion is too irritable for manipulation but may well respond to mobilization, particularly the bridging or manual traction technique described below. An antalgic posture indicates severity. In radiculopathy with minimal, stable neurological signs, manipulation is not contraindicated but may not be effective. Increasing unstable neurological signs are a contraindication as the prolapse could be increased.

A history of recent trauma has been identified as a risk factor in vertebrobasilar insufficiency due to damage to the lining of the vertebral artery, therefore manipulation is contraindicated. Past history of trauma, head injury, fracture and previous surgery are all relative contraindications and judgements will have to be made on individual cases.

The drug history will identify the contraindication of anticoagulation therapy to manipulation due to the risk of intraspinal bleed. The long-term use of systemic steroid medication predisposes the patient to osteoporosis; this and a known diagnosis of osteoporosis is a contraindication to manipulation. Patients considered susceptible to osteoporosis may be relatively contraindicated and individual judgements will need to be made. Caution should be exhibited with patients who have blood clotting disorders.

Patients with pyschosocial components, the so called 'yellow flags', may be unsuitable for manipulation and even the mobilization regime may present a relative contraindication, again judgements will need to be made on individual cases.

The treatment regime discussed below is contraindicated in the absence of patient consent. The patient should be given all details of their diagnosis together with the proposed treatment regime and a discussion of the risks and benefits should ensue to enable them to give their informed consent. Consent is the patient's agreement, written or oral, for a health professional to provide care. It may range from an active request by the patient for a particular treatment regime to the passive acceptance of the health professional's advice. The process of consent, within the context of the orthopaedic medicine, is 'fluid' rather than one instance in time when the patient gives their consent. The patient is constantly monitored and feedback is actively requested. The treatment procedures can be progressed or stopped at the patient's request or in response to adverse reactions. Reassessment is conducted after each technique and a judgement made about proceeding. The patient has a right to refuse consent and this should be respected and alternative treatment options discussed. For further information on consent, the reader is referred to the Department of Health web site *www.doh.gov.uk/consent*.

Safety recommendations for spinal manipulative techniques are included in the Appendix.

THE CERVICAL MOBILIZATION PROCEDURE

It is important to emphasize that the treatment techniques in this section will be described carefully in a step-by-step fashion to enable their application. However, the professional judgement and existing skill of the operator will allow each technique to be adapted.

The order of the techniques as they appear here merely provides a guide towards the development of skills at each stage and it is not necessarily an order of efficacy. It is important constantly to reassess the patient's comparable signs and to decide on the next step in the light of patient response. In this way the orthopaedic medicine approach can properly be integrated into existing practice as fresh decisions are made and the underlying hypothesis is modified. It is traditional to start each session with manual traction as this technique seems to achieve the greatest response; if progression is required then the other techniques are carried out, with a vertebrobasilar artery test conducted prior to the application of manipulation in each session of treatment.

Manipulation as such, defined as a minimal amplitude, high velocity thrust at the end of range, is only carried out if judgement deems it necessary. The mobilization procedure suggested is usually sufficient to reduce most uncomplicated cervical disc lesions, i.e. with no neurological signs or symptoms.

The enormous benefit of this cervical mobilization procedure outweighs the small risk of vertebrobasilar complications but that is not to take the risk lightly. The appropriate steps to minimize this risk, suggested in the guidelines below, should always be taken, but huge debate continues on the true incidence of complications from cervical manipulation, and it has been ascertained that the tests themselves carry a degree of risk. The reader is recommended to check for the most recent developments before applying the techniques, as safety issues are in a state of change and the most up-to-date guidelines should be adhered to.

The techniques involve traction, slight extension of the head and sometimes rotation, and these are the positions which have been implicated in causing compromise of the vertebral arteries. However, it should be emphasized that this is not the only area of danger in this region; the spinal cord is vulnerable to central disc herniation and these same positions assist centralization of the herniated disc material and aim to prevent further central displacement that could potentially endanger the cord.

It is not possible to say how many times each technique is to be attempted since the process of reassessment is the basis for each clinical decision and the circumstances vary in every clinical encounter. Nonetheless, a balance must be found between sidestepping the question and providing a recipe for treatment. Some guidance will be given in terms of expectations, with respect to the different states and stages of the conditions presented.

Generally, the more acutely painful lesions require gentle treatment, but reassurance and advice may be more appropriate in the early stages without the application of passive treatment. For the subacute or less irritable states, if the technique is helping, it is repeated; if no change occurs after a few attempts the next technique is chosen; if the patient's signs and symptoms are abolished, treatment should be stopped. Once improvement plateaus in each session, or if the progress is uncertain, the treatment is either modified to an alternative modality or ceases, with the patient being reassessed at the next session when a new status quo will have emerged.

In general, lesions producing central or bilateral pain should be treated with central techniques, i.e. manual traction, traction with leverage, anteroposterior glide. Lesions producing unilateral pain are treated with manual traction, progressing to rotational mobilizations under traction and manipulation if necessary. The monitoring that takes place during this step-by-step progression of forces is most important to safety.

Figure 8.36   Bridging technique.

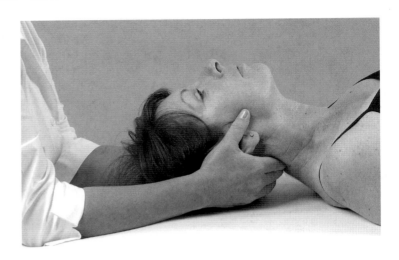

Bridging technique

The indication for use is the patient with a highly irritable lesion: an acute whiplash injury; the acute torticollis seen in Clinical Model 1; the antalgic posture of a wry neck seen in Clinical Model 2; an acute presentation of Clinical Model 3. Progression to manual traction may be made as the irritability of the lesion is reduced. It is a method of applying gentle traction and should not produce an increase in symptoms.

Position the patient supine on the couch a little way down from the top edge. Sit on a chair at the head of the couch and gently adjust the patient's position so that your forearms and elbows are fully supported, with your hands resting under the patient's neck (Fig. 8.36). Make a bridge with the fingers and rest them under the occiput. Tilt the hands into radial deviation, which tips the head slightly back, and pull, flexing your forearms by pulling yourself towards the patient, to apply minimal traction. Hold the pull for a few seconds, according to patient comfort. Gently release and repeat as required, gradually applying more traction as the tissues relax. This technique can be adjusted and applied to different spinal segmental levels.

The following mobilization procedure is applied to the cervical lesion that ideally falls into Clinical Model 2. Manual traction may also be appropriate in Clinical Models 1 and 3, the rotation techniques are not contraindicated for either, but the lesion is possibly too irritable and may be made worse. The patient who falls into Clinical Model 3 and displays root signs will probably not be helped by manipulation, but again it is not a strict contraindication provided the neurological signs are not severe or progressive.

Manual traction (Cyriax 1984)

This is always recommended as the first technique to be performed in each treatment session for the less irritable or subacute neck. It is generally comfortable for the patient and allows both you and the patient to become used to the handling techniques. It is often not necessary to progress beyond this stage if positive results are achieved. After each technique an increase in range and/or decrease in symptoms is to be expected.

Explain the technique and its intention to the patient. All mobilization techniques are carefully monitored by the operator for a change in symptoms. Patients are instructed to signal if they wish the manoeuvre to cease for any reason. It is important that patients appreciate that they have control over each manoeuvre – the final overpressure of the Grade C manipulation (see below) is the only exception to this – which is why feedback on discomfort should be obtained from the patient right up to the moment of its application.

Raise the couch approximately level with your hips. Position the patient in supine with their shoulders level with the head of the couch and supporting their head in your hands. An assistant is needed to apply counterpressure at the same time as you apply the manual traction by restraining the movement of the patient's shoulders, adopting a walk-standing position at the side of the couch. If no assistant is available, restraining Cyriax 'horns' or non-slip matting may be used.

Position one of your hands to cup the occiput or support just below the occiput, allowing the head to tip into slight extension; the cervical spine itself should remain in a neutral position. The other hand rests comfortably around the patient's chin, avoiding the trachea, and your forearm lies along the side of the face.

Place both feet directly under the patient's head and bend both your knees. Lean out with straight arms to apply the traction using body weight (Fig. 8.37). Perform the technique slowly, allowing the traction to establish for several seconds, then pull yourself back to the upright position and release the traction.

Sit the patient up slowly and re-examine the comparable signs, before deciding on the next manoeuvre.

Figure 8.37   Manual traction.

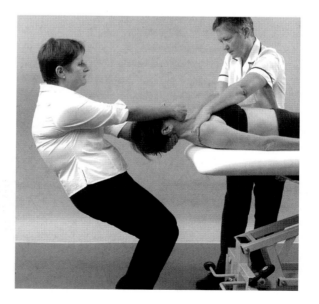

Assess the patient's body weight compared with your own. If you are much heavier than the patient do not apply maximum body weight. Less body weight can be achieved by positioning the feet a little further back but the arms should still be straightened.

A patient with dentures should leave them in situ with some padding placed between the teeth to help prevent discomfort and perhaps breakage.

This technique of manual traction is essential to most other manoeuvres and it is worthwhile practising it to gain confidence and competence.

A patient classified as Clinical Model 3 who experiences a reduction in signs and symptoms after the application of manual traction can be progressed to sustained mechanical traction as described below, since in the authors' clinical experience, manual traction provides a short temporary effect with this model.

Manual traction plus rotation (Cyriax & Cyriax 1983, Cyriax 1984)

The pain-free, or least painful, rotation is chosen first as this will be more comfortable for the patient. The hand holds are the same as above, with a right rotation requiring your right hand to be positioned around the chin (Fig. 8.38), and vice versa for a left rotation.

Apply the traction as above. Allow it to establish for a few seconds, then rotate into the least painful rotation by side flexing your body. Return to the mid-position and release the traction as above. Three variations of this technique can be applied, and each is a progression of the other.

- *Grade A*: mid-range rotation (Fig. 8.39)
- *Grade B*: to end of available range (Fig. 8.40). Here it is so important to understand the nature of end-feel and to be sensitive to any abnormal end-feel such as muscle spasm, which suggests the technique should be abandoned
- *Grade C*: manipulation, the final high velocity, minimal amplitude thrust is applied at end of range. (See reference to the 'Guidance for

Figure 8.38   Hand positioning for manual traction plus rotation to the right.

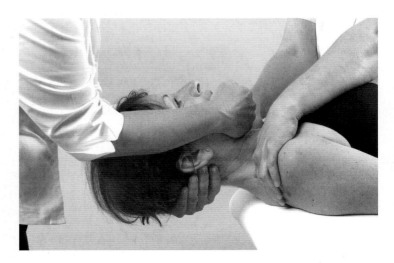

Figure 8.39   Manual traction plus rotation, Grade A.

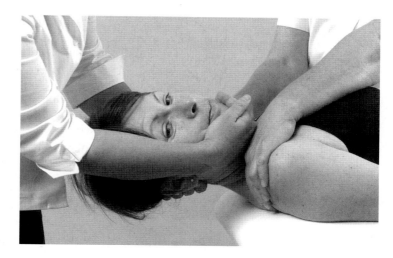

Figure 8.40   Manual traction plus rotation, Grade B, and position at which a Grade C manipulation is applied.

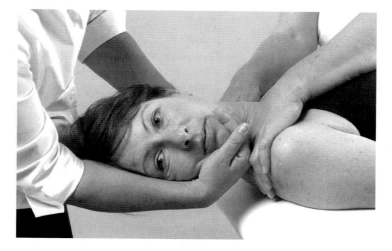

pre-manipulative testing of the cervical spine', Barker et al 2001, on page 311, before proceeding to manipulation.)

If these three stages have proved unsuccessful, the procedure is now repeated using the same routine into the more painful range of rotation. Under traction, this should not produce an increase in symptoms and any increase is an indication to stop. Again, progression is only made to the next step if necessary.

VERTEBROBASILAR ARTERY TESTING

In recent years, the potential risk to the cerebral blood flow from cervical manipulation techniques has received much publicity in relation to incidents and accidents following cervical manipulation (Krueger & Okazaki 1980, Weinstein & Cantu 1991, Sinel & Smith 1993, Rivett 1994,

Carey 1995, Sternbach et al 1995). Trauma to the vertebral artery leading to stroke is a rare but devastating complication of cervical manipulation. Potential risk and precipitating factors have been suggested by various authors, but the basis for these suggestions remain unclear. Initiation for the testing procedures seems to stem from cadaver studies conducted by Brown & Tatlow (1963) which showed the contralateral vertebral artery to be sometimes occluded on rotation, extension or combined rotation and extension. More recent studies have demonstrated conflicting results on the effect of position of the cervical spine on blood flow in the vertebral arteries, questioning the validity and clinical value of the pre-manipulative tests.

The Australian Physiotherapy Association was probably the first group to introduce a formal protocol for pre-manipulative testing of the cervical spine. The current guidance (see Fig. 8.41) was a joint venture between the Society of Orthopaedic Medicine and the Manipulation Association of Charted Physiotherapists, published in *Manual Therapy*, the *Journal of Orthopaedic Medicine* and, more recently, in *Physiotherapy* (Barker et al 2001). The guidance aims to guide the decision-making process towards safe application of cervical manipulation, to heighten awareness of the risks and complications, and to improve quality of care by informing of current best practice. The flow chart is reproduced below (Fig. 8.41) and is current at the time of writing, but the reader should ascertain the most up-to-date guidelines in case of revisions while in press.

Haldeman et al (1999) assessed the English language literature from 1966 to 1993 to determine potential precipitating events and risk factors, classifying vertebrobasilar dissection and occlusions as follows:

Traumatic: major trauma was identified in 37 cases such as road traffic accident, direct impact and sporting injuries, e.g. skiing, surfing and bungee jumping, and minor trauma was identified in 58 cases associated with activities of daily living such as sustained rotation and extension in painting the ceiling, sleeping in an awkward position, visit to the hairdresser, amusement park rides and looking over the shoulder while driving the car.

Spontaneous: 160 cases were identified, but it was difficult to highlight particular risk factors in this group as there was no preceding trauma.

Spinal manipulation: this was implicated in 115 cases, but most of these were extrapolated or generalized from retrospective case reports. In terms of experimental design, this evidence is considered to be the lowest ranked on which to base changes in clinical practice. Potential risk has been estimated at between 1 in 4 million and 1 in 1.3 million manipulations, but there is virtually no detailed information on the magnitude of forces applied or the type of manipulative procedure applied. Rotation has the highest number of associations and young adults were most commonly affected. This is unsurprising, since rotation is the commonest cervical manipulation used and the young adult group is the group most likely to be manipulated. The potential risk could perhaps be compared to alternative treatments such as the risk of a prolonged course of NSAIDs or the risk from neck surgery or general anaesthesia.

Figure 8.41   Guidance for
pre-manipulative testing of the
cervical spine – Flowchart.

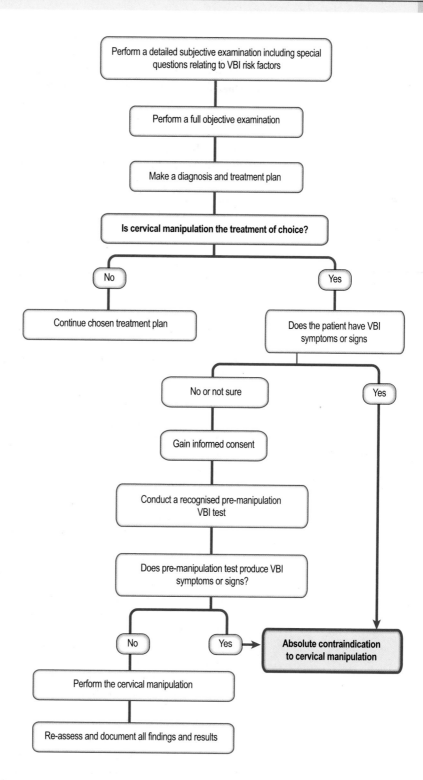

The vertebral artery is most vulnerable in its third section, the atlantooccipital region, where it takes two right-angled turns, one to pass behind the lateral mass of the atlas and the second to enter the foramen magnum. Here the artery is relatively fixed and immobile and manipulation involving rotation and/or extension has been implicated as a cause of vascular accident. The resultant shearing force on the arterial wall could lead to dissection, intramural haematoma and/or thrombus formation. The testing procedures commonly consist of rotation and extension which could be as hazardous as the manipulative techniques themselves, therefore the reliability and validity of the testing procedures has been questioned.

Rivett (1997) highlighted a case of a negative vertebral artery test despite complete occlusion. In contrast, Licht et al (2000) conducted a prospective study to assess vertebral artery blood flow in patients with positive pre-manipulative testing to investigate whether, despite the positive test, chiropractors would consider treating such patients if the subsequent Doppler ultrasound was normal. The majority of chiropractors surveyed agreed that they would proceed with the manipulation if the Doppler ultrasound was normal, despite the positive test. The study therefore concluded that a positive pre-manipulative test is not an absolute contraindication to cervical manipulation.

Rivett (1999) conducted a two-group experimental pilot study with a small sample of 20 subjects, to determine the effect of rotation or extension on vertebral artery and internal carotid blood flow (the sustained positioning was held for up to 60 seconds which is not comparable with the short duration that the position is assumed for the manipulative procedure). Some support for the reliability of pre-manipulative testing was demonstrated as significant changes occurred in blood flow in end-range positions involving contralateral rotation and extension. It was concluded that the screening procedures may be useful tests of the adequacy of the collateral circulation in preventing ischaemia if the blood flow through one of the vertebral arteries was critically reduced, say by cervical manipulation.

The benefit gained in pain relief and restoration of movement by an expertly applied manipulative technique should not be sacrificed in an attempt to be too cautious. Conflicting evidence of the risk versus the benefit can be found in the literature, Refshauge et al (2002) postulating that the risks outweigh the benefits while Jull et al (2002), in response, suggest that many of their arguments are biased or flawed and do not support their recommendations. The risk, no matter how small, does nevertheless exist and techniques involving traction and rotation have received criticism for being the most hazardous (Grant 1988). However, as discussed above, what is often not taken into account is that there are two potential danger areas within the cervical spine, the vertebral artery and the spinal cord. In attempting to reduce a disc lesion, traction is applied to assist centralization and to prevent further disc displacement into the vertebral canal where the prolapse could endanger the spinal cord.

Before embarking on any cervical technique the clinician is recommended to follow the guidance for safe practice as suggested below. The guidance has been devised to minimize the risk of complication following cervical mobilization techniques. Several points need to be considered before embarking on the testing regime.

Dizziness is one of the first symptoms of vertebrobasilar insufficiency, but it is also a symptom associated with cervical dysfunction, cervicogenic headaches, benign positional vertigo and inner ear problems. The vertebrobasilar artery system supplies the vestibular nuclei in the brainstem and the labyrinth of the inner ear (Grant 1988). A careful history will assist diagnosis. If benign postural vertigo is suspected, diagnosis can be confirmed by performing Hall–Pike positional testing which, if positive, demonstrates a characteristic torsional nystagmus when the head is reclined and turned to the affected side (Lempert et al 1995).

The test should not be considered in isolation, but in the context of the whole assessment procedure. Cervical traction is used as a technique by itself, or in conjunction with mobilization and manipulation. It is used to decompress the cervical joints, protecting the spinal cord from further posterior displacement of the disc during the technique. Traction is recommended as a first manoeuvre; it is relatively gentle and can be stopped immediately if adverse effects are noted or reported. It often achieves an increase in range and decrease in pain, making the addition of further techniques unnecessary. Manipulation is only applied when a regime of manual traction and traction with mobilization has failed to be effective. By progressing the treatment in this way, adverse vertebrobasilar artery symptoms should be picked up before a manipulation is applied.

GUIDANCE FOR PRE-MANIPULATIVE TESTING OF THE CERVICAL SPINE (BARKER ET AL 2001)

FLOWCHART (Fig. 8.41)

The guidance for pre-manipulative testing aims to identify patients with a potential risk of vascular accident if the vertebral artery is compromised. Rather than testing for vertebrobasilar insufficiency, it is probably a predictor of the ability of the collateral circulation to maintain perfusion of the brain should the vertebral artery (or arteries) be occluded. A detailed history, together with the objective examination, establishes a diagnosis. If manipulation is the treatment of choice, the clinician should discuss the risks and benefits of the proposed technique with the patient to gain informed consent. The flowchart (Fig 8.41) is self-explanatory, and it is currently advised that a recognized pre-manipulative test is conducted in each treatment session which is to include cervical manipulation. Some clinicians choose to apply the testing procedure prior to cervical mobilization, but this is an individual judgement and not currently mandatory. The guidance will be developed in the light of new research, but this guidance is current at the time of going to press. However the reader is advised to keep abreast of developments occurring in the intervening time.

Any recognized pre-manipulative testing procedure can be applied. The test described below places the patient's cervical spine in the simulated position for the manipulative procedures. However, this is a combined position, which is not exactly the same as the position for the individual techniques, nor can the manipulative thrust be simulated.

Figure 8.42   Vertebrobasilar artery test

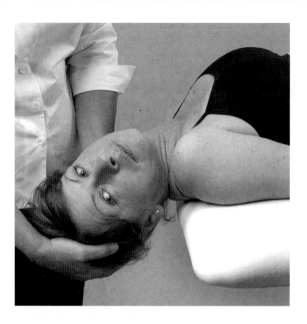

Position the patient in supine lying with the shoulders level with the end of the couch. Support the head comfortably. Place the head into a degree of extension, with side flexion and rotation of the cervical spine (Fig. 8.42). Keep the patient talking and the eyes open while maintaining the position for 30 s unless symptoms are evoked before this time. Allow the patient to rest in neutral before repeating the test to the other side.

The presence of dizziness, nausea, vomiting, sweating, pallor, blurred vision, dysarthria, fainting, tinnitus or paraesthesia in the head or arm constitutes a positive test.

The main symptoms and signs of a positive vertebrobasilar artery test can be remembered using the five Ds: dizziness, diplopia, drop attacks, dysarthria and dysphagia – a useful *aide-mémoire* attributed to Coman (Grant 1988).

If the test is found to be positive, slide the patient back onto the couch and leave lying in supine to recover. Help the patient to sit up steadily and check by questioning and observation that the symptoms have subsided before terminating the session, or continuing with a suitable alternative treatment modality.

Following the recommended guidance is the current basis for ensuring maximum safety and preparation for the unexpected. The clinician must take all due care while applying the test and the treatment techniques.

Anteroposterior glide under traction (Cyriax & Cyriax 1983, Cyriax 1984)

This technique is applied if the symptoms have centralized and the range of movement has increased, but extension remains slightly limited. The importance of fully reducing a disc prolapse is based on the hypothesis that a small central bulge, if left in situ, will gradually cause ligamentous traction and osteophyte formation, both of which have the potential to threaten the cord in later life. Therefore it aims to clear extension.

Place the couch a little lower than for the above manoeuvres. Position the patient supine on the couch as before, with an assistant ready to apply counterpressure. Stand sideways-onto the patient with both feet parallel and close to the couch, under the patient's head. One hand cups below the occiput and the forearm supports the weight of the head while cradling it against your abdomen. The other hand is positioned on the chin to be able to apply both traction and retraction (Fig. 8.43). Make a bridge by spreading your index finger and thumb. Apply the web to the chin and curl the remaining fingers so that they tuck around and under the chin (Fig. 8.44).

Lean out sideways as far as possible to apply traction. Once traction is established, bend your knees and apply pressure over the chin, taking the chin into maximum retraction to produce the anteroposterior glide while avoiding pressure from the knuckles against the larynx (Fig. 8.45). Allow the chin to return to neutral, avoiding protraction, and release the traction. Sit the patient up and reassess. If the manoeuvre has helped it can be repeated, this time using several retractions.

Figure 8.43 Anteroposterior glide under traction, starting position.

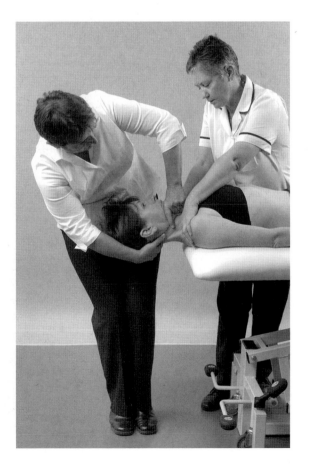

Figure 8.44 Anteroposterior
glide under traction, hand
position.

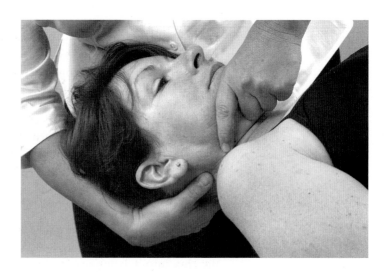

Figure 8.45 Anteroposterior
glide under traction, finishing
position.

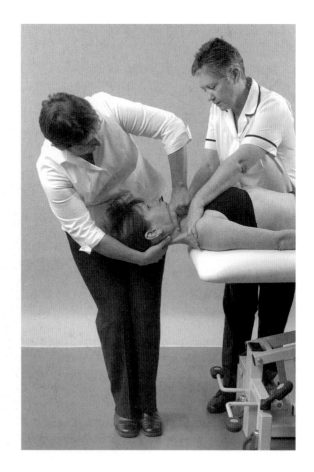

Lateral glide

This manoeuvre is used to relieve post-treatment soreness and to mobilize any residual tightness in the neck. It may be useful in mobilizing restricted side flexion in particular.

The couch is again slightly lower than hip height, as for the position for the anteroposterior glide under traction technique described above. No traction is applied with the lateral glide. An assistant, when available, stands parallel to the couch and the patient lies supine as above, but close to the assistant. The assistant grasps the patient's opposite arm with both hands and holds the patient close to prevent lateral movement of the thorax (Fig. 8.46).

Cup the patient's head in both hands, fingers around the occiput and thumbs parallel with the mandible. Your thenar eminences should support just in front of the ears, resting comfortably over the temporomandibular joint (Fig. 8.47). Bend your knees and position your abdomen against the patient's head but not enough to compress it. Apply the lateral glide by rocking from foot to foot, gradually increasing the pressure of your thenar eminences against the patient's head as the patient relaxes and more movement becomes available. To ensure that this is a rhythmical lateral

Figure 8.46   Lateral glide.

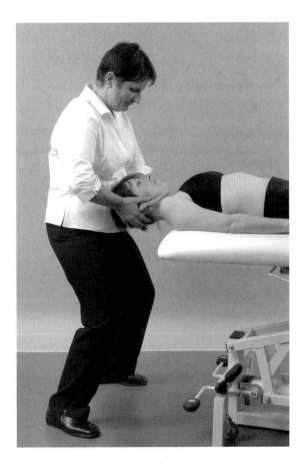

Figure 8.47 Lateral glide, hand position

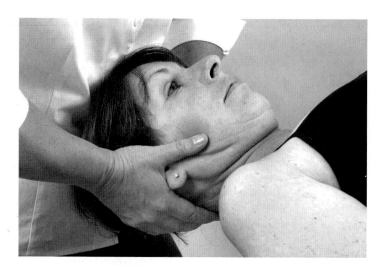

gliding movement without side flexion, keep the patient's nose straight and apply gentle pressure to the face as you move towards each side.

A slight upward movement of the patient's head may occur as your weight moves from each leg.

ADVANCED MANOEUVRES

These are stronger manoeuvres and it is definitely recommended that they should only be applied after attending an orthopaedic medicine course.

Traction with leverage (Cyriax & Cyriax 1983, Cyriax 1984)

The indication for this technique is that stronger traction is required for central or bilateral symptoms.

Position the patient in supine lying with the occiput level with the end of the couch. Cup the occiput and rest the back of your hand on the couch. Apply manual traction as described previously. At the end of the technique, bend your knees smartly to apply more traction, using your hand underneath as a pivot (Fig. 8.48). Maintain the traction as you straighten your knees, having applied the technique for a few seconds.

Manual traction plus rotation

This is the same technique as the rotation technique described previously, but it applies a different hand hold with the neck starting in a degree of rotation, which gives a stronger rotation overall.

Start with the patient's head turned into a small degree of rotation before applying the technique in order to secure a good grip. Cup your hand, pronate your forearm and place it comfortably on the side of the patient's face with the fingers under the chin, such that they face the direction of the rotation you are aiming towards (Fig 8.49). Stand with

Figure 8.48   Traction with leverage.

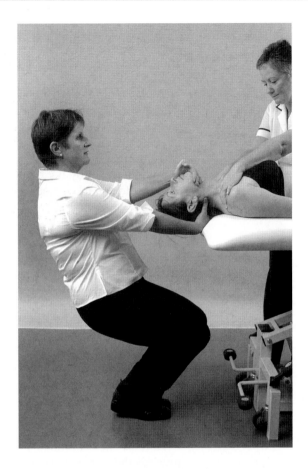

Figure 8.49   Manual traction plus rotation. The alternative hand position produces stronger rotation.

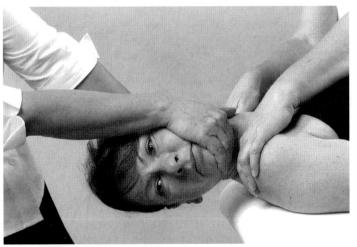

your feet rotated a little in that same direction. Apply the manual traction and rotation in the progression recommended for the rotation techniques described above. (See Guidance for pre-manipulative testing, Fig. 8.41, before proceeding to manipulation.)

Manual traction plus side flexion (Cyriax & Cyriax 1983, Cyriax 1984)

If the rotations have not cleared the symptoms, a side flexion technique can be applied.

Always start by side-flexing the patient away from the painful side.

Position the patient as for manual traction. An assistant stands on the side to which the neck will be side-flexed and moves the patient a little closer so that the patient's shoulder fits into the corner of the couch. The assistant then reaches over to place a hand over the patient's opposite shoulder to fix it by holding onto the top edge of the couch, so resisting the side flexion movement (Fig. 8.50).

If you will be moving towards the patient's left side flexion, place your left foot against the side of the couch, or against the assistant's extended right foot. Lean out sideways to give traction, taking your right foot off the floor (Fig. 8.51). After a short pause to allow the traction to take effect, swing your body backwards, pivoting on your left foot and applying side flexion to the patient's neck. Maintaining control, apply a smart thrust at the end of range (Grade C) and maintain traction as you swing your body back to the straight pull position, when you can steadily put your right foot to the floor and release the traction. The technique can be progressed through the Grade A (mid-range), Grade B (full range) and Grade C (manipulation) as described for the rotations above. (See Guidance for pre-manipulative testing, Fig. 8.41, before proceeding to manipulation.)

As you practise this technique you will find that the momentum of the movement will help achieve a smooth transition through the various stages.

Reverse the assistant's position and the instructions if side flexion towards the right side is indicated.

CERVICAL TRACTION

Cyriax did not advocate the use of cervical traction to the same extent as lumbar and was of the opinion that it was used 'far too often' (Cyriax

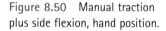

Figure 8.50 Manual traction plus side flexion, hand position.

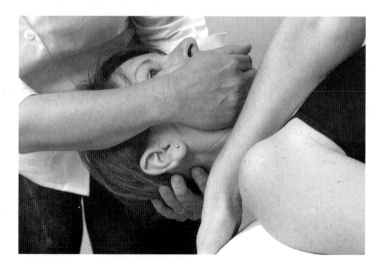

Figure 8.51   Manual traction plus side flexion.

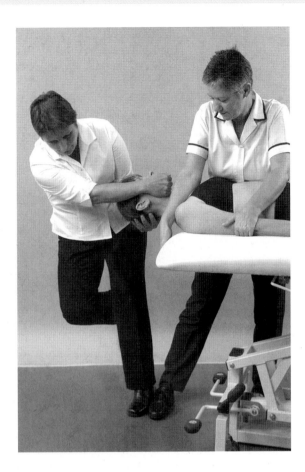

1982). A systematic review of the literature on the efficacy of traction for neck and back pain was presented by Van der Heijden et al (1995), but most of the selected studies proved to be of poor quality. No clear indications of the effectiveness or ineffectiveness of traction could be ascertained from this study.

Hickling (1972) described the application of sustained cervical traction in either sitting (cervical suspension) or lying, and various studies have been published to explore the merits or disadvantages of each. Cervical suspension, the application of vertical traction with the patient sitting, appeared to be the choice of Cyriax, although from the authors' experience while training at St Thomas's Hospital, where Cyriax's ideas under-pinned treatment techniques, traction in inclined supine lying (long traction) was used more frequently. Colachis & Strohm (1965) quoted the paper of Gartland which mentioned Krusen's list of advantages of cervical suspension over long or horizontal traction:

- Convenience of application
- Elimination of friction
- Accuracy of measurement
- Facilitation of manipulation

Stoddard (1954) was critical of cervical suspension since he observed that his patients found it difficult to relax in this position. He also believed that sustained traction impaired blood flow, and favoured intermittent traction. Deets et al (1977) mention that Maitland had the opposite view and preferred traction in sitting since his patients found it more comfortable. They also report that Crue found that greater foraminal separation was observed in the supine position than in sitting.

Colachis & Strohm (1965), in a study of 10 normal medical students, found that the separation of the cervical vertebrae under traction increased with the angle of flexion to the horizontal of the rope applying the pull. They found that the poundage applied had a comparatively greater effect on the joint separation and the maximum of 30 lb (14 kg) used in their investigation had the greatest effect. Judovitch (1952) studied radiographs of the cervical spine under different poundages of traction and found that 25 lb (11 kg) of vertical traction straightened the cervical lordosis, while at 45 lb (20.5 kg) a mean stretch of 5 mm was achieved in the cervical spine. Deets et al (1977) cite a further study of Colachis & Strohm which demonstrated that the greatest elongation of the posterior portion of the disc was observed with the angle of rope pull at 35° to the horizontal.

Hickling (1972) recounted Cyriax's suggestion that cervical suspension should be just sufficient to lift the patient's buttocks from the chair, implying that forces of near body weight were being applied. However, this was for a short duration of 1–5 min. In lying, average treatments ranged from 15 to 25 lb (7–11 kg), according to the size and overall response of the patient. The traction was applied horizontally or in slight flexion at an unspecified angle but with consideration for patient comfort and preference.

Readers must weigh up for themselves the pros and cons of applying traction in the sitting versus supine position. The characteristics of the individual patients encountered will form part of the decision-making process.

Another factor in the application of cervical traction is the length of time for which it should be applied. Colachis & Strohm (1965) noted that no further increase of intervertebral separation occurred after 7 s of sustained traction and Judovitch (1952) stated that the time of application should be decreased as greater forces were applied. Hickling (1972) suggested that traction of 15–25 lb (7–11 kg) should be continued for between 15 and 25 min. This recommendation is based on empirical findings and more work needs to be done to establish the optimum duration of treatment.

The literature is unclear in its support of either sustained or intermittent traction. Moeti & Marchetti (2001) used intermittent traction for patients with radicular symptoms and demonstrated that patients with symptoms of more than 12 weeks' duration had minimal improvement, and those with symptoms for less than 12 weeks had a better outcome. Improved circulation, reduction of adhesions and reduction of pain via presynaptic inhibition at spinal cord level have been suggested as possible mechanisms for improvement due to intermittent traction (Wong et al 1997). Chung et al (2002) used MRI to evaluate the reducibility of cervical disc herniation under traction on 29 patients and seven healthy volunteers. Using a traction device which essentially consisted of a portable inflatable 'accordion'-shaped neck collar to produce 30 lb of traction force over 10 min, an increase in length of the vertebral column was demonstrated in both groups, and 21 patients had complete or partial reduction of the disc herniation.

CONTRAINDICATIONS TO CERVICAL TRACTION

These are largely the same as for cervical manipulation and the reader is referred to the discussion of contraindications above.

Care should be taken in applying traction to the elderly and they must be thoroughly questioned for the presence of any contraindications.

Most traction beds and mobile traction equipment of modern design have the facility to apply cervical and lumbar traction.

A cervical harness is required to rest under the occiput and chin, with straps or cord passing to a spreader bar above the head. There are several types of harness which nowadays are made of washable materials, which also have the advantage of being pliable to give comfortable support. The simplest uses two padded rectangles which mould to the head as the traction is applied, but others are made of more substantial materials and have adjustable clasps to accommodate the differing shapes of patients.

The straps to the spreader bar should be long enough to give safe clearance above the head. A rope passes from the central point of the spreader bar via a pulley or pulleys to a fixing cleat in manually applied units, or directly into the housing of the automatic device.

Technique

Explain the technique carefully to the patient, mentioning possible after-effects such as stiffness or temporary increase in discomfort, and ask for consent to proceed.

If applying traction in the sitting position, use a firm chair with comfortable back support. Patients often like to have their arms resting on two or three pillows on their lap, both for support and to encourage relaxation.

Put the cervical harness in place under the jaw and occiput, providing extra padding if necessary, and place tissue between the patient and the harness, for reasons of hygiene. Attach the harness to the traction unit and place on the appropriate setting, considering the patient's size and general demeanour.

Discuss the treatment time with patients, explaining that the treatment aims to be as 'long and strong' as is comfortable, but they can call a halt to the treatment at any time. In practice, patients are usually comfortable with about 15 min traction at the first treatment and even on subsequent attendances 20 min is usually the maximum required.

Give patients sight of a clock and an alarm bell or buzzer and apply the traction steadily. Keep in close contact with the patient while the traction is being applied, since occasionally patients can become light-headed.

At the end of the treatment time release the traction slowly and observe the patients' response as you do so. Let patients sit for a moment or two while they roll the shoulders and relax the tissues, and allow them to get up when they feel ready. If applying traction in supine ensure that the patient is comfortable with one or two pillows under the head and knees as desired.

Apply the cervical harness in the same way as for sitting traction. Adjust the angle of pull and select the appropriate setting. Feedback from the patient will ensure that the traction is strong and comfortable. There is a convention that lesser weights are applied in traction in supine than in the sitting position, but for a longer time (Hickling 1972) On this basis, weights of 5–7 kg might be applied on the first treatment for 20 min, for example, increasing to 10 kg for 25–30 min at subsequent attendances.

Traction should be applied, preferably, on a daily basis but weekends can be excluded to allow any soft tissue discomfort from the application of the harness to subside. Patients may not be able to attend daily due to time or financial constraints and the pressures on outpatient departments may also deny this frequency. However, it is still appropriate to try the technique as frequently as possible since satisfactory results may still be achieved.

Improvement usually occurs after two to four treatments and the whole treatment episode may be continued over a 2- or 3-week period if necessary. If there is no change in the symptoms after four treatments the position, the weight, angle of pull or the time of application may be adjusted, but if there is still no change, the technique should be abandoned and another modality or course of action selected.

Advice on neck care and posture should be given to patients while they are undergoing treatment and an appropriate gentle exercise programme should be devised.

References

Aprill C, Dwyer A, Bogduk N 1989 Cervical zygapophyseal joint pain patterns II: a clinical evaluation. Spine 15:458–461

Barker S, Kesson M, Ashmore J et al 2001 Guidance for pre-manipulative testing of the cervical spine. Physiotherapy 87(6):3112–321

Beeton K, Jull G 1994 Effectiveness of manipulative physiotherapy in the management of cervicogenic headache: a single case study. Physiotherapy 80: 417–423

Bird H A 1995 Work related syndromes. In: Collected reports on the rheumatic diseases. Arthritis and Rheumatism Council for Research, London, p 162–164

Bogduk N 1986 The anatomy and pathophysiology of whiplash. Clinical Biomechanics 1:92–101

Bogduk N 1992 The anatomical basis for cervicogenic headache. Journal of Manipulative and Physiological Therapeutics 15:67–70

Bogduk N 1994 Innervation and pain patterns of the cervical spine. In: Grant R (ed) Physical therapy of the cervical and thoracic spine, 2nd edn. Churchill Livingstone, Edinburgh, p 65–76

Brown B St J, Tatlow W T 1963 Radiographic studies of the vertebral arteries in cadavers – effects of position and traction on the head. Radiology 81:80–88

Bush K, Chaudhuri R, Hillier S et al 1997 The pathomorphologic changes that accompany the resolution of cervical radiculopathy. Spine 22(2):183–186

Carey P F 1995 Suggested protocol for the examination and treatment of the cervical spine – managing the risk. Journal of the Canadian Chiropractic Association 39:35–40

Clark C 1994 Rheumatoid involvement of the cervical spine. Spine 19:2257–2258

Colachis S C, Strohm B R 1965 A study of tractive forces and angle of pull on vertebral interspaces in the cervical spine. Archives of Physical Medicine and Rheumatology 46:820–830

Connell M D, Wiesel S W 1992 Natural history and pathogenesis of cervical disc disease. Orthopedic Clinics of North America 23:369–380

Chung T-S, Lee Y-J, Kang S-W et al 2002 Reducibility of cervical disk herniation: evaluation at MR imaging during cervical traction with a nonmagnetic traction device. Radiology 225:895–900

Cyriax J 1982 Textbook of orthopaedic medicine, 8th edn. BaillièreTindall, London, vol 1

Cyriax J 1984 Textbook of orthopaedic medicine, 11th edn. BaillièreTindall, London, vol 2

Cyriax J, Cyriax P 1983 Illustrated manual of orthopaedic medicine. Butterworths, London

Deets D, Hands K L, Hopp S S 1977 Cervical traction. Physical Therapy 57:255–261

Department of Health 1995 Cervical spine instability in people with down syndrome. Chief Medical Officer's Update, 7. HMSO, London

Doherty M 1995 Fibromyalgia syndrome. In: Lewin I G, Seymour C A (eds) Collected reports on the rheumatic diseases. Arthritis and Rheumatism Council for Research, London, p 83–86

Frumkin L R, Baloh R W 1990 Wallenberg's syndrome following neck manipulation. Neurology 40:611–615

Grant R 1988 Dizziness testing and manipulation of the cervical spine. In: Grant R (ed) Physical therapy of the cervical and thoracic spines. Churchill Livingstone, Edinburgh, p 111–124

Haldeman S, Kohlbeck F, McGregor M 1999 Risk factors and precipitating neck movements causing vertebrobasilar artery dissection. Spine 24(8):785–794

@Refs:Hazelman B L 1995 Polymyalgia rheumatica and giant cell arteritis. In: Lewin I G, Seymour C A (eds) Collected reports on the rheumatic diseases. Arthritis and Rheumatism Council for Research, London, p 97–100

Herrick A L 1995 Reflex sympathetic dystrophy. In: Lewin I G, Seymour C A (eds) Collected reports on the rheumatic diseases. Arthritis and Rheumatism Council for Research, London, p 132–137

Hickling J 1972 Spinal traction technique. Physiotherapy 58:58–63

Hinton M A, Harris M B, King A G 1993 Cervical spondylolysis. Spine 18:1369–1372

Jenkins D G 1979 Clinical features of arm and neck pain. Physiotherapy 65:102–105

Judovitch B 1952 Herniated cervical disc. American Journal of Surgery 84:646–650

Jull G A 1994a Headaches of cervical origin. In: Grant R (ed) Physical therapy of the cervical and thoracic spine, 2nd edn. Churchill Livingstone, Edinburgh, p 261–285

Jull G 1994b Cervical headache – a review. In: Boyling J D, Palastanga N (eds) Grieve's Modern manual therapy, 2nd edn. Churchill Livingstone, Edinburgh, p 333–347

Jull G, Magarey M, Niere K et al 2002 Physiotherapy, a responsible profession to use cervical manipulation: response to Refshauge et al. Australian Journal of Physiotherapy 48:180–183

Kang J D, Georgescu H I, McIntyre-Larkin L et al 1995 Herniated cervical intervertebral discs spontaneously produce matrix metalloproteinases, nitric oxide, interleukin-6, and prostaglandin E2. Spine 20:2373–2378

Kleynhans A M, Terrett A G J 1985 The prevention of complications from spinal manipulative therapy. In: Glasgow E F, Twomey L T, Scull E R et al (eds) Aspects of manipulative therapy. Churchill Livingstone, Edinburgh, p 161–175

Krueger B R, Okazaki H 1980 Vertebral-basilar distribution infarction following chiropractic cervical manipulation. Mayo Clinic Proceedings 55:322–331

Kumar P, Clark M 2002 Clinical medicine, 5th edn. Baillière Tindall, London

Laslett M, van Wijmen P 1999 Low back and referred pain: diagnosis and a proposed new system of classification. NZ Journal of Physiotherapy 27(2):5–14

Lempert T, Gresty M A, Bronstein A M 1995 Benign positional vertigo – recognition and treatment. British Medical Journal 311:489–491

Licht P, Christensen H, Hoilund-Carlsen P 2000 Is there a role for pre-manipulative testing before cervical manipulation? Journal of Manipulative and Physiological Therapeutics 23(3):175–179

McKenzie R A 1981 The lumbar spine: mechanical diagnosis and therapy. Spinal Publications, Waikanae, New Zealand

McKinney L A 1989 Early mobilization and outcome in acute sprains of the neck. British Medical Journal 299:1006–1008

Mathews J A 1995 Acute neck pain – differential diagnosis and management. In: Lewin I G, Seymour C A (eds) Collected reports on the rheumatic diseases. Arthritis and Rheumatism Council for Research, Chesterfield, p 142–144

Matsuda Y, Sano N, Watanabe S et al 1995 Atlanto-occipital hypermobility in subjects with Down's syndrome. Spine 20:2283–2286

Mealy K, Brennan H, Fenelon G C C 1986 Early mobilization of acute whiplash injuries. British Medical Journal 292:656–657

Mendel T, Wink C S, Zimny M 1992 Neural elements in human cervical intervertebral discs. Spine 17:132–135

Mercer S, Bogduk N 1999 The ligaments and annulus fibrosus of the human adult cervical intervertebral discs. Spine 24(7):619–628

Mercer S, Bogduk N 2001 Joints of the cervical vertebral column. Physical Therapy 31(4):174–182

Mitchell J, McKay A 1995 Comparison of left and right vertebral artery intracranial diameters. Anatomical Record 242:350–354

Moeti P, Marchetti G 2001 Clinical outcome from mechanical intermittent cervical traction for the treatment of cervical radiculopathy: a case series. Journal of Orthopaedic and Sports Physical Therapy 31(4):207–213

Mooney V, Robertson J 1976 The facet syndrome. Clinical Orthopaedics and Related Research 115:149–156

Netter F H 1987 Musculoskeletal system, part I. Ciba Collection of Medical Illustrations, vol 8. Ciba-Giegy, New Jersey

Nilsson N 1995 The prevalence of cervicogenic headache in a random population sample of 20–59 year olds. Spine 20:1884–1888

Nordin M, Frankel V H 2001 Basic biomechanics of the musculoskeletal system, 3rd edn. Lippincott, Williams & Wilkins, Philadelphia

Oliver J, Middleditch A 1991 Functional anatomy of the spine. Butterworth Heinemann, Oxford

Ombregt L, Bisschop P, tar Veer H 2003 A system of orthopaedic medicine, 2nd edn. Churchill Livingstone, Edinburgh

Palastanga N, Field D, Soames R 2002 Anatomy and human movement, 4th edn. Butterworth Heinemann, Oxford

Pizzutillo P D, Woods M, Nicholson L et al 1994 Risk factors in Klippel–Feil syndrome. Spine 19:2110–2116

Prescher A 1998 Anatomy and pathology of the ageing spine. European Journal of Radiology 27:181–195

Pueschel S M, Moon A, Scola F H 1992 Computerised tomography in persons with Down syndrome and atlantoaxial instability. Spine 17:735–737

Refshauge K M, Parry S, Shirley D et al 2002 Professional responsibility in relation to cervical spine manipulation. Australian Journal of Physiotherapy 48:171–178

Riddle D L 1998 Classification and low back pain: a review of the literature and critical analysis of selected systems Physical Therapy 78(7):708–737

Rivett H M 1994 Cervical manipulation: confronting the spectre of the vertebral artery syndrome. Journal of Orthopaedic Medicine 16:12–16

Rivett D 1997 Preventing neurovascular complications of cervical manipulation. Physical Therapy Review 2:29–37

Rivett D 1999 Effects of pre-manipulative tests on vertebral artery and internal carotid artery blood flow – a pilot study. Journal of Manipulative Physiological Therapeutics 22(6):368–375

Saal J S, Saal J A, Yurth E F 1996 Nonoperative management of herniated cervical intervertebral disc with radiculopathy. Spine 21(16):1877–1883

Schoensee S K, Jensen G, Nicholson G et al 1995 The effect of mobilisation on cervical headaches. Journal of Orthopaedic and Sports Physical Therapy 21:184–196

Schwarzer A C, Aprill C N, Derby R et al 1994 Clinical features of patients with pain stemming from the lumbar zygapophysal joints. Spine 19:1132–1137

Sinel M, Smith D 1993 Thalamic infarction secondary to cervical manipulation. Archives of Physical Medicine and Rehabilitation 74:543–546

Sjaastad O 1992 Cervicogenic headache – the controversial headache. Clinical Neurology and Neurosurgery 94 (Suppl.):147S–149S

Sternbach G, Cohen M, Goldschmid D 1995 Vertebral artery injury presenting with signs of middle cerebral artery occlusion. Journal of Vascular Disease 46:843–846

Stoddard A 1954 Traction for cervical nerve root irritation. Physiotherapy 40:48–49

Tanaka N, Fujimoto Y, Howard S et al 2000 The anatomic relation among the nerve roots, intervertebral foramina and intervertebral discs of the cervical spine. Spine 25(3):286–291

Taylor J R, Twomey L T 1993 Acute injuries to cervical joints: an autopsy study of neck sprain. Spine 18:1115–1122

Taylor J R, Twomey L T 1994 Functional and applied anatomy of the cervical spine. In: Grant R (ed) Clinics in physical therapy of the cervical and thoracic spine, 2nd edn. Churchill Livingstone, Edinburgh, p 1–25

Toole J F, Tucker S H 1960 Influence of head position on cerebral circulation. Archives of Neurology 2:616–622

Van der Heijden G, Beurskens A, Assendelft W et al 1995 The efficacy of traction for back and neck pain: a systematic, blinded review of randomised clinical trial method. Physical Therapy 75(2):93–104

Walker D J 1995 Rheumatoid arthritis. In: Lewin I G, Seymour C A (eds) Collected Reports on the rheumatic diseases. Arthritis and Rheumatism Council for Research, Chesterfield, p 39–44

Walsh M T 1994 Therapist management of thoracic outlet syndrome. Journal of Hand Therapy Apr/May:131–144

Weinstein S M, Cantu R C 1991 Cerebral stroke in a semi-pro football player – a case report. Medicine and Science in Sports and Exercise 22:1119–1121

Williams P L 1998 Gray's Anatomy: the anatomical basis of medicine and surgery, 38th edn. Churchill Livingstone, Edinburgh

Wong A, Lee M-Y, Chang W et al 1997 Clinical trial of cervical traction modality with electromyographic biofeedback. American Journal of Physical Medicine and Rehabilitation 76(1):19–25

Zeidman S M, Ducker T B 1994 Rheumatoid arthritis: neuroanatomy, compression, and grading of deficits. Spine 19:2259–2266

Chapter **9**

The thoracic spine

SUMMARY

Thoracic pain is commonly encountered and provides a challenge in diagnosis, since referred pain from visceral problems can mimic pain of somatic origin, and vice versa. Disc lesions are considered by some to be a comparatively rare cause of thoracic pain, probably due to the supportive nature of this relatively stiff area brought about by the sternal and vertebral articulations of the ribs. While this might be so for the mid-thoracic region, lower thoracic disc lesions may be more common than previously thought.

This chapter sets out to explain the anatomy of the thoracic spine and highlights the somatic structures which are a common cause of pain. Pain patterns are discussed and the non-mechanical causes of thoracic back pain are presented to aid diagnosis and appropriate management.

The clinical examination procedure is outlined and interpreted, the contraindications are emphasized and the treatments used in orthopaedic medicine are described, with notes on the indications for their use.

ANATOMY

There are 12 thoracic vertebrae which gradually increase in size from above down, marking a transition between cervical and lumbar vertebrae. A typical thoracic vertebra is easily recognized by its costal facets, its heart-shaped superior surface and waisted vertebral body (Fig. 9.1). The *vertebral canal* in the thoracic region is round and smaller than that found in either the cervical or lumbar spine. Short *pedicles* pass almost directly backwards and thick, broad *laminae* overlap each other from above down.

The slope of the long *spinous processes* gradually increases downwards with the fifth to eighth spinous processes overlapping each other. The eighth spinous process is the longest, while the 12th is shorter, horizontal and similar to the lumbar spinous processes.

Long, rounded, club-like *transverse processes* are directed posterolaterally and slightly superiorly. Except for the 11th and 12th vertebrae, oval, anterior facets lie at the tips of all transverse processes. These facets articulate with the tubercles of the corresponding ribs.

Figure. 9.1 Typical thoracic vertebra. From Anatomy and Human Movement by N Palastanga D Field and R Soames. Reprinted by permission of Elsevier Ltd.

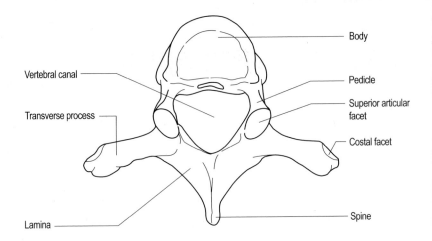

Flat *articular processes* project superiorly and inferiorly to form the thoracic zygapophyseal joints. Their direction facilitates the movement of rotation, that is coupled with side flexion, while also permitting a range of flexion and extension. Rotation is a particular feature of the thoracic spine and is facilitated by the direction of the articular facets and rotation of the fibres in the intervertebral discs. The shearing movement common to lumbar discs does not occur so readily in the thoracic spine (Kapandji 1974). The orientation of the articular facets changes at T11, marking a change from the rotational segment above and the non-rotational segment of the lumbar spine below.

The thoracic *intervertebral joints* consist of the vertebral body above and below and the *intervertebral disc*. These joints are supported by anterior and posterior longitudinal ligaments, supraspinous, interspinous and intertransverse ligaments and the ligamentum flavum that connects adjacent laminae internally. Further support is gained by the costovertebral joints and ligaments which directly involve the intervertebral disc.

Nakayama et al (1990), Maiman & Pintar (1992), Oppenheim et al (1993), Bogduk & Valencia (1994) and Boriani et al (1994) all share the opinion that disc lesions are relatively uncommon in the thoracic spine, in contrast to the claim that disc lesions account for a higher proportion of thoracic pain than is often realized (Cyriax & Cyriax 1983, Mellion & Ladeira 2001). The bony anatomy, including the primary kyphotic curve, and the surrounding ligamentous structures related to the costovertebral joints may have a stabilizing effect on the intervertebral disc, making displacement less likely in this region. The rib cage also exerts a stabilizing effect by restricting movement, particularly in the upper segment where the ribs are firmly attached anteriorly and posteriorly.

Movement in the thoracic spine is limited. This is due in part to the thoracic disc height relative to vertebral body height being less than in the cervical or lumbar spines with the ratio of disc diameter to height 2–3 times greater than in the lumbar spine. The acute angle of orientation of the annular fibres and the relatively small nucleus in the thoracic spine contribute to this lack of mobility. The angle of the zygapophyseal joints in the thoracic spine facilitates rotation while limiting flexion and anterior translation and having little influence on side flexion (Edmondston & Singer 1997). Little has been written about the structure and function of the thoracic disc, therefore they are not covered in depth here.

Twelve pairs of ribs normally attach posteriorly to the thoracic spine. The upper seven pairs are termed true ribs and attach anteriorly to the sternum. The lower five pairs consist of false and floating ribs, the false ribs attaching to the costal cartilage above.

A *typical rib* consists of a shaft and anterior and posterior ends. It is the posterior end that concerns us here. The posterior end of the rib typically has a *head, neck* and *tubercle* and articulates with the thoracic vertebrae, forming the posterior rib joints. The head of the rib is divided into two demifacets by a horizontal ridge that is attached to the disc via an intra-articular ligament. The lower facet articulates with its corresponding vertebra; the upper facet articulates with the vertebra above.

The tubercle of the rib is at the junction of the neck with the shaft and articulates with the transverse process of the corresponding vertebra. Just lateral to the tubercle the rib turns to run inferiorly forwards; this point is the *angle of the rib*.

A cervical rib may be present as an extension of the costal elements of the seventh cervical vertebra. It generally passes forwards and laterally into the posterior triangle of the neck where it is crossed by the lower trunk of the brachial plexus and the subclavian vessels. Compression of these structures may produce motor and sensory signs and symptoms.

POSTERIOR RIB JOINTS

Two joints, the costovertebral and costotransverse joints, attach the rib firmly to the vertebral column (Fig. 9.2). These assist stabilization of the intervertebral joint while being relatively unstable themselves. Minor subluxations of these joints may be responsible for the mechanical pattern of signs and symptoms associated with a thoracic pain. This minor instability may also account for the ease with which subluxations occur and can be reduced in this region.

The *costovertebral joint* is a synovial joint formed between the head of the rib and two adjacent vertebral bodies, except at the first, 11th and 12th ribs, where a joint is formed with a single vertebral body. The joint surfaces are covered by articular cartilage and surrounded by a fibrous capsule. The capsule is thickened anteriorly by the radiate ligament while the posterior aspect of the capsule blends with the nearby denticulation of the posterior longitudinal ligament. An intra-articular ligament divides the joint and attaches the transverse ridge of the rib head to the intervertebral disc.

The *costotransverse joint* joins the upper 10 ribs to the transverse processes of their corresponding vertebra. The joint is surrounded by a fibrous capsule that is reinforced posteriorly by the lateral costotransverse

Figure 9.2   Posterior rib joints. Costovertebral and costotransverse joints, horizontal section. From Anatomy and Human Movement by N Palastanga D Field and R Soames. Reprinted by permission of Elsevier Ltd.

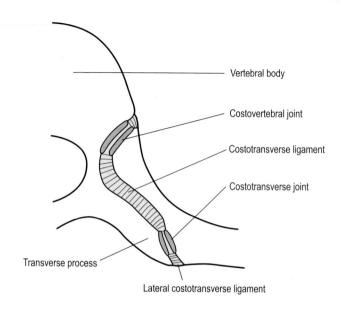

Vertebral body

Costovertebral joint

Costotransverse ligament

Costotransverse joint

Transverse process

Lateral costotransverse ligament

ligament. The joint is further stabilized by the costotransverse ligament that joins the transverse process to the neck of the rib, and the superior costotransverse ligament which connects the rib to the transverse process of the vertebra above. Movements occur concurrently at the costovertebral and costotransverse joints and are determined by the shape and direction of the articular facets. This amounts to small rotary and gliding movements in association with the 'bucket handle' action of the ribs during respiration.

Three thin musculotendinous layers occupy the intercostal space between adjacent ribs and may become symptomatic due to strain (Fig. 9.3). The *external intercostal muscle* is the most superficial, with fibres running in an oblique direction downwards and forwards. The *internal intercostal muscle* lies beneath with fibres running in the opposite direction, and the thinnest and deepest layer is formed by the *innermost (intimi) intercostal muscle*, which is thin and possibly absent, with fibres running in the same direction as the internal intercostal muscle.

DIFFERENTIAL DIAGNOSIS AT THE THORACIC SPINE

Orthopaedic medicine treatment techniques for the thoracic spine are aimed at reducing a mechanical lesion, i.e. subluxation of a posterior rib joint or herniations of the intervertebral disc.

Minor subluxation of the posterior rib joints

Subluxation of one or other of the posterior rib joints is a common cause of thoracic pain. The articulating surfaces of these joints are relatively

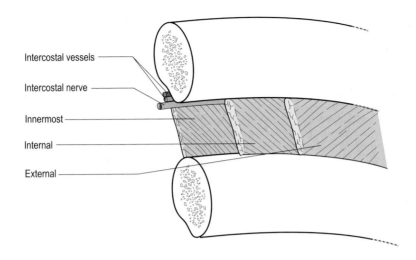

Figure 9.3   Layers of intercostal muscles. Adapted from Palastanga et al. (1994) with permission.

Intercostal vessels

Intercostal nerve

Innermost

Internal

External

shallow and unstable, rendering them susceptible to minor subluxations. The relatively trivial incidents that provoke thoracic mechanical pain and the relative ease with which it is reduced leads us to this hypothesis. Differential diagnosis of thoracic pain is difficult because of the numerous conditions that refer pain to the area and the lesions that mimic mechanical pain.

Patients present with a sudden onset of pain; the precipitating event is usually trivial and they often feel a pop or click. More gradual onset can be associated with working in rotated postures. The pain presents a typical mechanical picture of pain aggravated by movement and posture and eased by rest. In common with a thoracic disc lesion, a deep breath often provokes the pain, presumably because the 'bucket handle' action of the ribs during respiration translates aggravating movements to the rib joints at the spine.

On examination there is a non-capsular pattern of limited movement involving one rotation more than the other and these simple mechanical lesions usually respond rapidly to manipulation. Provided that there are no contraindications present (see below), the manipulative techniques described in this chapter can be applied. The usual postural and management advice should also be given to prevent recurrence, which is also a typical feature.

Thoracic disc lesions

It is important to reduce a thoracic disc displacement because of the potential for the displaced fragment to compromise the spinal cord. The thoracic vertebral canal is relatively small, therefore central prolapse poses the most threat.

In a review of the literature, Oppenheim et al (1993) reported an estimated annual incidence of one case of thoracic disc herniation per 1 million population. However, Mellion & Ladeira (2001) present a more current review of the literature which suggests that thoracic disc herniations are more common than previously thought and that in many cases, these may be asymptomatic. It is primarily a condition of middle age, occurring between the third and fifth decade, and affects the lower thoracic levels more frequently. This is probably because the lower thoracic spine is free of the restriction of the rib cage, making it more mobile, and the transition to the non-rotational lumbar spine produces greater torsional stresses here. The most common level reported was T11, 12, and 75% of thoracic disc lesions occurred below T8.

Positive diagnosis of a thoracic disc lesion is difficult. There is no regular pattern to the history, signs and symptoms, as found at the cervical and lumbar spine, and it is not possible to produce a clinical model on which to base differential diagnosis. Wilke et al (2000) reported a case of shoulder pain associated with a lower thoracic disc herniation. Central disc prolapse is most likely to compress the spinal cord and produce signs of myelopathy which include progressive paraparesis, increased reflexes, decreased sensation and bladder dysfunction. A posterolateral prolapse produces segmental signs and symptoms.

In a review of the literature, Mellion & Ladeira (2001) highlight degenerative change, traumatic incidents, lifting, rotation, falls, exercise, rugby tackles and road traffic accidents as precipitating factors for thoracic disc lesions. The onset may be sudden and severe or insidious and slowly progressive. Mellion & Ladeira mention that Cyriax was the first author to describe the clinical presentation of a thoracic disc lesion. They suggest it may give four classic presentations: intermittent thoracic back pain which may be aggravated by sitting and relieved by standing; acute thoracic 'lumbago' with the thoracic spine fixed in flexion following a bending or twisting motion; thoracic root pain and paraesthesia; and symptoms of spinal cord compression. Chest pain may be constant or intermittent and may be central, localized or diffuse, a band-like dermatomal chest pain is not uncommon and abdominal referral may occur. If accompanied by cord compression, complaints of bladder involvement, lower limb paraesthesia and gait disturbance may be reported and findings may include spastic muscle weakness, hyperreflexia and positive Babinski sign.

Mellion & Ladeira (2001) suggest that upper thoracic disc lesions are less common. Radiculopathies involving T1 share similarities with those occurring at C8, with numbness and weakness in the hand and pain in the arm and medial forearm. Weakness of the intrinsic hand muscles may be involved with T1, but this is an uncommon finding and the clinician must exclude non-mechanical causes such as Pancoast's tumour. Horner's syndrome (miosis and ptosis of the eye) is associated with T1 involvement but not C8. Presence of Horner's syndrome would therefore be contraindicated in manipulation or mobilization of the thoracic joints until the cause of the symptoms has been determined. Disc lesions at the T2 and 3 levels are even less common and there are few reports in the literature of the features of involvement of T3–T8; symptoms of nerve root involvement at these levels may produce intercostal neuralgia. If there is involvement of the dura mater or dural nerve root sleeve, their mobility will be impaired and signs provoked on flexion of the cervical spine and scapular approximation. T9–T11 may produce a dermatomal pattern of pain and can include the abdomen and groin, often being confused with visceral symptoms. These lower levels may also mimic lumbar presentations including low back and leg pain.

In summary, small uncomplicated thoracic disc lesions may present with sudden or gradual onset of pain that may be felt posteriorly, anteriorly or radiating laterally. Pressure on the dura mater produces multisegmental reference of pain. The pain should have a typical mechanical behaviour, i.e. aggravated by movement and posture and eased by rest. Dural symptoms of increased pain on a cough, sneeze or deep breath may be present.

On examination, a non-capsular pattern of limited movement will be found, with one rotation being significantly more painful or limited than the other. Dural signs of pain on neck flexion and/or scapular approximation may be present if the dura mater is compromised. If there are no neurological signs and signs of cord compression are absent the treatment techniques described in this chapter may be used. Alternatively, since lower thoracic displacements are more common, they may be treated using the techniques described for the lumbar spine.

Urgent surgical intervention is necessary for patients showing signs of spinal cord compression. Otherwise, uncomplicated thoracic disc lesions follow a path of recovery similar to that seen in cervical and lumbar disc lesions, responding to physical treatments and eventually stabilizing with time (Brown et al 1992).

OTHER CAUSES OF THORACIC PAIN AND ASSOCIATED SIGNS AND SYMPTOMS

Cervical disc lesions commonly refer pain into the thoracic region and this is particularly indicative of dural reference producing unilateral or bilateral scapular pain. The patient has a typical mechanical picture, with cervical movements increasing the pain felt in the thoracic region. Pain is not reproduced by thoracic movements. Minor chest wall pain may frequently be recognized as referred from the cervical spine, and Yeung & Hagen (1993) reported two cases of herniated C6–C7 disc producing major neuropathic chest wall pain which were treated surgically.

Arthritis presents with the capsular pattern of limited movement.
- *Degenerative osteoarthrosis* can affect the spinal joints, causing secondary signs and symptoms. Gross degenerative changes may produce central osteophytes that may cause gradual cord compression. Anterior and lateral lipping of the vertebral body, as well as wedging of mid-thoracic vertebrae, has been associated with degenerative osteoarthrosis of the thoracic spine (Osman et al 1994).
- *Inflammatory arthritis* can involve the thoracic spine. Rheumatoid arthritis commonly affects the costovertebral, costotransverse and zygapophyseal joints. Reiter's disease can affect the spinal joints, although it is more frequently seen in the lower limb joints. Ankylosing spondylitis, when it involves the thoracic cage, causes

---

Capsular pattern of the thoracic spine
- Equal limitation of rotations.
- Equal limitation of side flexions.
- Some limitation of extension.
- Usually full flexion.

a reduction in chest expansion. Thoracic pain and stiffness may be its presenting symptoms.

Serious non-mechanical conditions can affect the thoracic area and suspicions are alerted when the patient appears unwell, has a fever, night pain with or without night sweats, or reports an unexpected weight loss. The pain is not affected by movement or postures and is often unrelenting.

- *Malignant disease*, both primary and secondary, may be a cause of pain in the thoracic spine. Bronchial carcinoma accounts for 95% of all primary tumours of the lung and may present with a cough and chest pain (Kumar & Clark 2002). Tumours in the bronchus, breast, kidney and prostate commonly metastasize to bone. Intradura and extradural neoplasm, although relatively rare, may produce symptoms similar to nerve root irritation. Watanabe et al (1992) reported a case of benign osteoblastoma in the sixth thoracic vertebra presenting with thoracodorsal pain in a 19-year-old woman, increased by coughing and shifting sleeping positions. Hodges et al (1994) report a case of intraspinal, extradural synovial cyst at the level of T4–T5 in a 51-year-old woman experiencing intermittent mid-thoracic and lumbar pain after lifting.
- *Spinal infections* may include osteomyelitis or epidural abscess. The organism responsible may be *Staphylococcus aureus*, *Mycobacterium tuberculosis* or, rarely, *Brucella* (Kumar & Clark 2002).

Bone conditions can include acquired conditions or congenital abnormalities. These conditions may be asymptomatic and a chance finding on X-ray.

- *Scheuermann's disease* is vertebral osteochondritis, most commonly seen in males in the 12–18-year age group. It usually involves the lower thoracic vertebrae, often T9. The disc may move forwards between the cartilage end-plate and the anterior longitudinal ligament, producing wedging. It may produce minor thoracic backache and a local dorsal kyphosis may be evident on spinal flexion (Corrigan & Maitland 1989). Scheuermann's disease has been associated with Schmorl's nodes and degenerative lumbar disc disease in relatively young patients (Heithoff et al 1994).
- *Schmorl's nodes* are protrusions of the intervertebral disc into the cancellous bone of the vertebral body. This may produce an anterior prolapse, causing separation of a small fragment of bone, seen on X-ray as a limbus vertebra (Taylor & Twomey 1985).
- *Osteoporosis* is a reduction in bone mass that may present a problem in postmenopausal women, who lose bone density faster than men. It is common in the sixth and seventh decades of life. Pain is not due to the condition itself, but usually to secondary wedge compression fractures of the vertebral body (Turner 1991). The patient presents with moderate to severe episodes of thoracic back pain that gradually resolve over the course of approximately 6 weeks. Fracture produces wedging of the vertebral body on X-ray and a characteristic increase in thoracic kyphosis is seen.

Fracture may present with a history of trauma. The fracture may involve elements of the vertebra or the ribs. The position of the pain and local tenderness will give an indication to the site of possible fracture.

Visceral disease can produce local thoracic pain or pain referred to the thoracic region that mimics mechanical pain, making diagnosis difficult. In visceral conditions the patient is usually unwell, which will aid diagnosis, but this is not always so.

- *Angina* is usually felt in the chest and can be referred into the arms. If mild, it may mimic mechanical pain. The patient experiences increased pain with exertion, e.g. climbing stairs.
- *Pulmonary embolism, pleurisy, pneumothorax*, etc. all present with chest pain, but other distinguishing features will hopefully lead to diagnosis, which is often difficult.
- *Acute pancreatitis* produces abdominal pain localized to the epigastrium or upper abdomen, but pain may be referred to the mid- or low thoracic region.
- *Acute cholecystitis* can cause pain in the epigastrium and right hypochondrium, but pain may also be referred to the back and shoulder.
- The *testes* may refer pain to the lower thoracic area as they are supplied by nerves derived from the 10th and 11th thoracic spinal segments.

Shingles (herpes zoster) is related to a chickenpox virus infection affecting one posterior nerve root. The patient presents with a dermatomal reference of pain that may be present for some days before the typical rash appears. The rash consists of vesicles following a segmental course related to the affected nerve root.

Soft tissue conditions can produce thoracic pain.
- *Muscle lesions* are relatively common in the thoracic region, therefore resisted tests are included in the routine examination. Commonly the intercostal muscles are affected, particularly if there is a history of a fractured rib. Palpation determines the site of the lesion.
- *Tietze's syndrome* is a condition affecting the costochondral or chondrosternal joints. It is usually unilateral, affecting one, two or three joints that are tender to palpation. The cause is not known, but the condition may follow a respiratory condition that involves prolonged coughing. The condition is self-limiting and may be treated with physiotherapeutic pain-relieving modalities, non-steroidal anti-inflammatory drugs or injection of corticosteroid and local anaesthetic (Kumar & Clark 2002).
- *Epidemic myalgia (Bornholm disease)* is due to infection by the Coxsackie B virus. The features are an upper respiratory tract illness and fever followed by pleuritic and abdominal pain and muscular tenderness. It may occur in young adults in the late summer and autumn, but resolves spontaneously within a week (Kumar & Clark 2002).

COMMENTARY ON THE EXAMINATION

OBSERVATION

A general observation of the patient is made, assessing the *face, posture and gait*. Serious pathology should show in the face with the patient appearing tired and drawn. An assessment of the gait is important; the presentation of a disc lesion at the thoracic spine may present a serious threat to the spinal cord and signs of myelopathy may show in the gait pattern, which if severe will be spastic in nature.

HISTORY (SUBJECTIVE EXAMINATION)

The *age, occupation, sports, hobbies and lifestyle* of the patient will indicate possible lesions and any contributing factors to the condition that may need to be addressed to prevent recurrence. Mechanical lesions tend to be found in the middle-aged group. Osteoporosis can affect post-menopausal women. Serious conditions may present in both the very young and the elderly, and caution is required if these particular age groups present with symptoms mimicking a mechanical lesion. Habitual postures may have relevance to the symptoms, as will the patient's sports or hobbies.

The *site and spread* of symptoms may indicate the site of the lesion. The initial site of the symptoms may be different to the current situation and it may be helpful to know this. Mechanical lesions can produce central pain, anterior pain or both. Pain may radiate around the chest wall and this may be indicative of nerve root involvement. Progressively increasing and radiating pain is usually sinister. Symptoms may spread in a multisegmental distribution, indicating dural involvement, or separate satellite areas of pain may be related to visceral causes. Cardiac pain characteristically radiates from the chest into one or both arms. Mechanical lesions of the posterior rib joints produce relatively local pain, but movement may provoke sharp, shooting or twinging pain.

The nature of the *onset and duration* of the symptoms will assist differentiation of mechanical lesions from more serious pathology. Minor subluxation of the posterior rib joints usually has a sudden onset, with the patient recalling the exact time of onset. The mode of onset is usually trivial and is often associated with a popping or cracking sound. The duration is generally short; patients seek help as they realize the mechanical nature of the problem, having 'felt it go'. Minor subluxation may present gradually following the adoption of an awkward posture for some time. A disc lesion may have a gradual or sudden onset. A history of trauma may indicate possible fracture. More serious pathology generally starts insidiously for no apparent reason and the duration of the symptoms may be many weeks or months. Recurrent episodes may be indicative of mechanical instability or inflammatory arthritis.

The *behaviour* of the pain is important since mechanical lesions produce a recognizable pattern of behaviour. The pain is better for rest and worse for activity. Providing the mechanical lesion does not wake the patient on turning, night pain is not a feature and the patient is usually well-rested. The provoking activities are consistent and every time the patient repeats a particular aggravating movement, the pain is produced.

The 24 h pain pattern gives an indication of severity and irritability of the condition. Inflammatory symptoms are worse at night, but if the patient does get to sleep there is stiffness on waking which may take some time to wear off. This would be generally indicative of inflammatory arthritis. If night pain is a feature, the patient will look tired and this generally indicates serious pathology.

Other *symptoms* may indicate a mechanical lesion, be it either a minor posterior rib joint subluxation or minor disc lesion. A deep breath may aggravate the pain, and needs to be distinguished from such conditions as pleurisy and pulmonary embolism, for example. These conditions may also produce pain on a deep breath, but the subsequent findings on the objective assessment will confirm whether the lesion is mechanical. Although movements are small at the posterior rib joints, the length of the ribs produces a greater proportion of movement at the anterior ends. This movement may also be painful in an intercostal muscle strain. A cough or sneeze increasing the pain could be indicative of minor subluxation or, more commonly, dural irritation, and symptoms are generally increased with activity and relieved by rest.

As the vertebral canal in the thoracic spine is small, disc displacement can threaten the spinal cord and produce symptoms of myelopathy; these must be ruled out. The patient is asked about the presence of paraesthesia in the feet, weakness in the legs and difficulty in walking. A specific question must be asked about bladder and bowel function, to rule out myelopathy (Oppenheim et al 1993). If any impairment is noted, the patient should be referred for neurosurgical opinion.

Other joint involvement may give an indication of any polyarthritic condition.

Past medical history will give information concerning conditions that may be relevant to the patient's current complaint or reveal possible alternative diagnoses and contraindications to treatment. An indication of the patient's general health will indicate any systemic illness. It may be pertinent to take the patient's temperature. The patient should be asked about any recent unexplained weight loss.

On considering *medications*, the patient should be specifically asked about anticoagulants, long-term oral steroids, antidepressant medication and the current intake of analgesics, as an objective measure of pain control requirement.

INSPECTION

The patient should undress to underwear and an inspection carried out in a good light. A general inspection of the posture is made assessing *bony deformity*. Note the position of the head and neck, cervical, thoracic and lumbar curves. Is there any evidence of cervical protraction or dowager's hump, excessive or local thoracic kyphosis? Note the position of the scapulae and any evidence of scoliosis, whether structural or acquired.

Colour changes or *swelling* would not be expected unless associated with a history of recent trauma. The typical appearance of shingles may be seen or the mottled reddening (erythema ab igne) produced following prolonged application of excessive heat, giving an indication of the severity of the pain.

Muscle wasting may be seen in the scapular area associated with neuritis.

STATE AT REST

Before any movements are performed, the state at rest is established to provide a baseline for comparison.

The suggested sequence for the objective examination will now be given, followed by a commentary including the reasoning in performing the movements and the significance of the possible findings.

EXAMINATION BY
SELECTIVE TENSION
(OBJECTIVE
EXAMINATION)

Eliminate the Cervical Spine

- Active cervical extension (Fig. 9.4a)
- Active right cervical rotation (Fig. 9.4b)
- Active left cervical rotation (Fig. 9.4c)
- Active right cervical side flexion (Fig. 9.4d)
- Active left cervical side flexion (Fig. 9.4e)
- Active cervical flexion (a dural sign due to the upward migration of the dura mater in this area during cervical flexion) (Fig. 9.4f)

Dural Test

- Scapular approximation (Fig. 9.5)

Articular and Muscle Signs
Standing

- Active thoracic extension (Fig. 9.6)
- Active right thoracic side flexion (Fig. 9.7a)
- Active left thoracic side flexion (Fig. 9.7b)
- Active thoracic flexion (Fig. 9.8)
- Resisted thoracic side flexions (Figs 9.9 a,b)

Sitting

- Active thoracic right rotation (Fig. 9.10a)
- Active thoracic left rotation (Fig. 9.10b)
- Passive thoracic right rotation (Fig. 9.11a)
- Passive thoracic left rotation (Fig. 9.11b)
- Resisted thoracic right rotation (Fig. 9.12a)
- Resisted thoracic left rotation (Fig. 9.12b)
- Resisted thoracic flexion (Fig. 9.13)

Supine Lying

- Plantar response (Fig. 9.14)

Prone Lying

- Resisted thoracic extension (Fig. 9.15)

Palpation

- Spinous processes for pain, range and end-feel (Fig. 9.16)

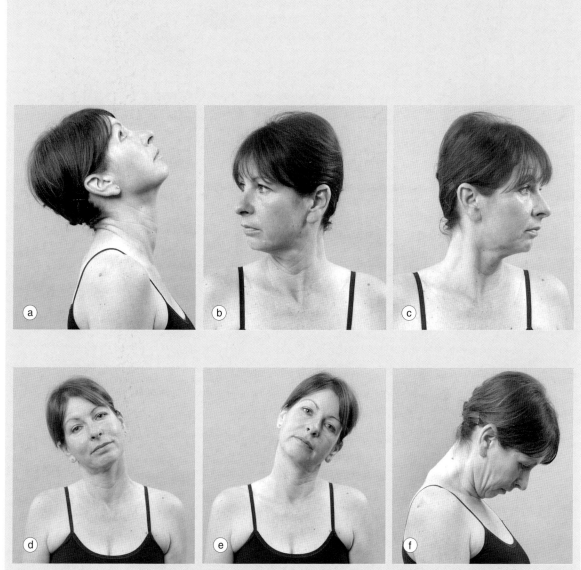

Figure 9.4   Six active cervical movements to eliminate the cervical spine as a cause of pain. (a) Extension; (b, c) rotations; (d, e) side flexions; (f) flexion.

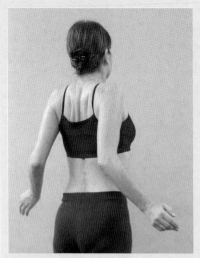

Figure 9.5   Dural test: scapular approximation.

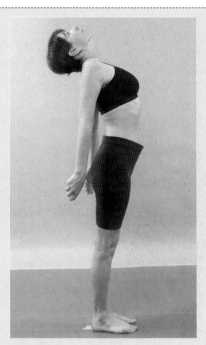

Figure 9.6   Active extension.

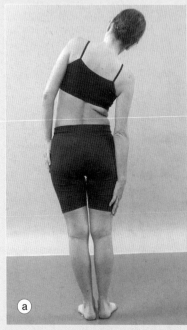

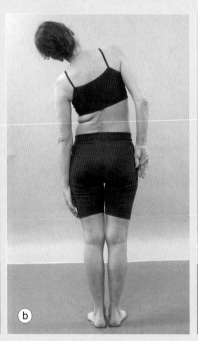

Figure 9.7   (a, b) Active side flexions.

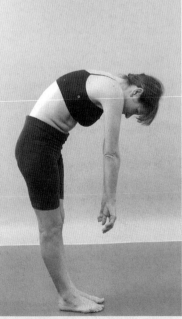

Figure 9.8   Active flexion.

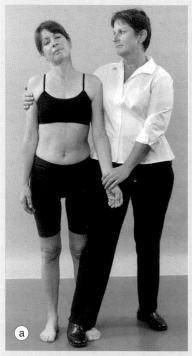

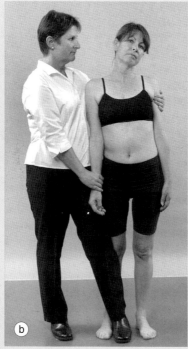

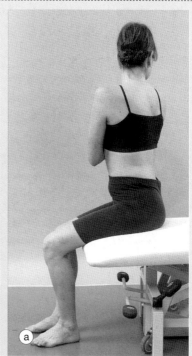

Figure 9.9   (a, b) Resisted side flexions.

Figure 9.10   (a) Active rotations.

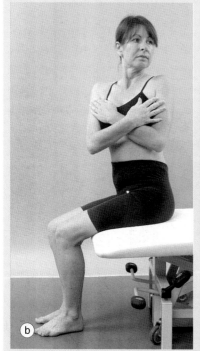

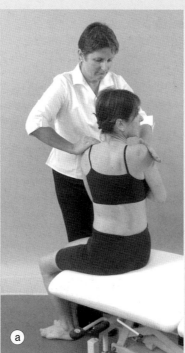

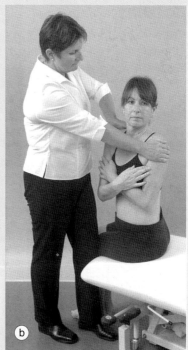

Figure 9.10   (b) Active rotations.

Figure 9.11   (a, b) Passive rotations.

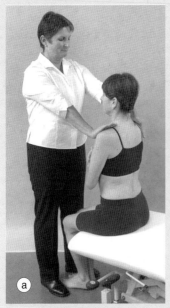
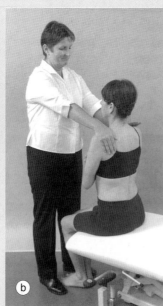

Figure 9.12   (a, b) Resisted rotations.

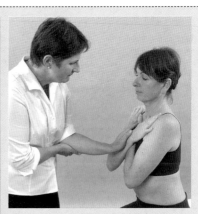

Figure 9.13   Resisted flexion.

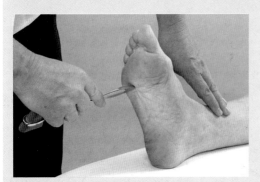

Figure 9.14   Plantar response.

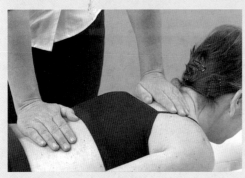

Figure 9.15   Resisted extension.

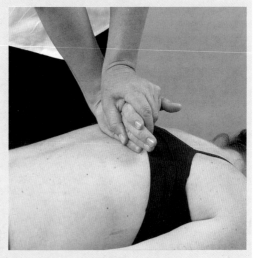

Figure 9.16   Palpation.

The cervical spine is a possible source of pain felt in the thoracic region and it must first be eliminated. If cervical flexion is the only movement to reproduce the thoracic pain, it is considered to be a dural sign for the thoracic spine since neck flexion draws the dura upwards (Fig. 9.4f). Scapular approximation is conducted as a dural test since it pulls on the dura via the T1 and 2 nerve roots and may be positive in a disc lesion at these levels (Fig. 9.5).

In common with other regions of the spine, the thoracic spine is considered to be an 'emotional' area and the movements are assessed actively to observe willingness to perform the movements, as well as assessing the articular signs for pain and limited range of movement. The capsular or non-capsular pattern will become evident through these movements.

Capsular pattern of the thoracic spine
- Equal limitation of rotations.
- Equal limitation of side flexions.
- Some limitation of extension.
- Usually full flexion.

Resisted side flexion is assessed looking for evidence of a muscle lesion. Resisted tests may also be applied if serious pathology or psychological factors are suspected.

The patient sits to fix the pelvis while the rotations are assessed for pain, range of movement, end-feel and the capsular pattern. End-feel, which is normally elastic, is particularly pertinent to the rotations since these movements may show minimal limitation and pain in minor subluxations of the posterior rib joints. Passive overpressure can be applied to any of the other movements if appropriate. Resisted flexion may also be assessed in this position.

The non-capsular pattern involves pain and/or limitation of at least one of the rotations.

The patient is positioned in supine lying to test for the Babinski reflex, the extensor plantar response, by stroking up the lateral border of the sole of the foot and across the metatarsal heads. If the response is extensor, i.e. upgoing, it is indicative of an upper motor neuron lesion; the normal response is flexor.

The patient is positioned in prone lying to complete the examination. Resisted extension is applied and the spinous processes are palpated assessing pain, range of movement and end-feel at each segmental level.

Any other tests can be added to this basic routine examination of the thoracic spine, including repeated, combined and accessory movements and neural tension testing as appropriate.

TREATMENT OF THORACIC LESIONS

Manipulation is the treatment of choice for thoracic mechanical lesions, either minor subluxation of the posterior rib joints or an uncomplicated thoracic intervertebral disc lesion. Central displacement can endanger the spinal cord and if present, the history and objective examination should reveal signs of spinal cord compression.

CONTRAINDICATIONS TO THORACIC MANIPULATION

It is impossible to be absolutely definitive about all contraindications to thoracic manipulation and nothing can substitute for a rigorous assessment of the presenting signs and symptoms and an accurate diagnosis. Signs and symptoms of spinal cord compression requires urgent neurosurgical referral; the ill patient should be investigated for the cause of the systemic illness. As mentioned above, Horner's syndrome is a contraindication to manipulation or mobilization of the thoracic joints until the cause of the symptoms has been determined, due to its association with more serious pathology. Anticoagulation therapy and blood clotting disorders are relative contraindications and medical advice may need to be sought. Prolonged corticosteroid therapy may predispose the patient to osteoporosis and a sensible selection of less aggressive techniques is advised in mechanical·lesions; however, pathological fracture will need to be excluded. Secondary tumour needs to be eliminated as a cause of pain in patients with a past history of primary tumour.

The treatment regime discussed below is contraindicated in the absence of patient consent. The patient should be given all details of their diagnosis together with the proposed treatment regime and a discussion of the risks and benefits should ensue to enable them to give their informed consent. Consent is the patient's agreement, written or oral, for a health professional to provide care. It may range from an active request by the patient for a particular treatment regime, to the passive acceptance of the health professional's advice. The process of consent, within the context of the orthopaedic medicine, is 'fluid' rather than one instance in time when the patient gives their consent. The patient is constantly monitored and feedback is actively requested. The treatment procedures can be progressed or stopped at the patient's request or in response to adverse reactions. Reassessment is conducted after each technique and a judgement made about proceeding. The patient has a right to refuse consent and this should be respected and alternative treatment options discussed. For further information on consent, the reader is referred to the Department of Health website: *www.doh.gov.uk/consent*.

Safety recommendations for spinal manipulative techniques are included in the Appendix.

INDICATIONS FOR THORACIC MANIPULATION

- Mechanical thoracic lesion, either a minor disc herniation or a minor subluxation of posterior rib joint
- A sudden or gradual onset of pain
- Central, unilateral, local or referred pain
- Non-capsular pattern, usually limitation and/or pain of at least one thoracic rotation
- No neurological signs
- No contraindications

THORACIC MANIPULATION TECHNIQUES

It is recommended that a course in orthopaedic medicine is attended before the treatment techniques described are applied in clinical practice (see Appendix).

As with the cervical spine, the treatment techniques in this section will be described carefully in a step-by-step fashion to enable their application. However, the professional judgement and existing skill of the operator will allow each technique to be adapted. The techniques described have been adapted from those originally described by Cyriax & Cyriax (1983) and Cyriax (1984). Clinically, minor subluxation of a posterior rib joint has been judged to be a more common lesion than thoracic disc lesion and hence the techniques are not carried out under traction. As with all manipulations, the comparable signs are reassessed after each manoeuvre and a decision made about the next. If the techniques fail to produce a reduction in signs and symptoms, they can be applied under traction (see below) (Cyriax & Cyriax 1983, Cyriax, 1984).

The position of the bed for each manoeuvre is a matter of personal choice. The extension thrust techniques are best conducted with the bed as low as possible.

Straight extension thrust

Position the patient comfortably in prone lying, preferably with the head in neutral, with the face positioned in the nose hole and the arms resting over the edge of the couch or at the patient's side. Palpate for the tender thoracic level. Apply the ulnar border of your hand, reinforced with the other hand, to the most tender spinous process, which will indicate the level of the lesion (Fig. 9.17). With the patient relaxed, apply downward pressure to test the end of range of the tissues. Remove all pressure and ask the patient to take a small breath in. Apply pressure downwards with straight arms, following the breath out. Apply a minimal amplitude, high velocity thrust once all the slack is taken up.

This technique is uncomfortable for the patient as the thrust is applied to the tender bony spinous process. The following manoeuvre is much more comfortable for the patient. Both techniques may have to be applied at one or two levels. It is common to find one, two or even three tender levels, in which case the most tender level is chosen first.

Figure 9.17 Straight
extension thrust.

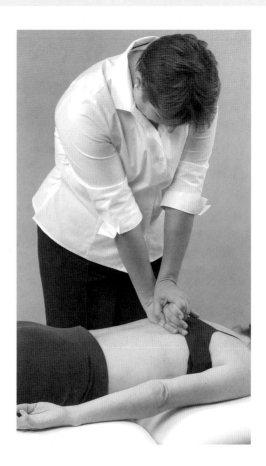

Extension with a rotational component

Position the patient as for the above manoeuvre and again locate the most tender spinous process by palpation. The technique can be applied in one of two ways but it may be necessary to do both if, on reassessment, the first manoeuvre is unsuccessful.

Position your hands as follows on either side of the spinous processes over the paraspinal muscle bulk, approximately over the underlying transverse processes.

1. Take the pisiform of your hand which is nearest to the patient's head and place it adjacent to the spinous process and on the side nearest to yourself at the painful level (fingers pointing caudally). The pisiform will now be resting over the transverse process (Figs 9.18–9.20). Place the trapeziofirst-metacarpal joint of your other hand adjacent to the spinous process on the level above, resting on the transverse process on the opposite side. With the patient relaxed, apply downward pressure to test the end of range of the tissues. Remove all pressure and ask the patient to take a small breath in. Follow the movement down as the patient breathes out; the position of your hands will automatically apply the rotation/extension thrust and further

Figure 9.18   Extension with a
rotational component.

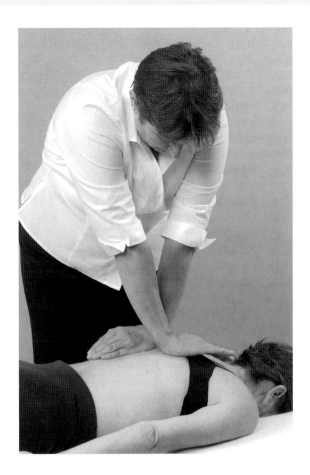

Figure 9.19   Extension with a
rotational component showing
hand position

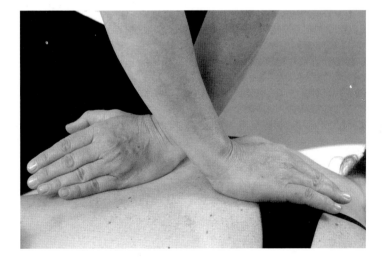

Figure 9.20 Extension with a rotational component, hand position demonstrated on spine.

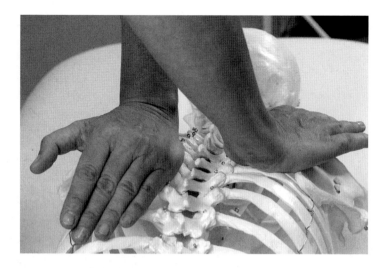

rotation of the hands is unnecessary. Apply a minimal amplitude, high velocity thrust through straight arms once all of the slack is taken up.

2. This technique is the reverse of that described above. Take the trapeziofirst-metacarpal joint of your hand which is nearest to the patient's head and place it adjacent to the spinous process at the painful level (fingers pointing caudally). The trapeziofirst-metacarpal joint will now be resting over the transverse process on the side opposite to yourself (Figs 9.21–9.23). Place the pisiform of your other hand on the level above, over the transverse process on the side nearest to yourself With the patient relaxed, apply downward pressure to test the end of range of the tissues. Remove all pressure and ask the patient to take a small breath in. Follow the movement down as the patient breathes out; the position of your hands will automatically apply the rotation/extension thrust and further rotation of the hands is unnecessary. Apply a minimal amplitude, high velocity thrust through straight arms once all of the slack is taken up.

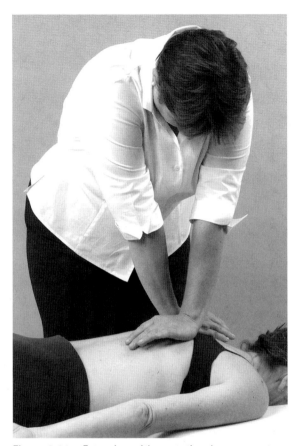

Figure 9.21   Extension with a rotational component; alternative position.

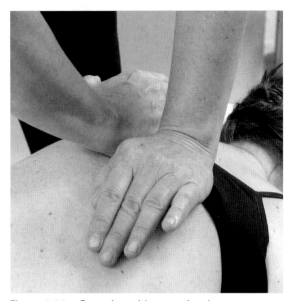

Figure 9.22   Extension with a rotational component showing alternative hand position

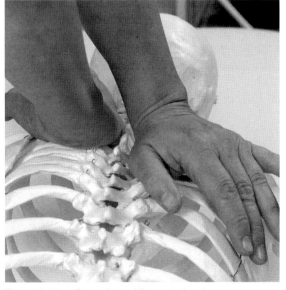

Figure 9.23   Extension with a rotational component, alternative hand position demonstrated on spine.

Sitting rotation

Position the patient astride the end of a narrow couch to fix the pelvis, with the patient's back towards you and the patient's arms folded across the chest. Stand close to the patient and bend your knees. Hug the patient so that the patient's shoulder fits into the front of your axilla (Fig. 9.24). Keep the patient as close as possible, while the heel of your other hand rests adjacent to the spinous process just above the painful level (Fig. 9.25). Ask the patient to rotate actively as far as possible. Rotate the spine a little further passively and straighten your knees to apply some traction to the patient's upper trunk (Fig. 9.26). Rotate a little further and apply a minimal amplitude, high velocity thrust towards rotation once all of the slack is taken up, by smartly rotating your body and pushing through the heel of your hand.

Figure 9.24   Sitting rotation, starting position.

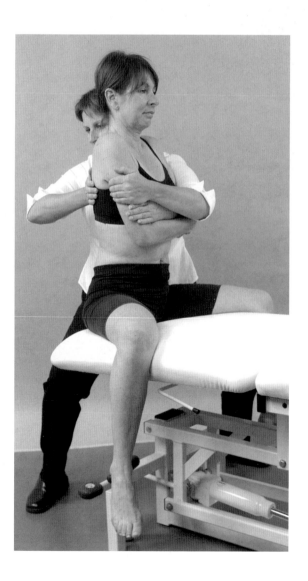

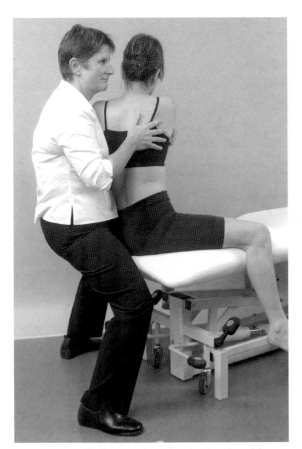

Figure 9.25   Sitting rotation, showing hand position just above painful level.

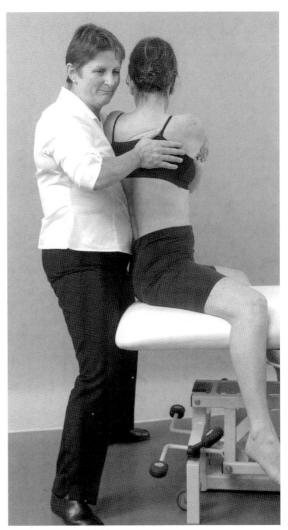

Figure 9.26   Sitting rotation, traction applied by straightening knees, before application of the Grade C manipulation.

Rotate the patient into the least painful rotation first. If that fails to improve symptoms, the technique can be repeated in the opposite direction.

Sitting extension thrust with a degree of traction

Position the patient in sitting on the side of the couch with the patient's hands, overlapping each other, behind his or her head. Stand on the couch behind the patient and place one knee at the painful level, with a pillow or padding placed between your knee and the patient's back. Wrap your hands over and below the patient's upper arms and lean the patient back

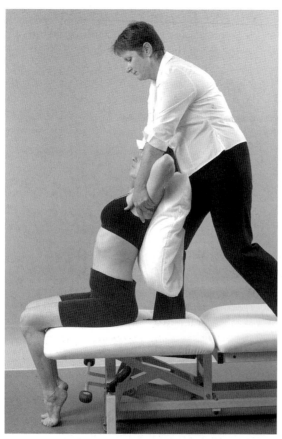

Figure 9.27   Sitting extension thrust, starting position

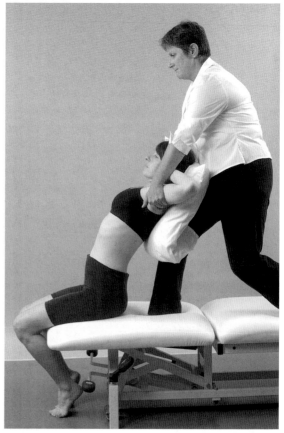

Figure 9.28   Sitting extension thrust with a degree of traction.

over your knee (Fig. 9.27), applying traction by moving your body weight backwards onto your other leg (Fig. 9.28). Once the patient has relaxed, extend the thoracic spine by applying a small amplitude, high velocity upward lift of your knee against the spine.

THORACIC TRACTION

Thoracic traction is difficult to apply and is not as effective as in the cervical and lumbar joints, probably due to the comparative rigidity of the spine and to the sternal and vertebral attachments of the ribs.

Cyriax devised a method of applying distraction before performing the straight extension and the extension with rotational component techniques, using two assistants to pull longitudinally through the patient's arms and legs before the technique is applied (Cyriax & Cyriax 1983, Cyriax 1984). In practice, two assistants are rarely readily available and the added benefit of the distraction is unproven. However, the added distraction may be considered for patients with symptoms that are resistant to other treatment techniques.

The higher and lower thoracic levels form part of the cervicothoracic and thoracolumbar transition levels respectively, and traction, or mobilization under traction, applied to the cervical and lumbar regions will affect these levels. For mid to lower thoracic levels the thoracic harness needs to be placed higher on the rib cage, which can lead to uncomfortable pressure in the axillae that is not well-tolerated by the patient.

If the history, signs and symptoms do warrant its use, it is applied on the same lines as for the lumbar spine.

Intercostal muscle strain (Cyriax 1984)

Generally, muscle lesions at the spinal joints are rare. However, it is not uncommon to find a lesion in the intercostal muscles. The onset of pain may follow a chest infection with prolonged coughing, overexertion or as the result of a fractured rib. Pain is felt locally and reproduced on resisted testing. Palpation reveals an area of tenderness in one intercostal space.

The lesion responds well to transverse friction massage. Position the patient in half-lying and locate the tender area (Fig. 9.29). Using an index or middle reinforced finger, direct the pressure up or down against the affected rib and apply transverse friction massage parallel to the rib, according to the general principles.

Figure 9.29   Friction of the intercostal muscles

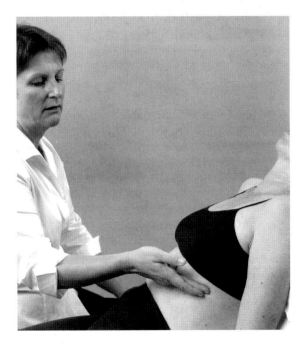

References

Bogduk N, Valencia F 1994 Innervations and pain patterns of the thoracic spine. In: Grant R (ed) Clinics in physical therapy, physical therapy of the cervical and thoracic spine, 2nd edn. Churchill Livingstone, Edinburgh, p 77–87

Boriani S, Biagini R, de Lure F et al 1994 Two-level thoracic disc herniation. Spine 19:2461–2466

Brown C W, Deffer P A, Akmakjian J et al 1992 The natural history of thoracic disc herniation. Spine 17:S97–S102

Corrigan B, Maitland G D 1989 Practical orthopaedic medicine. Butterworths, London;

Cyriax J 1984 Textbook of orthopaedic medicine, 11th edn. Baillière Tindall, London, vol 2

Cyriax J, Cyriax P 1983 Illustrated manual of orthopaedic medicine. Butterworths, London

Edmondston S J, Singer K P 1997 Thoracic spine: anatomical and biomechanical considerations for manual therapy. Manual Therapy 2(3):132–143

Heithoff K B, Gundry C R, Burton C V et al 1994 Juvenile discogenic disease. Spine 19:335–340

Hodges S D, Fronczak S, Zindrick M R et al 1994 Extradural synovial thoracic cyst. Spine 19:2471–2473

Kapandji I A 1974 The physiology of the joints, trunk and the vertebral column. Churchill Livingstone, Edinburgh, vol 3

Kumar P, Clark M 2002 Clinical medicine, 5th edn. Baillière Tindall, London

Maiman D J, Pintar F A 1992 Anatomy and clinical biomechanics of the thoracic spine. Clinical Neurosurgery 38:296–324

Mellion L R, Ladeira C 2001 The herniated thoracic disc: a review of the literature. Journal of Manual and Manipulative Therapy 9(3):154–163

Nakayama H, Hashimoto H, Hase H et al 1990 An 80 year old man with thoracic disc herniation. Spine 15:1234–1235

Oppenheim J S, Rothman A S, Sachdev V P 1993 Thoracic herniated discs – review of the literature and 12 cases. Mount Sinai Journal of Medicine 60:321–326

Osman A A, Bassiouni H, Koutri R et al 1994 Ageing of the thoracic spine: distinction between wedging on osteoarthritis and fracture in osteoporosis – a cross-sectional and longitudinal study. Bone 15:437–442

Palastanga N, Field D, Soames R 1994 Anatomy and human movement. Butterworth Heinemann, Oxford

Taylor J R, Twomey L T 1985 Vertebral column development and its relation to adult pathology. Australian Journal of Physiotherapy 31:83–88

Turner P 1991 Osteoporotic back pain – its prevention and treatment. Physiotherapy 77:642–646

Watanabe M, Kihara Y, Matsuda Y et al 1992 Benign osteoblastoma in the vertebral body of the thoracic spine – a case report. Spine 17:1432–1434

Wilke A, Wolf U, Lageard P et al 2000 Thoracic disc herniation: a diagnostic challenge. Manual Therapy 5(3):181–184

Yeung M, Hagen N 1993 Cervical disc herniation presenting with chest wall pain. Le Journal Canadien des Sciences Neurologiques 20:59–61

Chapter 10

The hip

SUMMARY

Degenerative osteoarthrosis of the hip, even before the development of X-ray changes, is frequently overlooked as a treatable condition when symptomatic relief can often be obtained by the mobilization or injection techniques described in orthopaedic medicine.

Pain in the hip region can be incorrectly attributed to the lumbar spine and/or sacroiliac joint, while the bursae in the area may not be considered, and can evade diagnosis. Groin strain and hamstring injury are familiar to the clinician,

though worthy of mention to enhance effective treatment.

This chapter describes the anatomy relevant to common lesions in the hip region to which orthopaedic medicine principles of treatment can be applied. A commentary follows, highlighting the relevant points of the history and suggesting a methodical sequence for objective examination. Lesions are then discussed with treatment alternatives and overall management.

ANATOMY

INERT STRUCTURES

The *hip joint* is a synovial joint formed between the head of the femur and the acetabulum of the innominate bone. The *head of the femur* is slightly more than half a sphere and faces anteriorly, superiorly and medially to articulate with the acetabulum forming a ball-and-socket joint. This articulation offers great stability and provides sufficient mobility for gait. The close packed position of the hip joint is full extension, with a degree of abduction and medial rotation (Hartley 1995, Williams 1998).

The *acetabulum* is deepened by the fibrocartilaginous acetabular labrum and all articular surfaces are covered by articular cartilage. The *fibrous capsule*, lined with synovium, surrounds most of the neck of the femur, attaching above to the acetabular rim, below to the intertrochanteric line anteriorly and 1 cm above the intertrochanteric crest posteriorly. Both the joint capsule and the articular cartilage tend to be thicker anterosuperiorly, which is the region of most stress in weight-bearing. Synovial plicae (folds or reflections of the synovial membrane) have been identified by Fu et al (1997), found mainly on the external surface of the lower medial part of the acetabular labrum (labral plicae) but also at the base of the ligament of the head of the femur and on the base of the femoral neck. The labral plicae may potentially be a source of pain if injured or thickened since, in the normal state, these have been seen to slip between the articular surfaces of the femoral head and acetabulum during medial rotation and to return to their original position during lateral rotation.

Three ligaments reinforce the articular capsule and control movement. All three are taut in extension and relaxed in flexion. The *iliofemoral ligament* has strong medial and lateral bands which form a Y-shape, passing from the anterior inferior iliac spine to the intertrochanteric line. The *pubofemoral ligament* passes from the superior pubic ramus to blend distally with the capsule and the medial border of the iliofemoral ligament. The *ischiofemoral ligament* passes from the ischium and winds superiorly and laterally to the upper part of the femoral neck, blending with the capsule of the hip joint and supporting it posteriorly.

The *psoas bursa* (L2–L3; Cyriax 1982) is 5–7 cm long and 2–4 cm wide in its normal collapsed state (Underwood et al 1988, Toohey et al 1990, Flanagan et al 1995, Zimmermann et al 1995). In 15% of cadaveric specimens, the psoas bursa was seen to communicate with the hip joint via an aperture between the iliofemoral and pubofemoral ligaments (Flanagan et al 1995). It may be a simple bursa or multiloculated with well-defined thin walls (Meaney et al 1992).

The psoas bursa lies beneath the musculotendinous junction of the iliopsoas muscle and the front of the capsule of the hip joint (Fig. 10.1). It cushions the iliopsoas tendon as it winds round the front of the hip joint to its posteromedial insertion on the lesser trochanter. It is related anteromedially to the femoral artery and anteriorly to the femoral nerve (Canoso 1981). Its point of location is just distal to the mid-point of the inguinal ligament, deep to the femoral artery.

The *gluteal bursa* (L4–L5; Cyriax & Cyriax 1983) is not a single entity, but for clinical purposes is considered to be so. At least four separate bursae lie between the different planes of the gluteal muscles as they attach to or pass over the greater trochanter, collectively forming the gluteal bursa.

Two bursae are associated with gluteus maximus: a large *trochanteric bursa* (Fig. 10.2) separating it from the lateral aspect of the greater trochanter and a gluteofemoral bursa lying between it and vastus lateralis (Williams 1998). The trochanteric bursa of gluteus medius lies between its tendon and the anterosuperior aspect of the greater trochanter. The trochanteric bursa of gluteus minimus separates its insertion from the medial part of the greater trochanter (Williams 1998). One further bursa may be present, the ischial bursa, lying between the ischial tuberosity and the lower part of gluteus maximus.

CONTRACTILE STRUCTURES

Anterior muscles are flexors of the hip, although they may also assist other hip movements. Some pass over the knee where they also have an effect. Resisted flexion of the hip tests mainly psoas major; with the knee flexed it is also testing rectus femoris.

Figure 10.1   Position of the
psoas bursa.

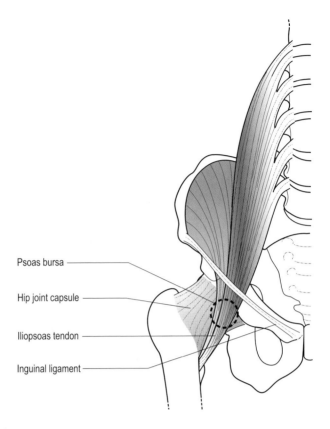

Psoas bursa

Hip joint capsule

Iliopsoas tendon

Inguinal ligament

Psoas major (ventral rami L1–L3) has its origin from the lumbar spine.
It descends to pass under the centre of the inguinal ligament receiving the
fibres of iliacus on its lateral side. The iliopsoas tendon crosses the front
of the hip joint where it is cushioned by the underlying psoas bursa. The
combined tendon winds posteriorly to insert into the lesser trochanter of
the femur.

Sartorius (femoral nerve L2–L3) passes from the anterior superior iliac
spine to cross the thigh medially, inserting into the upper medial aspect
of the tibia. It marks the lateral border of the femoral triangle.

Rectus femoris (femoral nerve L2–L4) is part of the quadriceps
mechanism and has its main effect at the knee. However, its origin above
the hip makes it a two-joint muscle and it also acts as a powerful hip
flexor, being most efficient when the knee is flexed (Kapandji 1987). It has
two heads of origin: a straight head from the anterior inferior iliac spine
and a reflected head from just above the acetabular rim. It joins the rest
of the quadriceps to insert into the patellar tendon.

Posterior muscles are extensors of the hip. Gluteus maximus acts
principally as a hip extensor while the hamstrings assist hip extension,
but their main effect is in flexing the knee. Since the hamstring muscles
run over two joints, their efficiency in extending the hip increases if the
knee is locked into extension (Kapandji 1987).

Figure 10.2 Position of trochanteric bursa.

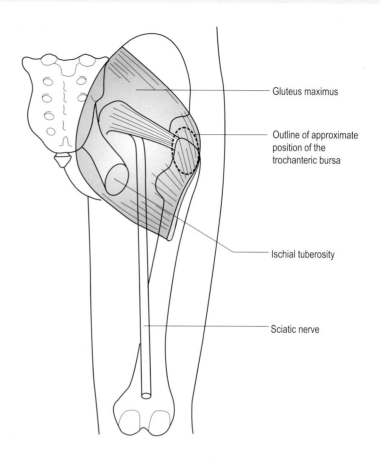

Gluteus maximus

Outline of approximate position of the trochanteric bursa

Ischial tuberosity

Sciatic nerve

Gluteus maximus (inferior gluteal nerve L5, S1–S2) is the largest and most superficial of the gluteal muscles. It passes from behind the posterior gluteal line on the blade of the ilium to the iliotibial tract and upper femur. The large trochanteric bursa separates the insertion of gluteus maximus from the lateral aspect of the greater trochanter.

Biceps femoris (sciatic nerve L5, S1–S2) is the lateral hamstring with two heads of origin. A long head arises from an inferomedial facet on the ischial tuberosity (which it shares with semitendinosus) and a short head from the lateral lip of the linea aspera. Its fibres converge into a fusiform muscle belly and its tendon of insertion attaches to the head of the fibula.

Semitendinosus and semimembranosus are the medial hamstrings. *Semitendinosus* (sciatic nerve L5, S1–S2) takes origin from the inferomedial facet on the ischial tuberosity. Its muscle belly ends in the middle of the thigh and its long tendon of insertion lies on semimembranosus before winding around to the medial aspect of the upper tibia. *Semimembranosus* (sciatic nerve L5, S1–S2) takes origin from the superolateral facet on the ischial tuberosity and has its main insertion onto the posterior aspect of the medial tibial condyle into the tuberculum tendinis.

Functionally, the small, deep muscles of the hip are responsible for lateral rotation.

Piriformis (L5, S1–S2) originates in the pelvis, exiting through the greater sciatic foramen to attach to the upper border of the greater trochanter.

Obturator externus (posterior branch of the obturator nerve L3–L4) and *obturator internus* (nerve to obturator internus L5, S1) pass posteriorly to the hip joint and insert into the medial surface of the greater trochanter and trochanteric fossa.

Gemelli (L5, S1) pass from the ischial spine and ischial tuberosity to the medial aspect of the greater trochanter.

Quadratus femoris (nerve to quadratus femoris L5, S1) passes from the ischial tuberosity to the quadrate tubercle in the middle of the trochanteric crest.

Lateral muscles are abductors and lateral rotators. Gluteus medius is the main hip abductor while medius and minimus together are responsible for maintaining the position of the opposite side of the pelvis in single-leg stance. Weakness of the hip abductors produces a positive Trendelenburg sign. Tensor fascia lata and the anterior fibres of gluteus medius and minimus also produce medial rotation and flexion because they lie anterior to the frontal plane of the hip joint. Lying posteriorly, some fibres of gluteus medius and minimus are responsible for lateral rotation and extension (Kapandji 1987).

Gluteus medius (superior gluteal nerve L5, S1) is partially overlapped by maximus and lies in a slightly deeper plane. It originates from the blade of the ilium between posterior and anterior gluteal lines and inserts into the lateral aspect of the greater trochanter.

Gluteus minimus (superior gluteal nerve L5, S1) is the deepest gluteal muscle and arises between the anterior and inferior gluteal lines, inserting into the medial part of the anterior trochanteric surface.

Tensor fascia lata (superior gluteal nerve L4–L5) arises from the anterior 5 cm of the outer lip of the iliac crest and the anterior superior iliac spine. It passes downwards and laterally to insert into the anterior border of the iliotibial tract. The adductor muscles originate in the pelvis and pass to the medial aspect of the thigh.

Functionally, the *medial muscles* are responsible for adduction of the hip. Medial rotation at the hip is a secondary function of gluteus medius, minimus and tensor fascia lata; adductor magnus, longus and pectineus may also contribute to this movement.

Gracilis (obturator nerve L2–L3) is the most medial hip adductor. It passes from the lower half of the body of the pubis, the inferior pubic ramus and the adjacent ischial ramus, to run vertically downwards to just below the medial tibial condyle.

Pectineus (femoral nerve L2–L3) passes from the pecten pubis running posterolaterally to a line joining the lesser trochanter to the linea aspera.

Adductor longus (obturator nerve L2–L4) is the most superficial adductor. It passes from the body of the pubis, in the angle between the crest and the symphysis pubis, to descend posterolaterally to the middle third of the linea aspera.

Adductor brevis (obturator nerve L3) lies deep to adductor longus, passing from the lower aspect of the body of the pubis and the inferior pubic ramus to its attachment on the femur, between the lesser trochanter and the linea aspera.

Adductor magnus (upper fibres, obturator nerve; lower fibres, tibial branch of the sciatic nerve, L2–L4) is the largest and deepest adductor muscle. It is considered to have two separate portions, one an adductor portion and the other a hamstring portion, each with its own separate nerve supply. It takes origin from the inferior pubic ramus, the adjacent ischial ramus and the inferolateral aspect of the ischial tuberosity. Its upper fibres pass mainly horizontally to the linea aspera of the femur and form the adductor part of the muscle. Its lower fibres pass more vertically to the adductor tubercle on the medial femoral condyle and are the hamstring part.

A GUIDE TO SURFACE MARKING AND PALPATION

PELVIC REGION

Palpate the *iliac crest*, which should be obvious in most people as no muscles attach to its superior border. The highest point of the crest lies just posterior to the mid-point and gives an approximate indication of the level of the spinous process of L4.

Palpate the *anterior superior iliac spine* which is subcutaneous and located at the anterior end of the iliac crest. It marks the lateral attachment of the inguinal ligament and the origin of the sartorius muscle.

Palpate the *posterior superior iliac spine* which is situated at the posterior end of the iliac crest. It is not as readily palpable as the anterior spine, but lies under a dimple in the upper buttock, approximately 4 cm lateral to the spinous process of S2. It gives attachment to the sacrotuberous ligament. Imagine a line drawn from the posterior superior iliac spine to the spinous process of S2; this line crosses the centre of the *sacroiliac joint* and gives an indication of the joint's position.

Consider the position of the *anterior and posterior inferior iliac spines* which lie below the superior spines and are not as readily palpable. The anterior inferior spine gives origin superiorly to the long head of rectus femoris and inferiorly to part of the iliofemoral ligament.

Locate the position of the *pubic tubercle* at the medial end of the inguinal crease, lying at the same level as the top of the greater trochanter. It marks the medial attachment of the inguinal ligament.

Palpate the bony *ischial tuberosity*, which lies in the buttock approximately 5 cm lateral to the midline just above the gluteal fold. In the sitting position, body weight is supported by the ischial tuberosities. Each is most easily palpated with the patient in side lying and the hip placed in flexion, to bring the ischial tuberosity out from under the bulk of gluteus maximus.

LATERAL ASPECT OF THE THIGH

In side lying palpate the *greater trochanter*, which is a large quadrangular bony prominence situated at the upper lateral shaft of the

Figure 10.3   Location of hip
joint for the injection by
grasping the greater trochanter.

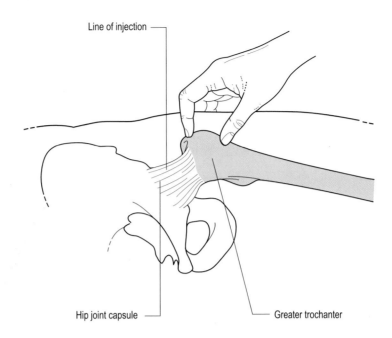

Line of injection

Hip joint capsule

Greater trochanter

femur, approximately one hand's-breadth below the iliac crest. Grasp the
greater trochanter with your thumb, index and middle fingers (Fig. 10.3),
lifting the leg passively into abduction to relax the iliotibial tract. The
greater trochanter will be a useful bony landmark for some of the
injection techniques around the hip.

ANTERIOR ASPECT OF THE THIGH

Consider the position of the *femoral triangle* on the anterior thigh
(Fig. 10.4). Place the leg into the FABER position – a combination of
*F*lexion, *AB*duction and *E*xternal (lateral) *R*otation of the hip – to give
you an indication of the borders of the triangle. The inguinal ligament
forms the base of the triangle, sartorius its lateral border and adductor
longus its medial border. Iliopsoas and pectineus lie in the floor of the
femoral triangle.

Consider the position of the *lateral femoral cutaneous nerve* of the thigh
(L2–L3) as it passes under or through the inguinal ligament, just medial
to the anterior superior iliac spine. It may be compressed here, causing a
condition called meralgia paraesthetica, which produces paraesthesia and
pain in the nerve's distribution on the lateral side of the thigh. It is found
in obese patients and those who wear tight fitting clothes or belts (Adkins
& Figler 2000).

Palpate for the *femoral artery* which passes down through the middle
of the triangle with the femoral vein situated medially and the femoral
nerve laterally. You will locate a strong pulse just distal to the mid-point
of the inguinal ligament.

Locating the femoral pulse will prove a useful landmark for the
structures passing deep to it. From superficial to deep these are the

Figure 10.4 Femoral triangle, also showing emerging lateral cutaneous nerve of thigh.

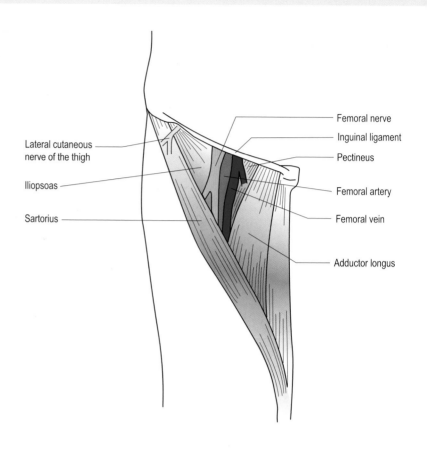

iliopsoas tendon, which is en route to its insertion into the lesser trochanter, the psoas bursa, and the hip joint.

POSTERIOR ASPECT OF THE BUTTOCK AND THIGH

Consider the position of the *sciatic nerve* in the buttock (Fig. 10.5). You can locate its approximate position by marking a point midway between the posterior superior iliac spine and the greater trochanter, which identifies the position of the nerve as it leaves the pelvis via the greater sciatic foramen, emerging under piriformis. Join this to another mark at a point just medial to the mid-point between the greater trochanter and the ischial tuberosity. This indicates the position of the nerve as it exits the buttock under the lower border of gluteus maximus (Williams 1998).

MEDIAL ASPECT OF THE THIGH

Place the leg into the FABER position to identify the thick, cordlike tendon of *adductor longus*. Palpate this tendon to appreciate its width and depth.

Figure 10.5   Approximate course of the sciatic nerve in the buttock and thigh.

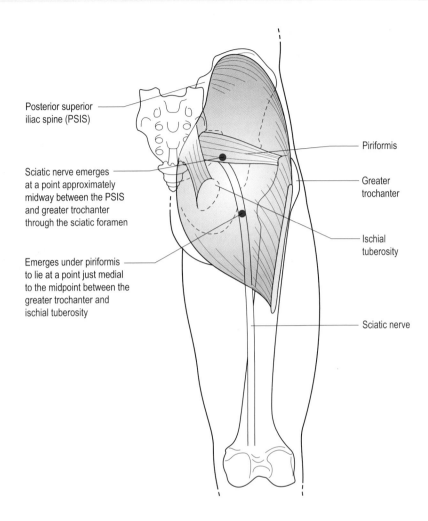

Posterior superior iliac spine (PSIS)

Sciatic nerve emerges at a point approximately midway between the PSIS and greater trochanter through the sciatic foramen

Emerges under piriformis to lie at a point just medial to the midpoint between the greater trochanter and ischial tuberosity

Piriformis

Greater trochanter

Ischial tuberosity

Sciatic nerve

COMMENTARY ON THE EXAMINATION

OBSERVATION

A general observation is made of the patient's *face and overall posture*, but particular attention is paid to the *gait*. Since the function of the hip joint is to support body weight, lesions involving the joint mechanics tend to cause alterations in the gait pattern. An uneven stride will indicate restricted movement, as found in arthritis, or may be due to pain on weight-bearing. Excessive lateral rotation on walking may indicate a slipped epiphysis in the young or may be present with pain or advanced capsular contracture in the elderly, indicating an arthrosis with a marked capsular pattern. A Trendelenburg gait will indicate weak abductor muscles.

Pain in the hip joint region may originate in the lumbar spine and a detailed history will help to eliminate a lesion in the area.

HISTORY (SUBJECTIVE EXAMINATION)

The *age, occupation, sports, hobbies and lifestyle* of the patient may alert the examiner to the possible cause of the lesion.

The age of the patient is relevant to conditions at the hip. Degenerative osteoarthrosis typically presents in the middle to older age group, although it is not uncommon to find it in younger athletes, especially road runners. Muscle lesions and bursitis affect the middle age group, while loose bodies can present as a complication of osteoarthrosis in the older group or as osteochondritis dissecans in adolescents.

Children can develop hip problems which if misdiagnosed can be potentially serious, and an orthopaedic opinion should always be sought. 'Irritable hip' is a non-specific diagnosis for groin pain, limited movement and a limp. Perthes disease affects boys aged 4–10 and is an osteochondritis of the femoral epiphysis. Slipped epiphysis is either sudden or gradual slipping of the superior epiphyseal plate which may produce a lateral rotation deformity. It tends to occur in overweight adolescents and is more common in boys, who present with pain on exercise. Transient synovitis is of unknown aetiology and affects children under 10 years. Juvenile chronic arthritis usually begins in other joints, but it can also affect the hip joints. Emms et al (2002) remind us that although it is well known that knee pain in children may be referred from the hip, it must not be forgotten that hip pathology may masquerade as knee pain in adult patients as well.

Occupation, sports, hobbies and lifestyle will certainly indicate the aggravating factors of the condition and allow the clinician to formulate a programme of treatment and advice, tailored to the patient's individual needs.

Specific sports-related conditions should be considered. Stress fracture of the femoral neck may be encountered in young adults who are involved in endurance and high intensity sports; initially anterior hip pain occurs late into the sporting activity but progresses to limit activity, occurring during any weight-bearing episode and even at rest. It should also be suspected in women with the female athletic triad of amenorrhoea, eating disorder and osteoporosis. Diagnosis is essential to prevent progression to avascular necrosis of the femoral head (O'Kane 1999, Adkins & Figler 2000).

Osteitis pubis, a poorly understood pathological condition involving the pubic bone and symphysis pubis, presents with groin pain which may be bilateral. The symptoms may be aggravated by exercise, twisting, turning and kicking. Pain is provoked by resisted adduction which is usually accompanied by weakness, and there is tenderness to palpation over the pubic tubercles and symphysis pubis (Brukner & Khan 2002). The so called 'sports hernias' should also be considered as a cause of anterior hip pain. These are thought to be responsible for activity-related hip pain, particularly in football, rugby and ice hockey players (O'Kane 1999).

The *site and spread* of pain may be local, indicating a superficial or less irritable lesion such as a muscle strain, or diffuse, indicating a larger lesion or gross inflammation.

Referred pain may originate from the lumbar spine. The sensory nerve supply to the hip joint is mainly through the femoral nerve L2–L3;

therefore the joint itself refers pain into these dermatomes depending on the size of the lesion. Part of the L2 and L3 dermatomes covers the upper buttock and a hip lesion may present as low back pain only.

Groin pain or pain referred to the knee in the child or adolescent without obvious cause must be considered serious and a specialist opinion sought for the possibility of the conditions mentioned above.

The *onset* of the symptoms may be gradual or sudden.

In osteoarthrosis the pain has a gradual onset, initially during weight-bearing activities, progressing to hip pain without weight-bearing, and present at rest (Cailliet 1990). A history of previous trauma such as fracture, which alters joint biomechanics, can predispose the joint to degenerative changes.

Relatively minor trauma can fracture the pelvis in the elderly, producing severe pain of sudden onset. Loose bodies present suddenly, as do traumatic muscular lesions. Muscles around the hip joint can be easily strained, since many are two-joint muscles, and a sudden explosive contraction such as that seen in sprinting may produce overstretching (Hartley 1995). Overuse or repetitive movements may produce chronic contractile lesions or bursitis.

The *duration* of symptoms indicates the stage of the lesion in the inflammatory process. Degenerative osteoarthrosis will present a typical history of gradually worsening episodes of pain. Bursitis tends to give a gradual onset of aching pain and therefore is often present for many months before the patient seeks treatment. A severe pain which gradually increases in intensity, and remains so, is indicative of a serious lesion. This, coupled with other findings in the history, may be indicative of the 'sign of the buttock' (see below).

The *symptoms and behaviour* need to be considered. The behaviour of the pain gives an indication of the nature of the lesion. For example, osteoarthrosis at the hip joint may be aggravated by activity or weight-bearing, or inflamed bursae and muscle sprains are worse with use and eased by rest.

The other symptoms described by the patient may give essential clues to diagnosis. Bursae produce pain on activities which squeeze or compress them, e.g. lying on the side or sitting. Loose bodies tend to produce twinging pain and a sensation of giving way on weight-bearing. Arthritis tends to produce morning pain and stiffness due to accumulation of intracapsular swelling overnight (Hartley 1995). Degenerative osteoarthrosis, in its early stage, often produces night pain. Unrelenting pain should be considered serious, especially if the patient is unwell with a fever, night sweats and rigors.

To determine if the pain is coming from the lumbar spine, the patient is questioned about the presence of paraesthesia and pain produced by a cough or sneeze.

An indication of *past medical history, other joint involvement* and *medications* may give a clue to diagnosis and will establish whether contraindications to treatment techniques exist. Patients should be asked about any unexpected recent weight loss, indicative of more serious lesions, such as secondary deposits which are common in the hip and pelvis (Paice

1995). Differential diagnosis should also consider the exclusion of hip pain associated with pathology of the abdominal and pelvic organs as well as femoral or inguinal hernias.

INSPECTION

An inspection of the general posture in weight-bearing will indicate any *bony deformity*. Look for general postural asymmetry which may be relevant, the position of the buttock creases, posterior superior iliac spines, anterior superior iliac spines, level of the iliac crests, any leg length discrepancy and the position of the feet.

Colour changes and *swelling* are not expected at the hip because it is such a deep joint, but they may be associated with trauma, bruising and abrasions. If redness and swelling are present in the buttock area without a history of trauma, the 'sign of the buttock' (see below) may be suspected.

Muscle wasting may be seen in the glutei associated with a lumbar lesion, or in the quadriceps associated with degenerative osteoarthrosis of the hip or a lumbar lesion.

STATE AT REST

Before any movements are performed, the state at rest is established to provide a baseline for subsequent comparison.

The suggested sequence for the objective examination will now be given, followed by a commentary including the reasoning in performing the movements and the significance of the possible findings.

Eliminate the Lumbar Spine

- Active lumbar extension (Fig. 10.6)
- Extension repeated with foot on stool if indicated (Fig. 10.7)
- Active lumbar right side flexion (Fig. 10.8)
- Active lumbar left side flexion (Fig. 10.9)
- Active lumbar flexion (Fig. 10.10)

Supine Lying

- Passive hip flexion (Fig. 10.11)
- Passive hip medial rotation for end-feel (Fig. 10.12)
- Passive hip lateral rotation (Fig. 10.13)
- Passive hip abduction (Fig. 10.14)
- Passive hip adduction (Fig. 10.15)
- Resisted hip flexion (Fig. 10.16)
- Resisted hip abduction (Fig. 10.17)
- Resisted hip adduction (Fig. 10.18)
- Resisted hip extension (Fig. 10.19)

Prone Lying

- Passive hip extension (Fig. 10.20)
- Passive hip medial rotation for range (Fig. 10.21)
- Resisted hip medial rotation (Fig. 10.22)
- Resisted hip lateral rotation (Fig. 10.23)
- Resisted knee flexion (Fig. 10.24)
- Resisted knee extension (Fig. 10.25)

Accessory Test for the Psoas Bursa

- Passive hip flexion and adduction (Fig. 10.26)

Accessory Test for the 'Sign of the Buttock'

- Straight leg raise (Fig. 10.27)

Palpation

- Once a diagnosis has been made, the structure at fault is palpated for the exact site of the lesion

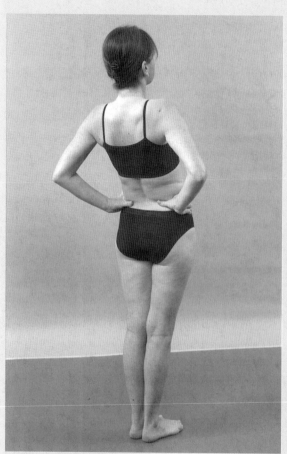

Figure 10.6   Active extension.

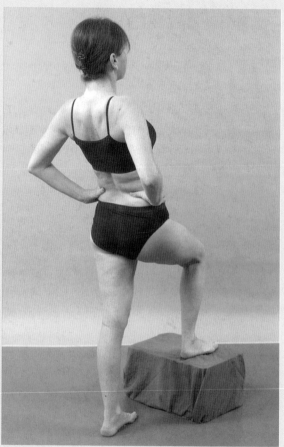

Figure 10.7   Active extension with hip flexed to differentiate between hip and lumbar spine as the cause of pain.

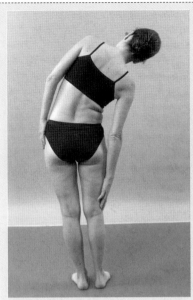

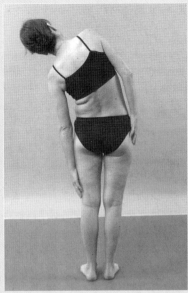

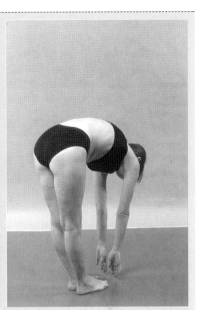

Figure 10.8   Active right side flexion.   Figure 10.9   Active left side flexion.   Figure 10.10   Active flexion.

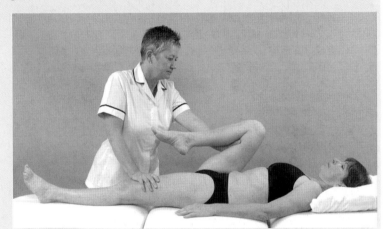

Figure 10.11   Passive flexion.

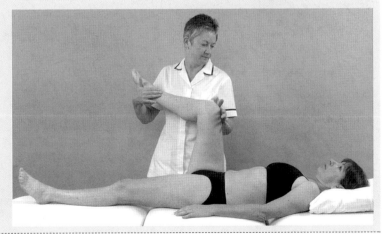

Figure 10.12   Passive medial rotation.

Figure 10.13   Passive lateral rotation.

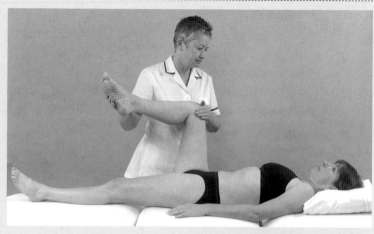

Figure 10.14   Passive abduction.

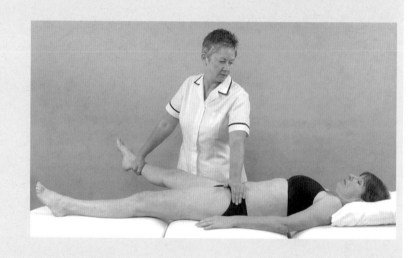

Figure 10.15   Passive adduction.

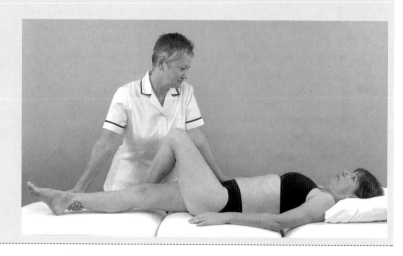

Figure 10.16   Resisted flexion.

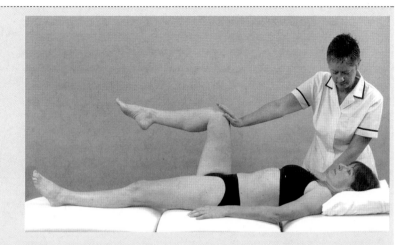

Figure 10.17   Resisted abduction.

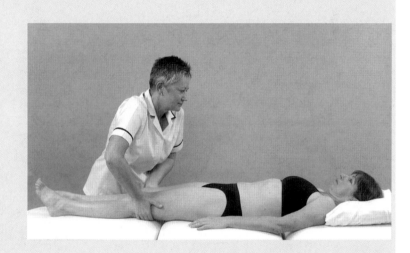

Figure 10.18   Resisted adduction.

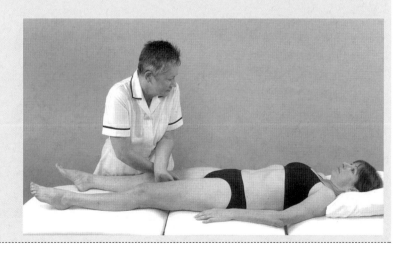

Figure 10.19   Resisted extension.

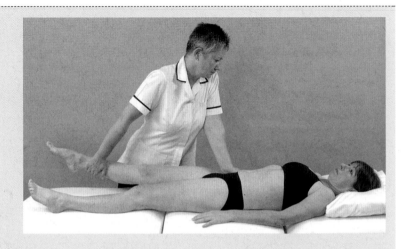

Figure 10.20   Passive extension.

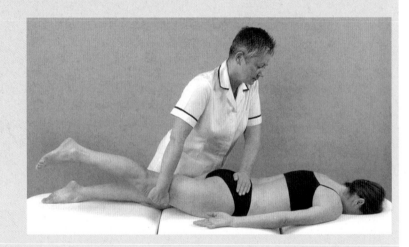

Figure 10.21   Passive medial rotation.

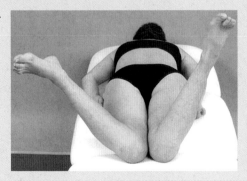

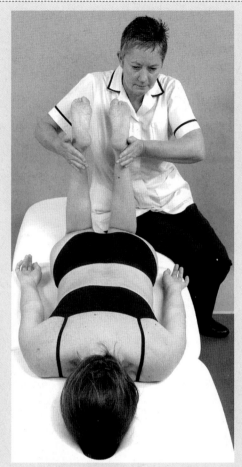

Figure 10.22   Resisted medial rotation.

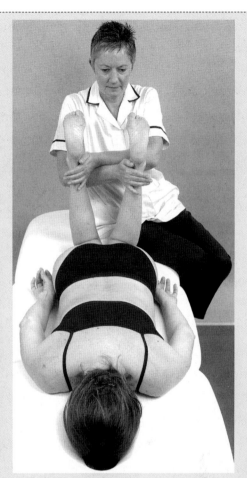

Figure 10.23   Resisted lateral rotation.

Figure 10.24   Resisted knee flexion.

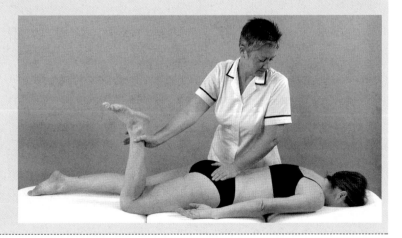

Figure 10.25   Resisted knee extension.

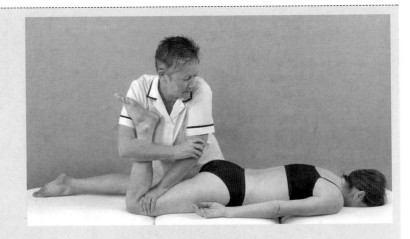

Figure 10.26   Combined flexion and adduction to compress the psoas bursa.

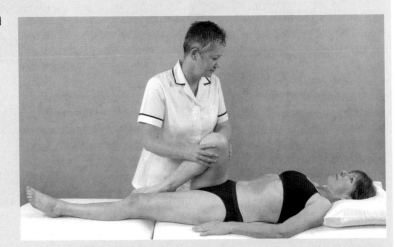

Figure 10.27   Straight leg raise: accessory test for 'sign of the buttock'

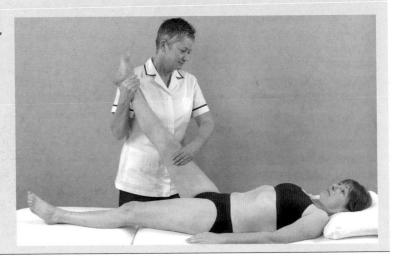

The routine for the examination of the hip is conducted in the above order as it allows all tests in each position of standing, supine and prone to be completed.

The lumbar spine is first assessed by the four active movements. If active lumbar extension reproduces the pain, it should be repeated with the hip joint eliminated by placing it into flexion with the foot up on a stool. If extension is still painful, the lesion lies in the lumbar spine and a more thorough investigation of this must then be made.

If serious hip pathology is suspected and to clear the lumbar spine, a straight leg raise is included ('sign of the buttock', see below). Tests for sacroiliac joint involvement may also be included at this stage, as indicated by the history, and are described in Chapter 14.

The passive hip movements test the inert structures for pain, range of movement and end-feel. Limited movement may be typical of the capsular pattern of limitation due to arthritis. Normally, passive flexion has a 'soft' end-feel while passive medial rotation, lateral rotation and extension have an 'elastic' end-feel. It is not possible to appreciate the end-feel of the capsule on passive abduction and adduction as the tension in the overlying soft tissue structures provides the end of range of these movements before the capsule can be stressed. A bursitis or a loose body in the joint produces a non-capsular pattern of movement.

The resisted movements test the contractile structures for pain and power. At the hip, muscle lesions are commonly found in the adductors, quadriceps and hamstrings, but positive resisted tests may also be an accessory sign in bursitis. Resisted flexion tests mainly psoas, but since the knee is flexed it also tests rectus femoris. Resisted abduction tests mainly gluteus medius, while resisted adduction tests the adductor muscles, particularly adductor longus. Resisted extension tests mainly gluteus maximus, but since the knee is extended, this also tests the hamstrings. Resisted rotation tests the medial and lateral rotators of the hip, resisted knee flexion tests the hamstring muscles and resisted knee extension tests the quadriceps muscle group.

Accessory tests can be applied if indicated. Combined hip flexion and adduction can be applied to compress the psoas bursa to confirm its diagnosis, and a straight leg raise can be included if the 'sign of the buttock' is suspected (see below).

> **Capsular pattern of the hip joint**
> - Most limitation of medial rotation.
> - Less limitation of flexion and abduction.
> - Least limitation of extension.

CAPSULAR LESIONS

The movements limited in the capsular pattern have a characteristically 'hard' end-feel. If, on examination, the capsular pattern exists at the hip joint, then an arthritis is present. The hip can be affected by degenerative osteoarthrosis, traumatic arthritis, rheumatoid arthritis and any of the spondyloarthropathies.

Arthritis at the hip is commonly degenerative osteoarthrosis, usually occurring over the age of 60 in 50% of the population (Kumar & Clark 2002). It may be subdivided into primary athritis which has no recognizable predisposing cause although subtle secondary factors may be present, or secondary arthritis due to predisposing factors including occupational overuse, previous fracture or altered biomechanics, e.g. leg length discrepancies, and congenital or developmental abnormalities. Men and women are equally affected (Dieppe 1995, Sims 1999). However, Kersnič et al (1997) suggest that as women have a significantly smaller femoral head radius and a larger acetabular diameter than men, contact stress on the articular surfaces is increased. The female femoral and pelvic shape may predispose women to osteoarthrosis, especially in association with increased body weight. Intrinsic factors such as altered biomechanics or extrinsic factors such as hardness of the floor, and the influence of sporting and leisure activities, may also contribute to degenerative change (Sims 1999).

Sims (1999) presents a hypothesis that the neuromuscular system plays a role in the development of degenerative osteoarthrosis. Strong contraction of the hip abductor mechanism prevents dropping of the contralateral pelvis in single leg standing which produces an increase of 4–5 times body weight distributed through the hip joint. This is further increased during fast walking and running. Any alteration in the abductor mechanism, therefore, may lead to an uneven distribution of stress, resulting in articular cartilage degeneration. Dynamic loading of the hip occurs during the impact of heel strike and may involve single or repetitive loads. The impact load through the hip can exceed 8 times body weight during a stumble (Bergmann et al, cited in Sims 1999). Abnormal loading may also occur as a result of alteration in the centre of gravity such as that which occurs during an antalgic gait pattern, for example. Although this reduces the compressive forces of the abductor muscles as the centre of gravity shifts towards the stance limb, the load is transferred to the superior aspect of the femoral head where it becomes concentrated, leading to cartilage destruction. An abnormal gait pattern may be the result of pathology anywhere in the lower limb kinetic chain, from the lumbar spine to the foot, and need not be confined to the hip. The articular surfaces of the hip are slightly incongruent such that the apex of the acetabulum is a non-contact area allowing lubrication of the articular cartilage. The joint becomes more congruent during the ageing process, so reducing lubrication and possibly contributing further to degenerative change.

McGory & Endrizzi (2000) detail a case report of adhesive capsulitis of the hip, a diagnosis based on clinical findings with no evidence of bony changes on X-ray. The patient concerned had a history of hypothyroidism and had previously been diagnosed with bilateral adhesive capsulitis of the shoulder. They postulate that the involvement of the three separate joints gives credibility to the theory that adhesive capsulitis is a systemic rather than a local condition. Adhesive capsulitis of the hip follows a similar course to that demonstrated at the shoulder, and also responds to manual treatment and/or injection in a similar way.

The pain of osteoarthrosis usually has a gradual onset and may be felt in the upper buttock, groin and anterior thigh, up to or beyond the knee. Pain is associated with activity in the early stages, but as the condition advances, pain is also present at rest. Joint stiffness and loss of movement, such as difficulty in reaching to put on shoes and socks, are also presenting factors. X-ray changes are not a good indicator of symptoms as joint pathology can be present long before symptoms present and vice versa.

After diagnosis, the condition may stabilize and the prognosis can be good. However, patients referred for surgery usually have a fairly rapid deterioration and severe symptoms progress over a period of 1–2 years. It seems that osteoarthrosis progresses with periods of exacerbation and periods of remission (Dieppe 1995).

Treatment for osteoarthrosis depends on the stage and activity of the disease as indicated by the severity/irritability of the lesion. It can be divided into early, middle and late stages (Stages I, II or III) for the application of appropriate treatment.

EARLY STAGE OSTEOARTHROSIS OF THE HIP (STAGE I)

This is usually the initial phase of diagnosis of the condition. The patient complains of buttock or groin pain associated with weight-bearing activities and the pain sometimes disturbs sleep. On examination, the patient has a mild capsular pattern of limited medial rotation, flexion and perhaps abduction, with extension not yet affected. The limited movements have an abnormal 'hard' end-feel due to muscle spasm, but some elasticity remains. The principle of treatment, applied during this early stage, is to stretch the capsular adhesions using a Grade B capsular stretching technique in conjunction with heat applied to the joint. The aim of treatment is to relieve pain, allowing a greater range of pain-free movement to be established.

Grade B mobilization for early osteoarthrosis (Saunders 2000)

The movements limited in the capsular pattern are stretched using Grade B mobilization. However, functional benefit is often gained by stretching flexion alone.

To stretch flexion, position the patient in supine lying with counter-pressure on the other leg to stabilize it and to ensure that maximum stretch is applied to the affected hip joint capsule (Fig. 10.28). Place one

Figure 10.28   Grade B mobilization, stretching flexion.

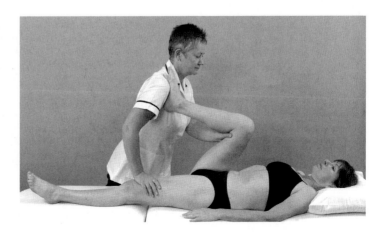

hand under the patient's lower thigh, to avoid involving the knee and to give a little distraction, which makes the manoeuvre more comfortable. Place the patient's foot against your shoulder to assist with stretching and to help guide the movement. After stretching flexion, slide the patient's leg over your shoulder and return the leg steadily to the bed under some distraction to reduce discomfort (Fig. 10.29).

To stretch extension, reverse the position described above for stretching flexion, with pressure applied to stretch extension of the affected leg (Fig. 10.30).

To stretch abduction, fix the good leg over the edge of the couch and position the affected leg in as much abduction as possible (Fig. 10.31). Increase this range of movement periodically.

To stretch medial rotation, position the patient in prone lying with the knee flexed to 90°. Fix the opposite buttock and apply the pressure carefully to the medial aspect of the knee. Take care with this manoeuvre as it may apply a strong torsion force to the neck of the femur and may also affect the knee (Fig. 10.32).

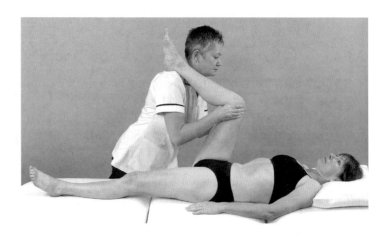

Figure 10.29   Grade B mobilization, returning leg under some distraction.

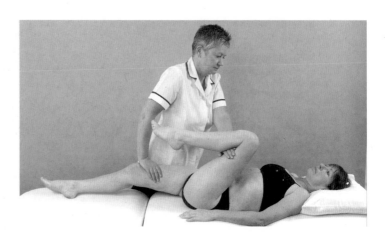

Figure 10.30   Grade B mobilization, stretching extension.

Figure 10.31   Grade B
mobilization, stretching
abduction.

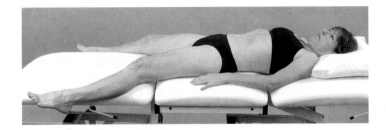

Figure 10.32   Grade B
mobilization, stretching medial
rotation.

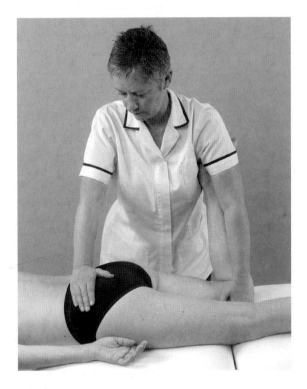

Treatment aims to provide symptomatic relief, but it relies on the patient continuing with a self-management programme.

Initially the patient is seen regularly to assess the effect of the capsular stretching and to teach the patient home management. Clinical judgement should be used to guide how long each session of stretching should last. The pain may be aggravated for 2–4 hours and this should be explained to the patient. Treatment continues until either a plateau is reached or patients are confident to continue with their own stretching exercises and management.

In this early stage of the disease the patient may experience anxiety over the diagnosis and possible prognosis. Treatment must also include education of the patient, reassurance to relieve anxiety and encouragement to empower the patient to manage the condition (Dieppe 1995). Advice should be given about appropriate exercise, encouraging regular use and mobilization to prevent the further deterioration which immobilization would induce. A balance must be achieved between sufficient weight-bearing and rest and avoiding prolonged overloading of the joint.

Although there is no evidence that diet changes the progressive nature of the disease, the overweight patient should be encouraged to lose weight. Obesity may increase the load on the weight-bearing surfaces, progressing the degenerative process more rapidly (Dieppe 1995). Sticks and other walking support may be appropriate to aid daily living.

Although capsular stretching in the early stage may relieve pain and increase the range of movement, the patient may also require assistance from analgesics. Paracetamol and low-dose ibuprofen may be appropriate in the early stages of the disease (Dieppe 1995). If non-steroidal anti-inflammatory drugs (NSAIDs) are needed to control pain they should be prescribed for short periods of time during acute phases of the disease. The risks of gastrointestinal disturbance and renal insufficiency from NSAIDs are well documented and patients with osteoarthrosis fall into the older age group which is particularly susceptible to these side-effects (Dieppe 1995, Rang et al 2003). Other forms of pain relief, such as acupuncture, may be effective (McIndoe et al 1995), although Klaber Moffett et al (1996) demonstrated no specific effectiveness for the use of pulsed short wave for osteoarthritic hip or knee pain.

MIDDLE STAGE OSTEOARTHROSIS OF THE HIP (STAGE II)

Here the patient's symptoms and signs indicate a progression of the disease. Pain may be present at rest as well as exacerbated by weight-bearing activities. On examination, a moderate to severe capsular pattern is found and the limited movements have a 'hard' end-feel. Capsular stretching may no longer provide benefit and the treatment of choice in the short term may be injection.

A lateral approach is advocated for reasons of safety. Leopold et al (2001) conducted a study of 30 cadaver hips to test the hypothesis that, using anatomical landmarks, the anterior and lateral injection approaches to the hip joint result in reproducibly correct intra-articular needle placement and avoid important periarticular neurovascular structures. The success rate of intra-articular injection was 60% using the anterior approach and 80% using the lateral approach. During the anterior approach the needle passed significantly closer to neurovascular structures than the lateral approach, which was never within 25 mm of any such structures. The study concluded that the lateral approach under fluoroscopy or ultrasound would be the safest and most effective method for injecting the hip joint.

Injection of the hip joint (Cyriax & Cyriax 1983, Cyriax 1984)

Suggested needle size: 20G × 3$^1/_2$ in (0.9 × 90 mm) spinal needle
Dose: 40 mg triamcinolone acetonide in a total volume of 5 ml

Position the patient in side lying with the painful leg uppermost and supported in a neutral position on a pillow. Locate the greater trochanter by grasping it between thumb, index and middle fingers; the index finger should be resting on the top of the trochanter. To test you are in the correct position, move the leg passively into some abduction (Fig. 10.33), to relax the iliotibial tract, and you should feel your index finger sink in over the top of the trochanter.

The capsule of the hip joint almost completely surrounds the neck of the femur. By inserting the needle just above the index finger, i.e. above the greater trochanter, and aiming vertically downward towards the neck of the femur, the needle should be intracapsular once you gently make contact with bone (Fig. 10.34). You will feel a resistance as the needle pierces first the fascia lata, then the capsule before reaching bone (Fig. 10.35). Deliver the injection as a bolus. The patient is advised to maintain a period of relative rest for approximately 2 weeks following injection.

Controversy exists concerning repeated steroid injections into weight-bearing joints and the risk of steroid arthropathy (Cameron 1995). Therefore, as a general precaution, repeated corticosteroid injections into the hip joint have not been recommended and it has been advised that no more than two a year should be given without monitoring the degenerative condition of the joint with X-ray investigation. However, Raynauld et al (2003) conducted a study on repeated injections into the knee joint and established no harmful effects (see Ch. 11).

Figure 10.33 Abducting the hip to locate the hip joint line.

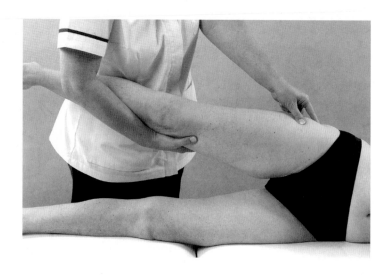

Figure 10.34 Injection of the hip joint.

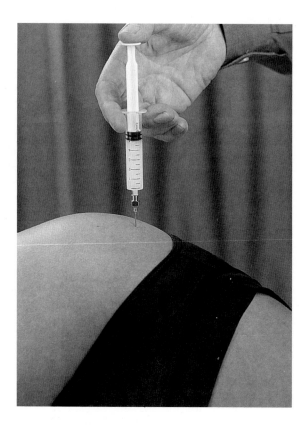

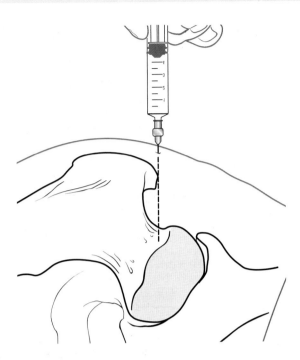

Figure 10.35   Injection of the hip joint showing direction of approach and needle position.

LATE STAGE OSTEOARTHROSIS OF THE HIP (STAGE III)

Conservative management no longer controls the patient's pain and functional disability may now be serious. Surgery is probably indicated, but there are no agreed criteria or guidelines for electing to perform hip surgery (Dieppe 1995). Pain, age and disability, as well as psychological factors, should all be taken into consideration by the patient and surgeon.

Injection may be given for pain relief during this stage, as described above.

RHEUMATOID ARTHRITIS

This may affect the hip joint and symptomatic relief may be gained from intra-articular injection, given as described above.

NON-CAPSULAR LESIONS

LOOSE BODY

A loose body in the hip joint causes twinges of pain felt in the groin or radiating down the front of the leg. These twinges may be associated with a momentary sensation of locking or giving way and an inability to weight-bear. This history suggests a loose body in the joint which periodically becomes impacted between the joint surfaces. The loose body may be associated with the rare condition osteochondritis dissecans in adolescents, but most commonly occurs secondary to the onset of degenerative osteoarthrosis at the joint (Cyriax & Cyriax 1983). Differential diagnosis should exclude labral tears which are found in the young adult. Labral pathology is often associated with traumatic incidents which may be minor twisting or hyperextension injuries. Pain is usually felt in the groin with clicking, locking and/or giving way (O'Kane 1999, Hickman & Peters 2001).

Signs of a loose body consist of a non-capsular pattern, commonly with pain at the end of range of full passive hip flexion and lateral rotation. If the range of movement demonstrates limitation, a springy end-feel may be appreciated. The principle of treatment applied is to reduce the loose body using strong traction together with Grade A mobilization. If successful, the loose body will be moved to a position within the joint where it no longer causes these typical symptoms.

Two mobilization techniques will be described (Cyriax & Cyriax 1983, Cyriax 1984).

Loose body mobilization technique 1

Position the patient in supine on the couch with an assistant applying counterpressure at the anterior superior iliac spines; padding may make it more comfortable for the patient. The assistant must start by applying pressure in an anterior–posterior direction and be prepared to change to apply cephalad pressure towards the end of the manoeuvre.

Your choice of manoeuvre with either lateral or medial rotation will depend on the physical findings during examination and the least painful rotation is attempted first: this is usually medial rotation.

Mobilization 1a: with medial rotation

Stand on the end of the couch, with your feet close together and parallel to the edge. Face the direction of medial rotation and apply a butterfly grip with the thumbs parallel on the lateral aspect of the lower leg, taking care to avoid undue pressure around the malleoli (Fig. 10.36). The

Figure 10.36 Loose body mobilization 1a for the hip, showing hand position for mobilization into medial rotation.

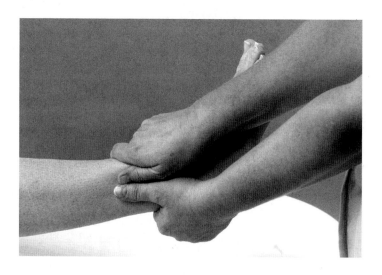

Figure 10.37   Loose body mobilization 1a for the hip, showing body positioning and assistant's counterpressure.

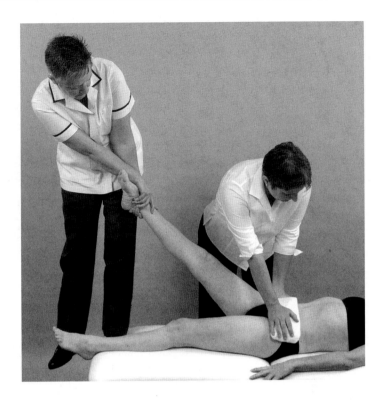

hands are wrapped comfortably around the talus and calcaneum to provide anchorage points and pull the ankle into a degree of dorsiflexion, to prevent undue movement at the ankle joint. The forearm rests against the lateral border of the patient's foot, helping to direct the movement towards medial rotation.

Next, take your distal leg off the couch and lean out to apply traction with your elbows straight (Fig. 10.37). Maintain the traction throughout the rest of the manoeuvre, which is to rotate the patient's leg back and forth towards medial rotation while simultaneously stepping down off the couch, which automatically takes the hip from flexion, towards extension. Re-examine the patient and decide on the next manoeuvre.

Mobilization 1b: with lateral rotation

The manoeuvre is exactly the same as that described above, but in reverse.

Face the movement of lateral rotation and rotate the patient's leg under strong traction, back and forth towards lateral rotation (Figs 10.38 and 10.39).

Figure 10.38   Loose body mobilization 1b for the hip, showing hand position for mobilization into lateral rotation.

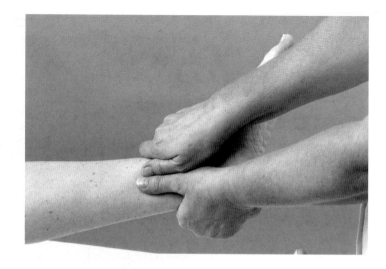

Figure 10.39   Loose body mobilization 1b for the hip, showing body positioning and assistant's counterpressure.

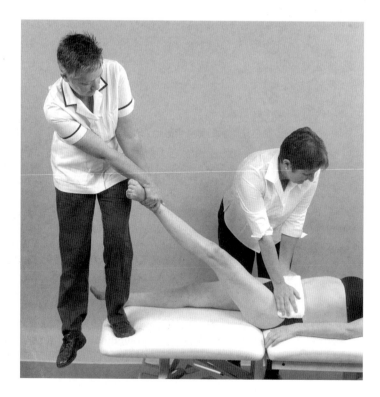

Mobilization 2a: with medial rotation

Loose body mobilization technique 2 (Cyriax & Cyriax 1983, Cyriax 1984)

Position the patient in supine on the couch. An assistant applies counter-pressure to the anterior superior iliac spines. Padding may make it more comfortable for the patient (Fig. 10.40). Alternatively a seat belt can be used to maintain the patient's position on the couch.

Put your caudal foot up on the couch, beside and below the patient's buttock. Flex the patient's knee so that the crook of their knee (popliteal fossa) is placed over your thigh (Fig. 10.41). Take care to avoid pressure on the gastrocnemius muscle as it is uncomfortable.

Place one hand on the lateral aspect of the patient's knee and the other on the medial aspect of the patient's ankle. An assistant comfortably anchors the patient's pelvis on the bed. To apply traction, plantarflex your foot on the couch to lift the patient's leg while simultaneously pushing down on the patient's ankle. Maintain this traction as you rotate the patient's leg smartly towards medial rotation, using the patient's leg as a lever. Re-examine the patient and decide on the next manoeuvre. Alternatively the patient's leg may be rotated smartly to and fro as for mobilization.

Mobilization 2b: with lateral rotation

The manoeuvre is exactly the same as that described above, but reverse the hand positions to enable the patient's leg to be smartly rotated towards lateral rotation (Fig. 10.42). Alternatively the patient's leg may be rotated smartly to and fro as for mobilization.

Figure 10.40 Loose body mobilization 2a for the hip, showing assistant's hand position.

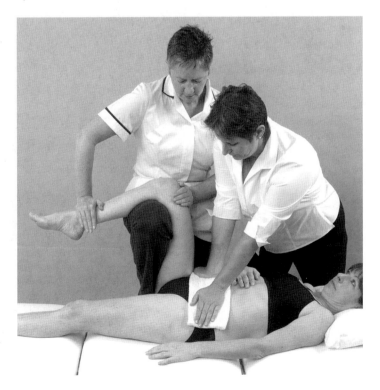

Figure 10.41 Loose body mobilization 2a for the hip, showing application of traction before the thrust into medial rotation.

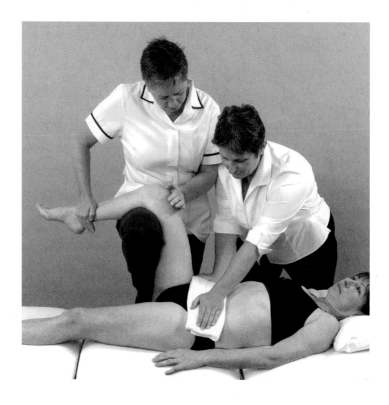

Figure 10.42 Loose body mobilization 2a for the hip, showing application of traction and the thrust into lateral rotation.

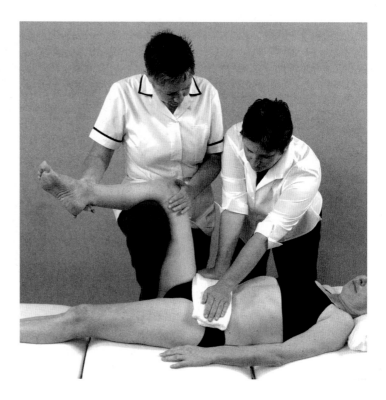

BURSITIS

Psoas, trochanteric or occasionally ischial bursitis may be a cause of pain at the hip, although they are difficult to diagnose definitively and may be overlooked. Both present a muddled clinical picture and may be misdiagnosed as a tendinopathy. However, because of the close anatomical relationship of bursae to tendons, bursitis may coexist with tendinopathy.

The patient commonly presents with a gradual onset of pain, often with no obvious cause. Although it is possible to induce a bursitis by direct trauma, it is usually the result of overuse activity, with the pain increased by activity and better for rest.

On examination, a muddled clinical picture emerges of a non-capsular pattern with some resisted tests and some passive tests reproducing the pain. This may mimic that of tendinopathy. Tendinopathy usually produces a predictable clinical picture of pain on the appropriate resisted test and pain on passive stretching in the opposite direction. In contrast, a bursitis may produce pain when passively squeezed under a contracted muscle or tendon and thus this muddle emerges.

Psoas bursitis

Psoas bursitis commonly produces a local groin pain, but can cause pain to be referred into the L3 dermatome. It has a gradual onset of pain with the patient unable to recall the precipitating factors. It may be associated with overuse or repetitive movements and exacerbated by hip flexion movements, e.g. bending to put on shoes and socks, rising from sitting with hips flexed, walking up stairs or hills, brisk walking, jogging or kicking (Broadhurst 1995b). The pain may produce a shortened gait stride and, through underuse, a secondary capsulitis.

Primary effusion of the bursa is possible, but its communication with the hip joint makes it a reservoir for joint effusion. Therefore psoas bursitis is often associated with hip joint involvement, especially rheumatoid arthritis (Armstrong & Saxton 1972, Meaney et al 1992).

On examination, a non-capsular pattern exists with a combination of passive hip flexion and adduction, squeezing the bursa and producing pain, which may be used as a comparable sign. Other signs could include pain on passive lateral rotation, passive extension and resisted flexion of the hip. However, clinically, resisted flexion is usually found to be painfree (Cyriax 1982).

Some enlarged bursae have been reported to produce a palpable mass in the groin, causing extrinsic pressure on adjacent neurovascular structures (Underwood et al 1988, Toohey et al 1990, Meaney et al 1992). On diagnostic scanning these enlarged bursae have been shown to contain solid components consisting of various debris, e.g. cellular debris, osteocartilaginous plaques, fibrin, clot and calcium deposits (Meaney et al 1992).

Differential diagnosis should exclude other hip joint pathology and lumbar spine involvement, as well as so-called 'Gilmore's groin', a disruption of the external oblique aponeurosis causing dilatation of the superficial inguinal ring, torn conjoined tendon and dehiscence between the inguinal ligament and torn conjoined tendon. Males are more commonly affected. It presents as a gradual onset of groin pain in athletes, particularly footballers. The pain is increased by sporting activity, on getting out of bed, especially the day after a game, and on sudden movement, e.g. sprinting or coughing. On examination there are no physical findings. Diagnosis is made by the examining doctor inverting the scrotum and examining the superficial inguinal ring. On the symptomatic side the ring is dilated and tender and there may be a cough impulse. This condition may require surgical repair (Gilmore 1995).

Treatment for psoas bursitis is a large-volume, low-dose local anaesthetic plus an appropriate amount of corticosteroid.

Injection of the psoas bursa (Cyriax & Cyriax 1983, Cyriax 1984)

Suggested needle size: 20G × 3¹/₂ in (0.9 × 90 mm) spinal needle
Dose: 20 mg triamcinolone acetonide in a total volume of 10 ml

---

Position the patient in supine on the couch. Locate the psoas bursa by palpating for the femoral pulse just distal to the mid-point of the inguinal ligament. This is the surface marking point for the position of the psoas bursa; mark this point. Move approximately 5 cm laterally and 5 cm distally, marking both of these points. If you draw an imaginary line to connect these three points you will form an inverted right-angled triangle (Fig. 10.43). This now gives you the angle of insertion which is to follow the direction of the hypotenuse, aiming to pass deeply, in order to traverse under the neurovascular bundle in the femoral triangle, to reach the deeply located psoas bursa (Fig. 10.44).

Figure 10.43 Surface markings for injection of psoas bursitis.

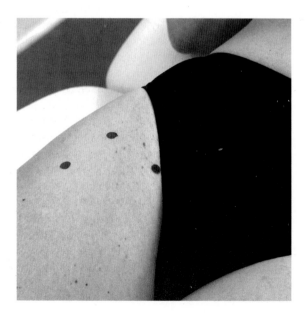

Figure 10.44   Injection of psoas bursitis.

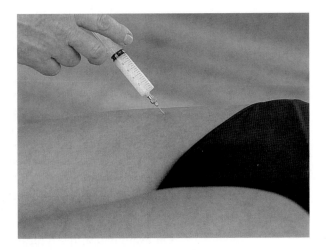

Figure 10.45   Injection of psoas bursitis showing direction of approach and needle position.

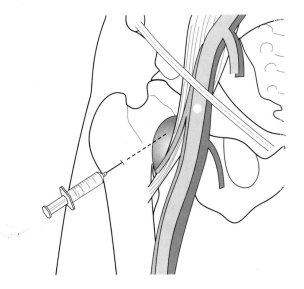

Once the needle tip makes contact with bone it should be located in the region of the hip joint anteriorly. Withdraw it slightly into the overlying psoas bursa and inject at this point (Fig. 10.45). It may be possible to inject as a bolus but, more commonly, a peppering technique is required to cover the extent of this large bursa, fanning out to cover an area approximately the size of a golf ball (Cyriax & Cyriax 1983). The patient is advised to maintain a period of relative rest for approximately 2 weeks following injection.

Trochanteric bursitis

Trochanteric bursitis involves inflammation of the bursae associated with the gluteal muscles and their insertion into the greater trochanter. Although several bursae around the hip region are prone to inflammation, trochanteric bursitis is the most common (Adkins & Figler 2000).

The cause is occasionally traumatic through direct injury, but more commonly due to overuse through occupational or sporting activities. It may be associated with a tight iliotibial band where the bursa may be irritated by direct friction, or secondary to altered biomechanics of gait, leg length discrepancy, low back pain or sacroiliac dysfunction (Haller et al 1989, Collée et al 1991, Norris 1998, Caruso & Toney 1994). It is common in obese, middle-aged women (Rasmussen & Fano 1985, Allwright et al 1988, Gerber & Herrin 1994). It may also be secondary to arthritis of the hip joint and it is not uncommon to find the bursa tender after total hip replacement (Dennison & Beverland 2002).

The pain is usually a diffuse ache or burning pain felt over the lateral aspect of the hip and/or referred down the lateral aspect of the leg.

Aggravating factors are walking, climbing stairs, standing for prolonged periods, crossing the legs in sitting and lying on the affected side.

On examination the typical muddled clinical picture of bursitis may emerge with some or all of the following involved: a non-capsular pattern of pain on passive hip flexion, abduction and lateral rotation as the bursa is squeezed – these movements in combination may be positive (FABER test), passive adduction which may compress the bursa and resisted abduction which may produce the pain as the bursa is compressed by the contraction of adjacent muscles (Little 1979, Cyriax & Cyriax 1983, Dennison & Beverland 2002). Frequently, diagnosis depends on the typical history of presentation and pain referral, an absence of physical signs, and tenderness to palpation of the greater trochanter.

Karpinski & Piggott (1985) suggested a greater trochanteric pain syndrome, to cover all symptoms of pain and tenderness felt at the greater trochanter, in association with pain on resisted abduction.

Palpation will reveal the area of inflammation, typically over the superolateral aspect of the greater trochanter. Care should be taken in palpation, to compare with the unaffected side, as trigger points are commonly found in the buttock, which can be misleading. Differential diagnosis should include iliotibial band syndrome, with which trochanteric bursitis can coexist. Iliotibial band syndrome presents with a similar pattern of lateral hip and/or knee pain, but is painful on provocative testing using Ober's test as follows: with the patient in side lying, the hip neutral and the knee flexed, extend the hip and adduct the femur. Iliotibial band tightness and/or lateral thigh pain will be demonstrated as the knee will extend as the femur is adducted (Adkins & Figler 2000, Brukner & Khan 2002).

Once diagnosis is established, the treatment of choice is an injection of low-dose, large-volume local anaesthetic with an appropriate amount of corticosteroid.

Injection of the trochanteric bursa

Suggested needle size: 21G × 1½ in (0.8 × 40 mm) or 21G × 2 in (0.8 × 50 mm) green needle
Dose: 20 mg triamcinolone acetonide in a total volume of 3–5 ml

Figure 10.46   Injection of the trochanteric bursa.

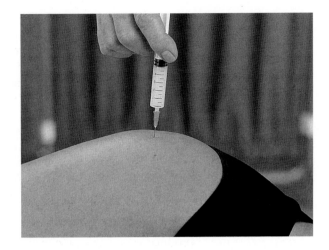

Figure 10.47   Injection of the trochanteric bursa showing direction of approach and needle position.

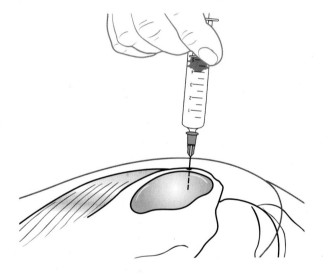

Position the patient comfortably in side lying and palpate for the area of tenderness over the superolateral aspect of the greater trochanter where gluteus maximus inserts into the iliotibial tract (Fig. 10.46). Deliver the injection by a peppering technique, covering the area of tenderness (Fig. 10.47). The patient is advised to maintain a period of relative rest for approximately 2 weeks following injection.

Gluteal bursitis

Injection of the more common trochanteric bursa has been described above, but any of the bursae associated with the gluteal muscles may be affected. The patient presents with a muddle of signs as described above and palpation will indicate the area involved. Once the area of tenderness has been identified it can be injected using a peppering technique following the principles given above.

Ischial bursitis

An ischial bursitis (weaver's bottom) involves the ischial bursa of gluteus maximus. It produces pain on prolonged sitting, especially on hard surfaces; the pain is relieved by standing. Pain may be reproduced near the end of range of the straight leg raise (Broadhurst 1995a). It is a rare cause of buttock pain but the principles of treatment can be applied.

Complicated bursitis

Septic bursitis has been described, more commonly occurring in the olecranon and prepatellar bursae, where *Staphylococcus aureus* was usually the infective organism (Hoppmann 1993, Zimmermann et al 1995). A case of tuberculosis of the trochanteric bursa has also been described (Rehm-Graves et al 1983). It has also been reported as a cause of hip pain associated with rheumatoid arthritis (Raman & Haslock 1982). Pain referred from the lumbar spine and sacroiliac joint may produce a similar pattern of signs and symptoms and has been described by Traycoff (1991) as pseudotrochanteric bursitis. Occasionally bursitis may be complicated by calcification, making it resistant to normal conservative management (Gerber & Herrin 1994).

SIGN OF THE BUTTOCK

The sign of the buttock is pain produced on straight leg raise which increases on flexing the knee and hip (Cyriax & Cyriax 1983). An empty end-feel is appreciated as more range of movement is available, but any attempt to produce more hip flexion is abruptly stopped by voluntary muscle spasm and the patient puts out the hand to stop the movement.

A positive sign indicates a major lesion in the buttock or hip region. The history will usually reveal an unwell patient, who looks ill and may have a fever with night sweats and rigors. The pain may be unrelenting in the buttock, hip or leg. It is not eased by rest and therefore night pain is a feature.

On examination, a non-capsular pattern of movement at the hip, and often the lumbar spine, is discovered. Pain may be increased by lumbar flexion and resisted tests at the hip, but the cardinal feature of this condition is the positive sign of the buttock.

Possible causes of the sign of the buttock are neoplasm of the upper femur or ilium, fracture of the sacrum, ischiorectal abscess, sepsis, either septic bursitis or arthritis, or osteomyelitis of the upper femur (Cyriax & Cyriax 1983). Urgent medical attention and further investigation are required.

CONTRACTILE LESIONS

The mode of onset of contractile lesions around the hip may be sudden through strain, gradual through overuse or traumatic through direct injury, causing muscle contusion. Lesions commonly affect the hamstrings, quadriceps and adductor longus muscles. Less common lesions of the psoas and sartorius are not described, although the principles of diagnosis and treatment would equally apply to any muscle lesion in the region.

HAMSTRINGS

The hamstrings act to extend the hip and flex the knee and commonly present as strained, perhaps due to their relative weakness in comparison to the quadriceps (Sutton 1984). As two-joint muscles, they are susceptible to injury, because there is a greater potential for overuse.

The onset is usually sudden, e.g. a sudden stretch or a rapid contraction against resistance such as the ballistic action of sprinting which produces acute pain, further increased by activity, swelling and bruising. Precipitating factors include altered posture, poor condition, inadequate warm-up and fatigue (Sutton 1984, Worrell 1994). The patient may report tightness or pain in the posterior thigh some time before the acute onset. Gradual onset due to overuse is possible, but chronic hamstring strain is more commonly the result of a previous acute episode which may have healed during a period of relative immobilization. Consequent tightness or shortening of the muscle belly makes it vulnerable.

On examination the patient has pain on resisted knee flexion and pain on passive straight leg raising. In most clinic situations, testing for hamstring strain is conducted statically in a non-weight-bearing position. In reality the hamstrings function, and are most often injured, in dynamic weight-bearing situations. This is an important point to remember for full rehabilitation of any muscle lesion in the region.

Palpation reveals the site of the lesion, with muscle belly strains commonly occurring deeply in the mid-thigh region. Chronic overuse strain occurs at the origin from the ischial tuberosity. Treatment of the origin may be by deep transverse frictions or injection.

Figure 10.48 Palpation of ischial tuberosity prior to application of transverse frictions.

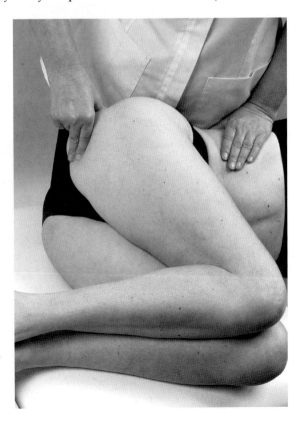

Transverse frictions to the origin of the hamstrings

Position the patient into side lying on the unaffected side with the hips and knees flexed to 90° to expose the ischial tuberosity from under the lower border of gluteus maximus (Fig. 10.48). Frictions can then be applied transversely across the fibres using the fingers of one hand reinforced with the other hand to maintain pressure back against the origin, and rocking body weight downwards and upwards through straight arms. Start gently, then apply deep transverse frictions for 10 min after the analgesic effect is achieved. Relative rest is advised where functional movements may continue, but no overuse or stretching until the muscle is pain-free on resisted testing.

An alternative position involves positioning the patient in prone lying with the knee supported over the edge of the bed on a stool to place the hip and knee into flexion and to expose the ischial tuberosity (Fig. 10.49). Apply transverse frictions by using one thumb reinforced with the other, directed firstly up against the ischial tuberosity and then transversely across the fibres.

Figure 10.49   Transverse frictions to the origin of the hamstrings, alternative position.

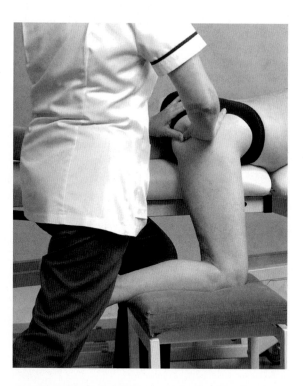

Injection of the origin of the hamstrings

Suggested needle size: 23G × 1 in (0.6 × 25 mm) blue needle (or as appropriate for the patient)
Dose: 20 mg triamcinolone acetonide in a total volume of 1.5 ml

Use either position adopted for transverse frictions of the hamstrings' origin. Locate the area of tenderness over the ischial tuberosity and insert the needle perpendicular to it (Fig. 10.50). Deliver the injection by a peppering technique into the teno-osseous junction (Fig. 10.51). The patient is advised to maintain a period of relative rest for approximately 2 weeks following injection.

Figure 10.50   Injection of the origin of the hamstrings.

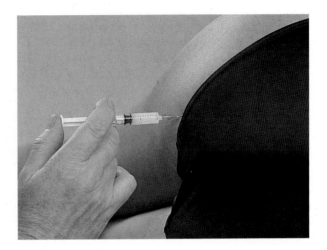

Figure 10.51   Injection of the origin of the hamstrings showing direction of approach and needle position.

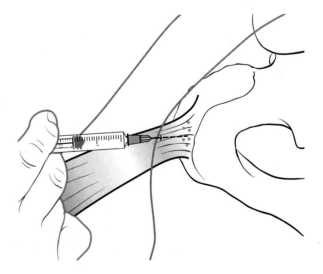

Transverse frictions for acute muscle belly

In the first 3–5 days following injury (depending upon the irritability of the lesion), protection, rest, ice, compression and elevation are used to control the early inflammatory phase. Treatment is conducted on a daily

Figure 10.52   Transverse frictions to the hamstring muscle bellies.

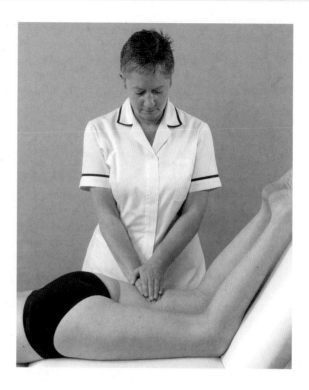

basis and transverse frictions applied gently to maintain the muscle belly function. Position the patient in prone lying with the knee flexed, to place the muscle belly in the shortened position; this allows the muscle fibres to be moved transversely by the frictions (Fig. 10.52). Apply the transverse frictions gently and, once some analgesia has been achieved, apply approximately six deeper sweeps. Follow this immediately with Grade A mobilization, encouraging an active muscle contraction within the pain-free range to broaden the fibres. Teach the patient to use a normal heel–toe gait, with the aid of crutches if necessary.

After approximately 5 days (again, depending upon irritability) the depth of transverse frictions and Grade A mobilizations can be increased until a full range of pain-free movement is achieved. Treating an acute muscle belly lesion in this way should avoid shortening of the muscle fibres and the need to apply stretching techniques.

Transverse frictions for chronic muscle belly

Apply the transverse frictions with the muscle belly in a relaxed position and once the analgesic effect is achieved, apply deeper transverse frictions for 10 min (Fig. 10.52 and 10.53). Follow this with vigorous Grade A exercises to maintain the mobility gained.

It is important that the hamstrings are not undertreated and, to prevent recurrence of symptoms, transverse frictions should be continued for approximately 1 week after cessation of symptoms. If the muscle is tight, traditional stretches can be applied once the resisted tests are pain-free.

Figure 10.53 Transverse frictions to the hamstring muscle bellies, alternative technique (chronic).

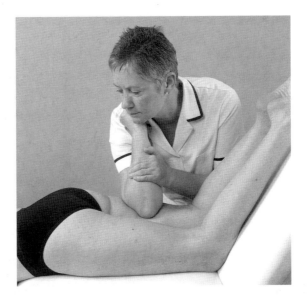

Rehabilitation following hamstring lesions

In either the acute or the chronic situation, once the hamstrings have been rendered pain-free by transverse frictions and Grade A mobilizations, a full rehabilitation programme can be implemented, including stretching to lengthen the muscle if appropriate. Attention should be paid to the dynamic rather than the static function of the hamstrings. Weight-bearing activities and rehabilitation under speed are important considerations (Coole & Gieck 1987).

QUADRICEPS

The mechanism of injury of the quadriceps is similar to that of the hamstrings and the principles of treatment and rehabilitation can be applied in much the same way. The patient presents with anterior thigh pain, pain on resisted knee extension and pain on resisted hip flexion (if rectus femoris is involved). As a two-joint muscle, rectus femoris is the most susceptible to injury. Palpation reveals the site of the lesion, which may be within the tendon of rectus femoris from the anterior inferior iliac spine, or in the belly of the muscle, usually mid-thigh (see Ch. 11).

Transverse frictions to the origin of rectus femoris (Cyriax & Cyriax 1983, Cyriax 1984)

Position the patient in half lying to allow the hip flexors to relax. Locate the origin of rectus femoris and apply two fingers to the tendon (Fig. 10.54). Push down onto the tendon and apply transverse frictions across the fibres. Since the lesion is usually chronic, 10 min transverse frictions are applied after the analgesic effect is achieved. Relative rest is advised where functional movements may continue, but no overuse or stretching until the muscle is pain-free on resisted testing.

Figure 10.54 Transverse frictions to the origin of rectus femoris.

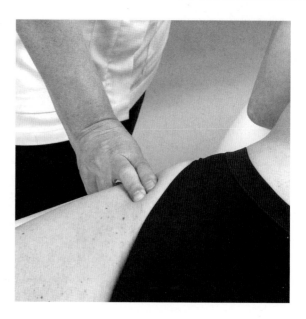

ADDUCTOR LONGUS

Adductor longus is the most common adductor muscle to be strained at the hip. It is sometimes known as a 'rider's strain' due to overuse of adductor longus in working a horse while riding.

The patient has groin or medial thigh pain, with pain on resisted adduction and passive abduction. The lesion is in one of two sites: either the origin from the pubis or the musculotendinous junction. Treatment of the origin is by either transverse frictions or injection. The musculotendinous junction usually responds well to transverse frictions and injection is not usually necessary.

Transverse frictions to adductor longus

Teno-osseous site

Position the patient in supine with the leg in a degree of abduction and lateral rotation, supported on a pillow. With an index finger reinforced by the middle finger, locate the area of tenderness at the teno-osseous junction (Fig. 10.55). Apply the frictions firstly in a direction down onto the bone, then transversely across the fibres, for 10 min after gaining analgesia. This may be an embarrassing treatment for the patient and it may be more appropriate to teach patients to do the transverse frictions themselves.

Musculotendinous site

Position the patient as above and locate the area of tenderness at the musculotendinous junction. The transverse frictions may be imparted by a pinching manoeuvre (Fig. 10.56) (Cyriax & Cyriax 1983, Cyriax 1984), or by pressure directed firstly down against the tendon and then transversely across the fibres (Fig. 10.57). Apply the transverse frictions for 10 min after gaining analgesia.

Relative rest is advised where functional movements may continue, but no overuse or stretching until the muscle is pain-free on resisted testing.

Figure 10.55   Transverse frictions to the origin of adductor longus.

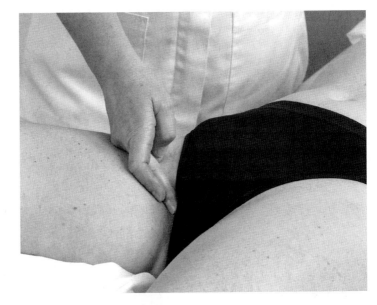

Figure 10.56   Transverse frictions to adductor longus, musculotendinous site.

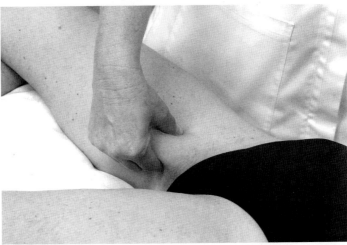

Figure 10.57   Transverse frictions to adductor longus, musculotendinous site, alternative hand position.

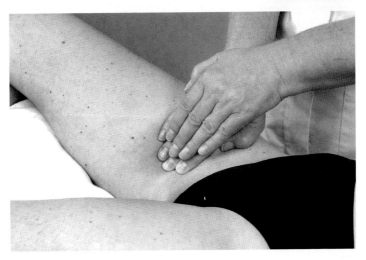

Injection of the origin of adductor longus (Cyriax & Cyriax 1983)

Suggested needle size: 23G × 1¹/₄ in (0.6 × 30 mm) blue needle
(depending on size of the patient)
Dose: 20 mg triamcinolone acetonide in a total volume of 1.5 ml

Position the patient as for the transverse frictions. Insert the needle into the origin of adductor longus, which is situated in the angle between the symphysis and the obturator crest (Fig. 10.58). Once in the tenoosseous junction and in contact with bone, deliver the injection by the peppering technique (Fig. 10.59). The patient is advised to maintain a period of relative rest for approximately 2 weeks following injection.

Figure 10.58 Injection of the origin of adductor longus.

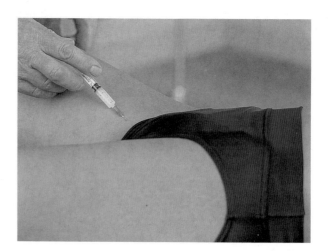

Figure 10.59 Injection of the origin of adductor longus showing direction of approach and needle position.

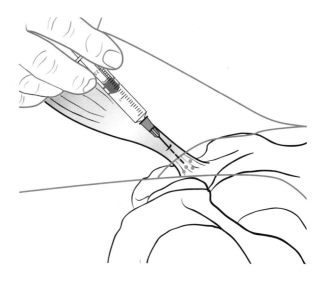

References

Adkins S B, Figler R A 2000 Hip pain in athletes. American Family Physician 61(7):2109–2118

Allwright S J, Cooper R A, Nash P 1988 Trochanteric bursitis: bone scan appearance. Clinical Nuclear Medicine 13:561–564

Armstrong P, Saxton H 1972 Ilio-psoas bursa. British Journal of Rheumatology 45:493–495

Broadhurst N 1995a Ischial bursitis. Australian Family Physician 24:1121

Broadhurst N 1995b Iliopsoas tendinopathy and bursitis. Australian Family Physician 24:1303

Brukner P, Khan K 2002 Clinical sports medicine, 2nd edn. McGraw Hill, Sydney

Cailliet R 1990 Soft tissue pain and disability, 2nd edn. F A Davis, Philadelphia

Cameron G 1995 Steroid arthropathy – myth or reality? Journal of Orthopaedic Medicine 17:51–55

Canoso J J 1981 Bursae, tendons and ligaments. Clinics in Rheumatic Diseases 7:189–221

Caruso F A, Toney M A O 1994 Trochanteric bursitis – a case report of plain film, scintigraphic and MRI correlation. Clinical Nuclear Medicine 19:393–395

Collée G, Dijkmans B A C, Vandenbroucke J P et al 1991 Greater trochanteric pain syndrome trochanteric bursitis in low back pain. Scandinavian Journal of Rheumatology 20:262–266

Coole W, Gieck J H 1987 An analysis of hamstring strains and their rehabilitation. Journal of Orthopaedic and Sports Physical Therapy 9:77–85

Cyriax J 1982 Textbook of orthopaedic medicine, 8th edn. Baillière Tindall, London, vol 1

Cyriax J 1984 Textbook of orthopaedic medicine, 11th edn. Baillière Tindall, London, vol 2

Cyriax J, Cyriax P 1983 Illustrated manual of orthopaedic medicine. Butterworths, London

Dennison J, Beverland D E 2002 An audit of trochanteric bursitis in total hip arthroplasty and recommendations for treatment. Journal of Orthopaedic Nursing 6(1):5–8

Dieppe P 1995 Management of hip osteoarthritis. British Medical Journal 311:853–857

Emms N W, O'Connor M, Montgomery S C 2002 Hip pain can masquerade as knee pain in adults. Age and Ageing 31:67–69

Flanagan F L, Sant S, Coughlan R J et al 1995 Symptomatic enlarged iliopsoas bursae in the presence of a normal plain hip radiograph. British Society for Rheumatology 34:365–369

Fu Z, Peng M, Peng Q 1997 Anatomical study of the synovial plicae of the hip joint. Clinical Anatomy 10(1):235–238

Gerber J M, Herrin S O 1994 Conservative management of calcific trochanteric bursitis. Journal of Manipulative and Physiological Therapeutics 17:250–252

Gilmore O J A 1995 Gilmore's groin. Physiotherapy in Sport 18:14–15

Haller C C, Coleman P A, Estes N C et al 1989 Traumatic trochanteric bursitis. Kansas Medicine 90:17–22

Hartley A 1995 Practical joint assessment – lower quadrant, 2nd edn. Mosby, London

Hickman J M, Peters C L 2001 Hip pain in the young adult. American Journal of Orthopaedics 30(6):459–467

Hoppmann R A 1993 Diagnosis and management of common tendinopathy and bursitis syndromes. Journal of South Carolina Medical Association 89:531–535

Kapandji I A 1987 The physiology of the joints: lower limb, 5th edn. Churchill Livingstone, Edinburgh, vol 2

Karpinski M R K, Piggott H 1985 Greater trochanteric pain syndrome. Journal of Bone and Joint Surgery 67B:762–763

Kersnič B, Iglič A, Kralj-Iglič V et al 1997 Increased incidence of arthrosis in women could be related to femoral and pelvic shape. Archives of Orthopaedic and Trauma Surgery 116(6–7):345–347

Kesson M, Atkins E, Davies I 2003 Musculoskeletal injection skills. Butterworth Heinemann, Oxford

Klaber Moffett J A, Richardson P H, Frost H et al 1996 A placebo controlled double blind trial to evaluate the effectiveness of pulsed short wave therapy for osteoarthritic hip and knee pain. Pain 71(2):121–127

Kumar P, Clark M 2002 Clinical medicine, 5th edn. Baillière Tindall, London

Leopold S S, Battista V, Oliverio J A 2001 Safety and efficacy of intra-articular hip injection using anatomic landmarks. Clinical Orthopaedics and Related Research 391:192–197

Little H 1979 Trochanteric bursitis: a common cause of pelvic girdle pain. Canadian Medical Association Journal 120:456–458

McGory B J, Endrizzi D P 2000 Adhesive capsulitis of the hip after bilateral adhesive capsulitis of the shoulder. American Journal of Orthopaedics 29(6):457–460

McIndoe A K, Young K, Bone M E 1995 A comparison of acupuncture with intra-articular steroid injection as analgesia for osteoarthritis of the hip. Acupuncture in Medicine 13:67–70

Meaney J F, Cassar-Pullicino V N, Ethrington R et al 1992 Ilio-psoas bursa enlargement. Clinical Radiology 45:161–168

Norris C M 1998 Sports injuries: diagnosis and management for physiotherapists, 2nd edn. Butterworth Heinemann, Oxford

O'Kane J W 1999 Anterior hip pain. American Family Physician 60(6):1687–1696

Paice E 1995 Pain in the hip and knee. British Medical Journal 310:319–322

Raman D, Haslock I 1982 Trochanteric bursitis – a frequent cause of 'hip' pain in rheumatoid arthritis. Annals of the Rheumatic Diseases 41:602–603

Rang H P, Dale M M, Ritter J M et al 2003 Pharmacology, 5th edn. Churchill Livingstone, Edinburgh

Rasmussen K-J E, Fano N 1985 Trochanteric bursitis: treatment by corticosteroid injection. Scandinavian Journal of Rheumatology 14:417–420

Raynauld J-P, Buckland-Wright C, Ward R et al 2003 Safety and efficacy of long-term intraarticular steroid injection in osteoarthritis of the knee. Arthritis and Rheumatism 48(2):370–377

Rehm-Graves S, Weinstein A J, Calabrese L H et al 1983 Tuberculosis of the greater trochanter bursa. Arthritis and Rheumatism 26:77–81

Sims K 1999 The development of hip osteoarthritis: implications for conservative management. Manual Therapy 4(3):127–135

Sutton G 1984 Hamstrung by hamstring strains: a review of the literature. Journal of Orthopaedics and Sports Physical Therapy 5:184–195

Toohey A K, LaSalle T L, Martinez S et al 1990 Iliopsoas bursitis: clinical features, radiographic findings, and disease associations. Seminars in Arthritis and Rheumatism 20:41–47

Traycoff R B 1991 'Pseudotrochanteric bursitis': the differential diagnosis of lateral hip pain. Journal of Rheumatology 18:1810–1812

Underwood P L, McLeod R A, Ginsburg W W 1988 The varied clinical manifestations of iliopsoas bursitis. Journal of Rheumatology 15:1683–1685

Williams P L 1998 Gray's Anatomy: the anatomical basis of medicine and surgery, 38th edn. Churchill Livingstone, Edinburgh

Worrell T W 1994 Factors associated with hamstring injuries – an approach to treatment and preventative measures. Sports Medicine 17:338–345

Zimmermann B, Mikolich D J, Ho G 1995 Septic bursitis. Seminars in Arthritis and Rheumatism 24:391–410

Chapter **11**

The knee

SUMMARY

Knee injuries are largely in the province of sport. Developments in arthroscopic techniques have done much to facilitate diagnosis and repair. Initial diagnosis is crucial to appropriate management, particularly of the ligamentous and contractile lesions.

This chapter presents the anatomy of the knee relating to commonly encountered lesions. The commentary which follows explores the relevant points of history, aiding diagnosis, and the suggested method of objective examination adheres to the principles of selective tension. The lesions, their treatment and management are then discussed.

ANATOMY

INERT STRUCTURES

The lower end of the femur consists of two large femoral condyles which articulate with, and transfer weight to, corresponding surfaces on the tibial condyles at the tibiofemoral joint. The two femoral condyles are separated posteriorly and inferiorly by the intercondylar notch or fossa. The anterior aspect of the femur bears an articular surface for the patella to form the patellofemoral joint.

The lateral femoral epicondyle gives attachment to the proximal end of the *lateral (fibular) collateral ligament*. Below this lies a smooth groove which contains the tendon of popliteus in full flexion of the knee. The medial femoral condyle displays a prominent *adductor tubercle* on the medial supracondylar line and just below this the medial epicondyle gives origin to the *medial (tibial) collateral ligament*. Posteriorly, the heads of gastrocnemius originate from the femoral condyles.

The tibia has an expanded upper end which overhangs the shaft posteriorly. The upper weight-bearing surface bears two shallow tibial condyles divided by the intercondylar area. Below the posterolateral tibial condyle lies an oval facet for articulation with the head of the fibula at the *superior (proximal) tibiofibular joint*. Anteriorly lies the prominent *tibial tuberosity* which gives insertion to the infrapatellar tendon (ligamentum patellae). *Gerdy's tubercle* lies anterolaterally and marks the insertion of the iliotibial tract (Kapandji 1987, Burks 1990).

The upper end of the fibula is expanded to form the head, which articulates with the tibia on its superomedial side, at the superior tibiofibular joint. The apex of the head of the fibula gives attachment to the lateral collateral ligament and the biceps femoris tendon. The common peroneal nerve winds round the neck of the fibula.

From Here →

The *patella*, the largest sesamoid bone in the body, lies within the quadriceps tendon and articulates with the lower end of the femur at the *patellofemoral joint*. It is a flat triangular-shaped bone with its base uppermost and apex pointing inferiorly. It has anterior and posterior surfaces and upper, medial and lateral borders. Its anterior surface shows vertical ridges produced by fibres of the quadriceps which pass over it. This surface is separated from the skin by a synovial-lined potential space, the subcutaneous *prepatellar bursa*. It contains minimal fluid and is only obvious when inflamed (Pope & Winston-Salem 1996).

Rectus femoris and vastus intermedius insert into the base of the patella, and the roughened posterior aspect of the apex gives attachment to the proximal end of the *infrapatellar tendon (ligamentum patellae)*. A subcutaneous *superficial infrapatellar bursa* lies between the infrapatellar tendon and the skin; a *deep infrapatellar bursa* lies deep to the distal portion of the infrapatellar tendon and the underlying tibia and has no communication with the knee joint (LaPrade 1998). It is located by palpation on the lateral side of the infrapatellar tendon in extension, just proximal to the tibial tubercle; a point of access for injection (LaPrade 1998). Several fat pads are interposed between the knee joint capsule and synovial lining. The *infrapatellar fat pad of Hoffa* lies between the infrapatellar tendon and the knee joint and may be subjected to trauma or impingement (Jacobson et al 1997).

The vastus medialis and lateralis muscles send tendinous insertions to the medial and lateral borders of the patella in the form of *quadriceps expansions* (or the *patella retinacula*). The lateral expansion receives a distinct extension from the iliotibial tract and the quadriceps expansions together are responsible for transverse stability of the patella. The medial quadriceps expansion blends with the anterior fibres of the medial collateral ligament.

to Here →

The posterior articulating surface of the patella is covered with thick articular cartilage which is divided by a vertical ridge into medial and lateral articular facets for articulation with the femur, with an 'odd' facet on the medial side.

The knee joint consists of the tibiofemoral, patellofemoral and superior tibiofibular joints. The former two articulations exist within the same capsule but each has a different function:

- *Tibiofemoral joint*: involved in weight-bearing activities
- *Patellofemoral joint*: the joint of the extensor mechanism of the knee

The *tibiofemoral joint* is a synovial hinge joint between the convex condyles of the femur and the slightly concave articular surfaces of the tibia. Mobility is not normally compatible with stability in a joint, but the incongruent joint surfaces of the knee make it a mobile joint, while the shape of the articular surfaces and the interaction of muscles, tendons and strong ligaments all contribute to stability.

Two semilunar cartilages, the *menisci*, deepen the tibial articulating surface and contribute to the congruency of the joint. The menisci facilitate load transmission, shock absorption, lubrication and stability (Bessette 1992). The peripheral rim of each meniscus is attached to deep fibres of the capsule which secure it to the edge of the tibial condyles. These deep capsular fibres are known as the *coronary ligaments* (*corona*, Latin = around) or meniscotibial ligaments. They are strong, but lax enough to allow axial rotation to occur at the meniscotibial surface. The lateral coronary ligaments are longer than the medial to allow for the greater excursion of the lateral meniscus (Burks 1990).

The menisci are composed of collagen fibres. The superficial collagen fibres are oriented radially and the deep fibres are circumferential (Bessette 1992). The orientation of the collagen fibres facilitates dispersion of compressive loads by the circumferential fibres and resistance to longitudinal stresses by the radial fibres; the fibre orientation at the surface of the meniscus is a random meshwork thought to be important for distributing shear stress (Greis et al 2002). Injury usually involves rotational strains and may result in longitudinal or transverse splitting of the fibrocartilage, or separation of the thinner inner part of the meniscus from the thicker outer portion, forming a 'bucket handle' lesion.

The *medial meniscus* is the larger of the two and is almost semicircular in shape. Its periphery has a definite attachment to the deep part of the medial collateral ligament, which forms part of the fibrous capsule of the knee joint. The *lateral meniscus* is almost circular but it is separated from the capsule of the knee joint at its periphery by the tendon of popliteus, from which it receives an attachment. Posteriorly, the lateral meniscus contributes a ligamentous slip to the posterior cruciate ligament, known as the *posterior meniscofemoral ligament*.

The fibrous capsule of the knee joint is strongly supplemented by expansions from the tendons that cross it, plus ligamentous thickenings and independent ligamentous reinforcements. The medial collateral ligament, in particular, provides a strong integral reinforcement of the capsule, attaching also to the medial meniscus. The anterior capsule is reinforced by the quadriceps expansions and an extension from the iliotibial band. Independent ligaments such as the lateral collateral ligament and cruciates also have a strong stabilizing effect on the joint.

The cylindrical *fibrous capsule* is invaginated posteriorly and lined with synovial membrane. The synovium is reflected upwards anteriorly under the quadriceps, approximately three fingers' breadth, to form the *suprapatellar bursa*. The articularis genu muscle connects vastus intermedius and the upper part of the suprapatellar bursa, maintaining the bursal cavity during extension of the knee. *Plicae* (folds of synovium that protrude inwards) exist in the knee joint and may be responsible for symptoms. Three are usually recognized: the superior plica, thought to be an embryological remnant of the division between the suprapatellar bursa and the joint; the inferior plica, located in the intercondylar notch anterior to the anterior cruciate ligament; and a medial plica, a vertical fold, varying from a small ridge to a cord-like structure adjacent to the medial border of the patella (Boles & Martin 2001).

Numerous bursae are associated with the knee, facilitating the function of the tendons which are running more or less parallel to the bones, to exert a lengthwise pull across the joint (Palastanga et al 2002). Posteriorly, a bursa sits under each head of origin of gastrocnemius. Laterally, bursae lie either side of the lateral collateral ligament, cushioning it from biceps femoris and popliteus, as well as between popliteus and the lateral femoral condyle. Medially, the *pes anserine bursa* sits between the distal medial collateral ligament and the tendons of sartorius, gracilis and semitendinosus, known collectively as the pes anserinus. The semimembranosus bursa lies between the tendon of semimembranosus and the medial tibial condyle of the tibia and a variable number of small bursae lie deep to the medial collateral ligament.

The ligaments of the knee provide a dynamic guide during movement and act as a passive restraint to abnormal translations (Barrack & Skinner 1990). Each ligament is orientated in a direction to produce stability, and force is dissipated at the insertion by a gradual transition from ligament, to fibrocartilage, to bone (Woo et al 1990).

The *medial collateral ligament* is a strong, broad, flat band lying posteriorly over the medial joint line. The posteromedial position of the medial collateral ligament means that its anterior border may be palpated running perpendicular to and approximately halfway along the medial joint line, the ligament itself lying roughly two and a half fingers' width behind this point. Passing from the medial femoral epicondyle just distal to the adductor tubercle, it descends vertically across the joint line and runs forwards to its attachment on the medial condyle and shaft of the upper tibia approximately 5 cm below the joint line, posterior to the pes anserinus insertion. As the ligament crosses over the knee joint its anterior fibres blend with fibres of the medial patellar retinaculum (El-Dieb et al 2002). It is the primary static stabilizer of the medial aspect of the knee joint and is assisted by the quadriceps expansions and the tendons of sartorius, gracilis and semitendinosus, which cross over its lower part, and from which it is separated by the pes anserine bursa.

The medial collateral ligament is composed of superficial and deep layers. The superficial part of the ligament, often referred to as the tibial collateral ligament, consists of fibres which pass directly from the femur to the tibia (Staron et al 1994, Schweitzer et al 1995). These fibres are relatively strong and provide 80% of the resistance to valgus force (Schenck & Heckman 1993). Under the superficial medial collateral ligament the capsule is thickened to form the deep medial collateral ligament which is firmly anchored to the medial meniscus (Pope & Winston-Salem 1996). This part of the ligament is relatively weaker. The capsule is further thickened by superior fibres, the meniscofemoral ligaments, which attach the meniscus to the femur, and inferior fibres, the meniscotibial ligaments, more commonly known as the coronary ligaments, which attach the meniscus to the tibia (Burks 1990, Staron et al 1994).

The primary stabilizing role of the medial collateral ligament is to support the medial aspect of the knee joint preventing excessive valgus movement. Its secondary stabilizing role is in preventing lateral rotation of the tibia, anterior translation of the tibia on the femur and hyperextension of the knee. Most of the ligament is taut in full extension preventing hyperextension, but it also remains taut throughout flexion (Pope & Winston-Salem 1996). Mechanisms of injury commonly include a rotation stress to the knee and the ligament is often injured together with the anterior cruciate ligament and medial meniscus. Valgus injuries occur through direct impact to the lateral aspect of the knee.

The *lateral collateral ligament* in isolation is a shorter, cord-like ligament separated from the capsule of the knee joint by the tendon of popliteus. It is approximately 5 cm long and roughly the size of half a pencil (Evans 1986, Palastanga et al 2002). It runs from the lateral femoral epicondyle to the head of the fibula where it blends with the insertion of biceps femoris to form a conjoined tendon which is an important lateral stabilizer. However, the lateral collateral ligament may be more complex than that. Anatomically it is closely related to the underlying *iliotibial band* which is similar in width and direction to the medial collateral ligament and may indeed provide dynamic stability to the lateral aspect of the knee joint. Posteriorly the lateral collateral ligament has a relationship with the arcuate popliteal ligament and the popliteus tendon (Pope & Winston-Salem 1996). Its primary stabilizing role is to restrain varus movement, supporting the lateral aspect of the knee (Burks 1990), with a secondary stabilizing role in controlling posterior drawer and lateral rotation of the tibia. Injuries to the lateral collateral ligament complex are not as common as those to the medial aspect, but if they do occur, they are more disabling and difficult to diagnose. Mechanisms of injury include a varus force applied to the knee in flexion and/or medial rotation, an unusual position for the knee accounting for the relative rarity of this injury (El-Dieb et al 2002).

The *oblique popliteal ligament* is an extension of semimembranosus which partially blends with and strengthens the posterior capsule. The *arcuate popliteal ligament* is a Y-shaped thickening of the posterolateral capsule passing from the head of the fibula to arch over the tendon of popliteus.

The *cruciate ligaments* are strong intracapsular, but extrasynovial, ligaments said to be about as thick as a pencil (Evans 1986). They are called cruciate (*crus*, Latin = cross) because of the way they cross in the intercondylar fossa and are named anterior or posterior by their tibial attachments. Their primary stabilizing role is to resist anterior and posterior translation of the tibia under the femur. Their secondary stabilizing function is to act as internal collateral ligaments controlling varus, valgus and rotation (Schenck & Heckman 1993).

The *anterior cruciate ligament* passes from the anterior tibial intercondylar area upwards, posteriorly and laterally, twisting as it goes, to attach to the posteromedial aspect of the lateral femoral condyle. Anatomically it can be divided into two parts: an anteromedial band which is taut in flexion and a posterolateral band which is taut in extension. Functionally, the ligament has a stabilizing effect throughout the range of movement (Katz & Fingeroth 1986, Perko et al 1992). Its primary stabilizing role resists anterior translation and medial rotation of the tibia on the femur. A secondary stabilizing role relates it to the collateral ligaments in resisting valgus, varus and hyperextension stresses (Evans 1986). A study by Butler et al (1980) showed the anterior cruciate ligament to provide 86% of the total resisting force to anterior translation, with other ligaments and capsular structures making up the remaining secondary restraint (Katz & Fingeroth 1986). The most common mechanism of injury to the anterior cruciate ligament is lateral rotation combined with a valgus force applied to the fixed tibia. Less common mechanisms may include hyperextension, medial rotation in full extension or anterior translation produced by direct injury to the calf. Most tears occur within the ligament itself, with 20% involving either bony attachment (El-Dieb et al 2002).

The *posterior cruciate ligament* passes upwards, anteriorly and medially from the posterior intercondylar area to attach to the anterolateral aspect of the medial femoral condyle. The ligament is said to be twice as strong and less oblique than the anterior cruciate ligament and its close relationship to the centre of rotation of the knee joint makes it a principal stabilizer (Palastanga et al 2002). As well as controlling posterior translation of the tibia on the femur, it seems to have a role in producing and restraining rotation of the tibia, since posterior translation occurs with concomitant lateral rotation of the tibia. Injury to the posterior cruciate ligament is not as common as to its anterior partner. Forced posterior translation of the tibia on the flexed knee, the typical 'dashboard' injury, is the most common mechanism of injury, but it may also be injured in forced hyperextension (El-Dieb et al 2002).

The main function of the knee joint is weight-bearing; therefore symptoms are usually produced on weight-bearing activities. During the gait cycle, the forces across the tibiofemoral joint amount to two to five times body weight according to position and activity. However, the forces may increase to 24 times body weight during activities such as jumping (Palastanga et al 2002).

The range of movement at the knee joint is greatest in the sagittal plane with an active range from 0° extension to 140° of flexion. Approximately 5–10° of passive extension is usually available and up to 160° of passive flexion, which is halted when the calf and hamstring muscles approximate and the heel reaches the buttock. During flexion and extension, the menisci stay with the tibia so that these movements occur between the femoral condyles rolling and sliding over the menisci.

Active and passive axial rotation occur with the knee joint in flexion and the range available is greatest at 90° of flexion. Active lateral rotation amounts to approximately 45° and medial rotation of 35°, with a little more movement in each direction available passively. During axial rotation, the menisci now stay with the femur and rotation occurs between the femoral condyles and the menisci rolling and gliding over the tibial condyles. The coronary ligaments are lax enough to permit this movement.

A few degrees of automatic, involuntary rotation occurs to achieve the locked or unlocked positions of the knee. During the last 20° or so of knee extension, lateral rotation of the tibia on the femur occurs to produce the terminal 'screw-home' or 'locking' phase of the knee. This achieves the close packed position of the knee joint, where it is most stable, and rotation and accessory movements are impossible to perform on the normal extended knee. The knee is unlocked by the action of popliteus medially rotating the tibia on the femur.

The locking mechanism of the knee occurs because the medial femoral condyle is slightly longer than the lateral and the shape of the tibial condyles allows the lateral femoral condyle to glide more freely and over a greater distance than the medial. The ligaments around the knee contribute to stability in extension when most fibres are under tension.

Helfet's test (Nordin & Frankel 2001) ensures that the locking mechanism of the knee is intact. The test is performed as follows:

Position the patient in high sitting and mark the middle of the patella. Assess the position of the tibial tuberosity in respect to this midline mark and it should lie just medial to it. Extend the knee and repeat the observations. The tibial tuberosity should now lie just lateral to the midline mark, confirming that lateral rotation of the tibia has occurred.

The *patellofemoral joint* is the joint between the posterior aspect of the patella and the anterior surface of the femur. It is the joint of the extensor mechanism of the knee and therefore gives rise to symptoms on antigravity activities. The patella performs two important biomechanical functions at the knee (Nordin & Frankel 2001):

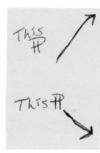

- It produces anterior displacement of the quadriceps tendon throughout movement, assisting knee extension by increasing the lever arm of the quadriceps muscle force
- It increases the area of contact between the patellar tendon and the femur, distributing compressive forces over a wider area

The articular cartilage on the back of the patella is said to be the thickest in the body, at 5–6 mm thick (Evans 1986). It is divided into areas for articulation with the medial and lateral femoral condyles in varying degrees of flexion and extension. The patella glides caudally approximately 7 cm and rotates as the knee moves from full extension to full flexion. The patella eventually sinks into the intercondylar groove in full knee flexion (Nordin & Frankel 2001).

Patellofemoral symptoms may arise from instability, maltracking, malalignment, subluxation and dislocation, which may lead to eventual chondromalacia patellae and osteoarthrosis of the joint. There is a tendency for the patella to slip laterally, particularly as the knee moves towards full extension, and this is counteracted by:

- The high lateral border of the patellar groove on the femur
- The active muscle pull of the oblique fibres of vastus medialis
- The medial quadriceps expansion

The *superior tibiofibular joint* is a synovial plane joint between the lateral tibial condyle and the head of the fibula; it communicates with the knee joint in 10% of adults (Bozkurt et al 2003). The joint capsule is reinforced by anterior and posterior tibiofibular ligaments. Small accessory movements are possible at this joint which is mechanically linked to the inferior tibiofibular joint and dissipates torsional stress applied to the ankle. It is therefore influenced by movements at the ankle joint (Bozkurt et al 2003).

CONTRACTILE STRUCTURES

The contractile structures at the knee consist of muscles which originate from the hip region and insert at the knee, or originate at the knee and insert below the ankle. The muscles will be described in relationship to the knee and the reader is referred to the chapters on the hip and ankle for further discussion of the muscle groups.

Quadriceps femoris (femoral nerve L2–L4) is composed of four muscles: rectus femoris, vastus lateralis, vastus medialis and vastus intermedius, uniting around the patella to form the *infrapatellar tendon*, which passes from the apex of the patella to insert into the tibial tuberosity.

Rectus femoris originates above the hip joint and inserts into the base of the patella (upper border) with fibres continued over and on each side of the patella contributing to the infrapatellar tendon.

Vastus lateralis passes down from the upper anterolateral femur to form a broad tendon which eventually tapers as it inserts into the lateral border of the patella as the lateral quadriceps expansion. Vastus lateralis contributes to the main quadriceps tendon, passing over the patella, as well as blending with fibres of the iliotibial tract to form a lateral extension and to support the anterolateral joint capsule.

Vastus medialis passes from the upper anteromedial femur downwards, to join the common quadriceps tendon and the medial border of the patella as the medial quadriceps expansion. The lower fibres, which form the medial expansion, run more horizontally and have their origin from adductor magnus, with which they share a nerve supply. These fibres are commonly known as the vastus medialis obliquus (VMO).

Vastus intermedius is the deepest part of the quadriceps and inserts with rectus femoris into the base of the patella as the *suprapatellar tendon*.

Quadriceps femoris is the main extensor muscle of the knee joint. Vastus medialis is believed to be particularly active during the later stages of knee extension, when it exerts a stabilizing force on the patella to prevent it slipping laterally. Although quiet in standing, the quadriceps femoris muscle contracts strongly in such activities as climbing.

The *hamstrings* (sciatic nerve L5, S1–S2), comprising biceps femoris, semimembranosus and semitendinosus, are responsible for flexion of the knee and medial and lateral rotation of the knee when flexed in the mid-position.

Biceps femoris inserts into the head of the fibula, splitting around the lateral collateral ligament as it does so, with which it forms a conjoined tendon. *Semimembranosus* has its main attachment into the posterior aspect of the medial tibial condyle, but sends slips onto blend with other structures to support the posteromedial capsule. *Semitendinosus* curves around the medial tibial condyle to the upper surface of the medial tibia together with sartorius and gracilis to form the *pes anserine tendon complex*. These tendons blend with the medial capsule, lending it some support. The pes anserine tendon complex is responsible for flexion of the knee and medial rotation of the tibia on the femur (Valley & Shermer 2000).

The *iliotibial tract* inserts into Gerdy's tubercle on the anterolateral aspect of the upper tibia and blends with the lateral capsule and the lateral quadriceps expansion; functionally it is related to the lateral collateral ligament. Tensor fascia lata, acting with gluteus maximus, tightens the tract and assists extension of the knee.

Popliteus (tibial nerve L4–L5, S1) originates within the capsule of the knee joint as a tendon arising from the groove on the lateral aspect of the lateral femoral condyle. It separates the lateral collateral ligament from the fibrous capsule of the knee joint and, as it passes downwards, backwards and medially, it sends tendinous fibres to the posterior horn of the lateral meniscus. It forms a fleshy, triangular muscle belly and attaches to the posterior aspect of the tibia above the soleal line. Popliteus is the primary medial rotator of the knee, medially rotating the tibia on the femur and unlocking the knee joint from the close packed position. Some consider that, through its attachment to the lateral meniscus, it pulls the meniscus backwards during rotatory movements, possibly preventing it from being trapped (Safran & Fu 1995). Its complex attachment to the lateral meniscus, arcuate ligament, posterior capsule and lateral femoral condyle provides an appreciable role in dynamic stability, particularly in preventing forwards displacement of the femur on the tibia (Burks 1990, Safran & Fu 1995, El-Dieb et al 2002).

Gastrocnemius (tibial nerve S1–S2) arises by two heads from the posterior aspect of the medial and lateral femoral condyles and together with soleus and plantaris forms the triceps surae. As well as its action at the ankle, gastrocnemius is a strong flexor at the knee, but is unable to act strongly at both joints simultaneously.

A GUIDE TO SURFACE MARKING AND PALPATION

ANTERIOR ASPECT
(Fig. 11.1)

Locate the *patella* at the front of the knee and identify its base (upper border), apex (lower border), medial and lateral borders. With the knee extended and relaxed you should be able to shift the patella from side to side to palpate the insertion of the *quadriceps expansions* under the edge of each border. Tilt the base and apex to locate the *suprapatellar* and *infrapatellar tendons* respectively.

Follow the *infrapatellar tendon* down to its insertion onto the tibial tuberosity, which lies approximately 5 cm below the apex of the patella in the flexed knee.

Palpate and mark in the *knee joint line* with the knee in flexion. The anterior articular surface of each femoral condyle and the anterior articular margins of the tibia should be palpable at either side of the patella. Both can be followed round onto the medial and lateral aspects, but it is not possible to palpate the joint line posteriorly since it is covered by many musculotendinous structures.

Figure 11.1   Anterior aspect of the knee.

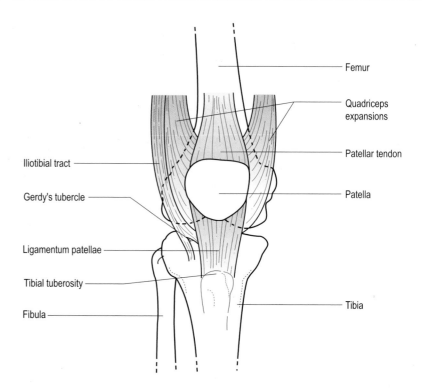

- Femur
- Quadriceps expansions
- Patellar tendon
- Patella
- Iliotibial tract
- Gerdy's tubercle
- Ligamentum patellae
- Tibial tuberosity
- Fibula
- Tibia

With the knee joint flexed, the apex of the patella marks the approximate position of the joint line. In extension, the apex of the patella lies approximately one finger's breadth above the joint line. This information may provide a useful guide if the joint is very swollen, making it difficult to palpate the joint line.

The *quadriceps muscle* forms the major anterior muscle bulk. On static contraction of this muscle, locate rectus femoris, which forms the central part of the muscle bulk. Vastus lateralis forms an obvious lateral muscle bulk, while vastus medialis terminates in oblique fibres which form part of the medial quadriceps expansion.

LATERAL ASPECT (Fig. 11.2)

On the anterolateral surface of the tibia, approximately two-thirds of the way forward from the head of the fibula to the tibial tuberosity, palpate for *Gerdy's tubercle*, which gives attachment to the *iliotibial tract*. The tract should be obvious as the quadriceps contracts.

Palpate the *head of the fibula* just below the posterior part of the lateral condyle of the tibia where it forms the proximal tibiofibular joint. The common peroneal nerve can be rolled over the neck of the fibula.

Place the leg into the FABER position of *flexion*, *ab*duction and *ex*ternal (lateral) rotation, and palpate the lateral aspect of the knee joint line. You should be able to roll the cord-like *lateral collateral ligament* under your fingers.

Figure 11.2   Lateral aspect of the knee.

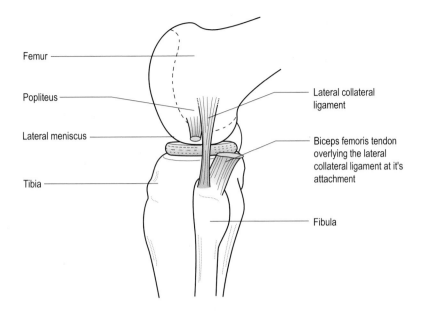

Femur

Popliteus

Lateral meniscus

Tibia

Lateral collateral ligament

Biceps femoris tendon overlying the lateral collateral ligament at it's attachment

Fibula

Figure 11.3   Medial aspect of the knee.

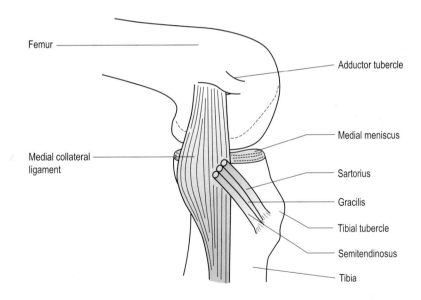

Femur

Medial collateral ligament

Adductor tubercle

Medial meniscus

Sartorius

Gracilis

Tibial tubercle

Semitendinosus

Tibia

MEDIAL ASPECT (Fig. 11.3)

Palpate the medial epicondyle of the femur and locate the prominent *adductor tubercle* on the upper part of the condyle. Deep palpation is necessary and the tubercle will feel tender to palpation.

Move directly distally from the adductor tubercle until you are over the joint line and see if you can identify, by palpation, the anterior edge of the *medial collateral ligament*. This ligament is approximately 8–10 cm long (Williams 1998, Palastanga et al 2002) and two and a half fingers' wide as it broadens to cross the joint line. Its anterior border may be palpated in most people and is usually in line with or just behind the central axis of the joint.

Visualize the position of the *sartorius, gracilis and semitendinosus* tendons (the pes anserine complex) as they cross the lower part of the medial collateral ligament to their insertion on the upper part of the medial tibia.

POSTERIOR ASPECT (Fig. 11.4)

Resist knee flexion and palpate the *hamstrings*, which form the muscle bulk of the posterior thigh. The point at which the medial and lateral hamstrings separate can be identified, with biceps femoris forming the lateral wall of the popliteal fossa and semitendinosus lying on semimembranosus forming the medial wall.

Biceps femoris can be followed down to its insertion onto the head of the fibula.

On the medial side of the popliteal fossa, *semitendinosus* can be felt as an obvious tendon. Medial to it is *gracilis*, made more prominent by adding resisted medial rotation. Deeper to this is *semimembranosus*, remaining more muscular as it blends into its aponeurotic attachment.

Posteriorly, locate the two heads of *gastrocnemius* as they originate above the knee joint from the medial and lateral femoral condyles.

Figure 11.4   Posterior aspect of the knee.

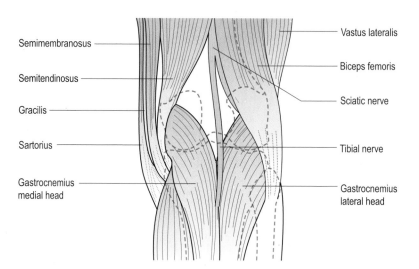

Semimembranosus

Semitendinosus

Gracilis

Sartorius

Gastrocnemius medial head

Vastus lateralis

Biceps femoris

Sciatic nerve

Tibial nerve

Gastrocnemius lateral head

COMMENTARY ON THE EXAMINATION

OBSERVATION

A general observation is made of the patient's *face and overall posture*, but as the knee is a weight-bearing joint, particular attention is paid to the *gait* pattern. Note if an antalgic posture or gait has been adopted; a limp will be evident during gait if the patient has an abnormal stride length or is not weight-bearing evenly. Toeing in or out, together with abnormalities of foot posture, should also be noted.

HISTORY (SUBJECTIVE EXAMINATION)

A detailed history is required at the knee since it gives important diagnostic clues, including typical injury patterns, which may be confirmed by clinical examination. It also assists in the identification of lesions which may be better suited for specialist referral.

The *age, occupation, sports, hobbies and lifestyle* of the patient are particularly relevant.

Some conditions affect certain age groups. Knee pain in children is commonly referred from the hip and it is necessary to carry out a thorough examination of both joints. Meniscal lesions are unusual in children and increase in incidence from adolescence onwards. A gradual onset of knee pain in adolescents may be related to patellofemoral joint syndromes or Osgood–Schlatter's disease which presents as a localized pain felt over the tibial tuberosity due to traction apophysitis of the tibial tubercle.

The young adult, particularly male, may present with traumatic meniscal lesions associated with rotational injury during sporting activities (Greis et al 2002). Females tend to present with instability, subluxation or episodes of dislocation of the patella.

Rheumatoid arthritis may affect the knee and onset usually occurs between the ages of 30 and 40. Degenerative osteoarthrosis affects the older age group, but may occur earlier if predisposed by previous injury or through overuse in sporting activity. It is important to remember that osteoarthrosis can affect both the patellofemoral and tibiofemoral joints. Degenerative meniscal lesions occur more commonly in males in the 4th to 6th decades and can develop in association with degenerative joint disease (Greis et al 2002).

The lifestyle of the patient will reflect whether occupational or recreational activities are a contributing factor to their condition. Sport in particular may be responsible for traumatic incidents to the relatively unstable knee, especially in positions of flexion. Progressive microtrauma may be the result of incorrect training or overtraining, muscle imbalances or poor joint biomechanics.

The *site* of the pain indicates whether it is local or referred. Superficial structures tend to give local pain and point tenderness; therefore lesions of the medial collateral ligament, coronary ligaments or the tendinous insertions of the muscles around the knee give reasonably accurate localization of pain. Acutely inflamed lesions or deep lesions, such as of the tibiofemoral joint, menisci or cruciate ligaments, produce a vague, more widely felt, deep pain, with the patient unable to accurately localize the lesion.

The *spread* of pain generally indicates the severity of the lesion. While referred pain is expected distally to the site of the lesion, the knee as a central limb joint may also produce some proximal pain in the thigh. Pain referred from the hip or lumbar spine can be felt at the knee and both may need to be eliminated as a cause of pain.

Anterior knee pain is a description of the symptoms felt by the patient, although the term is often misused as a diagnosis. It usually indicates patellofemoral joint involvement, but must not be considered to be due to it exclusively.

The anatomy at the knee makes the structures susceptible to direct and indirect trauma. The menisci and ligaments are often the sites of acute lesions, while the contractile structures are susceptible to overuse as well as acute trauma. The superior tibiofibular joint is mechanically linked to its inferior counterpart and influenced by mechanisms of injury at the foot and ankle.

The *onset* of the pain is extremely relevant to lesions at the knee. Trauma is a common precipitating cause and the sudden nature of the injury makes it easily recalled by the patient. A direct injury can cause muscular contusion and commonly involves the quadriceps. A direct blow to the patella, such as a fall on the flexed knee, may result in fracture, or may cause contusion of the periosteum or involvement of the prepatellar bursa. A direct blow to the anterior aspect of the upper tibia or, again, a fall on the flexed knee, can injure the posterior cruciate ligament.

In contact sports such as rugby and football, the lateral side of the knee is vulnerable to impact, which may result in excessive valgus strain affecting the medial collateral ligament. Injury may be produced by excessive forces applied to the flexed knee while the foot is fixed, e.g. skiing injuries. The medial collateral ligament, anterior cruciate ligament and medial meniscus may be affected. The position of the coronary ligaments involves them in rotational injuries. Major ligamentous rupture, particularly of the anterior cruciate ligament, is usually accompanied by a 'pop' or tearing sound as the patient feels the ligament 'go' (Edwards & Villar 1993).

Hyperextension injuries can affect any of the ligaments, since all are taut in extension, but the anterior cruciate ligament and medial collateral ligament are most commonly affected. Recalling the exact onset of the injury, the forces involved and the position of the leg at the time of injury will give an idea of the likely anatomy involved in the lesion.

Muscle injuries are common around the knee, as the major muscle groups span two joints and may affect the origin, insertion or mid-belly. Strain results from eccentric contraction (attempting to contract when the muscle is on the stretch), when the muscle is unable to overcome the resistance. Explosive sprinting action affects the hamstrings and the quadriceps, and rectus femoris particularly may be affected by kicking against strong resistance. A direct blow to the quadriceps may cause severe haematoma. Patellar instability, subluxation or dislocation affects the medial quadriceps expansions, vastus medialis or the medial capsule.

Repetitive minor injury results in microtrauma, making the onset of the lesion difficult to recall, and the examiner will have to be aware of contributing factors such as overtraining, training errors, foot posture and faulty knee joint biomechanics. Lateral knee pain due to iliotibial band friction syndrome is common in long-distance runners. Infrapatellar tendinopathy is common in activities associated with jumping and the bursae can be inflamed if any structures passing over them are overused.

The *duration* of the symptoms will indicate the stage in the inflammatory process reached, or the recurrent nature of the condition. Different treatment approaches depend on the acute, subacute or chronic nature of a ligamentous sprain or muscle belly strain. Overuse lesions around the knee tend to be chronic in nature and are present for some considerable time before the patient seeks treatment.

Recurrent episodes of pain and swelling may be due to instability and derangement of the joint. Patellar subluxation, meniscal lesions or partial ligamentous tears may produce pain and joint effusion after use. Degenerative osteoarthrosis may be symptom-free until overuse triggers a synovitis with increased pain and swelling.

The *symptoms and behaviour* need to be considered. The behaviour of the pain and the symptoms described by the patient are very relevant to diagnosis at the knee. Immediate pain after injury indicates a severe lesion but pain developing or increasing slowly over several hours may indicate less serious pathology. The ability to continue with the sport or activity after the onset of pain is often indicative of minor ligamentous sprain, whereas major ligament disruption and muscle tears, meniscal lesions or cruciate rupture often result in the patient being totally incapacitated.

Total rupture of a ligament may produce severe pain at the time of injury but, following the initial injury, pain may not be a particular feature since the structure is totally disrupted. Partial ligamentous rupture continues to produce severe pain on movement.

The quality of the pain may indicate severity, but it is important to remember the subjective nature of pain. Aggravating factors can be activity, which indicates a mechanical or muscular lesion, or rest, which indicates a ligamentous lesion with an inflammatory component.

Postures such as prolonged sitting may affect the patellofemoral joint in particular. A pseudo-locking effect often occurs when the patient first gets up to weight-bear. This is not the same as true locking of the knee joint, but is a stiffness experienced by the patient which usually resolves after a few steps. It is thought to be due to excessive friction from changes in the articular cartilage of the patella. Walking, squatting and using stairs all aggravate patellofemoral conditions, particularly going downstairs, when the forces acting on this joint are increased to approximately three times body weight.

The tibiofemoral joint, as the weight-bearing joint, usually produces symptoms on weight-bearing activities, i.e. the stance phase of walking or running or prolonged standing. Pain produced on deep knee bends, rising from kneeling and rotational strains may indicate a meniscal lesion.

The other symptoms described by the patient give important clues to diagnosis. Swelling may be a symptom and it is important to know if it is constant or recurrent or provoked by activity. Swelling occurring within 2 h of injury is indicative of haemarthrosis; the joint may feel warm to touch and the swelling may be tense. Structures responsible for a haemarthrosis are those with a good blood supply, the anterior cruciate ligament being the commonest cause of a haemarthrosis. Amiel et al (1990) quoted a study by Noyes in which over 70% of patients presenting with acute haemarthrosis of the knee had an acute tear of the anterior cruciate ligament. The forces required for rupture of the posterior cruciate ligament are great and therefore the posterior capsule usually tears as well with blood escaping into the calf, where swelling and bruising may have been noticed by the patient.

Swelling which develops over 6–24 h is synovial in origin due to traumatic arthritis. Structures with a relatively poor blood supply tend to produce this traumatic arthritis, e.g. meniscal lesions, the deep part of the medial collateral ligament involving the capsule of the knee joint and subluxation or dislocation of the patella.

Activity may provoke swelling in conditions such as degenerative joint disease, chronic instability or internal derangement. This may be confirmed after the objective examination which may stir up the condition. Localized swelling may indicate bursitis, e.g. prepatellar bursitis, Baker's cyst (synovial effusion into the gastrocnemius or semimembranosus bursa due to effusion in the knee joint) or meniscal cyst, which more commonly affects the lateral meniscus.

The presence of an effusion may affect the gait pattern and limit full extension. Reflex inhibition of the quadriceps muscle and an inability to lock the knee gives a feeling of insecurity on weight-bearing with the patient complaining of a sensation of 'giving way'. Giving way on weight-bearing may also be due to a loose body or meniscal lesion; it is momentary and occurs together with a twinge of pain. Muscle imbalances, particularly involving VMO, may produce a feeling of apprehension as the knee feels as if it will give way. This may occur when weight-bearing after sitting for prolonged periods or walking downstairs.

True locking of the knee is indicative of a meniscal lesion and usually occurs in conjunction with a rotary component to the injury. It has a tendency to recur. The locking may resolve spontaneously over several hours or days or it may need to be manipulatively unlocked. Locking usually occurs at 10–40° short of full extension (Hartley 1995). Meniscal lesions occurring in isolation may present with acute pain and swelling and the patient may report locking or catching. Degenerative meniscal lesions occur in older patients who present with an atraumatic history, mild swelling, joint line pain and mechanical symptoms (Greis et al 2002). A ruptured anterior cruciate ligament can cause locking as the ligamentous flap catches between the joint surfaces. True locking must be distinguished from the pseudo-locking associated with the patellofemoral joint after prolonged sitting.

Provocation of pain on the stairs is important. The patellofemoral joint characteristically produces more pain on coming downstairs, due to the greater joint reaction force, although the pain may also have been provoked while walking upstairs.

Clicking, snapping or catching may be due to internal derangement. Grating and pain associated with crepitation are usually indicative of degenerative changes of the tibiofemoral joint, patellofemoral joint, or both.

To exclude symptoms arising from the lumbar spine, the patient should be questioned about paraesthesia and pain provoked by coughing or sneezing.

Other joint involvement should be explored to ascertain the possibility of inflammatory joint disease. *Past medical history* should exclude serious pathology, and questions about *medications* will highlight any contraindications to treatment. If degenerative osteoarthrosis is considered a factor in the diagnosis, the patient can be questioned about significant weight gain. It has been suggested that obesity is a cause of osteoarthrosis in the knee (Felson et al 1988, Felson & Chaisson 1997).

INSPECTION

The knee should be fully extended in standing. If not, some compromise of the terminal screw home or locking mechanism exists, or an effusion with limited extension is present as part of the capsular pattern.

The knee should be inspected in both the weight-bearing and non-weight-bearing positions. In standing the normal slight valgus tibiofemoral angle should be obvious.

The whole lower limb is inspected for leg length discrepancy and obvious **bony deformity** such as genu valgum, varum, recurvatum or 'wind-swept' knees (one varus, one valgus). The posture of the feet is important. Overpronation or a tight Achilles tendon may be related to the knee symptoms and a detailed biomechanical assessment is then required. Position of the pelvis and obvious spinal deformities may be important to note if relevant to symptoms.

The position, shape and size of the patellae are noted if relevant to the presenting symptoms. Patellar alignment is measured by the Q-angle – the angle between the line of the quadriceps muscle (anterior superior iliac spine to the mid-point of the patella) and the patellar tendon (mid-point of the patella to the tibial tuberosity). An angle of between 15 and 20° is considered normal for patellar alignment and tracking, and less or more than this can be considered to be a malalignment (Norris 1998).

Colour changes may be present, especially if the condition is acute, when the joint looks red due to inflammatory changes. Direct trauma may produce bruising and acute muscle lesions may show bruising, particularly in the quadriceps and hamstring muscles. Distal colour changes may be indicative of circulatory problems.

In standing, all muscle groups are inspected for *wasting*. The quadriceps wastes rapidly due to reflex inhibition if pain, swelling or degenerative change are present. In patellofemoral problems wasting of the oblique fibres of vastus medialis may be obvious.

Loss of the dimple on the medial aspect of the knee will indicate the presence of *swelling*, drawn out of the suprapatellar bursa by gravity. Minor swelling may not be obvious and may only be apparent on testing by palpation in the supine position.

STATE AT REST

Before any movements are performed, the state at rest is established to provide a baseline for subsequent comparison.

The suggested sequence for the objective examination will now be given, followed by a commentary including the reasoning in performing the movements and the significance of the possible findings.

EXAMINATION BY SELECTIVE TENSION (OBJECTIVE EXAMINATION)

Supine Lying

- Palpation for heat (Fig. 11.5), swelling (Fig. 11.6) and synovial thickening (Fig. 11.7)
- Passive knee flexion (Fig. 11.8)
- Passive knee extension, once for range (Fig. 11.9a), once for end-feel (Fig. 11.9b)
- Passive valgus stress (Fig. 11.10a, b)
- Passive varus stress (Fig. 11.11)
- Passive lateral rotation (Fig. 11.12a)
- Passive medial rotation (Fig. 11.12b)
- Posterior drawer test (Figs 11.13–11.15)
- Anterior drawer test (Fig. 11.16)
- Lachman test (Fig. 11.17)

Provocation Tests for the Menisci (Saunders 2000)

- Flexion, lateral rotation and valgus (Fig. 11.18)
- Flexion, lateral rotation and varus (Fig. 11.19)
- Flexion, medial rotation and valgus (Fig. 11.20)
- Flexion, medial rotation and varus (Fig. 11.21)

Prone Lying

- Resisted knee extension (Fig. 11.22)
- Resisted knee flexion (Fig. 11.23)

Palpation

- Once a diagnosis has been made, the structure at fault is palpated for the exact site of the lesion

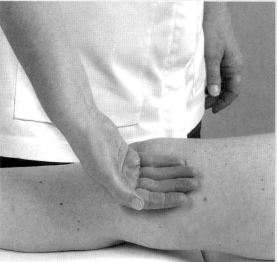

Figure 11.5   Palpation for heat.

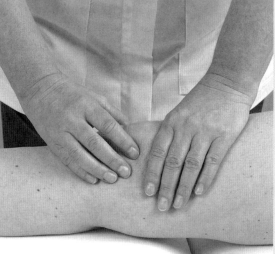

Figure 11.6   Palpation for swelling.

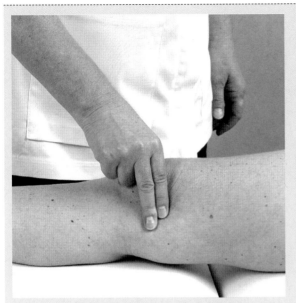

Figure 11.7   Palpation for synovial thickening.

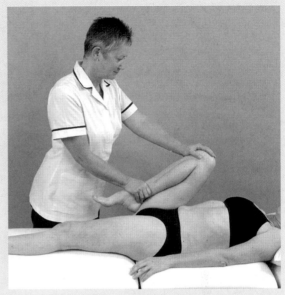

Figure 11.8   Passive flexion.

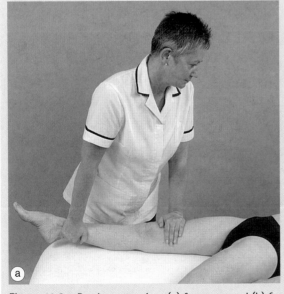

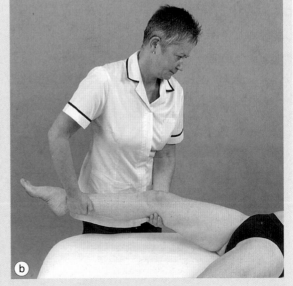

Figure 11.9   Passive extension: (a) for range and (b) for end-feel.

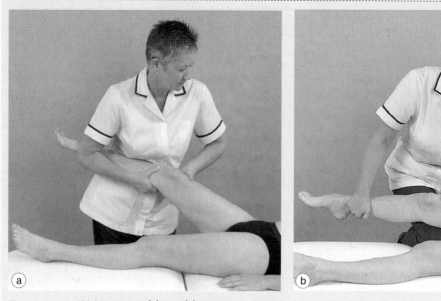

Figure 11.10   Valgus stress (a) and (b) alternative position.

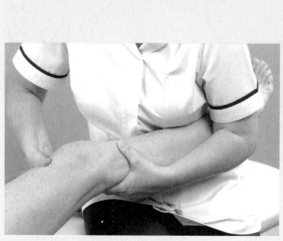

Figure 11.11   Varus stress.

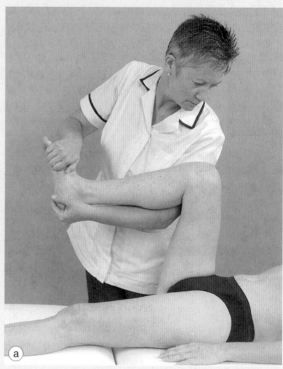

Figure 11.12   Passive (a) lateral and (b) medial rotation.

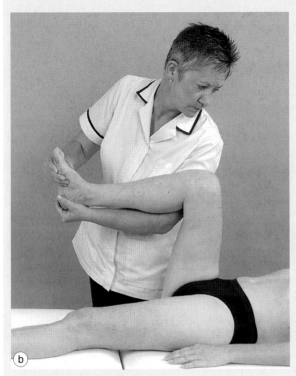

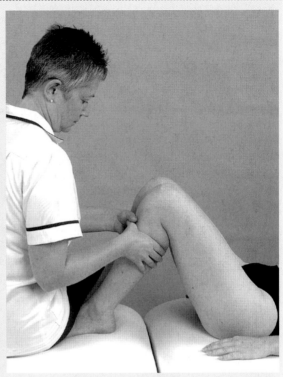

Figure 11.12   cont.

Figure 11.13   Posterior drawer test.

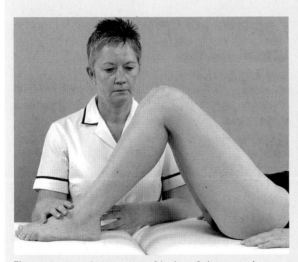

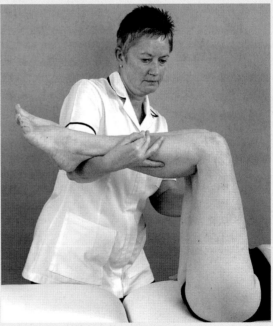

Figure 11.14   Assessment of laxity of the posterior cruciate ligament.

Figure 11.15   Assessment of laxity of the posterior cruciate ligament, alternative position.

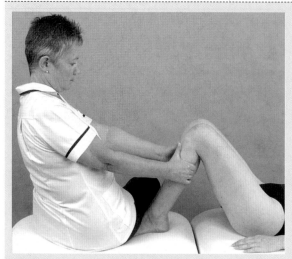

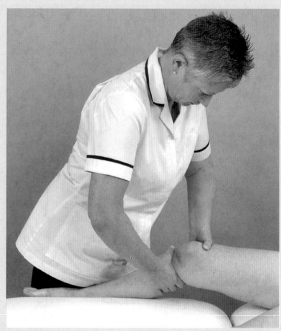

Figure 11.16   Anterior drawer test.

Figure 11.17   Lachman test.

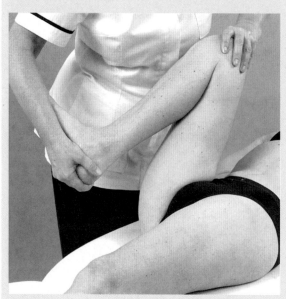

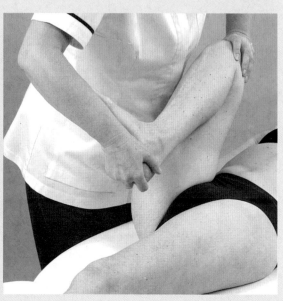

Figure 11.18   Flexion, lateral rotation and valgus.

Figure 11.19   Flexion, lateral rotation and varus.

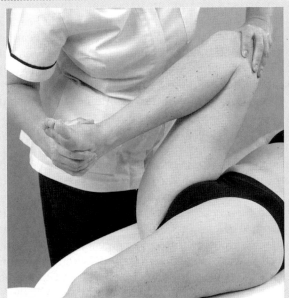

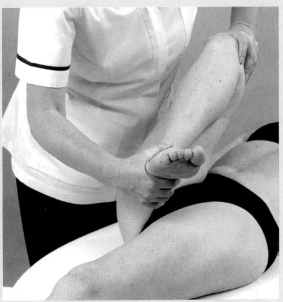

Figure 11.20   Flexion, medial rotation and valgus.

Figure 11.21   Flexion, medial rotation and varus.

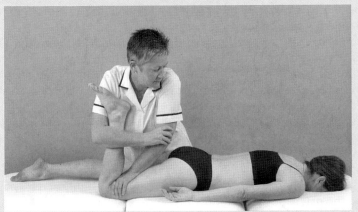

Figure 11.22   Resisted knee extension.

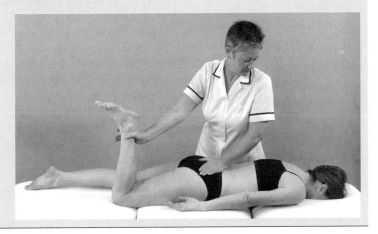

Figure 11.23   Resisted knee flexion.

The combined history and examination are important at the knee. The symptoms described by the patient result from functional weight-bearing activities but the knee is examined clinically in a non-weight-bearing position. Lesions vary from simple contusions, muscle strains and ligament sprains to arthritis and major ligamentous rupture and instability. It is important to be able clinically to diagnose lesions at the knee, but also to appreciate the limits of clinical examination and determine when onward referral for specialist opinion is necessary.

The acute knee should be examined as soon as possible after injury, before effusion causes pain, apprehension and limited movement. Effusion makes it difficult to test accurately for ligamentous instability and to apply provocative meniscal tests. The acute knee is usually managed conservatively until the traumatic arthritis subsides. Residual instability which fails to respond to conservative management or internal derangement due to meniscal lesions can be dealt with surgically at a later date, and neither is usually considered to be an emergency.

Palpation tests are conducted for signs of activity within the joint. Temperature changes are assessed using the dorsal aspect of the same hand and comparing like with like. Inflammatory conditions will show an increase in *heat* compared with the other side. It may be necessary to repeat this test at the end of the examination to assess if an inflammatory response has been triggered by the examination, giving an indication of the irritability of the lesion.

Several tests exist for *swelling* and the choice is left to the reader on the basis of personal opinion on effectiveness and preference. A sensitive test for minor swelling involves placing the finger and thumb of one hand on either side of the patella just below the bony periphery. The web between the index finger and thumb of the other hand applies compression to the suprapatellar bursa which squeezes fluid out into the joint cavity and, if positive, is felt to part the finger and thumb of the other hand. Other tests involve wiping the fluid from one side of the joint to the other, compression of the suprapatellar bursa and the front of the joint just below the patella to assess fluctuation of fluid, or pressing down on the patella to assess for the presence of a patellar 'tap'.

Synovial thickening is assessed by palpation of the medial and lateral femoral condyles. Thickening of the synovium is normal here because of the presence of synovial plica and the medial plica is more obvious to palpation. Assessment for excessive thickening of the synovium is confirmed if the tissue feels 'boggy' to the touch. Hill et al (2001) regard synovial thickening as a contributor to pain in the osteoarthritic knee and an indication of the severity of the disease.

The position of the patella should be assessed to see if it is shifted, tilted or rotated with respect to the other side. It should be emphasized here that the orthopaedic medicine approach has limited relevance to patellofemoral malalignment syndromes. The interested reader is referred to other excellent texts on this subject.

The primary passive movements of flexion and extension are performed to assess the tibiofemoral joint. Pain, range of movement and end-feel are noted, which will indicate the presence of the capsular or

---

Capsular pattern at the knee joint

- More limitation of flexion than extension.

non-capsular pattern. Bijl et al (1998) found an indication of the capsular pattern of the knee, but could not recommend it as a valid test for arthritis. In contrast, Fritz et al (1998) found evidence for the existence of a capsular pattern to support the identification of patients with knee joint arthrosis or arthritis. Passive flexion normally has a soft end-feel and passive extension a hard end-feel. The thigh is fixed above the knee and the foot is lifted to assess the range of hyperextension present, normally 5–10°. A further test is conducted for the end-feel of extension whereby the leg is lifted into approximately 10° of flexion and dropped into extension to assess for the normal, bony hard end-feel. This is sometimes known as the 'bounce home' test and an abnormally 'soft' or 'springy' end-feel indicates the end of range has not been reached due to a meniscal lesion, loose body or joint effusion. The presence of the non-capsular pattern indicates a ligamentous lesion or a loose body in the joint, or possibly a meniscal problem.

The secondary passive movements at the knee are applied to assess the ligaments. It is important to compare the two limbs since, although joint motion varies considerably within the population, there is very little variation between right and left in a normal subject (Daniel 1990). The tests depend on the muscles being relaxed and the eye, feel and experience of the examiner, who is looking for an excessive range of movement compared with the asymptomatic knee and an abnormal soft end-feel with no definite end point if laxity is present.

Secondary passive movements are applied to the knee in a loose packed position of 20–30° of flexion since no passive or accessory movements should be present with the knee in full extension. If movement can be detected in the close packed position, serious ligamentous disruption is present, with accompanying damage to capsular components. Minor ligamentous laxity may be subclinical; therefore recognition of such symptoms from the history leads to onward referral for more detailed assessment of ligamentous laxity.

The intention here is to list the ligaments that need to be tested, with the figures providing illustrations of suggested testing methods. The methods are not proposed as the 'best' way of testing and will not be described in detail within the text. The interested reader is referred to the fuller descriptions of these and other methods to be found in textbooks devoted to the knee and sports injuries.

Butler et al (1980) referred to the concept of primary and secondary ligament restraints to movement in a specific direction. A ligament may act as a primary restraint in one direction and as a secondary restraint in another. Rupture of a primary restraint results in excessive movement; rupture of the secondary restraint to that movement, with the primary restraint intact, does not result in increased movement. Rupture of both primary and secondary restraint produces a much greater increase in movement. For example, rupture of the anterior cruciate ligament (primary restraint) produces some increase in anterior translation, rupture of the medial collateral ligament (secondary restraint) produces no detectable increase in anterior translation and rupture of both (primary and secondary restraints) results in a much greater increase in movement.

Orthopaedic medicine treatment techniques will be directed at simple ligamentous sprains, but it is important to recognize more serious ligament disruption or intra-articular derangement due to a meniscal lesion in order to make the appropriate onward specialist referral.

Valgus and varus stresses are applied to the knee in approximately 20–30° of flexion and assess the primary stabilizing function of the medial and lateral collateral ligaments, respectively. The range of movement available is noted and compared with the asymptomatic knee. The end-feel is assessed, which is normally firm elastic.

Axial rotation should be tested at 90° of knee flexion as the range of movement is greatest in this position. Passive lateral rotation is usually 45° and assesses the medial coronary ligaments, and passive medial rotation is usually 35° and tests the lateral coronary ligaments.

The posterior and anterior drawer tests are both performed with the knee at 90° of flexion. The neutral position of the resting knee must be established compared with the contralateral normal knee.

The posterior drawer test is applied first for the posterior cruciate ligament, since a deficient posterior cruciate ligament could give a false-positive to anterior translation. As the tibia is pushed posteriorly, the thumbs rest over the anterior joint line to assess the 'sag-back' or step created anteriorly by the excessive posterior drawer. Isolated rupture of the posterior cruciate ligament is a rare lesion, but the posterior drawer test is a sensitive and specific test for the posterior cruciate ligament (Rubinstein et al 1994, Palastanga et al 2002, Malanga et al 2003).

The anterior drawer test assesses the anterior cruciate ligament, although it is considered an insensitive and poor diagnostic indicator of lesions of this ligament, especially in the acute knee (Katz & Fingeroth 1986, Malanga et al 2003). The haemarthrosis and traumatic arthritis 'splint' the knee, making it difficult to place the knee in 90° of flexion, and pain produces protective spasm in the hamstrings preventing anterior tibial translation. In a chronic knee, the secondary stabilizing role of an intact medial collateral ligament may prevent anterior translation at 90° of knee flexion.

The Lachman test is a clinical test with a high diagnostic accuracy to determine anterior cruciate laxity (Katz & Fingeroth 1986, Smith & Green 1995, Malanga et al 2003). The Lachman test may be difficult to perform especially if the limb is large or the patient unable to relax sufficiently. Several modifications have been made to the Lachman test since it was first described by Torg et al in 1976, including a 'drop leg' Lachman test described by Adler et al (1995) and a reversed Lachman test described by Cailliet (1992).

Similarly, the pivot-shift test has several methods of application (see Malanga et al 2003). It is essentially a dynamic test to determine the degree of instability related to anterior cruciate ligament injury. However, it may also be difficult to apply in the acute knee.

Four provocation tests are applied if the history indicates a meniscal lesion. Each meniscus is put under compression and stress during combined movements of flexion, valgus, varus and both rotations.

Other traditional tests for a meniscal lesion include the 'bounce home' test of passive knee extension for end-feel, the McMurray's test which takes the leg from a position of flexion towards extension, with medial or lateral rotation of the tibia, and Apley's grind or compression test. There is mixed support for the various meniscal tests in the literature. Joint line tenderness seems to be the best clinical indicator of medial meniscus injury and there are reports of the low specificity and sensitivity rates associated with the McMurray's test (Malanga et al 2003). Negative clinical testing is not conclusive evidence that a meniscal lesion does not exist. If the history is indicative, or the patient is experiencing recurrent episodes of locking and/or giving way, referral should be made for specialist opinion with arthroscopy, in modern practice the 'gold standard' for diagnosis at the knee (Curtin et al 1992).

The resisted tests are applied looking for pain and power. Resisted knee extension tests the quadriceps and resisted knee flexion the hamstrings. Having established that there is no pain on testing the muscles in the mid-position, accessory provocation tests may be included to provoke minor contractile lesions. The quadriceps and hamstrings can be tested in varying degrees of knee flexion and extension, and isotonically. The hamstring muscles may be tested in conjunction with medial or lateral rotation to isolate the lesion to the medial or lateral hamstrings. Popliteus may be assessed by testing resisted knee flexion in conjunction with resisted medial rotation of the tibia (Fig. 11.24).

Figure 11.24   Resisted knee flexion and medial rotation of the tibia.

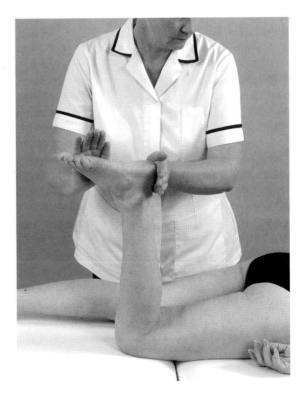

CAPSULAR LESIONS

Capsular pattern at the knee joint
- More limitation of flexion than extension.

The presence of the capsular pattern indicates arthritis and the history indicates the cause of the arthritis. The possibilities are an acute episode of degenerative osteoarthrosis, inflammatory arthritis such as rheumatoid arthritis or traumatic arthritis.

Traumatic arthritis is usually a secondary response to a ligamentous lesion at the knee. As a capsular ligament, damage to the medial collateral ligament produces a secondary traumatic arthritis; a ruptured cruciate ligament may also produce a haemarthrosis.

Symptomatic osteoarthrosis and inflammatory arthritis may benefit from an intra-articular injection of corticosteroid. Treatment for traumatic arthritis should be directed to the cause of the lesion, i.e. the ligamentous injury.

Injection of the knee joint (Cyriax & Cyriax 1983, Cyriax 1984)

Suggested needle size: 21G × 1¹/₂ in (0.8 × 40 mm) green needle
Dose: 30 mg triamcinolone acetonide in a total volume of 4 ml

---

Position the patient comfortably in supine lying with the knee supported in extension. Glide the patella medially, pressing down on the lateral edge to lift the medial border (Fig. 11.25). Insert the needle halfway along the medial border of the patella, aiming laterally and slightly posteriorly, parallel with the articular surface of the patella (Fig. 11.26). Once the needle is intra-articular, deliver the injection as a bolus. The patient is advised to maintain a period of relative rest for approximately 2 weeks following injection. Chakravarty & Pharoah (1994) demonstrated that 24 h of complete bed rest following injection of the knee joint for rheumatoid arthritis produced a more prolonged benefit.

Figure 11.25 Injection of the knee joint.

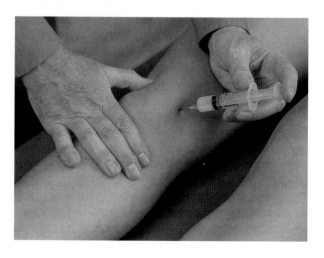

Figure 11.26 Injection of the knee joint showing direction of approach and needle position.

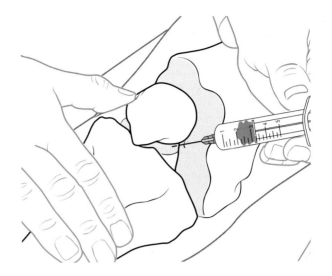

Controversy exists over repeated corticosteroid injections into weight-bearing joints and its association with the development of steroid arthropathy, with opposing views being supported (Parikh et al 1993, Cameron 1995). Raynauld et al (2003) conducted a randomized, double blind, placebo-controlled trial to determine the efficacy of long-term intraarticular corticosteroid injection (40 mg triamcinolone acetonide every 3 months) in osteoarthritis of the knee. The 1- and 2-year follow-up showed no difference in the loss of joint space over time between the corticosteroid injection group and the saline injected group. There was a trend in the corticosteroid group to show greater symptomatic relief, with pain and stiffness significantly improved. The authors concluded that there was no significant deleterious effect on the anatomical joint structure in either group, indicating that repeated intra-articular injections are safe.

NON-CAPSULAR LESIONS

LOOSE BODY

From the history, symptoms of momentary giving way on weight-bearing accompanied by twinges of pain indicate a possible loose body in the knee joint. The loose body may be a fragment of cartilage or bone associated with degenerative osteoarthrosis in the older adult, or a flap of meniscus which may momentarily give way or lock on weight-bearing.

Osteochondritis dissecans may affect the knee in adolescents, usually between the ages of 15 and 20 years. A small fragment of bone becomes demarcated from a condyle and detaches to form a loose body. Pain, swelling, locking and giving way are the symptoms. On examination, a non-capsular pattern is present with a small limitation of flexion or extension, but not both. The end-feel is characteristically springy.

If the joint should lock, it is usually temporary and it unlocks spontaneously. A joint which requires manipulative unlocking probably requires referral for specialist opinion and possibly arthroscopy.

It may be possible to have a loose body impinged between the joint surfaces in degenerative osteoarthrosis. If the loose fragment impinges on the medial side of the joint, the patient presents with signs of an intrinsic medial collateral sprain, but in the absence of trauma. The capsular pattern of degenerative osteoarthrosis is present with a non-capsular pattern superimposed; the patient complains of increased pain on the valgus stress. The primary lesion should be treated and the secondary ligamentous sprain should therefore subside.

The treatment of choice to reduce a loose body is strong traction together with Grade A mobilization, theoretically aiming to move the loose body to another part of the joint and to restore full, pain-free movement.

The strong traction is applied to the joint and a medial or lateral movement is applied simultaneously with a movement from flexion towards extension.

Loose body mobilization technique 1 (Saunders 2000)

This technique may only be applied to a relatively fit patient, but it enables the technique to be applied single-handedly.

Position the patient in supine lying with the legs hanging over the end of the couch, the thighs supported. Arrange the couch so that it is as high as it will go and elevate the head end of the couch. Run your hand down the posterior aspect of the ankle, grasping the calcaneum and pulling the ankle into dorsiflexion. Place the other hand on top of the talus in order to rotate the leg into either medial or lateral rotation (Figs 11.27 and 11.28) (position your hands such that the hand on top of the foot will be pulling, not pushing, into rotation). Bend your knees and straighten your arms to apply traction (Fig. 11.29). Once traction is established, straighten your knees to extend the patient's knee, smartly rotating the leg at the same time (Fig. 11.30).

Figure 11.27   Loose body mobilization for the knee 1; hand position for mobilization into medial rotation.

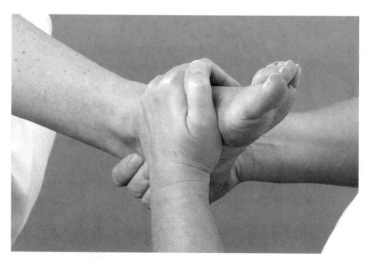

Figure 11.28   Loose body mobilization for the knee 1; hand position for mobilization into lateral rotation.

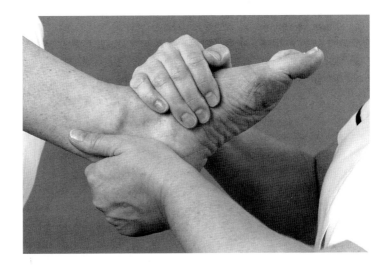

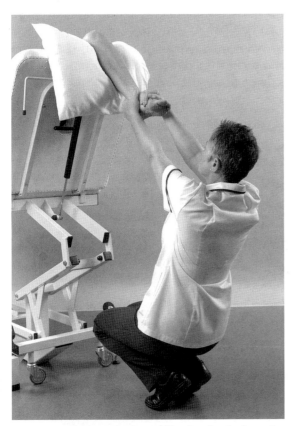

Figure 11.29   Loose body mobilization for the knee 1; starting position applying traction.

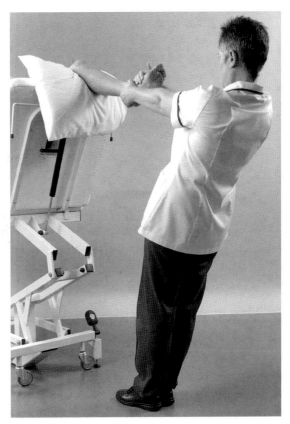

Figure 11.30   Loose body mobilization for the knee 1; ending the manoeuvre, avoiding full extension of the patient's knee.

Reassess the patient for an increase in range and a change in the end-feel. If the technique has helped, it can be repeated; if not, change your hand position to effect the opposite rotation. The basis of this technique is traction, rotation and a movement towards extension of the knee. It can be modified to suit the patient or operator and you are encouraged to be inventive with the technique. It can be applied with the patient sitting over the edge of the bed, or a 'seat belt' may be applied to help the traction.

Loose body mobilization technique 2 (Cyriax & Cyriax 1983, Cyriax 1984)

This technique requires an assistant. Position the patient in prone lying with the knee flexed to 90°. Stand adjacent to the patient's flexed knee, placing your foot distal to the patient, on the couch. Place the web between your index finger and thumb of one hand around the calcaneum to pull the ankle into dorsiflexion; the other hand wraps comfortably around the dorsum of the foot. Lift the patient's foot onto your flexed knee (Fig. 11.31a) and plantarflex your foot to raise the knee from the couch (Fig. 11.31b). Ask the assistant to apply the traction to the knee joint by placing two hands behind the knee joint and applying body weight to the thigh (Fig. 11.31c). Once traction is established, remove your foot from the couch and place it to the side (Fig. 11.31d). Maintain the traction as you smartly rotate the lower leg, simultaneously moving from flexion towards extension (Fig. 11.31e). Reassess and repeat as necessary.

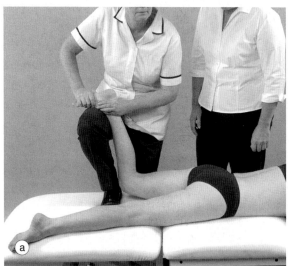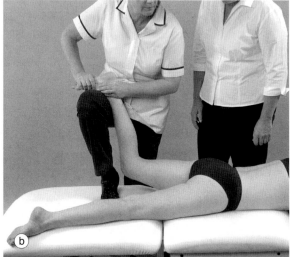

Figure 11.31   Loose body mobilization for the knee 2:
a) starting position
b) plantarflexing foot to raise knee
c) assistant applying counter-pressure through thigh to apply distraction at the knee
d) Grade A mobilization applied whilst moving towards extension and maintaining distraction
e) completion of the manoeuvre.

Figure 11.31   Cont'd

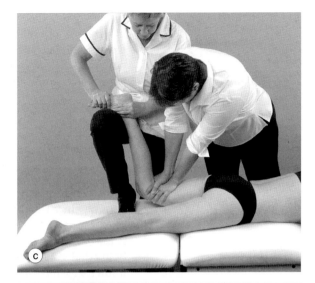

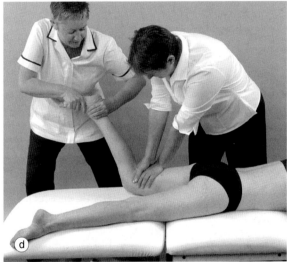

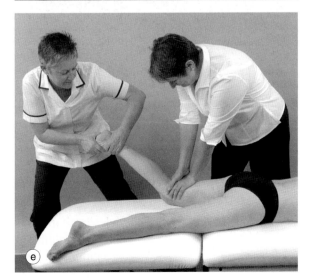

MEDIAL COLLATERAL LIGAMENT SPRAIN

The medial collateral ligament is the ligament most vulnerable to injury at the knee, but the following principles of treatment may also be applied to the lateral collateral ligament if it is the site of the lesion. As the lateral collateral ligament is not associated with the joint capsule, the acute effusion common to medial collateral sprain will probably be absent.

The collateral and cruciate ligaments function together to control and stabilize the knee. The medial collateral ligament is anatomically related to the medial meniscus and functionally related to the anterior cruciate ligament. Injury may result in 'O'Donaghue's unhappy triad', affecting all three structures (Evans 1986, Staron et al 1994). If tears of the medial meniscus and anterior cruciate ligament are confirmed by MRI or arthroscopy, subtle signs of medial collateral ligament sprain should be sought, since the three conditions usually coexist (Staron et al 1994).

Rupture of the cruciate ligaments or a meniscal lesion produces an acute effusion which can be managed conservatively as for the acute phase of medial collateral ligament sprain. Once the acute phase has settled, a full assessment of the knee can be carried out, including assessment for ligamentous laxity and the provocative meniscal tests. A decision may then be taken concerning onwards referral for specialist opinion.

Ligament injuries are graded 1–3 according to the amount of laxity and the end-feel (Daniel 1990, Schenck & Heckman 1993, Hartley 1995). The following is applied to the medial collateral ligament, but it should be noted that assessment for laxity on the acute knee will not be possible due to the effusion and painful muscle spasm:

Grade I

In a Grade I injury there is stretching and microfailure of some fibres of the ligament, pain, tenderness and swelling at the site of the injury, possibly a mild capsular pattern as the medial collateral ligament is an integral part of the capsule, no notable clinical instability and a firm elastic end-feel.

Grade II

Grade II injury is associated with moderate–major tearing of the ligament fibres, some exceeding their elastic limit, pain and tenderness at the site of injury, moderate to severe swelling, movement limited in the capsular pattern, a minor degree of ligamentous laxity noted clinically and a relatively firm elastic end-feel with a definite end-point.

Grade III

Grade III injury is diagnosed when there is macrofailure, or complete rupture of the ligament, swelling, possibly haemarthrosis and a capsular pattern of limited movement, severe pain at the time of injury, but relatively little since, definite ligamentous laxity noted, and the joint may click as it returns to the neutral position. There is a soft end-feel with no definite end-point.

Not all major ligamentous ruptures require surgical reconstruction, and decisions are based on the lifestyle of the patient. A good functional recovery from ligamentous laxity may be achieved by strengthening the dynamic stabilizers of the knee, the hamstrings and quadriceps muscles while maintaining control with appropriate braces. If haemarthrosis is present in the early acute knee, this will need to be aspirated.

From the history, medial collateral ligament sprain is possible if the knee is subjected to excessive valgus rotation of the flexed knee or a hyperextension force. A combination of trauma may occur and, as already stated, the medial collateral ligament can be damaged in association with the anterior cruciate ligament and medial meniscus.

Acute medial collateral ligament sprain

Initially, the lesion is accompanied by a secondary traumatic arthritis which presents with a capsular pattern of limited movement. It may be difficult to apply provocative stress tests to either the ligament or menisci to assess associated damage. The history of the mechanism of the injury, the position of the leg and the forces applied will indicate medial collateral ligament sprain. The valgus test will produce pain to confirm diagnosis, but the grade of sprain will be difficult to ascertain initially since the reflex muscle spasm and effusion effectively splint the knee. Presence of haemarthrosis indicates possible anterior cruciate ligament damage and the Lachman test can at least be applied to this acute knee. Haemarthrosis and the presence of a positive Lachman test may indicate onward referral for specialist opinion.

The acute situation is managed conservatively with daily treatment initially, consisting of PRICE (see Ch. 4). Gentle transverse frictions are started as early as possible, depending on the irritability of the lesion, to gain some movement of the ligament over the underlying bone. This is followed by Grade A mobilization to maintain the function of the ligament.

The patient is encouraged to maintain a normal gait pattern with the aid of crutches if necessary. Once it is judged that the tensile strength of the healing ligament has improved, the depth of transverse frictions is gradually increased and the range of active pain-free movement becomes greater, aiming to apply a directional stress to encourage alignment of fibres. The regime continues until a full range of pain-free movement is restored, always guided by reassessment for a reduction or exacerbation of symptoms. Other exercises are incorporated as appropriate, aiming towards full rehabilitation of the patient.

Transverse frictions for acute sprain of the medial collateral ligament (Cyriax & Cyriax 1983, Cyriax 1984)

Position the patient in half lying with enough pillows to support the knee in the maximum amount of extension that can be achieved without causing pain. Palpate for the site of the lesion, which may be difficult to locate due to the swelling. However, the commonest site of sprain is at the joint line and this can be located by following the advice given in the surface marking and palpation section earlier in the chapter. Place two or three fingers across the site of the lesion and gently apply transverse frictions to achieve an analgesic effect (Fig. 11.32). Once some analgesia and depth are achieved, apply deeper transverse frictions for approximately six sweeps, aiming to move the ligament fibres over the underlying bone in imitation of its normal function. Follow this immediately with Grade A active mobilization towards extension.

Figure 11.32 Transverse friction massage of the acute medial collateral ligament sprain in extension.

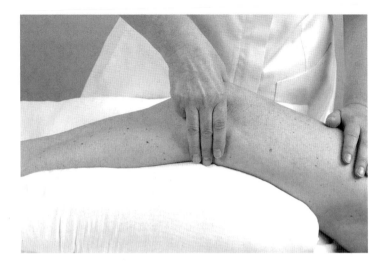

Next, support the knee in the maximum amount of flexion that can be achieved without pain, and repeat the friction technique as above (Fig. 11.33). Follow this immediately with Grade A active exercises towards flexion.

On a daily basis, the pain and swelling reduce and the range of movement increases. The knee should not be pushed towards extension as the medial collateral ligament is taut in extension and may become overstretched.

The usual exercises for maintenance of muscle strength should be included together with gait re-education and, eventually, full rehabilitation according to the patient's needs. Treating the ligament in this way maintains its mobility, length and function and should avoid the need to stretch.

An uncommon complication of medial collateral ligament sprain is Stieda–Pellegrini's syndrome (also known as Pellegrini–Stieda syndrome

Figure 11.33 Transverse friction massage of the acute medial collateral ligament sprain in flexion.

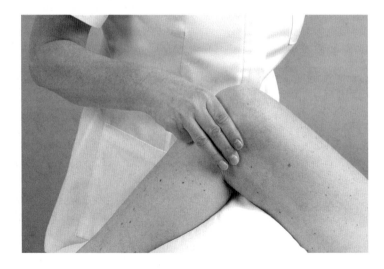

or Pellegrini–Stieda disease) and this should be considered if the range of movement at the knee fails to improve as expected (Cyriax 1982). It is believed that, following trauma to the medial collateral ligament, calcium is deposited in the ligament, usually near the superior medial femoral condyle (Wang & Shapiro 1995). Active movement of the knee joint is continued and corticosteroid injection may be appropriate if the pain persists.

Chronic medial collateral ligament sprain

The patient has a past history of sprain to the ligament which may have largely settled without treatment. However, activity still causes pain and transient swelling around the ligament. On examination, the patient may have end-range pain or limitation of movement of passive flexion, extension or both.

The valgus stress test produces the pain, as may hyperextension and passive lateral rotation – movements which tighten the ligament. Assessment should be made for instability and any associated structural damage of the cruciate ligaments and/or menisci.

The ligament has developed adhesions which interfere with the normal gliding function of the ligament. The principle of treatment is to rupture the unwanted adhesions with a Grade C manipulation, once the ligament has been prepared by deep transverse frictions. Following manipulative rupture, the patient is instructed to mobilize vigorously in order to maintain the movement gained through manipulation.

Grade C manipulation for chronic sprain of the medial collateral ligament (Cyriax and Cyriax 1983, Cyriax 1984)

The ligament is prepared for the manipulation with transverse frictions to achieve the analgesic effect. If passive extension is limited, position the patient in half lying with the knee in maximum extension and locate the site of the lesion by palpation, commonly at the joint line. Apply the transverse frictions with the index finger reinforced by the middle finger and the thumb placed on the opposite side of the knee for counterpressure (Fig. 11.34). Direct the pressure down onto the ligament and sweep

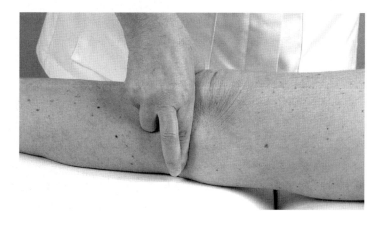

Figure 11.34 Transverse friction massage of the chronic medial collateral ligament sprain in extension.

transversely across the fibres, keeping the finger parallel to the upper border of the tibia. Treatment is applied until the analgesic effect is achieved.

The Grade C manipulation follows immediately after achieving the analgesic effect. Place one hand just above the knee to maintain the thigh on the couch. Wrap the other hand around the posterior aspect of the heel. Lean on the thigh, lifting the lower leg and, once end-range extension is achieved, apply the overpressure by a minimal amplitude, high velocity thrust applied by side flexing your body (Fig. 11.35).

If flexion is limited, next place the knee in maximum flexion. The direction of the transverse frictions will have to be adjusted to run parallel to the upper tibia, remembering that the ligament moves backwards a little in flexion (Fig. 11.36).

Figure 11.35   Grade C manipulation into extension.

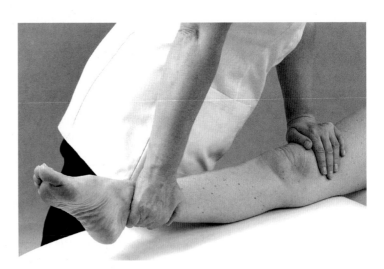

Figure 11.36   Transverse friction massage of the chronic medial ligament sprain in flexion.

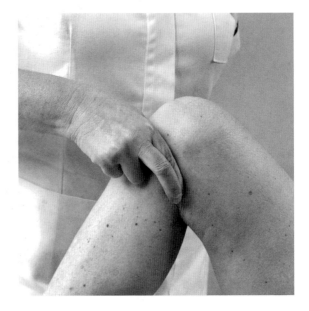

Figure 11.37   Grade C
manipulation into flexion:
a) starting position
b) completion of the
manoeuvre.

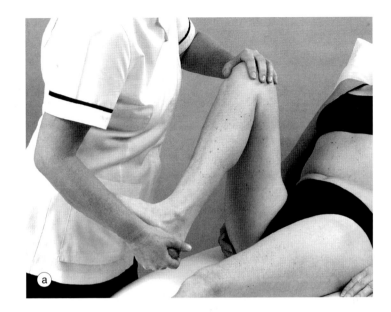

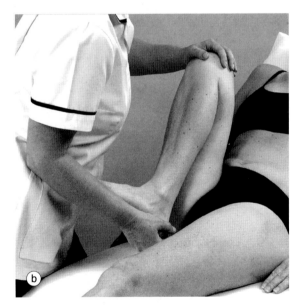

The Grade C manipulation follows immediately after achieving the analgesic effect by applying an overpressure towards flexion with the knee placed into lateral rotation, to achieve full range since the insertion of the medial collateral ligament sweeps forward. Place the hip and knee in maximum flexion. Cup the heel into your hand and pull the leg into lateral rotation by resting your forearm along the medial border of the foot (Fig. 11.37a). Maintain the lateral rotation and take the leg into maximum passive flexion. A minimal amplitude, high velocity thrust is applied into flexion (Fig. 11.37b). The technique can be modified to apply the thrust in the direction of the lateral rotation, or to add a valgus stress if assessment of the patient shows movement to be limited in these directions.

Treatment of chronic collateral ligament sprain is expected to be successful in two or three treatment sessions. It is important that the patient exercises the knee vigorously to maintain the mobility of the ligament.

CORONARY LIGAMENTS

The patient presents with a history of rotational strain and on examination there is pain on the appropriate passive rotation. The coronary ligaments may be involved in a hyperextension injury since the menisci move forwards during extension of the tibiofemoral joint. The longer lateral coronary ligaments are less vulnerable to trauma than the shorter medial coronary ligaments and the attachment of the medial meniscus to the deep part of the medial collateral ligament makes the medial aspect of the joint more susceptible to injury.

A sprain of the medial coronary ligaments will be discussed, but if the lesion lies in the lateral coronary ligaments, the same principles apply.

An effusion may be present depending on the severity of the lesion, but this is not usually as obvious as that occurring with injury to the collateral or cruciate ligaments. Medial coronary ligament sprain produces pain on passive lateral rotation of the tibia with the tibiofemoral joint at 90° of flexion. Pain may also be provoked by passive extension as the menisci move forwards on the tibia. Palpation confirms the site of the lesion, which is usually on the superior surface of the anteromedial aspect of the medial meniscus where the coronary ligaments attach the meniscus to the tibial plateau. It is essential that full palpation is conducted, including through the medial collateral ligament, to determine the extent of the lesion.

Transverse frictions to the coronary ligaments

The treatment of choice is transverse frictions. Position the patient comfortably in half lying with the knee in flexion and lateral rotation to expose the medial tibial condyle. Place an index finger reinforced by the middle finger on top of the edge of the medial meniscus at the site of the lesion in the medial coronary ligaments. Consider the position of the coronary ligaments that act as oblique 'staples' between the medial meniscus and the edge of the tibial plateau. Direct the pressure down onto the ligaments and sweep transversely across the fibres (Fig. 11.38). The transverse frictions are given for 10 min after the analgesic effect is achieved. Since the ligaments do not span the joint line, exercises or mobilization are not appropriate.

The ligaments may be injected, using the same position as for the transverse frictions and applying the general principles with regard to dosage, a peppering technique and advising relative rest for up to 2 weeks (Figs 11.39 and 11.40).

Figure 11.38   Transverse friction massage of the medial coronary ligaments.

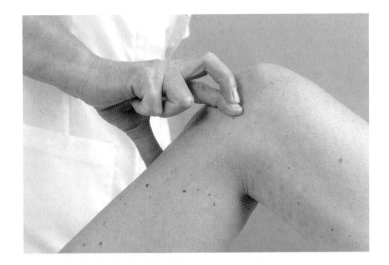

Figure 11.39   Injection of the medial coronary ligaments.

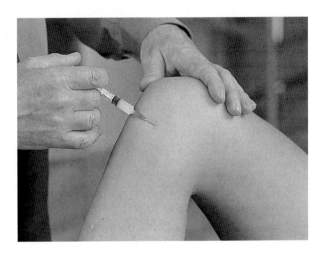

Figure 11.40   Injection of the medial coronary ligaments showing direction of approach and needle position.

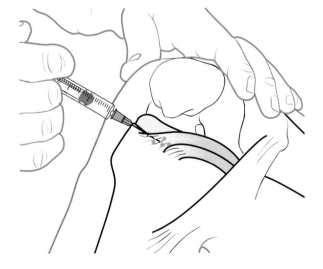

BURSITIS

Overuse or excessive friction can affect any of the bursae around the knee. The patient presents with pain localized to the site of the lesion and there may be local swelling. The prepatellar and infrapatellar bursae are commonly involved and, if swelling is a problem, the bursa can be drained. Bursitis may respond to locally applied electrotherapy or an injection of corticosteroid into the bursa. Before injecting the bursa, however, it is important to be sure that no infection is present, since septic bursitis is possible in the superficial bursae.

Pes anserinus syndrome may involve the tendons and/or bursa, but the condition may mimic medial collateral ligament sprain. Pain and tenderness occur 5–6 cm below the medial joint line; this is aggravated by activity and there may be slight swelling and crepitus over the bursal area. Treatment consists of locally applied anti-inflammatory modalities or applying the principles of corticosteroid injection (Safran & Fu 1995, Kesson et al 2003).

Excessive friction may cause iliotibial band syndrome involving the iliotibial tract and the underlying bursa. It particularly occurs in long-distance runners and cyclists and is often associated with tightness of the iliotibial tract (Safran & Fu 1995). Pain is felt laterally, 2–3 cm proximal to the knee joint. Aggravating factors are downhill running and climbing stairs. Local anti-inflammatory modalities may be applied together with a change in training techniques. General principles of treatment may be applied.

Injection of the bursae associated with the patella (Kesson et al 2003)

Suggested needle size: 21G × 1¹/₂ in (0.8 × 40 mm) green needle
Dose: 10 mg triamcinolone acetonide in a total volume of 2 ml

---

Position the patient with the knee supported in extension. Palpate for the tender area of the bursa and mark a point for insertion. Insert the needle into the mid-point of the tender area and inject as a bolus. Injection of the superficial infrapatellar bursa is illustrated in Figures 11.41 and 11.42, but the same principles can be applied to any bursa involved and the interested reader is referred to Kesson et al (2003).

Figure 11.41   Injection of the superficial infrapatellar bursa.

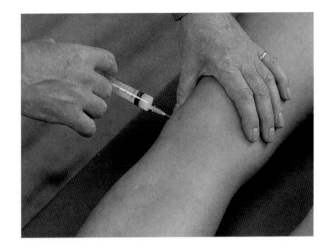

Figure 11.42   Injection of the superficial infrapatellar bursa showing direction of approach and needle position.

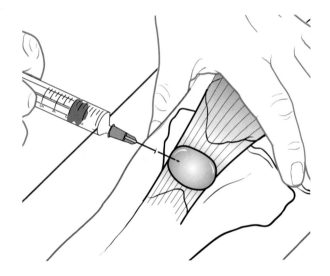

CONTRACTILE LESIONS

QUADRICEPS

Direct trauma to the quadriceps muscle belly causes swelling and superficial bruising which eventually tracks down the leg. Known in sporting circles as 'cork thigh', it has the potential to develop myositis ossificans traumatica, particularly if the contusion is accompanied by gross limitation of knee flexion (Norris 1998).

Transverse frictions to the quadriceps muscle belly

Position the patient in sitting with the knee straight to place the muscle belly in a shortened position. Locate the site of the lesion and, using the fingers, apply transverse frictions (Fig. 11.43). After the analgesic effect is achieved, apply six effective sweeps to the acute, irritable lesion and 10 min of deep transverse frictions for the chronic, non-irritable lesion, followed up by active Grade A exercises.

Figure 11.43 Transverse friction massage to the quadriceps muscle belly.

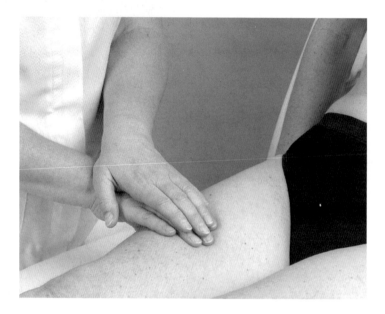

TENDINOPATHY OF THE MEDIAL AND LATERAL QUADRICEPS EXPANSIONS

The patient usually presents with a gradual onset of pain felt locally at the front of the knee associated with overuse. On examination there is pain on resisted knee extension and tenderness located at the medial, lateral or both borders of the patella. Often the lesion lies at the 'corners' of the patella.

Transverse frictions to the quadriceps expansions (Cyriax & Cyriax 1983, Cyriax 1984)

Having established the site of the lesion, deep transverse frictions are applied to the chronic lesion. Position the patient comfortably with the knee supported and relaxed in extension. Push and hold the patella to one side. Use the middle finger reinforced by the index finger and rotate the forearm to direct the pressure up and under the edge of the patella (Figs 11.44 and 11.45). Sweep transversely across the fibres in a superior–inferior direction and continue treatment for 10 min after the analgesic effect has been achieved. It may be necessary to treat several areas around the patella. Relative rest is advised where functional movements may continue, but no overuse or stretching until the structure is pain-free on resisted testing.

Figure 11.44   Transverse friction massage of the quadriceps expansions, medial.

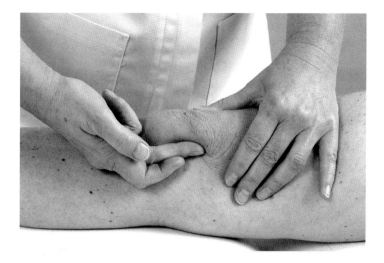

Figure 11.45   Transverse friction massage of the quadriceps expansions, lateral.

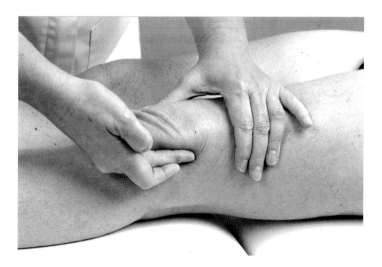

Overuse lesions of the quadriceps expansions may be secondary to malalignment or abnormal tracking of the patella. Treatment may be incorporated into a regime of corrective taping and re-education of the oblique portion of vastus medialis.

PATELLAR TENDINOPATHY

There are two sites for patellar tendinopathy:

- At the apex of the patella (infrapatellar tendon)
- At the base of the patella (suprapatellar tendon)

The most common is infrapatellar tendinopathy and it may be associated with repetitive jumping actions ('jumper's knee'). The repetitive overuse results in microfailure and fraying of the tendon fibres and areas of focal degeneration (Curwin & Stanish 1984).

The symptoms and signs are similar to those described for tendinopathy of the quadriceps expansions, but the site of the lesion will be located to either the infra- or suprapatellar tendons. Treatment may be deep transverse frictions or corticosteroid injection followed by relative rest. Infrapatellar fat pad inflammation (Hoffa's disease) produces symptoms that mimic infrapatellar tendinopathy, but pain is produced by gentle squeezing of the fat pad at either side of the patella (Curwin & Stanish 1984).

Transverse frictions to the infrapatellar and suprapatellar tendons (Cyriax & Cyriax 1983, Cyriax 1984)

Position the patient comfortably with the knee relaxed and supported in extension. Apply the web space between your index finger and thumb of one hand to the base of the patella, tilting the apex. Using the middle finger of the other hand reinforced by the index, supinate the forearm to direct the pressure up under the apex of the patella and sweep transversely across the fibres of the infrapatellar tendon (Fig. 11.46). Ten minutes' transverse frictions are applied after the analgesic effect is achieved. Relative rest is advised where functional movements may continue, but no overuse or stretching until the structure is pain-free on resisted testing.

Figure 11.46   Transverse frictions of the infrapatellar tendon.

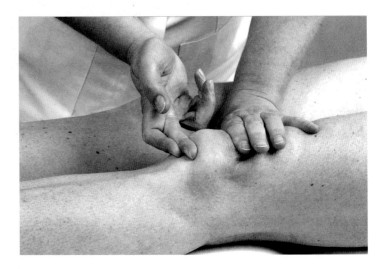

Injection of the infrapatellar and suprapatellar tendons (Cyriax & Cyriax 1983, Cyriax 1984)

Suggested needle size: 23G × 1 in (0.6 × 25 mm) blue needle
Dose: 20 mg triamcinolone acetonide in a total volume of 1.5 ml

Position the patient as described for the transverse frictions technique, applying pressure to the base of the patella with your stabilizing hand, to make the apex accessible (Fig. 11.47). Insert the needle just distal to the apex of the patella and advance until contact is made with bone. Deliver the injection by a peppering technique, fanning out to deposit two parallel rows of droplets of corticosteroid across the full width of the teno-osseous junction (Fig. 11.48). Note that the injection is delivered at the teno-osseous junction at the tendon–bone interface and not the body of the tendon, which is contraindicated. The patient is advised to maintain a period of relative rest for approximately 2 weeks following injection.

Figure 11.47   Injection of the infrapatellar tendon.

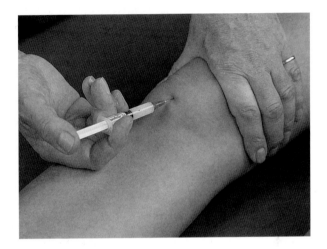

Figure 11.48   Injection of the infrapatellar tendon showing direction of approach and needle position.

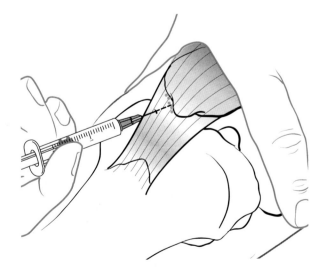

For treatment of suprapatellar tendinopathy, the above principles are applied with the base of the patella tilted upwards (Figs 11.49–11.51).

Figure 11.49   Transverse friction massage of the suprapatellar tendon.

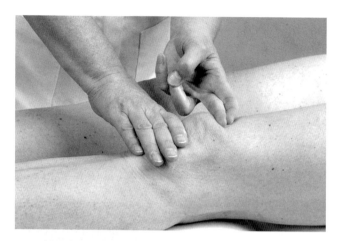

Figure 11.50   Injection of the suprapatellar tendon.

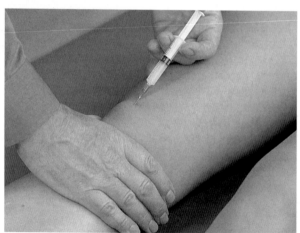

Figure 11.51   Injection of the suprapatellar tendon showing direction of approach and needle position.

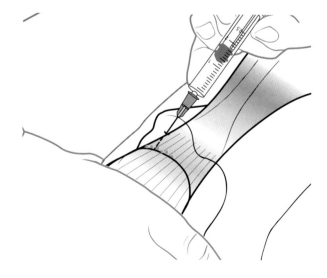

TENDINOPATHY OF THE INSERTIONS OF THE HAMSTRING MUSCLES

The patient presents with pain localized to the posterior aspect of the knee following a history of overuse. Pain is reproduced by resisted knee flexion and the site of tenderness is located medially or laterally according to the tendons involved. Principles of treatment can be applied using either deep transverse frictions or corticosteroid injection via a peppering technique. Relative rest is advised where functional movements may continue, but no overuse or stretching until the structure is pain-free on resisted testing.

Lesions of the hamstrings muscle belly and the tendon of origin are discussed in Chapter 10. Lesions of gastrocnemius are discussed in Chapter 12.

References

Adler G G, Hoekman R A, Beach D M 1995 Drop leg Lachman test. American Journal of Sports Medicine 23:320–323

Amiel D, Kuiper S, Akeson W H 1990 Cruciate ligaments. In: Daniel D, Akeson W H, O'Connor J J (eds) Knee ligaments: structure, function, injury and repair. Lippincott, Williams & Wilkins, Philadelphia, pp 365–376

Barrack R L, Skinner H B 1990 The sensory function of knee ligaments. In: Daniel D, Akeson W H, O'Connor J J (eds) Knee ligaments: structure, function, injury and repair. Lippincott, Williams & Wilkins, Philadelphia, pp 95–112

Bessette G C 1992 The meniscus. Orthopaedics 15:35–42

Bijl D, van Baar M E, Oostendorp R A B et al 1998 Validity of Cyriax' concept of capsular pattern for the diagnosis of osteoarthritis of hip and/or knee. Scandinavian Journal of Rheumatology 27:347–351

Boles C A, Martin D F 2001 Synovial plicae in the knee. American Journal of Roentgenology 177:221–227

Bozkurt M, Yilmaz E, Atlihan D et al 2003 The proximal tibiofibular joint. Clinical Orthopaedics and Related Research 406:136–140

Burks R T 1990 Gross anatomy. In: Daniel D, Akeson W H, O'Connor J J (eds) Knee ligaments: structure, function, injury and repair. Lippincott, Williams & Wilkins, Philadelphia, pp 59–75

Butler D L, Noyes F R, Grood E S 1980 Ligamentous restraints to anterior–posterior drawer in the human knee. Journal of Bone and Joint Surgery 62A:259–270

Cailliet R 1992 Knee pain and disability, 3rd edn. F A Davis, Philadelphia

Cameron G 1995 Steroid arthropathy – myth or reality? Journal of Orthopaedic Medicine 17:51–55

Chakravarty K, Pharoah P D 1994 A randomized controlled study of post-injection rest following intra-articular steroid therapy for knee synovitis. British Journal of Rheumatology 33(5):464–468

Curtin W, O'Farrell D, McGoldrick F et al 1992 The correlation between clinical diagnosis of knee pathology and findings in arthroscopy. Irish Journal of Medical Science 161:135–136

Curwin S, Stanish W D 1984 Jumper's knee. Tendinitis – its etiology and treatment. Collamore Press, Massachusetts

Cyriax J 1982 Textbook of orthopaedic medicine, 8th edn. Baillière Tindall, London, vol 1

Cyriax J 1984 Textbook of orthopaedic medicine, 11th edn. Baillière Tindall, London, vol 2

Cyriax J, Cyriax P 1983 Illustrated manual of orthopaedic medicine. Butterworths, London

Daniel D M 1990 Diagnosis of a ligament injury. In: Daniel D, Akeson W H, O'Connor J J (eds) Knee ligaments: structure, function, injury and repair. Lippincott, Williams & Wilkins, Philadelphia, pp 3–10

Edwards D, Villar R 1993 Anterior cruciate ligament injury. Practitioner 237:113–117

El-Dieb A, Yu J S, Huang G-S et al 2002 Pathologic conditions of the ligaments and tendons of the knee. Radiologic Clinics of North America 40:1061–1079

Evans P 1986 The knee joint. Churchill Livingstone, Edinburgh

Felson D T, Anderson J J, Naimark A et al 1988 Obesity and knee osteoarthritis. Annals of Internal Medicine 109(1):18–24

Felson D T, Chaisson C 1997 Understanding the relationship between body weight and osteoarthritis. Baillière's Clinical Rheumatology 11(4):671–681

Fritz J M, Delitto A, Efhard R E et al 1998 An examination of the selective tissue tension scheme with evidence for the concept of the capsular pattern of the knee. Physical Therapy 78(10):1046–1056

Greis P E, Bardana D D, Holmstrom M C et al 2002 Meniscal injury, I. Basic science and evaluation. Journal of American Academy of Orthopaedic Surgeons 10(3):168–176

Hartley A 1995 Practical joint assessment – lower quadrant, 2nd edn. Mosby, London

Hill C L, Gale D G, Chaisson C R et al 2001 Knee effusions, popliteal cysts and synovial thickening: association with knee pain. Journal of Rheumatology 28(6):1330–1337

Jacobson J A, Lenchik L, Ruhoy M K et al 1997 MR imaging of the infrapatellar fat pad of Hoffa. Radiographics 17(3):675–691

Kapandji I A 1987 The physiology of the joints: lower limb, 5th edn. Churchill Livingstone, Edinburgh, vol 2

Katz J W, Fingeroth R J 1986 The diagnostic accuracy of ruptures of the anterior cruciate ligament comparing the Lachman test, the anterior drawer sign, and the pivot shift test in acute and chronic knee injuries. American Journal of Sports Medicine 14:88–91

Kesson M, Atkins A, Davies I 2003 Musculoskeletal injection skills. Butterworth Heinemann, Oxford

LaPrade R F 1998 The anatomy of the deep infrapatellar bursa of the knee. American Journal of Sports Medicine 26(1):129–132

Malanga G A, Andrus S, Nadler S F et al 2003 Physical examination of the knee: a review of the original test description and scientific validity of common orthopaedic tests. Archives of Physical Medicine and Rehabilitation 84:592–603

Nordin M, Frankel V H 2001 Basic biomechanics of the musculoskeletal system, 3rd edn. Lippincott, Williams & Wilkins, Philadelphia

Norris C M 1998 Sports injuries: diagnosis and management for physiotherapists, 2nd edn. Butterworth Heinemann, Oxford

Palastanga N, Field D, Soames R 2002 Anatomy and human movement, 4th edn. Butterworth Heinemann, Oxford

Parikh J R, Houpt J B, Jacobs S et al 1993 Charcot's arthropathy of the shoulder following intra-articular corticosteroid injections. Journal of Rheumatology 20:885–887

Perko M M J, Cross M J, Ruske D et al 1992 Anterior cruciate ligament injuries, clues for diagnosis. Medical Journal of Australia 157:467–470

Pope T L, Winston-Salem N C 1996 MR imaging of the knee ligaments. Journal of the Southern Orthopaedic Association 5(1):46–62

Raynauld J-P, Buckland-Wright C, Ward R et al 2003 Safety and efficacy of long-term intraarticular steroid injection in osteoarthritis of the knee. Arthritis and Rheumatism 48(2):370–377

Rubinstein R A, Shelbourne K D, McCarroll J R et al 1994 The accuracy of the clinical examination in the setting of posterior cruciate ligament injuries. American Journal of Sports Medicine 22:550–557

Safran M R, Fu F H 1995 Uncommon causes of knee pain in the athlete. Orthopedic Clinics of North America 26:547–559

Saunders S 2000 Orthopaedic medicine course manual. Saunders, London

Schenck R C, Heckman J D 1993 Injuries of the knee. Clinical Symposia 45:2–32

Schweitzer M E, Tran D, Deely D M et al 1995 Medial collateral ligament injuries: evaluation of multiple signs, prevalence and location of associated bone bruises, and assessment with MR imaging. Radiology 194(3):825–829

Smith B W, Green G A 1995 Acute knee injuries: part I. History and physical examination. American Family Physician 51:615–621

Staron R B, Haramati N, Feldman F et al 1994 O'Donaghue's triad: magnetic resonance imaging evidence. International Skeletal Society 23:633–636

Torg J S, Conrad W, Kalen V 1974 Clinical diagnosis of anterior cruciate ligament instability in the athlete. American Journal of Sports Medicine 4:84–93

Valley V T, Shermer C D 2000 Use of musculoskeletal ultrasonography in the diagnosis of pes anserine tendinopathy: a case report. Journal of Emergency Medicine 20(1):43–45

Wang J C, Shapiro M S 1995 Pellegrini–Steida syndrome. American Journal of Orthopaedics 24(6):493–497

Williams P L 1998 Gray's Anatomy: the anatomical basis of medicine and surgery, 38th edn. Churchill Livingstone, Edinburgh

Woo S L-Y, Wang C, Newton P O et al 1990 The response of ligaments to stress deprivation and stress enhancement. In: Daniel D, Akeson W H, O'Connor J J (eds) Knee ligaments: structure, function, injury and repair. Lippincott, Williams & Wilkins, Philadelphia, pp 337–350

Chapter **12**

The ankle and foot

SUMMARY

Sprained ankle is a commonly encountered traumatic lesion in primary care. Mismanagement leads to a chronic persistent condition and likely recurrence. Other lesions of the foot and ankle have been attributed to faulty biomechanics which may also lead to adaptive postures in the lower limb and spine, with consequent problems.

This chapter confines itself to common lesions in the ankle and foot arising from arthritis, trauma or overuse and begins with a presentation of the relevant anatomy and palpation techniques to aid their identification. Points from the history are considered and a logical sequence of objective examination is given, followed by discussion of lesions and suggestions for treatment and management.

ANATOMY

INERT STRUCTURES

The *inferior tibiofibular joint* is the articulation between the fibular notch on the lateral aspect of the tibia and the distal end of the fibula. It is considered to be a syndesmosis because the firm union of the two bones is largely due to the interosseous membrane. Anterior and posterior ligaments reinforce the joint.

The deep part of the posterior ligament is the *inferior transverse tibiofibular ligament* which passes under the posterior ligament from the tibia into the malleolar fossa of the fibular. It is a thickened band of yellow elastic fibres forming part of the articulating surface of the ankle joint.

The firm union of the inferior tibiofibular joint is significant to the mortise of the ankle joint and a major factor in its inherent stability. When the ankle joint is in dorsiflexion, the close packed position, the elastic nature of the inferior tibiofibular joint ligament allows the joint to yield and separate, accommodating the wider anterior aspect of the trochlear surface of the talus. In plantarflexion the ligament recoils as the narrower posterior aspect of the talus moves into the mortise, approximating the malleoli to maintain a pinch-like grip on the talus.

Dorsiflexion and plantarflexion of the ankle will induce small accessory movements in the inferior tibiofibular joint which in turn affect the superior tibiofibular joint. Injuries of the syndesmosis usually involve forced dorsiflexion, causing widening or diastasis of the ankle mortise (Edwards & DeLee 1984, Boytim et al 1991, Marder 1994). However, isolated injuries are uncommon and damage usually occurs in association with other major ligamentous disruption and fracture.

The *ankle joint (talocrural joint)* is a uniaxial, synovial hinge joint between the mortise, formed by the distal ends of the tibia and fibula, including both malleoli, and the dome of the talus. Its function is complex, with the talocrural, subtalar and inferior tibiofibular joints working in concert to allow coordinated movement of the rear foot (Hertel 2002). It bears more weight per unit area than any other joint, and any malalignment or instability may lead to degenerative changes (Sartoris 1994). The joint surfaces are covered with hyaline cartilage and surrounded by a fibrous capsule which attaches to the margins of the articulating surfaces. The capsule is lined with synovium and reinforced by strong collateral ligaments. The congruity of the articular surfaces during loading of the joint, the static ligamentous control and the dynamic control of the musculotendinous units all contribute to the stability of the ankle joint (Hertel 2002).

The collateral ligaments are roughly triangular in their attachments, radiating downwards from the malleoli to a wide base. Each has anterior and posterior components which link with the talus, and a central component that links with the calcaneum.

Movement at the ankle joint occurs about a transverse axis in a sagittal plane and amounts to approximately 20° of dorsiflexion and 35° of plantarflexion, allowing the foot to adjust to the surface on which it is placed. Dorsiflexion achieves the close packed position of the ankle joint and no movement of the talus in the mortise should be possible in this position. In full plantarflexion, the loose packed position, a small amount of side-to-side movement of the talus should be possible.

The *medial collateral (deltoid) ligament* forms a strong multiligamentous complex spreading out in a fan shape over the medial aspect of the ankle joint. It forms a continuous line of attachment from the navicular in front, along the sustentaculum tali to the talus behind. The origins and insertions of the various parts of the ligament are contiguous and therefore not clearly demarcated, but it is generally accepted to have deep and superficial fibres. The superficial fibres cross the ankle and subtalar joints, while the deep fibres cross the ankle joint (Boss & Hintermann 2002).

As the medial collateral ligament offers such strong support to the medial aspect of the ankle joint, traumatic injuries more commonly cause fracture and disruption of the syndesmosis rather than ligamentous injury. Most strain on the ligament occurs with a dorsiflexion and eversion stress. Biomechanical problems in the foot can, however, lead to a gradual onset overuse lesion of the medial collateral ligament and treatment should be directed to the cause.

The *lateral collateral ligament* consists of three separate bands which leave the ligament deficient in its support of the lateral aspect of the ankle

Figure 12.1   Lateral collateral ligament of the ankle.

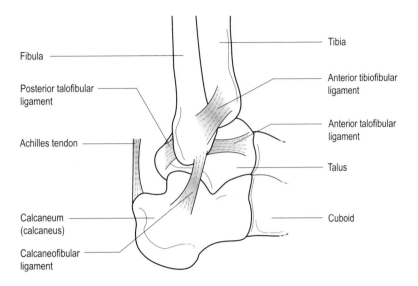

joint. Consequently forced inversion of the plantarflexed foot commonly affects the lateral collateral ligament (Liu & Jason 1994, Lee & Maleski 2002).

The components of the lateral collateral ligament are as follows (Fig. 12.1):

- The *anterior talofibular ligament* is an integral part of the capsule of the ankle joint. It arises from the anterior border and tip of the lateral malleolus and passes deeply and anteromedially across the ankle joint to the neck of the talus in the sinus tarsi. It is a wide, flattened band approximately the width of the patient's index finger. In the anatomical position, the ligament runs almost parallel to the transverse axis of the foot, while in plantarflexion it runs more parallel to the vertical axis of the leg. In this position, the ligament is most likely to be sprained particularly if the foot is inverted (Kannus & Renstrom 1991, Kumai et al 2002). It is the most vulnerable of the three components to forced plantarflexion or inversion injury (Hertel 2002)
- The *calcaneofibular ligament* is a narrow cord, separate from the capsule of the ankle joint. It arises from the apex of the lateral malleolus and passes obliquely inferoposteriorly, under the peroneal tendons, to attach to the calcaneum just behind the peroneal tubercle. Here it is closely related to the overlying peroneal sheath containing the tendons of peroneus longus and brevis (Marder 1994, Miller & Bosco 2002). This component of the ligament crosses both the ankle and subtalar joints and is vulnerable to varus stress; it is most taut in dorsiflexion
- The *posterior talofibular ligament* is a strong, thick band arising from the posterior border of the lateral malleolus and passing

horizontally and posteromedially to the posterior aspect of the talus. Clinically, it is rare to find involvement of this ligamentous component

The contribution of the individual lateral ligaments to ankle joint stability is not constant, but depends on the position of the ankle and foot in space. Ligamentous stabilization is most critical in the unloaded ankle as this is when injury tends to occur as initial contact is made with the ground during the gait cycle. During weight-bearing, stability is maintained by the bony congruency of the mortise. The anterior talofibular ligament has the weakest tensile strength with a load to failure two to three and a half times lower than that for the calcaneofibular ligament which is rarely injured in isolation (Boruta et al 1990, Miller & Bosco 2002).

The foot consists of 26 bones and 57 joints which enable it to act as a rigid structure for weight-bearing, e.g. pointing in ballet, or to be converted into a flexible structure for mobility, e.g. gait activities (Nordin & Frankel 2001). The foot supports body weight and controls posture by maintaining the centre of gravity. It assists propulsion and lift, as well as restraining gait activities and acting as a shock absorber. To provide this variety of functions, arches have developed together with the joints, ligaments and muscles, all contributing to functional activities. The main joints and ligaments of the arches, of clinical concern in orthopaedic medicine, will be described briefly here.

The *subtalar (talocalcaneal) joint* is a synovial joint between the talus and underlying calcaneum, which works in conjunction with the ankle and mid-tarsal joints to form a functional component. These joints together allow the foot to adapt to the surface of stance and to act as a shock absorber. They allow adjustment of the arches of the foot and, in conjunction with muscle activity, provide spring and propulsion to gait. During walking, the subtalar joint adapts to the side-to-side slope of the ground, accompanied by secondary rotation of the tibia (Evans 1990).

The subtalar joint consists of separate anterior and posterior joint cavities divided by the sinus tarsi (a narrow tunnel running obliquely forwards and laterally between the talus and the calcaneum). Interosseous and cervical ligaments stabilize the subtalar joint and form a barrier between the two joint capsules; they have been described as the 'cruciate ligaments of the subtalar joint' (Hertel 2002). This division of the subtalar joints has implications for injection of the joint which will be discussed below.

Movements at the subtalar joint are complex due to the shape of the articulating facets, which allow a degree of play to occur simultaneously in three planes. The calcaneum 'pitches', 'turns' and 'rolls' (Kapandji 1987) under the talus, enabling these accessory movements to contribute to the functional movements of the joint. This results in triplanar motion of the talus around a single oblique axis. The subtalar joint, therefore, is a uniaxial joint with one degree of freedom of movement, supination, which achieves a varus position of the calcaneum, and pronation, which achieves a valgus position of the calcaneum (Levangie & Norkin 2001).

The *mid-tarsal (transverse tarsal) joints* consist of the calcaneocuboid joint laterally and the talocalcaneonavicular joint medially. These joints adapt the posture of the foot, keeping the sole of the foot in contact with the ground whatever the slope of the surface or the position of the leg. Together they act as a shock absorber as well as providing elasticity and spring to gait.

The *calcaneocuboid joint* is supported by the *dorsal calcaneocuboid ligament* which is a capsular ligament that runs along the dorsolateral aspect of the joint and the *plantar calcaneocuboid* (the short plantar) and the *long plantar ligaments* (Levangie & Norkin 2001, Palastanga et al 2002). The dorsal calcaneocuboid ligament is sometimes involved in an inversion sprain of the ankle as it resists inversion and adduction of the mid-tarsal joint. The *talocalcaneonavicular joint* is supported by the *spring ligament* (otherwise known as the plantar calcaneonavicular ligament) which spans the gap between the calcaneum and navicular below the talar head. Consequentially, this joint can be visualized as a ball and socket joint. The facet on the head and lower surface of the neck of the talus forms the ball, the osseoligamentous socket being formed by the navicular anteriorly, the sustentaculum tali and calcaneum posteriorly and the spring ligament, which links the sustentaculum tali and navicular, supporting the head of the talus.

Movements at the mid-tarsal joint (calcaneocuboid and talocalcaneonavicular joint complex) do not occur in isolation (Levangie & Norkin 2001, Palastanga et al 2002). Accessory movements at the mid-tarsal joints consist of dorsiflexion and plantarflexion, abduction and adduction, and inversion and eversion.

A series of arches, ligaments and muscles satisfies the requirements of the foot to be able to provide both strength and mobility.

- The medial and lateral longitudinal arches are supported posteriorly by the calcaneum and anteriorly by the metatarsal heads. The talus forms the summit of the arch. The *medial longitudinal arch* is the larger of the two and has a dynamic role for gait. It consists of the calcaneum, talus, navicular, the cuneiforms and three medial metatarsals. It absorbs and transmits weight backwards through the calcaneum and forwards to the metatarsal heads, while providing elasticity for propulsion. The *lateral longitudinal arch* has a static role for weight-bearing. It is lower than the medial, making contact with the ground throughout its length to support load in standing. The main supporting mechanism for the longitudinal arches is the plantar fascia. Acting as a cable between the heel and the toes, it locks the joints of the foot and prevents the arches from collapsing during weight-bearing
- The *transverse arch* is formed by the distal row of tarsal bones and the bases of the metatarsals, and acts to support and transmit body weight. As body weight is applied, the metatarsal bones separate and flatten slightly

The arches of the foot depend on ligamentous and muscular support. The important ligaments are the long and short plantar ligaments, plantar aponeurosis and the spring ligament (plantar calcaneonavicular ligament). The intrinsic muscles of the foot maintain the arches, together with some of the long muscles of the leg. Tibialis anterior supports the medial arch, while peroneus longus supports the lateral arch.

The *plantar fascia* is a strong aponeurosis on the plantar surface of the foot which, together with the mid-tarsal ligaments and intrinsic and extrinsic muscles, withstands loading during weight-bearing. It consists of three variably developed components known as central, medial and lateral cords. The central cord is biomechanically the most important, arising from the medial side of the medial calcaneal tuberosity and consisting of longitudinally arranged fibres of collagen and elastin. The fibres pass distally into the forefoot, widening and thinning before dividing into five distinct bands that extend into the toes (Karr 1994, Yu 2000). At its insertion into the calcaneal tuberosity (the enthesis) it has a thickened 'cuff' similar in appearance to the rotator cuff of the shoulder (Yu 2000). This strong connecting cable passing between the pillars of the longitudinal arch has very little ability to lengthen, but under loading gives slightly to act as a shock absorber.

CONTRACTILE STRUCTURES

The numerous tendons crossing the ankle joint complex contribute to dynamic stability as well as producing movement of the various joints. The lateral muscles have a role in controlling supination and the anterior muscles probably slow the plantarflexion component of supination, acting to prevent injury to the lateral ligaments (Hertel 2002). As tendons cross the ankle joint, they change their direction from running vertically to horizontally. Several retinacula prevent the tendons from bowstringing under activity, while synovial sheaths protect the tendons as they pass under the retinacula.

The talus provides attachment for ligaments and many tendons pass over it, although it does not itself give insertion to any contractile unit.

All anterior muscles of the lower leg are supplied by the deep peroneal nerve and their principal function is dorsiflexion of the ankle and extension of the toes.

Tibialis anterior (L4–L5) takes origin from the upper two-thirds of the lateral tibial shaft and adjacent interosseous membrane. It becomes tendinous in its lower third, passing across the anteromedial aspect of the ankle joint to insert into the medial aspect of the medial cuneiform and the base of the first metatarsal. Its function is to dorsiflex the ankle during the swing-through phase of gait and to invert the foot. It raises the medial longitudinal arch and works in conjunction with other muscles to counteract gravity and to control foot placement. This tendon runs a relatively straight course and is not a common cause of pain. However, hill running or irritation from tight-fitting boots, for example, may cause lesions of tibialis anterior (Frey & Shereff 1988, Chandnani & Bradley 1994).

Extensor hallucis longus (L5, S1) takes origin from the middle of the anteromedial border of the fibula and passes downwards and medially to a tendon which inserts into the base of the distal phalanx of the hallux.

Functionally it dorsiflexes the ankle and extends the hallux to enable the big toe and foot to clear the ground during the swing-through phase.

Extensor digitorum longus (L5, S1) takes origin from the upper two-thirds of the anterior aspect of the fibula and passes downwards under the extensor retinacula, dividing into four tendons which insert into the dorsal digital expansions of the lateral four toes. Functionally, it assists dorsiflexion of the ankle and extends the lateral four toes, to clear the ground during the swing-through phase.

Peroneus tertius (L5, S1), a divorced part of extensor digitorum longus, arises from the lower anterolateral aspect of the fibula and inserts into the base of the fifth metatarsal. It functions as a weak dorsiflexor of the ankle and an evertor of the foot.

The peroneal muscles pass under two rectinacula to reach the lateral side of the foot. The principal function of the lateral muscles is to evert the foot, controlling side-to-side movements in standing and acting as the primary lateral dynamic stabilizers of the ankle (Frey & Shereff 1988). Peroneus longus, together with tibialis anterior, forms a stirrup for the foot, maintaining and supporting the arches. Both peroneus longus and brevis are supplied by the superficial peroneal nerve.

Peroneus longus is the main evertor of the foot and draws the medial side of the foot down, as in plantarflexion and eversion. Peroneus brevis also produces eversion and plantarflexion (Palastanga et al 2002).

Peroneus longus (L5, S1–S2), the more superficial of the two peroneal tendons, arises from the head and upper lateral two-thirds of the fibula. It becomes tendinous just above the ankle and passes behind the lateral malleolus in a sheath common to it and peroneus brevis. Continuing on, it crosses the lateral surface of the calcaneum, passing below the peroneal tubercle, where it leaves peroneus brevis. It occupies a groove on the lateral and plantar surfaces of the cuboid and crosses the sole of the foot obliquely to insert into the lateral side of the base of the first metatarsal and adjacent medial cuneiform.

Peroneus brevis (L5, S1–S2) arises from the lower lateral surface of the fibula. It lies in front of peroneus longus as the tendons pass behind the lateral malleolus in the common sheath. It crosses the calcaneum above the peroneal tubercle to insert into the base of the fifth metatarsal.

Generally, the more superficial posterior muscles are concerned mainly with plantarflexion of the ankle, while the deep muscles flex the toes. Both groups are supplied by the tibial nerve.

Gastrocnemius (S1–S2) is the most superficial of the posterior muscles and gives the calf its characteristic shape. It has two heads of origin from the appropriate posterior femoral condyle. The medial head is larger, extends more distally and is a common site for muscle belly injuries. The two muscle heads come together in a broad tendon which is joined on the anterolateral side by soleus, forming the Achilles tendon. Functionally, gastrocnemius flexes the knee and plantarflexes the ankle.

Soleus (S1–S2) lies deep to gastrocnemius, arising from the upper posterior aspect of the fibula and soleal line of the tibia. The muscle fibres blend into a membranous tendon which lies deep to the gastrocnemius, allowing both muscles to function individually. These tendon fibres then merge with the Achilles tendon.

Plantaris (S1–S2) arises from the posterior aspect of the lateral supracondylar ridge of the femur and descends medially to blend with the Achilles tendon. Its function is to assist gastrocnemius.

Gastrocnemius, soleus and plantaris form a functional group known as *triceps surae*; as well as functioning together they also have independent functions. Gastrocnemius works with plantaris to flex the knee and plantarflex the foot, providing propulsion to the push-off phase of gait. Soleus works continuously as a postural muscle through its slow-twitch muscle fibres which maintain the upright posture (McMinn et al 1995). In standing, the ankle is in a loose packed position with the centre of gravity falling anterior to the joint. Soleus counteracts the tendency for body weight to move forwards over the stationary foot (Williams 1998).

The *Achilles tendon* is a long tendon which receives the fibres of gastrocnemius and soleus. The insertion of the Achilles tendon is cushioned by two bursae – the retrocalcaneal bursa on its deep surface and the subcutaneous Achilles bursa on its superficial surface (Smart et al 1980). The tendon fibres twist as they pass down to their insertion into the middle of the posterior surface of the calcaneum. This twist in the tendon fibres is understood to be responsible for the tendon's elastic properties, the stored energy providing propulsion to lift the heel during walking, running and jumping activities (Norris 1998). The tendon has a zone of relatively poor vascularity 2–6 cm above its insertion and is prone to overuse, degeneration and rupture, particularly at this site (Smart et al 1980, Chandnani & Bradley 1994).

Tibialis posterior (L4–L5) arises from the upper posterolateral surface of the tibia. It passes behind the medial malleolus in its own sheath, crosses the deltoid ligament and inserts into the tuberosity of the navicular. It sends tendinous slips onto every tarsal bone except the talus. Functionally it is the main invertor of the foot, working with tibialis anterior. It gives support to the arches of the foot through its many tendinous insertions. It decelerates subtalar pronation after heel contact (Blake et al 1994). Activities which involve rapid changes in direction (e.g. soccer, tennis, hockey) place increased stress on tibialis posterior and make it vulnerable to injury in these situations (Frey & Shereff 1988).

Flexor digitorum longus (S2–S3) arises from the middle of the posterior surface of the tibia and passes downwards, becoming tendinous above the ankle joint. Behind the medial malleolus it is medial to tibialis posterior and occupies the groove under the sustentaculum tali. Dividing into four tendons, it inserts into the base of the distal phalanx of the lateral four toes. Functionally, flexor digitorum longus works with the lumbricals to keep the pads of the toes in contact with the ground, increasing the weight-bearing surface. It also acts to assist plantarflexion during the toe-off phase of gait, and repeated push-off activity may cause injury to this tendon (Frey & Shereff 1988).

The *lumbricals* (S2–S3) arise from flexor digitorum longus tendons and insert into the dorsal digital expansions. They flex the metatarsophalangeal joints and extend the interphalangeal joints; this counteracts the clawing tendency of the flexor digitorum longus. Together they maintain the medial arch.

Flexor hallucis longus (S2–S3) arises from the lower posterior surface of the fibula and passes behind the medial malleolus and under the sustentaculum tali to insert into the base of the distal phalanx of the big toe. It functions to provide the final thrust for toe-off and is important in supporting the medial longitudinal arch. Activities which involve repeatedly pushing off from the forefoot (e.g. ballet) may cause lesions in this tendon (Frey & Shereff 1988).

A GUIDE TO SURFACE MARKING AND PALPATION

MEDIAL ASPECT (Fig. 12.2)

Palpate the short, thick, *medial tibial malleolus*, appreciating that the apex, anterior and posterior borders are all subcutaneous. Compare this with the longer, slender, *lateral fibular malleolus* which tends to project further distally and lie slightly more posteriorly.

It is difficult to palpate the tendons lying behind the medial malleolus, but from medial to lateral they are *t*ibialis posterior, flexor *d*igitorum longus and flexor *h*allucis longus (*Tom*, *Dick* and *Harry*). You can palpate the *posterior tibial pulse* by applying light pressure behind the medial malleolus, approximately halfway between it and the Achilles tendon.

Consider the triangular *medial (deltoid) collateral ligament* which fans down from the medial malleolus to attach by a broad base from the navicular in front, to the talus behind.

Palpate the *sustentaculum tali* lying approximately one thumb's width directly below the medial malleolus, where it feels like a horizontal, bony shelf.

Figure 12.2   Medial aspect of the ankle.

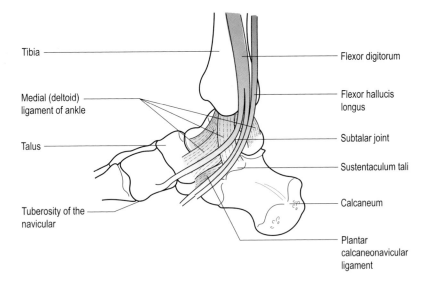

Move directly forwards from the sustentaculum tali to the next palpable bony bump, the *tuberosity of the navicular*. This gives insertion to *tibialis posterior* and lies at the level of the lip of a slip-on shoe. Move directly forwards from the navicular to palpate the *medial cuneiform* and the *base of the first metatarsal*.

ANTERIOR ASPECT (Fig. 12.3)

Place the ankle joint into plantarflexion and inversion, making the *talus* both visible and palpable anterior to the lateral malleolus. Palpate along from the anterior aspect of the lateral malleolus and the lower margin of the tibia to the anterior aspect of the medial malleolus to identify the *joint line of the ankle*.

Move to the front of the lateral malleolus and feel the depression on the lateral side of the talus; this marks the entrance to the *sinus tarsi* (the

Figure 12.3   Anterior aspect of the ankle.

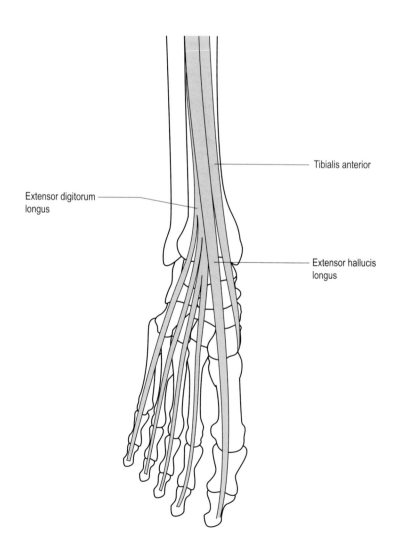

Tibialis anterior

Extensor digitorum longus

Extensor hallucis longus

Figure 12.4   Posterior
structures of the ankle.

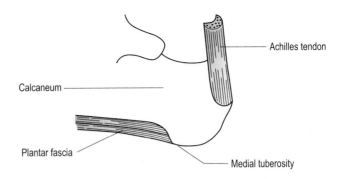

narrow tunnel which runs between the talus and calcaneum in front of the subtalar joint).

Palpate the *tibialis anterior, extensor hallucis longus, extensor digitorum longus and peroneus tertius tendons* (from medial to lateral) as they cross the ankle joint anteriorly.

Palpate the *dorsalis pedis pulse* approximately halfway between the malleoli on the dorsum of the foot, just lateral to the tendon of extensor hallucis longus.

POSTERIOR ASPECT (Fig. 12.4)

Palpate the *calcaneum*, the largest of the tarsal bones, which forms the bony prominence of the heel.

Palpate the *medial tuberosity of the calcaneum*, which can be located at the posteromedial edge of the plantar surface of the calcaneum; deep palpation may be necessary. This marks the insertion of the middle cord of the plantar fascia (Fig. 12.5).

Figure 12.5   Plantar fascia.

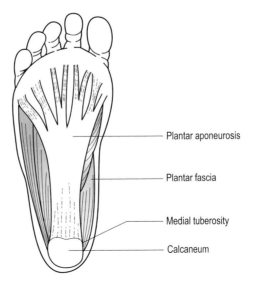

Locate the insertion of the *Achilles tendon* into the middle third of the posterior surface of the calcaneum. Palpate the Achilles tendon, appreciating its thickness, and follow it up to the two fleshy bellies of the gastrocnemius; the medial belly should be felt to extend further distally than the lateral.

LATERAL ASPECT
(Fig. 12.6)

Palpate the *lateral malleolus*. Move approximately one finger's width below it and slightly anteriorly to locate the *peroneal tubercle*. This tubercle varies in size and position so may not be obvious. It divides the tendons of peroneus longus and brevis.

Consider the individual components of the lateral collateral ligament which take origin from the lateral malleolus. The *anterior talofibular ligament* is approximately the width of an index finger and it passes deeply, anteromedially to the talus. Its fibres run roughly parallel to the sole of the foot and it may be palpated in the region of the sinus tarsi. The *calcaneofibular ligament* passes obliquely downwards and backwards, under the peroneal tendons. The *posterior talofibular ligament* passes horizontally backwards to attach to the posterior talus; it is difficult to palpate.

Palpate the *base of the fifth metatarsal* and appreciate its prominent tubercle which gives attachment to peroneus brevis. Placing a thumb vertically behind the base of the fifth metatarsal will indicate the approximate position of the calcaneocuboid joint line. Placing another thumb or finger transversely across the tip of the thumb forms a T and the cross-bar of the T is resting over the dorsal aspect of the joint, indicating the approximate position of the *dorsal calcaneocuboid ligament*.

Position your hand to resist eversion of the foot, to aid identification of the two lateral tendons, *peroneus longus and brevis*. Behind the lateral malleolus, peroneus brevis lies in front of longus. They divide at the peroneal tubercle, with brevis running above the tubercle and longus below.

Figure 12.6   Structures of the lateral aspect of the ankle.

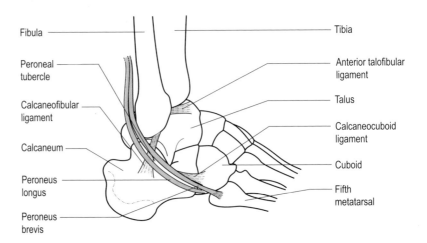

Fibula

Peroneal tubercle

Calcaneofibular ligament

Calcaneum

Peroneus longus

Peroneus brevis

Tibia

Anterior talofibular ligament

Talus

Calcaneocuboid ligament

Cuboid

Fifth metatarsal

COMMENTARY ON THE EXAMINATION

OBSERVATION

Before proceeding with the history, a general observation of the patient's *face, posture and gait* will alert the examiner to abnormalities, particularly of the gait pattern. A limp usually indicates abnormal weight-bearing, but a 'short leg' can produce a limp through functional discrepancies of hyperpronation and a flattened medial arch (Kannus 1992).

The most common injury to the ankle involves the lateral ligaments, but other injuries include lesions of the contractile units, subluxation of the peroneal tendons (through partial or complete rupture of the retinaculae), damage to the subtalar and mid-tarsal joints and injury to the various neurovascular structures crossing the region (Marder 1994, Lee & Maleski 2002). Fractures and dislocations at the ankle are outside the scope of this book.

HISTORY (SUBJECTIVE EXAMINATION)

The *age, occupation, sports, hobbies and lifestyle* of the patient may give an indication of the cause of the lesion and alert the examiner to possible biomechanical or postural problems.

The *site and spread* of pain help to localize the lesion, but as a peripheral joint, pain is usually well-localized. The presence of paraesthesia in the foot or pain in the calf or shin could suggest a more proximal lesion.

The *onset* of the symptoms may be sudden, due to trauma, or gradual, associated with overuse or arthritis. If the onset is traumatic in nature, the mechanism of injury should be deduced, particularly to give an indication of the ligaments involved. A 'snap' or 'popping' sensation at onset may indicate rupture of tendon, ligament or a fracture.

A minor injury is indicated by minimal pain and localized swelling, with the ability to continue weight-bearing activities. More severe injuries will produce diffuse swelling and an inability to weight-bear, suggesting ligamentous rupture or fracture.

The *duration* of symptoms indicates the stage of the lesion in the inflammatory process. A history of recurrent episodes indicates possible instability, requiring in-depth biomechanical assessment.

The *symptoms and behaviour* need to be considered. The behaviour of the pain indicates the nature of the lesion: mechanical lesions are eased by rest and aggravated by activity and weight-bearing.

Other symptoms described by the patient could include the ankle giving way; this is a symptom of ligamentous instability or possible loose body in the joint. A clicking or snapping sensation on the lateral aspect of the ankle could be due to disruption of the peroneal retinaculum, allowing subluxation of the tendons.

An indication of *past medical history, other joint involvement* and *medications* will aid diagnosis and establish whether contraindications to treatment techniques exist. Rheumatoid arthritis may affect the small joints of the foot.

INSPECTION

This should be conducted in both weight-bearing and non-weight-bearing postures.

Bony deformity and functional abnormalities, of the medial arch in particular, will usually manifest themselves in the weight-bearing position.

Check the height of the medial and longitudinal arches. Pes planus is a structural flat foot which is visible in both weight-bearing and non-weight-bearing positions, while a functional flat foot is only observed on weight-bearing.

The presence of functional flat foot can be generally estimated by looking for a difference in the height of the medial longitudinal arch in the non-weight-bearing and weight-bearing positions. Estimate the distance between the tuberosity of the navicular and the ground, first in a non-weight-bearing sitting position and secondly in the standing weight-bearing position (Evans 1990).

Observe the position of the Achilles tendon from behind for any deviations in the normal straight alignment, which would indicate postural deformity. Also notice if there is any angulation of the forefoot relative to the hindfoot.

Although it is important to note postural abnormalities of the foot, this should be kept relevant to the patient's presenting signs and symptoms. A detailed biomechanical assessment is not necessary for uncomplicated lesions, but recurrent symptoms or failure to resolve the patient's symptoms may require referral to a podiatrist or physiotherapy specialist in lower limb biomechanics.

It is worth inspecting the patient's shoes for abnormal areas of weight-bearing. This is particularly relevant to athletes and should include their training shoes. In a normal gait pattern, wear is seen on the lateral side of the heel and the medial side of the forefoot (Kannus 1992). Camber running or worn-out or incorrect training shoes can alter angles of contact between the foot and the ground and be an external cause of overuse (Evans 1990). Advice will need to be given regarding the type of shoe best suited to the patient's activities (Anthony 1987). Abnormal callus formation indicates abnormal weight-bearing.

Colour changes such as cyanosis, erythema or pallor may indicate circulatory involvement and a change in colour in transferring from the weight-bearing to the non-weight-bearing position should be further investigated by palpating for the presence of arterial pulses (Figs 12.7 and 12.8). Bruising is often associated with a recently sprained ankle or gastrocnemius muscle belly lesion and tracks peripherally. A severe sprain of the ankle can cause traction injury of the superficial peroneal nerve and vascular structures. Consideration should be given to these possibilities if changes in skin colour persist (Acus & Flanagan 1991).

Muscle wasting may be seen in the calf or peroneal muscles.

Swelling and any bruising on the lateral aspect of the ankle may be diffuse, indicating a moderate or major ligamentous lesion. Often a rounded mottled egg-shell-like swelling lies in front of the lateral malleolus: this is known as the *signe de la coquille d'oeuf* (Litt 1992).

Minor swelling may be indicated by loss of the hollows behind the malleoli. Local swellings and ganglia should also be noted.

Figure 12.7   Palpation for dorsalis pedis pulse.

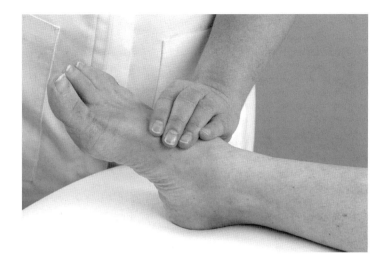

Figure 12.8   Palpation for posterior tibial artery.

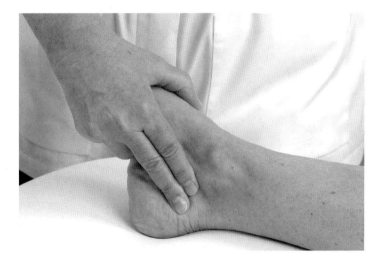

PALPATION

As peripheral joints, the ankle and foot are palpated for signs of activity. The presence of *heat* is assessed (Fig. 12.9) and *synovial thickening* is palpated most easily along the anterior joint line (Fig. 12.10). *Swelling* is usually observed, but it is also possible to palpate for swelling, particularly around the malleoli. If the history indicates major ligament sprain, the malleoli and talus can be palpated for any focal areas of tenderness which may indicate a fracture (Lee & Maleski 2002).

Figure 12.9   Palpation for heat.

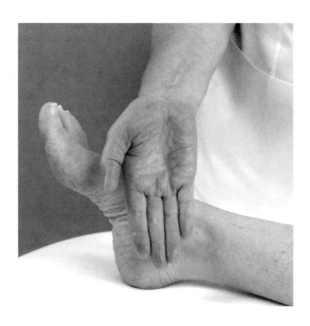

Figure 12.10   Palpation for synovial thickening.

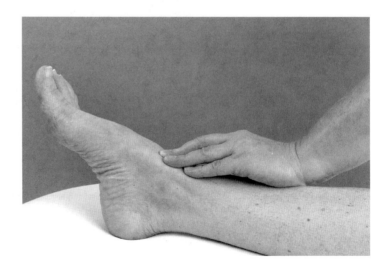

STATE AT REST

Before any movements are performed, the state at rest is established to provide a baseline for subsequent comparison. The suggested sequence for the objective examination will now be given, followed by a commentary including the reasoning in performing the movements and the significance of the possible findings.

EXAMINATION BY SELECTIVE TENSION (OBJECTIVE EXAMINATION)

Ankle Joint

- Passive dorsiflexion (Fig. 12.11)
- Passive plantarflexion (Fig. 12.12)

Subtalar Joint

- Passive varus of the calcaneum to produce supination (Fig. 12.13)
- Passive valgus of the calcaneum to produce pronation (Fig. 12.13)

Mid-Tarsal Joints

- Passive dorsiflexion and plantarflexion (Figs 12.14 and 12.15)
- Passive abduction and adduction (Figs 12.16 and 12.17)
- Passive eversion and inversion (Figs 12.18 and 12.19)

Gross Ligament Tests

- Passive inversion for lateral collateral ligament (Fig. 12.20)
- Passive eversion for medial (deltoid) ligament (Fig. 12.21)

Contractile Structures

- Resisted dorsiflexion (Fig. 12.22)
- Resisted plantarflexion (Fig. 12.23)
- Resisted inversion (Fig. 12.24)
- Resisted eversion (Fig. 12.25)

Accessory Ligament Tests

- Drawer test for the anterior talofibular ligament (Fig. 12.26)
- Talar tilt test for the calcaneofibular ligament and integrity of the mortise (Fig. 12.27)
- Test for the dorsal calcaneocuboid ligament (Fig. 12.28)

Toes

- Passive and resisted testing of the toes is not performed routinely, but is included if appropriate

Palpation

- Once a diagnosis has been made, the structure at fault is palpated for the exact site of the lesion

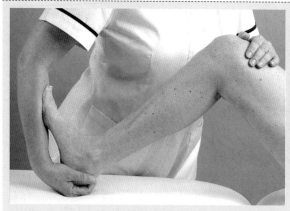

Figure 12.11   Passive ankle dorsiflexion.

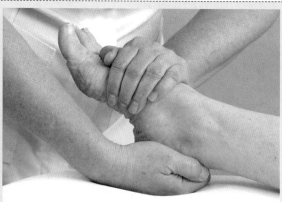

Figure 12.12   Passive ankle plantarflexion.

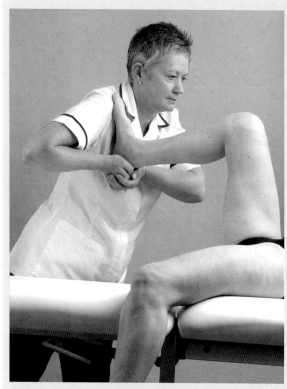

Figure 12.13   Hand position for varus and valgus stress subtalar joint: valgus stress shown.

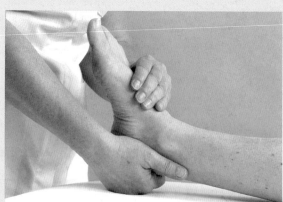

Figure 12.14   Passive mid-tarsal dorsiflexion.

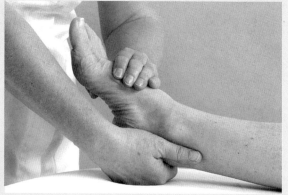

Figure 12.15   Passive mid-tarsal plantarflexion.

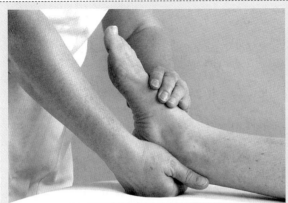

Figure 12.16   Passive mid-tarsal abduction.

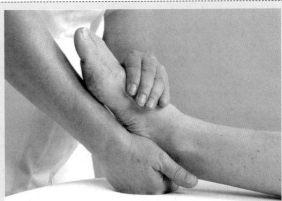

Figure 12.17   Passive mid-tarsal adduction.

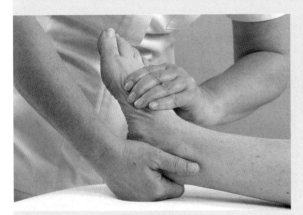

Figure 12.18   Passive mid-tarsal eversion.

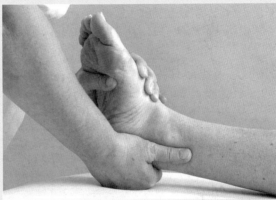

Figure 12.19   Passive mid-tarsal inversion.

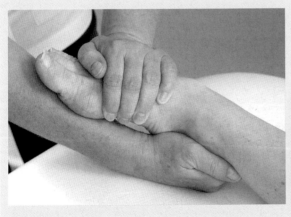

Figure 12.20   Passive inversion for lateral collateral ligament.

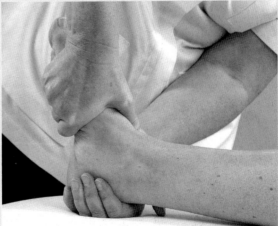

Figure 12.21   Passive eversion for medial (deltoid) ligament.

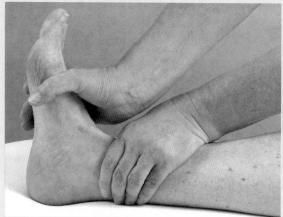

Figure 12.22   Resisted dorsiflexion.

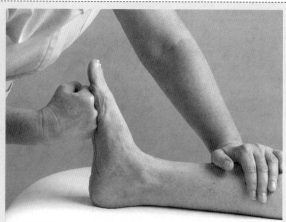

Figure 12.23   Resisted plantarflexion.

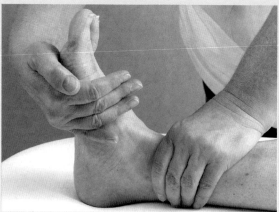

Figure 12.24   Resisted inversion.

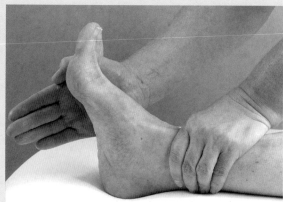

Figure 12.25   Resisted eversion.

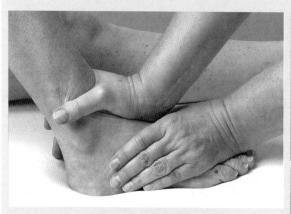

Figure 12.26   Drawer test for the anterior talofibular ligament.

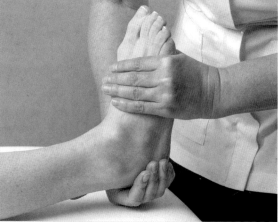

Figure 12.27   Talar tilt test for calcaneofibular ligament and integrity of the mortise.

Figure 12.28   Test for the dorsal calcaneocuboid ligament.

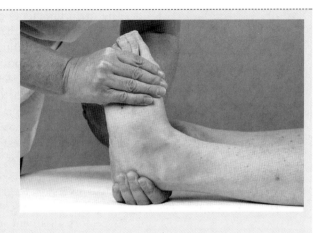

Capsular pattern of the ankle joint
- More limitation of plantarflexion than dorsiflexion.

Capsular pattern of the subtalar joint
- Increasing limitation of supination.
- Eventual fixation of the joint in pronation.

Capsular pattern of the mid-tarsal joints
- Limitation of adduction and inversion.
- Forefoot fixes in abduction and eversion.

Capsular pattern of the first metatarsophalangeal joint
- Gross limitation of extension.
- Some limitation of flexion.

The objective examination is carried out in non-weight-bearing with the patient positioned comfortably in supine lying. The joints are examined first, assessing the range of movement, pain and end-feel. Passive dorsiflexion normally has a hard end-feel and to achieve end range it must be performed with the knee in flexion to take the tension off the gastrocnemius muscle complex, which spans both the knee and ankle joints. Passive plantarflexion normally has a firm elastic end-feel due to tension in the tissues on the dorsal aspect of the foot. The presence of the capsular pattern should be noted.

Although individual passive movements can be produced at the ankle joint, it is difficult to produce isolated passive movements at the subtalar and mid-tarsal joints. To assess the small range of movement available at the subtalar joint, grasp the calcaneum with both hands. Flex the knee to allow relaxation of the gastrocnemius complex and push the ankle joint into the close packed position. The varus and valgus stress is then applied to the calcaneum through the heels of both hands, using body weight. The amount of passive movement available at the subtalar joint is limited to a few degrees of supination and pronation and the normal end-feel is hard for both.

To assess movements occurring at the mid-tarsal joints, pull down on the calcaneum to place the ankle joint into dorsiflexion. Place fingers and thumb on either side of the first metatarsal, around the narrow, lateral aspect of the foot, and move the mid-tarsal joint through its range of passive movements, plantarflexion and dorsiflexion, abduction and adduction, inversion and eversion. These movements are minimal, and difficult to produce in isolation.

Assessing passive movements of the toes is not part of the routine ankle examination, but the movements can be applied as necessary to assess for the presence of the capsular pattern.

Capsular pattern of the
other metatarsophalangeal
joints (may vary)
- More limitation of
  flexion than extension.
- Joints fix in extension.

Capsular pattern of the
interphalangeal joints
- Joints fix in flexion.

The main ligaments are tested by two gross composite movements, passive inversion for the lateral collateral ligament and passive eversion for the medial collateral ligament. Should it be necessary, the ligaments can be assessed individually, and accessory tests can be applied for joint instability (see below).

The contractile structures are assessed by resisted tests for pain and power. The joints are placed in the mid-position and maximum resistance applied. Resisted dorsiflexion tests mainly tibialis anterior and resisted plantarflexion tests gastrocnemius and the Achilles tendon. Testing the gastrocnemius group in lying may not produce symptoms and the test may need to be repeated in standing against the resistance of body weight. Resisted inversion tests mainly tibialis posterior and resisted eversion tests the peroneal muscles.

Accessory ligament and instability tests are applied if appropriate. The gross ligament test of passive inversion mainly tests the anterior talofibular ligament which crosses the ankle joint and is taut in plantarflexion. It is the most common ligamentous injury found at the ankle. It is further assessed by the *drawer test* which assesses its integrity (Marder 1994). Flex the leg to allow the foot to rest on the couch. Position yourself to view movement of the fibula on the lateral side of the ankle. Place one hand over the talus to fix it and the other just above the ankle joint. Apply pressure backwards against the fibula and tibia, comparing the degree of posterior movement of the fibula with the other side. Increased posterior movement of the fibula is a positive sign and indicates laxity or rupture of the anterior talofibular ligament. There is no standardized score for assessing abnormal displacement on the anterior drawer test, with some texts suggesting a grading system of 1–3 in excessive movement relative to the contralateral ankle. A 'suction sign' or dimple may be observed on the lateral aspect of the ankle if the anterior talofibular ligament is ruptured (Lee & Maleski 2002).

In a cadaver study, Beumer et al (2003) were unable to demonstrate significant displacement during various clinical tests, including the anterior drawer test, suggesting that syndesmotic injury is unlikely to be detected by such tests. However, the mean age of the 17 cadaver specimens was 78.4 years which may have had a bearing on ankle mobility and this was not addressed in the study. They conclude that pain rather than increased displacement should be considered as the outcome measure of these tests, but admit that how increased displacement relates to pain has not been demonstrated. Fujii et al (2000) similarly used elderly cadavers to assess the accuracy of the anterior drawer and talar tilt tests and although both tests demonstrated reasonable displacement of the hindfoot, neither was sufficient accurately to diagnose specific ligament involvement. It was concluded that these conventional stress tests are not sensitive due to a substantial amount of difference between movement of the cadaver specimens, examiner agreement and positions of the ankle for the tests. To our knowledge, these ligament tests have not been evaluated in vivo.

The calcaneofibular ligament crosses both the ankle joint and the subtalar joint. Injury to this ligament does not often occur in isolation, but is usually in conjunction with the anterior talofibular ligament. The calcaneofibular ligament resists varus stresses to the calcaneum in dorsiflexion. Combined rupture of these ligaments results in an increased *talar tilt* (Boruta et al 1990, Wilkerson 1992, Marder 1994). With the knee straight, passively dorsiflex the ankle (this allows it to fall just short of the close packed position) and apply a strong varus stress to the calcaneum; compare the range of movement with the other side. This test may also be graded 1–3 relative to the contralateral ankle and again dimpling may be observed (Lee & Maleski 2002).

Disruption of the inferior tibiofibular joint may be due to a forced dorsiflexion injury which can cause widening (diastasis) of the ankle mortise (Marder 1994). In clinical practice, such an injury would usually only occur in conjunction with other major ligamentous damage, but the talar tilt test can also be applied to test the integrity of the mortise. Apply the talar tilt test as above (it can only be accurately applied if the lateral collateral ligaments are intact). If there is any widening of the mortise, pain and excessive movement will be appreciated. A 'click' may be felt as the talus tilts excessively in the enlarged mortise (Cyriax & Cyriax 1983).

The *dorsal calcaneocuboid ligament* crosses the calcaneocuboid joint, part of the mid-tarsal complex, and may be involved in a lateral collateral ligament sprain or injured in isolation. To assess its involvement, apply passive adduction and inversion of the mid-tarsal joints looking for increased pain.

CAPSULAR LESIONS

The presence of a capsular pattern at any of the joints in the ankle and foot indicates arthritis. The history will have established the cause of the arthritis.

Osteoarthrosis is uncommon at the ankle unless predisposed by fracture, repetitive postural overuse or instability caused by recurrent sprain. An alteration in lower limb biomechanics may predispose any of the joints to degenerative osteoarthrosis. Localized degenerative osteoarthrosis of the subtalar joint may follow fractures of the talus or calcaneum (Evans 1990). Occasionally, a lateral ligament sprain produces a traumatic arthritis in the subtalar and mid-tarsal joints and, if unresolved, the joint can be injected with corticosteroid. Rheumatoid arthritis is more common in the smaller joints of the foot. Arthritis and gout of the first metatarsophalangeal joint cause a loss of the functional range of extension essential to gait activities. Corticosteroid injection may be given for symptomatic osteoarthrosis or the principles of mobilization may be applied. Rheumatoid arthritis may respond to corticosteroid injection.

> **Capsular pattern of the ankle joint**
> - More limitation of plantarflexion than dorsiflexion.

> **Injection of the ankle joint**
>
> Suggested needle size: 23G × 1 in (0.6 × 25 mm) blue needle or a 21G × 1¹/₂ in (0.8 × 40 mm) green needle
> Dose: 20 mg triamcinolone acetonide in a total volume of 3 ml

Position the patient in supine with the foot resting on the couch. This places the ankle in a degree of plantarflexion and opens the joint. Several needle entry points are possible and it may be necessary to palpate for a suitable opening over either malleolus, or between the tibialis anterior and extensor hallucis longus tendons, which avoids the dorsalis pedis artery (Fig 12.29). Having selected a needle entry point, give the injection as a bolus (Fig. 12.30). The patient is advised to maintain a period of relative rest for approximately 2 weeks following injection.

Injection of the subtalar joint (Cyriax & Cyriax 1983, Cyriax 1984)

Suggested needle size: 23G × 1 in (0.6 × 25 mm) blue needle
Dose: 10 mg triamcinolone acetonide in a total volume of 2 ml

Capsular pattern of the subtalar joint
- Increasing limitation of supination.
- Eventual fixation of the joint in pronation.

The subtalar joint is divided into two compartments by an interosseous ligament. Locate the joint line immediately above the sustentaculum tali and insert the needle approximately halfway along the joint line, angling it posteriorly to inject the posterior compartment first (Figs 12.31a and 12.32a). Then withdraw the needle a little and reinsert it anteriorly to inject the anterior compartment (Figs 12.31b and 12.32b). Give the injection as a bolus. The patient is advised to maintain a period of relative rest for approximately 2 weeks following injection.

Injection of the mid-tarsal joint (Cyriax & Cyriax 1983, Cyriax 1984)

Suggested needle size: 23G × 1 in (0.6 × 25 mm) blue needle
Dose: 10 mg triamcinolone acetonide in a total volume of 1.5 ml

The injection site will depend on which of the joints are affected, the talocalcaneonavicular joint, calcaneocuboid joint or both. Locate the appropriate joint line dorsally by palpation, avoiding the tendons and the

Figure 12.29   Injection of the ankle joint.

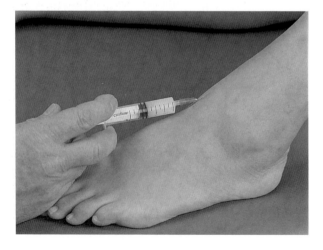

Figure 12.30   Injection of the ankle joint showing direction of approach and needle position.

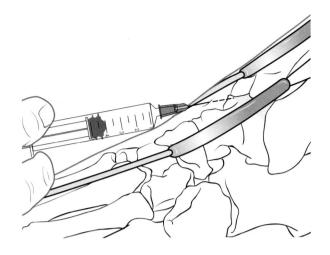

Figure 12.31   (a, b) Injection of the subtalar joint.

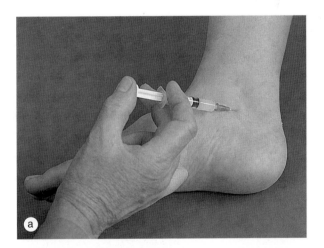

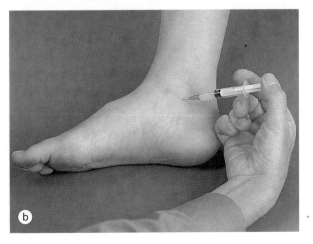

Figure 12.32 (a, b) Injection of the subtalar joint showing direction of approach and needle position.

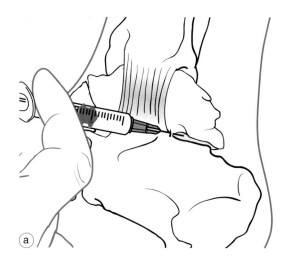

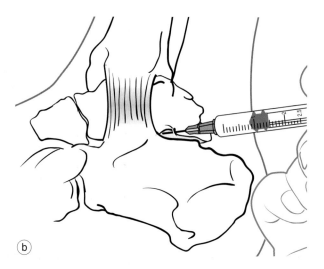

Figure 12.33   Injection of the midtarsal, calcaneocuboid joint.

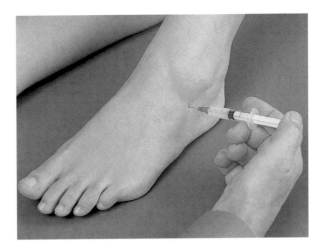

Figure 12.34   Injection of the midtarsal, calcaneocuboid joint showing direction of approach and needle position.

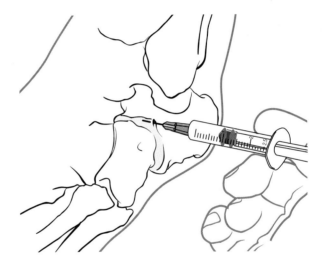

Capsular pattern of the mid-tarsal joints
- Limitation of adduction and inversion.
- Forefoot fixes in abduction and eversion.

Capsular pattern of the first metatarsophalangeal joint
- Gross limitation of extension.
- Some limitation of flexion.

dorsalis pedis artery if injecting the talocalcaneonavicular joint medially. (Figs 12.33 and 12.34 demonstrate injection of the calcaneocuboid joint.) Insert the needle and, once intracapsular, give the injection as a bolus. The patient is advised to maintain a period of relative rest for approximately 2 weeks following injection.

Figure 12.35 Injection of the first metatarsophalangeal joint.

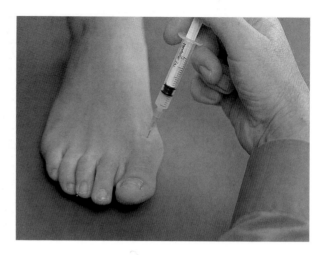

Figure 12.36 Injection of the first metatarsophalangeal joint showing direction of approach and needle position.

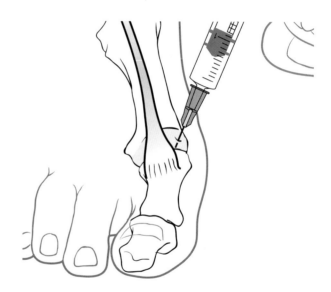

Injection of the first metatarsophalangeal joint (Cyriax & Cyriax 1983, Cyriax 1984)

Suggested needle size: 25G × ⁵/₈ in (0.5 × 16 mm) orange needle
Dose: 10 mg triamcinolone acetonide in a total volume of 0.5 ml

Identify the joint line dorsally by palpation and distract it to allow easier access; choose a point of entry to one side of the extensor tendon (Fig. 12.35). The injection is given as a bolus (Fig. 12.36). The patient is advised to maintain a period of relative rest for approximately 2 weeks following injection.

Figure 12.37 Injection interphalangeal joint.

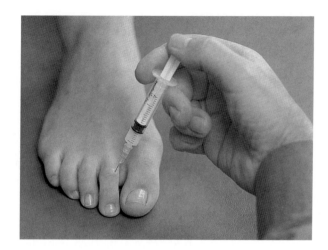

Figure 12.38 Injection interphalangeal joint showing direction of approach and needle position.

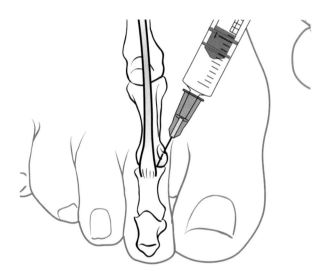

Capsular pattern of the other metatarsophalangeal joints (may vary)
- More limitation of flexion than extension.
- Joints fix in extension.

Capsular pattern of the interphalangeal joints
- Joints fix in flexion.

Injection of the other metatarsophalangeal and interphalangeal joints

Suggested needle size: 25G × ⁵/₈ in (0.5 × 16 mm) orange needle
Dose: 10 mg triamcinolone acetonide in a total volume of 0.5 ml

Identify the joint line dorsally by palpation. Insert the needle avoiding the extensor tendons, and give the injection as a bolus (Figs 12.37 and 12.38). The patient is advised to maintain a period of relative rest for approximately 2 weeks following injection.

NON–CAPSULAR LESIONS

LATERAL COLLATERAL LIGAMENT SPRAIN

Sprain of the lateral collateral ligament is the most common ankle injury, accounting for approximately 85–90% of ankle sprains (Stanley 1991, Liu & Jason 1994). The basic mechanism for lateral ligament sprain is a forced inversion injury (Sartoris 1994, Kerkhoffs et al 2002). Injury occurs commonly in sport, when a player may land on another player's foot, stumble on uneven ground; or, apart from sport, the patient may simply have tripped or slipped. The most common predisposition factor to suffering a lateral ligament injury is a history of at least one previous strain and an estimated 55% of patients do not seek treatment for a sprained ankle (Hertel 2002).

Diagnosis of sprain can be made on clinical grounds and X-ray investigation is only necessary if there is clear clinical evidence of fracture, e.g. marked bony tenderness to palpation (Auletta et al 1991, Litt 1992). The fibular end of the ligament is more likely to be involved in avulsion fractures than the talar end, which is protected by greater bone density (Kumai et al 2002). Forced inversion may cause avulsion of lateral structures or undisplaced fracture of the lateral malleolus, while impactive forces may stress medial structures (Sartoris 1994).

Lateral collateral ligament sprains most commonly involve the anterior talofibular ligament, with more severe injuries also involving other ligaments and structures on the lateral side of the ankle (Black et al 1978, Litt 1992, Liu & Jason 1994, Hertel 2002). Lateral collateral ligament sprains are graded according to the severity of the signs and symptoms (Boruta et al 1990, Stanley 1991, Litt 1992, Wilkerson 1992, Liu & Jason 1994, Kerkhoffs et al 2002).

Grade I   This is mild stretching of the ligament and surrounding structures. The patient presents with mild swelling and tenderness over the ligament, little or no haemorrhage, some limitation of movement and some difficulty in weight-bearing. On examination, no clinical instability is noted and prognosis is good. The injury takes approximately 8–10 days to resolve with early mobilization.

Grade II   This is partial rupture of the anterior talofibular ligament with mild instability of the joint. The patient presents with moderate to severe swelling, bruising, pain, local tenderness, a limited range of movement and great difficulty in weight-bearing. There is limitation of movement in the capsular pattern and a mild degree of ligamentous instability may be detected clinically. Prognosis remains good, the injury taking approximately 15–21 days to resolve with early mobilization.

Grade III   This is complete rupture of the anterior talofibular and calcaneofibular ligaments and lateral capsule with gross instability of the joint. The patient presents with diffuse swelling and marked evidence of haemorrhaging. There is severe pain and tenderness, loss of movement and great difficulty with weight-bearing. It may be difficult to assess for ligamentous laxity clinically as this may be masked by the swelling and the protective reflex muscle spasm produced by the pain.

Both operative and non-operative treatment options could be considered, but with conservative management prognosis is still good, providing the patient is not required to function at high levels of performance (Stanley 1991, Karlsson & Lansingeer 1992, Liu & Jason 1994). Recurrent sprains of the ankle with clinical laxity may need stress X-ray to measure the laxity before proceeding to eventual surgical repair. In general, surgical intervention for grade III sprains is only considered in the élite athlete, or where recurrent injury has failed to respond to conservative management and is producing functional disability. Otherwise, all grades of sprain are treated conservatively (Karlsson & Lansingeer 1992, Liu & Jason 1994, Ogilvie-Harris & Gilbart 1995).

Early mobilization is the key to the restoration of function in all grades of ligamentous sprain, giving a better overall result and a faster rate of recovery (Brooks et al 1981, Roycroft & Mantgani 1983, Stanley 1991, Ogilvie-Harris & Gilbart 1995, Shrier 1995). Non-steroidal anti-inflammatory drugs and ice, used early on in the inflammatory phase, seem to achieve an earlier recovery, but do not alter the overall outcome (Ogilvie-Harris & Gilbart 1995). Corticosteroid injection is not recommended for acute ankle sprains since collagen synthesis may be suppressed (Boruta et al 1990). Kerkhoffs et al (2002) present a review of randomized controlled trials in the literature to evaluate the effectiveness of immobilization as the treatment for acute sprained ankle in adults. Overall, results were better with functional treatment rather than immobilization, with a higher percentage of patients returning to work and sport, a reduced incidence of persistent swelling, limited movement and instability and higher patient satisfaction rates. Functional treatment is therefore the treatment of choice for acute sprained ankle.

Treatment is directed at all components involved in the sprain and depends on the stage reached in the inflammatory process.

Acute lateral collateral ligament sprain

A complete examination of the ankle and foot is not usually possible following an acute lateral collateral ligament sprain as the swelling and muscle spasm prevent movement. The history will indicate the mechanism of the injury and the amount of heat and swelling will give an indication of the severity. Any movement, active or passive, particularly into inversion, will be painful and pain is experienced on weight-bearing leading to an antalgic gait. The principles of treatment for acute ligament sprain are applied.

Protection, rest, ice, compression and elevation (PRICE) are applied immediately after the onset. Ice applied during the first 3 days after injury has been shown to shorten the recovery period. It is generally applied for 15–20 min three times daily (Hocutt et al 1982, Stanley 1991, Swain & Holt 1993).

Gentle transverse frictions are begun as early as possible, according to the irritability of the lesion, together with Grade A mobilization, aiming to maintain mobility. Treatment is delivered on a daily basis during the early acute phase and the patient is encouraged to maintain a normal heel–toe gait, possibly with the aid of crutches. Ankle supports or tape may be applied to provide compression during the early acute phase (O'Hara et al 1992).

From days 3 to 5 onwards, again dependent upon irritability, there should be sufficient tensile strength in the wound to allow an increasing depth of transverse frictions and a greater range of Grade A mobilization to be applied. Treatment continues until a full range of pain-free movement is attained.

Depending on the severity of the injury, the patient should be relatively pain-free and walking normally within 8–21 days, if seen within a day or two from the onset. Functional rehabilitation should involve muscle balance, peroneal strengthening and proprioceptive work to reestablish normal balance and coordination (Cornwall & Murrell 1991, Karlsson & Lansingeer 1992). Progression to running, sprinting, jumping, figure-of-eight running, twisting and turning follows, depending on the functional requirements of the patient. The lateral ligaments require the support of the peroneal tendons to resist inversion stresses; rehabilitation aims to restore muscle strength and to re-establish the protective reflexes (Boruta et al 1990).

Transverse frictions to the lateral collateral ligament components (Cyriax & Cyriax 1983, Cyriax 1984)

The anterior talofibular ligament is usually involved at its fibular end, but palpation will establish the exact site of the lesion which may also be at the talar insertion or across the joint line.

Stand on the patient's good side, placing an index finger reinforced by the middle finger onto the anterior edge of the lateral malleolus. Direct the transverse frictions back against the malleolus and sweep transversely across the fibres (Fig. 12.39). In the acute case begin the transverse frictions

Figure 12.39 Transverse frictions to the anterior talofibular ligament, acute sprain.

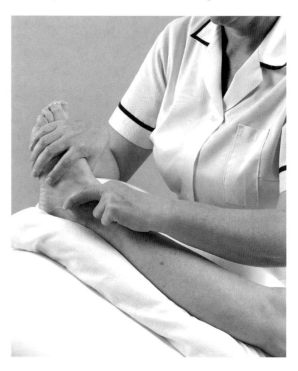

very gently to gain some analgesia. Progress to apply the transverse frictions more deeply and, once on the ligament, apply approximately six effective sweeps to achieve movement. The transverse frictions are followed immediately by Grade A mobilization together with gait correction.

If the calcaneofibular ligament is involved, the transverse frictions are directed up under the apex of the lateral malleolus and immediately followed by Grade A mobilization.

Treatment of any involvement of the peroneal tendons will be covered under contractile lesions.

Chronic lateral collateral ligament sprain

There is a history of a past sprained ankle which may have resolved without treatment. The patient complains of pain and some swelling on the lateral side of the ankle after exertion. Symptoms of recurrent giving way may indicate mechanical instability (ankle movement beyond the physiological limit which occurs due to anatomical changes such as ligamentous laxity) or functional instability (a subjective feeling of instability which occurs due to neuromuscular and proprioceptive deficits which provide dynamic control) (Tropp 2002). Provocative tests such as the drawer and talar tilt tests, as described above, can provide an indication of mechanical instability. The treatment approach for residual chronic ankle instability should be based on mechanical correction and functional rehabilitation, with an emphasis on proprioceptive reducation, muscle balance, postural control and taping may be appropriate for sporting activities. The importance of continuing rehabilitation for several months after the symptoms of acute ligamentous injury have subsided is paramount in preventing chronic recurrence (Hertel 2002). Surgery is only considered if rehabilitation fails (Liu & Jason 1994).

On examination there is usually pain on full passive inversion, indicating involvement of the anterior talofibular ligament. Pain on passive dorsiflexion with a varus stress to the calcaneum (talar tilt test) indicates involvement of the calcaneofibular ligament. Pain on passive adduction and inversion applied to the mid-tarsal joints indicates involvement of the dorsal calcaneocuboid ligament.

The ligament fibres have become adherent to the underlying bone and the principle of treatment is to rupture the unwanted adhesions with one Grade C manipulation at each session, once the ligament has been prepared by deep transverse frictions. Following manipulative rupture, the patient is instructed to mobilize vigorously, in order to maintain the movement gained through manipulation. Functional or structural instability is addressed by proprioceptive exercises and balance work (Lentell et al 1990). Treatment is usually successful and requires approximately one to three sessions.

Transverse frictions to the lateral collateral ligament components involved in a chronic sprain (Cyriax & Cyriax 1983, Cyriax 1984)

Transverse frictions to the anterior talofibular (Fig. 12.40) and calcaneofibular ligament (Fig. 12.41) are applied as described above. If the dorsal calcaneocuboid ligament is involved, the transverse frictions are applied from a position on the patient's good side; it is delivered by the index finger, reinforced by the middle finger, directed onto the ligament, which is located over the dorsal aspect of the calcaneocuboid joint (Fig. 12.42). The transverse frictions are applied to all involved ligaments to gain the analgesic effect, prior to the Grade C manipulation, which follows immediately.

Figure 12.40 Transverse frictions to the anterior talofibular ligament, chronic sprain.

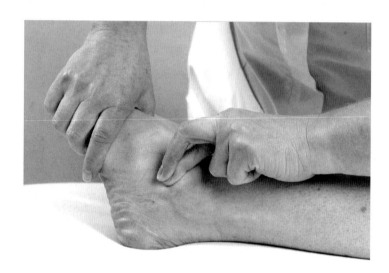

Figure 12.41 Transverse frictions to the calcaneofibular ligament.

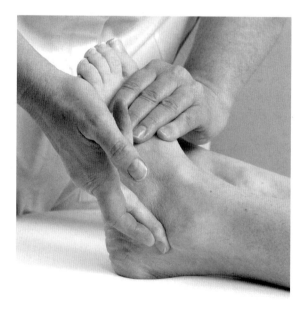

Figure 12.42 Transverse frictions to dorsal calcaneofibular ligament.

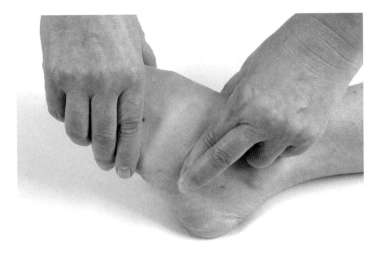

Grade C manipulation for chronic lateral collateral ligament sprain (Cyriax & Cyriax 1983, Cyriax 1984)

With the patient lying supine, stand at the foot of the couch. The treatment described is for the left ankle:

- Grasp the patient's left calcaneum with your left hand and pull it into varus to achieve a degree of supination at the subtalar joint (Fig. 12.43). Keep your thumb alongside the palm of your hand to avoid pressing against the lower leg which will tend to block the movement and is uncomfortable for the patient
- With a 'flipper' grip, wrap your right hand around the base of the first metatarsal (Fig. 12.44) and pull the foot into maximum plantarflexion (Fig. 12.45a). Be careful not to put your thumb round onto the sole of the foot, as this is uncomfortable for the patient and makes the technique less efficient
- Maintain the maximum plantarflexion while you step to the left, turning your body to the left through 90° to achieve maximum inversion (Fig. 12.45b, c)
- This step and turn also automatically pulls the forefoot into maximum adduction and inversion, taking up the slack (Fig. 12.46)
- Apply a minimal amplitude, high velocity thrust by a sharp adduction movement of your right arm

The increased range of movement must be maintained by vigorous exercise.

Figure 12.43 Grade C manipulation: calcaneum grasped and placed into varus.

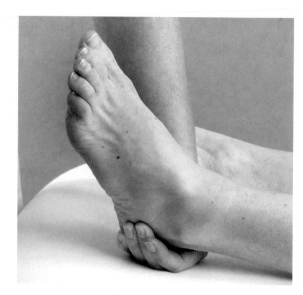

Figure 12.44 'Flipper' grip hand hold.

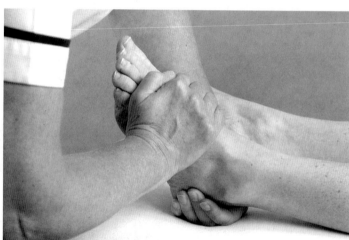

Figure 12.45 (a) Pulling foot into maximum plantarflexion.

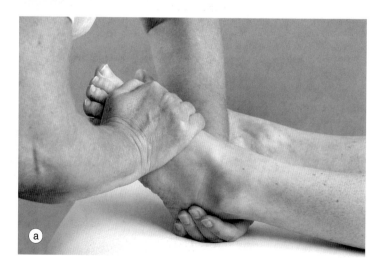

Figure 12.45   (b,c) Pulling foot into inversion and adduction.

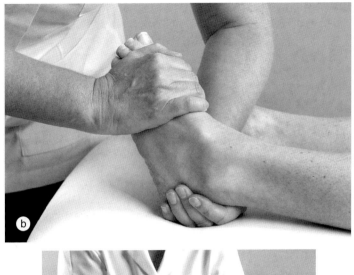

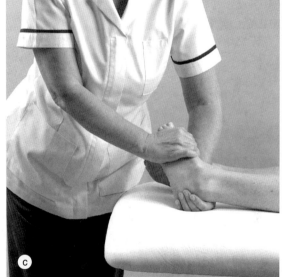

Figure 12.46   Grade C manipulation: body turned pulling the forefoot into maximum inversion and adduction before application of the final thrust.

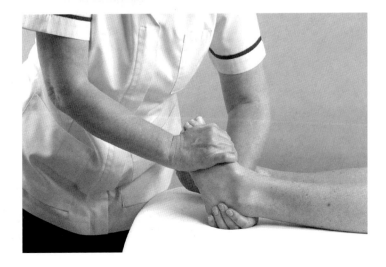

MEDIAL COLLATERAL LIGAMENT SPRAIN

Eversion sprains of the ankle represent 5–15% of all ankle injuries and are not common, as the medial collateral ligaments are 20–50% stronger than the lateral ligaments. The mechanism of injury involved is eversion with possible damage to the syndesmosis, or fracture of the malleoli, as well as injury to the medial ligament (Roberts et al 1995, Lee & Maleski 2002).

The treatment principles are applied as for the acute and chronic stages of the lateral collateral ligament if the injury is traumatic. The various directions of the ligament fibres need to be borne in mind, to be able to apply the frictions transversely. A Grade C manipulation is not applied in the chronic stage, due to the multidirectional nature of the fibres.

A secondary medial ligament sprain may develop through postural overuse. This is especially evident with flattening of the medial arch in the elderly. A biomechanical assessment of the foot may be indicated, together with orthotic correction to address the cause.

RETROCALCANEAL BURSITIS

The retrocalcaneal bursa is described as saddle-shaped, horseshoe-shaped or shaped like an inverted boomerang. It lies between the distal end of the Achilles tendon, near its insertion, and the superoposterior surface of the calcaneum (Stephens 1994, Bottger et al 1998). It rests against the Achilles fat pad superiorly and blends with the Achilles tendon posteriorly (Frey et al 1992).

An abnormally large bony bump (exostosis), known as Haglund's deformity, may be present on the superoposterior surface of the calcaneum; this may predispose towards retrocalcaneal bursitis. Soft tissue swellings are often associated with Haglund's deformity and are known as 'pump bumps' (Stephens 1994).

Objectively it is difficult to diagnose a retrocalcaneal bursitis differentially from an Achilles tendinopathy, with which it may coexist. It presents with posterior heel pain and a muddle of signs which may include pain on passive dorsiflexion which squeezes the inflamed bursa under the stretched Achilles tendon and/or passive plantarflexion which may squeeze the bursa between the Achilles tendon and the calcaneum. Swelling and tenderness to palpation may be present, just anterior to the insertion of the Achilles tendon. Retrocalcaneal bursitis may be a manifestation of rheumatoid arthritis or one of the spondyloarthropathies such as Reiter's disease (Hutson 1990, Frey et al 1992, Baxter 1994).

Frey et al (1992) demonstrated the existence of the retrocalcaneal bursa on X-ray using an injection of contrast medium. The normal bursa contains approximately 1 ml of fluid. Patients suffering from retrocalcaneal bursitis accepted less of the contrast medium than normal subjects, leading the authors to propose that this was due to inflammatory fluid, thickened oedematous bursal walls, hypertrophic synovial infoldings and pain. Bottger et al (1998) demonstrated the normal retrocalcaneal bursa to be 1 mm in an anterior–posterior dimension, 6 mm in the transverse dimension and 3 mm in the craniocaudal dimension; bursal dimensions greater than these were seen in symptomatic subjects.

Treatment consists of a local corticosteroid injection.

Injection of the retrocalcaneal bursa

Suggested needle size: 23G × 1 in (0.6 × 25 mm) blue needle
Dose: 10 mg triamcinolone acetonide in a total volume of 0.75 ml

Position the patient in the prone position with the foot in a degree of plantarflexion over a pillow. Palpate for the tender area anterior to the distal end of the Achilles tendon and insert the needle from either the medial or lateral aspect, running parallel to the anterior aspect of the Achilles tendon (Figs 12.47 and 12.48). Give the injection as a bolus if

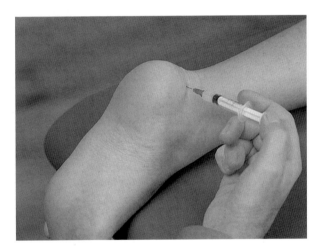

Figure 12.47   Injection of the retrocalcaneal bursa.

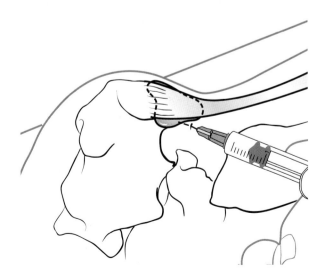

Figure 12.48   Injection of the retrocalcaneal bursa showing direction of approach and needle position.

possible, or pepper it if you feel the resistance of the synovial folds. The patient is advised to maintain a period of relative rest for approximately 2 weeks following injection.

SUBCUTANEOUS ACHILLES BURSITIS

The subcutaneous Achilles bursa lies between the skin and insertion of the Achilles tendon. It may be an adventitious bursa developing as a result of external friction (Gibbon & Cassar-Pullicino 1994). Inflammation of this bursa presents with subcutaneous swelling and tenderness over the heel and may be due to abnormal pressure from heel counters. Treatment consists of relative rest and advising the patient about footwear, with particular regard to the height and rigidity of the heel counter (Stephens 1994).

PLANTAR FASCIITIS

Plantar fasciitis produces a typical history of a gradual onset of pain felt over the medial plantar aspect of the heel at the enthesis of the central cord into the calcaneal tuberosity (Yu 2000). Its particular characteristic is pain under the heel when the foot is first put to the floor in the morning, easing after a few steps have been taken (Kibler et al 1991, Karr 1994). It is worse after prolonged periods of standing and on initial exercise, easing as the foot warms up.

Plantar fasciitis usually occurs in middle age, with obesity as a predisposing factor (Gibbon & Cassar-Pullicino 1994). It may be precipitated by an alteration in footwear, e.g. wearing flip-flops or other similar unsupporting shoes, or seen as a relatively common injury in the running athlete, where it constitutes approximately 10% of running injuries seen (Kibler et al 1991).

Postural foot deformity such as pes planus and overpronation lowers the medial longitudinal arch and may overstretch the plantar fascia. Tightness of the Achilles tendon limits dorsiflexion and may contribute to the overpronation (Evans 1990, Karr 1994). Due to the constant-length phenomenon, extension of the toes increases the height of the longitudinal arch – the 'windlass' effect of the plantar fascia (Canoso 1981, Sellman 1994) – so that activities involving long-term tip-toe standing, e.g. high heels, may excessively stress the plantar fascia. It may also be associated with rheumatoid arthritis or the spondyloarthropathies.

Diagnosis is made on the typical history and the absence of other findings on examination of the foot and ankle. Passive extension of the toes, with the foot in dorsiflexion, may reproduce the pain by its 'windlass' effect on the plantar fascia and tenderness to palpation is usually found over the medial calcaneal tuberosity.

The mechanism of the lesion is thought to be repetitive microtrauma through overloading of the longitudinal arch, which produces focal tears and fascial and perifascial inflammation at the insertion of the plantar fascia at the bone–fascia interface (the enthesis) (Kibler et al 1991, Karr 1994, Gibbon & Cassar-Pullicino 1994). It may be a traction injury occurring through repeated intrinsic muscle contraction against a stretched plantar fascia during the push-off phase of gait, the plantar fascia acting as an aponeurotic attachment for the first layer of the plantar muscles. Both mechanisms could possibly lead to the development of calcaneal spurs (Gibbon & Cassar-Pullicino 1994).

Differential diagnosis should exclude fat pad syndrome which tends to occur acutely following a fall onto the heel or chronically through poor heel cushioning (Brukner & Khan 2002). The patient will experience pain on palpation of the heel and treatment is aimed at addressing the cause, advice on footwear and activity modification.

Plantar fasciitis usually responds to conservative management. However, if this fails, surgery may be an option, with careful consideration paid to maintaining the load-bearing capacity of the longitudinal arch (Kulthanan 1992, Kim & Voloshin 1995). Tissue examined at the time of surgery has shown a hypercellular inflammatory response, reactive fibrosis and degenerative areas (Kibler et al 1991).

The chronic nature of the condition produces changes in the strength of the plantarflexors with loss of range of dorsiflexion and there may be alterations in the length of the stride (Kibler et al 1991, Chandler & Kibler 1993). All components of dysfunction should be considered when planning a rehabilitation programme.

Treatment of plantar fasciitis is local corticosteroid injection or transverse frictions. Either treatment is combined with rest from overuse activities and a full rehabilitation programme which may include intrinsic muscle exercises and correction of foot posture, if appropriate.

Although unusual, cases of spontaneous rupture of the plantar fascia have been reported, particularly among athletes. It usually occurs during rapid acceleration as the foot forcibly pushes against the ground, or may occur over time in association with sustained activity such as walking. The patient may report specific injury and a snapping sensation together with the appearance of a painful lump. The plantar fascia may be tender to palpation and bruising may be evident. Occasionally infection may occur, but this is usually associated with systemic disease such as diabetes mellitus with heel ulcerations, or extension from a surrounding soft tissue infection or through penetration by a foreign object. The calcaneum is the most commonly infected tarsal bone (Yu 2000).

Injection of the plantar fascia (Cyriax & Cyriax 1983, Cyriax 1984)

Suggested needle size: 21G × 1¹/₂ in (0.8 × 40 mm) or 21G × 2 in (0.8 × 40 mm) green needle
Dose: 20 mg triamcinolone acetonide in a total volume of 1.5 ml

Position the patient in prone lying with the knee flexed and the lower leg resting on a pillow. Hold the foot in dorsiflexion to apply some tension to the plantar fascia. Insert the needle at the medial border of the heel, anterior to the point of tenderness, and angled posteriorly towards the site of tenderness (Figs 12.49 and 12.50). Deliver the injection to the origin of the plantar fascia by a peppering technique, with the needle

Figure 12.49　Injection of the plantar fascia.

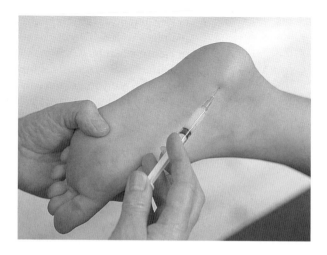

Figure 12.50　Injection of the plantar fascia showing direction of approach and needle position.

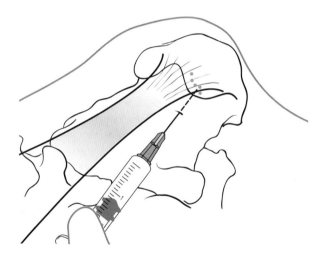

point in contact with bone at the anterior edge of the medial tubercle. The patient is advised to maintain a period of relative rest for approximately 2 weeks following injection.

Dasgupta & Bowles (1995) conducted bone scans on 15 patients with a diagnosis of plantar fasciitis, to localize the inflammatory focus. In 80% of patients, an area was localized to the medial aspect of the plantar surface of the calcaneum. An accurately placed injection into this area abolished the pain and tenderness. An accurate injection technique is important to prevent the need for repeated injection, as cases of plantar fascia rupture associated with corticosteroid injection have been reported (Sellman 1994).

Transverse frictions to the plantar fascia

Position the patient in supine lying with the foot held in dorsiflexion and the toes in extension, supported on a pillow, the leg in some lateral rotation. Standing on the affected side, direct the pressure posteromedially against the origin of the plantar fascia, either with one thumb alone or with one thumb reinforced by the other, and friction transversely across the fibres, the big toe may be extended to access the plantar fascia (Fig. 12.51). Maintain the transverse frictions for 10 min after achieving the analgesic effect. It is important to assess foot posture and to instruct the patient in intrinsic foot exercises. Care should be taken when teaching intrinsic foot exercises to avoid any clawing of the toes, which reinforces the activity of the long plantar flexors. Relative rest is advised where functional movements may continue, but no overuse or stretching until the structure is pain-free on resisted testing.

Other techniques including taping and supports may be applied, and a heel raise or cushion may help to reduce the stretch or pressure on the plantar fascia.

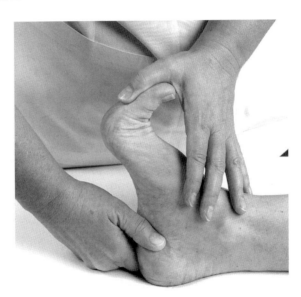

Figure 12.51 Transverse frictions to the plantar fascia.

LOOSE BODIES

Although relatively rare, loose bodies can occur in the ankle or subtalar joints. They may be due to degenerative changes in the joint or be associated with fragmented spurs on the tibial or talar side, or by avulsion from the dome of the talus or either malleolus (Scranton et al 2000). The patient presents with a history of twinging pain with giving way or a momentary inability to weight-bear; this symptom may also be indicative of mechanical ankle instability due to ligamentous laxity. On examination, a non-capsular pattern may be present. The principle of treatment for a loose body is applied – strong traction and Grade A mobilization. The direction selected for the mobilization is not important.

Figure 12.52 Loose body mobilization technique for ankle joint.

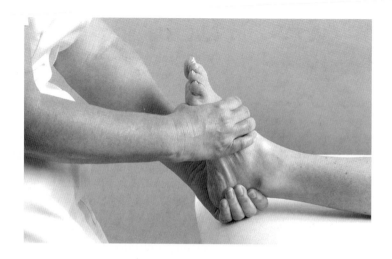

Loose body mobilization technique for ankle joint (Cyriax & Cyriax 1983, Cyriax 1984)

Position the patient in supine with the foot level with the end of the couch. Grasp the calcaneum and hold it to act as a fulcrum. Grasp the dorsum of the foot with the web of the other hand and lean back to apply strong traction. Allow the traction to establish, then apply a circumduction movement with the hand placed around the dorsum of the foot (Fig. 12.52).

Loose body mobilization technique for subtalar joint (Cyriax 1984)

Position the patient prone with the foot just off the end of the couch. Cross your thumbs over the posterosuperior aspect of the calcaneum and wrap your hands around the talus anteriorly. Lean back to apply strong traction and apply a varus and valgus movement to the calcaneum with the heels of your hands by rotating your body from side to side (Fig. 12.53).

Figure 12.53 Loose body mobilization technique for subtalar joint.

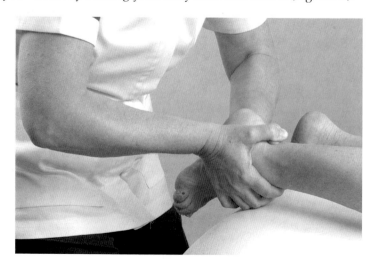

CONTRACTILE LESIONS

The following contractile lesions have been chosen for discussion since they occur relatively commonly in clinical practice. However, the principles of diagnosis and treatment can be applied to any other lesion.

PERONEAL TENDINOPATHY

Peroneal tendinopathy may be a chronic overuse injury, e.g. walking or training on unaccustomed surfaces, predisposed by altered foot biomechanics, or have an acute onset as tenosynovitis if the tendons are involved in an inversion sprain of the ankle. A few cases of rupture of the peroneus longus tendon secondary to repetitive inversion injury or forced eversion injury against resistance have been reported, presenting as chronic lateral ankle instability (Patterson & Cox 1999).

On examination pain is felt on the lateral side of the ankle on resisted eversion of the foot. Acute tenosynovitis may also produce pain on passive inversion. The exact site of the lesion is determined by palpation and may be at the musculotendinous junction, the tendons above, behind or below the malleolus, or at the insertion of peroneus brevis into the base of the fifth metatarsal. Disruption of the retinacula may cause snapping of the peroneal tendons due to subluxation or dislocation which may be obvious. However, to confirm this the ankle should be actively dorsiflexed and everted against resistance, which dynamically recreates the subluxation or dislocation of the tendons (Lee & Maleski 2002).

Transverse frictions are applied with the tendons on the stretch if the lesion involves the tendons in their common sheath behind or below the malleolus. If the lesion lies in the common sheath below the malleolus, corticosteroid injection can be applied as an alternative treatment modality.

Transverse frictions to the peroneal tendons (Cyriax & Cyriax 1983, Cyriax 1984)

Stand on the patient's good side and apply treatment to the appropriate site:

Musculotendinous junction

Locate the site of the lesion and apply the transverse frictions with the index finger, reinforced by the middle finger (Fig. 12.54). Maintain downward pressure as the frictions are applied transversely across the fibres.

Above the malleolus

Three fingers are required to cover the extent of the lesion (Fig. 12.55). Maintain downward pressure over the tendons as the transverse frictions are applied.

Behind the malleolus

Here the tendons run in a common sheath so they must be put on a stretch. Use the middle finger reinforced by the index and apply the transverse frictions by pronation and supination of the forearm (Fig. 12.56).

Figure 12.54   Transverse frictions to the peroneal tendons, musculotendinous junction.

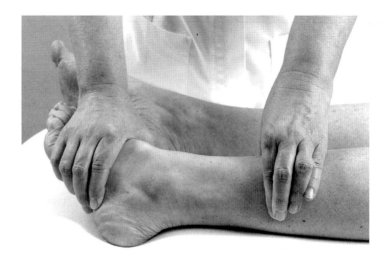

Figure 12.55   Transverse frictions to the peroneal tendons, above the malleolus.

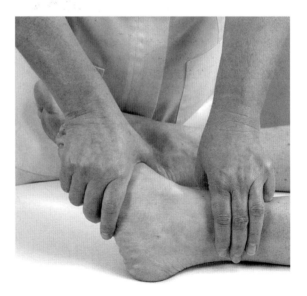

Below the malleolus   Two fingers are required to cover the extent of the lesion (Fig. 12.57). The tendons here continue in their common sheath, therefore they are treated on the stretch. Maintain downward pressure over the tendons as the transverse frictions are applied.

Figure 12.56 Transverse frictions to the peroneal tendons, behind the malleolus.

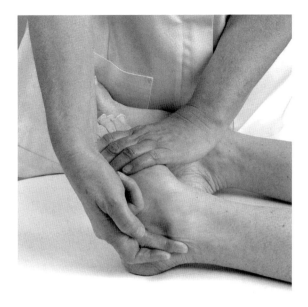

Figure 12.57 Transverse frictions to the peroneal tendons, below the malleolus.

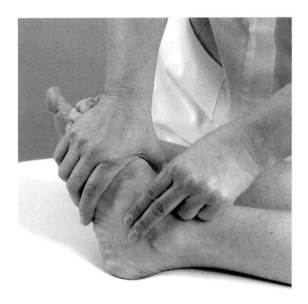

At the insertion of peroneus brevis into the base of the fifth metatarsal

An index finger, reinforced by the middle, is applied to the insertion and the frictions are delivered transversely across the fibres (Fig. 12.58).

Acute lesions are frictioned gently for approximately six effective transverse sweeps after achieving the analgesic effect. Chronic lesions require deep transverse frictions for approximately 10 min after achieving the analgesic effect. Relative rest is advised where functional movements may continue, but no overuse or stretching until the structure is pain-free on resisted testing.

Figure 12.58   Transverse frictions to the insertion of peroneus brevis into the base of the fifth metatarsal.

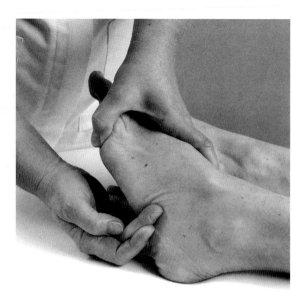

Injection technique for tenosynovitis of the peroneal tendons in the common sheath

Suggested needle size: 23G × 1 in (0.6 × 25 mm) blue needle
Dose: 10 mg triamcinolone acetonide in a total volume of 1 ml

Locate the peroneal tubercle, which indicates the distal end of the common sheath. Insert the needle into the sheath at the point of diversion of the tendons, aiming the needle towards the malleolus, parallel to the tendons (Fig. 12.59). Give the injection as a bolus into the sheath (Fig. 12.60). The patient is advised to maintain a period of relative rest for approximately 2 weeks following injection.

Injection technique for tendinopathy at the teno-osseous junction of peroneus brevis at the base of the fifth metatarsal

Suggested needle size: 25G × ⅝ in (0.5 × 16 mm) orange needle
Dose: 10 mg triamcinolone acetonide in a total volume of 1 ml

Locate the base of the fifth metatarsal and mark the tender point. Deliver the injection by a peppering technique at the teno-osseous junction

Figure 12.59   Injection
technique for tenosynovitis of
the peroneal tendons in the
common sheath.

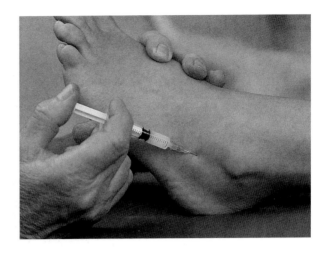

Figure 12.60   Injection
technique for tenosynovitis of
the peroneal tendons in the
common sheath.

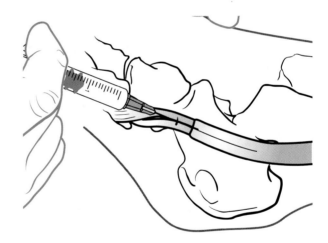

(Figs 12.61 and 12.62). The patient is advised to maintain a period of relative rest for approximately 2 weeks following injection.

The peroneal muscles act as dynamic stabilizers of the ankle joint and contract eccentrically to prevent inversion sprains (Shrier 1995). If the peroneal tendinopathy or tenosynovitis is the result of an inversion sprain, proprioception is most likely to have been altered; this may lead to functional instability and recurrent giving way. Rehabilitation must include peroneal strengthening and proprioceptive re-education, once the tendinopathy has been appropriately managed.

Figure 12.61   Injection technique at the teno-osseous junction of peroneus brevis: base of the fifth metatarsal.

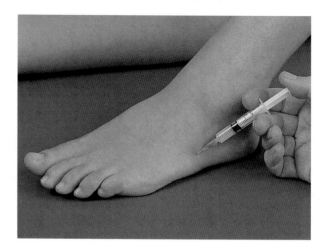

Figure 12.62   Injection technique at the teno-osseous junction of peroneus brevis: base of the fifth metatarsal, showing direction of approach and needle position.

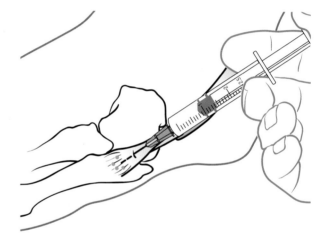

ACHILLES TENDINOPATHY

The Achilles tendon is the longest tendon in the body; it is up to 1.5 cm wide and less than 1 cm in anteroposterior thickness (Chandnani & Bradley 1994). It has the capacity to withstand high tensional forces with forces of 12.5 times body weight recorded (Alfredson & Lorentzon 2000). It consists of approximately 95% type I collagen fibres and elastin embedded in a matrix of proteoglycans and water. These fibres adopt a wavy 'crimp' configuration at rest and the primary response to tendon and fibre elongation is straightening out of the collagen fibre crimp. It is not surrounded by a true synovial sheath, but by a paratenon, a thin gliding membrane, which permits free movement of the tendon within the surrounding tissues. The blood supply is from the musculotendinous junction, the teno-osseous junction and the surrounding paratenon (Paavola et al 2002). Lesions of the Achilles tendon usually occur about 2–6 cm proximal to its insertion, which is the zone considered to be of relatively poor vascularity (Lagergren & Lindholm 1958, Smart et al 1980, Chandnani & Bradley 1994). Lesions can also exist at the musculotendinous and teno-osseous junctions. Differential diagnosis should include retrocalcaneal or superficial bursitis, impingement between the posterior part of the calcaneum and the Achilles tendon (Haglund's deformity), calcification or avulsion fracture, or occasionally mixed pathology (Alfredson & Lorentzon 2000).

A combination of pain in the Achilles tendon, swelling and impaired performance, together with pain on resisted plantarflexion, provides a clinical diagnosis of Achilles tendinopathy (Paavola et al 2002). Lesions of the Achilles tendon can be a tendonitis, an early acute condition, which may be reversible, responding to conservative treatment; or a tendinosis, i.e. focal degenerative lesions within the tendon itself which may be irreversible (Williams 1986, Mahler & Fritschy 1992, Paavola et al 2002). Partial or complete rupture may also exist. The condition has been considered to be a continuum of a degenerative process which may eventually progress to total rupture (Fox et al 1975, Read & Motto 1992). Lesions are common in older athletes, particularly those who participate in middle- or long-distance running, but also occur in the general population, often in those with a sedentary lifestyle (Alfredson & Lorentzon 2000, Paavola et al 2002).

Several aetiological mechanisms are suggested in the various texts for Achilles tendinopathy: altered biomechanics, overpronation, incorrect or worn out footwear, pressure from heel counters, one off incidents of direct trauma, inappropriate or changes in training surfaces, excessive training, training errors or indirect trauma, muscle weakness and/or imbalance, reduced flexibility, joint stiffness, male gender, obesity or leg length discrepancy. Achilles tendinopathy may also be associated with rheumatoid arthritis and the spondyloarthropathies (Smart et al 1980). As the fibres of gastrocnemius and soleus do not insert into the Achilles tendon in a parallel direction, abnormal shear stresses may be set up, creating an area of weakness and making it susceptible to injury (Frey & Shereff 1988).

Leadbetter (cited in Paavola et al 2002) suggests a mechanical theory, called the 'tendinosis cycle' for tendon degeneration, as the failure of the tendon to adapt to excessive changes in load either during a single incident or over a prolonged period of time. When the tendon is subjected to 4–8% repeated strain, it is unable to bear further tension. Injury occurs as the tendon tissue becomes fatigued and it is overwhelmed by repetitive microtrauma and thus unable to repair the fibre damage. The structure of the tendon is therefore disrupted and collagen fibres begin to slide past one another, weakening and breaking the collagen cross-links. Alfredson & Lorentzon (2000) emphasize that no inflammatory cells are seen histologically in tendinosis, but increased amounts of interfibrillar gel and glycosaminoglycans with changes in the collagen fibre structure. However, inflammation may affect the paratendinous structures leading to scar tissue development and this will need to be addressed during the treatment programme (Brukner & Khan 2002).

Patients present with a history of a gradual onset of pain felt locally at the back of the heel. They may or may not recall the causative factors. In the early phase of the condition pain usually follows strenuous activity, whereas in the more chronic condition, pain occurs during all activities and can be present at rest (Paavola et al 2002). The pain is worse when the foot is first put to the floor in the morning, easing after several steps (the different location of the pain distinguishes it from plantar fasciitis). Pain is increased by activity and the tendon itself may show some thickening. It is tender to palpation. Crepitus may be present, due to movement of the tendon within the paratenon which may be filled with fibrin exudate (Paavola et al 2002).

On examination, pain is felt on resisted plantarflexion, which should be performed against gravity with body-weight resistance to reproduce the symptoms in minor or chronic lesions. If the history indicates Achilles tendinopathy, but pain cannot be reproduced on examination, the patient may have to perform some sort of provocative exercise to produce symptoms before assessment to allow accurate diagnosis.

Rupture of the Achilles tendon rarely occurs if the tendon is healthy, but may occur if there is existing tendinosis with fibrous degeneration (Smart et al 1980). Rupture, whether partial or complete, may occur through indirect violent trauma, e.g. push-off with knee extension during weight-bearing as in sprinting, unexpected forced dorsiflexion, e.g. missing a step or stumbling, or forced dorsiflexion of the plantarflexed foot, as in falling from a height. It is accompanied by a sudden onset of pain (Smart et al 1980, Mahler & Fritschy 1992). Partial rupture and tendinosis may coexist, however, or possibly be regarded as the same condition (Alfredson & Lorentzon 2000).

Total rupture presents with a history of intense pain at the time of injury, but little pain following injury. Function is disrupted and the patient is unable to tip-toe stand. A gap may be palpable immediately after injury, and the ***Thompson's test*** may be positive. Position the patient in prone lying with the foot hanging off the couch and squeeze the bulk of the calf muscle. If intact, the Achilles tendon plantarflexes the foot. ***Matles test*** is a further aid to diagnosis of rupture, particularly if chronic. The patient is placed in prone lying and requested to flex the knee to 90°. Normally the foot should be slightly plantarflexed in this position and the test is positive if the foot falls into a neutral or a dorsiflexed position (Frey & Shereff 1988, Lee & Maleski 2002).

X-ray can be used to confirm complete rupture of the Achilles tendon. Kager's triangle is a triangular space filled with fatty tissue bordered posteriorly by the inner contour of the Achilles tendon, anteriorly by the deep flexor tendons and inferiorly by the upper border of the calcaneum (Grisogono 1989, Cetti & Andersen 1993). In total rupture, Kager's triangle loses its normal contours on the X-ray picture (Smart et al 1980). Ultrasound and magnetic resonance imaging have since become much more commonly used to confirm diagnosis.

The condition is treated by immobilization in plaster, usually after surgical repair, followed by early mobilization to achieve rapid recovery and to return to normal strength (Saw et al 1993).

Treatment of Achilles tendinopathy

Conservative treatment is advocated by most authors as the initial treatment strategy; however, sparse scientific evidence exists to support the various treatments on offer (Alfredson & Lorentzon 2000). Treatment should be accompanied by education of the patient in activity modification, particularly addressing the causative factors. A full explanation should be given of the prognosis and expected recovery time, which may well be in excess of 3 months (Brukner & Khan 2002). Return to sporting activity should be gradual and heel raises may be necessary to reduce the load on the tendon.

Alfredson et al (1998) and Alfredson & Lorentzon (2000) report on a specially designed heavy load eccentric calf muscle training programme over a 12-week period as a treatment for chronic Achilles tendinosis. All 15 patients included in the study had no pain during running and jogging after the 12-week training period and had returned to their pre-injury activity level. On a 2-year follow-up one patient was shown to have experienced a recurrence of symptoms and progressed to surgery while the rest remained pain-free. The authors could not fully explain the good results, but suggested that it could be due to loading-induced hypertrophy and increased tensile strength of the tendon, or to a stretching effect and lengthening of the muscle–tendon unit. A further explanation suggested that as the training programme was painful to perform, with severe pain being experienced during the early stage of the programme, pain perception within the tendon may have been altered. Brukner & Khan (2002) suggest that eccentric exercises can potentially cause damage if performed inappropriately or excessively; careful instruction and monitoring of the patient are therefore necessary.

The usual PRICE regime for acute injuries is adopted as necessary and the choice of electrotherapy modalities or cryotherapy is at the discretion of the therapist. The orthopaedic medicine approach involves the application of transverse frictions, but this is integrated into the programme of care for the patient. Other mobilization techniques such as specific soft tissue mobilizations (Hunter 1998) can also be included in this programme.

Transverse frictions to the Achilles tendon (Cyriax & Cyriax 1983, Cyriax 1984)

The most common sites for Achilles tendinopathy are the anterior aspect, the sides of the tendon and the insertion into the calcaneum. The affected site is identified by palpation.

Anterior aspect of the tendon

Position the patient in prone lying with the foot plantarflexed on a pillow. Push the relaxed Achilles tendon laterally with a finger, placing your middle finger reinforced by the index against the exposed anterolateral surface of the tendon (Fig. 12.63). Apply the transverse frictions by a pronation and supination movement of your forearm. Repeat the same procedure with the tendon pushed medially to gain access to the anteromedial side (Fig. 12.64).

Sides of the tendon

Position the patient in prone lying with the foot resting on a pillow over the edge of the couch. Rest your leg against the patient's foot to place it

Figure 12.63 Transverse frictions to the anterolateral aspect of the Achilles tendon

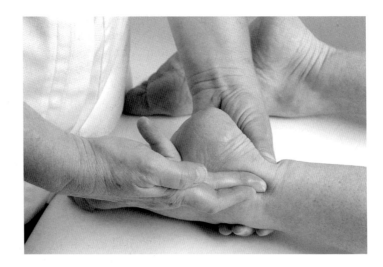

Figure 12.64 Transverse frictions to the anteromedial aspect of the Achilles tendon into the calcaneum.

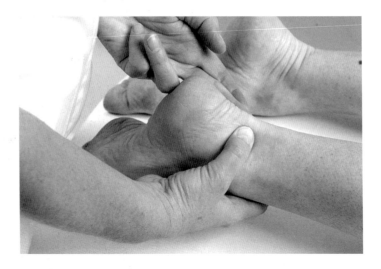

in a degree of dorsiflexion, applying enough tension to the Achilles tendon to stabilize it for treatment. Grasp the tendon between your fingers and thumb, depending on the extent of the lesion, and friction transversely across the fibres (Fig. 12.65).

Insertion of the Achilles tendon into the calcaneum

Position the patient in prone lying, with the head of the couch slightly elevated, preferably with a pillow under the foot to relax it into plantarflexion. This puts you into a good position and allows you to hold the calcaneum firmly as you apply transverse frictions to the insertion of the tendon into the middle third of the calcaneum. Make a ring formed by the index fingers, one reinforced by the other, and the thumbs. Rest your index fingers on the calcaneum and wrap your thumbs around the heel (Fig. 12.66). Direct the pressure through your index fingers down onto the insertion and impart the transverse frictions transversely across the fibres.

Figure 12.65   Transverse frictions to the sides of the Achilles tendon.

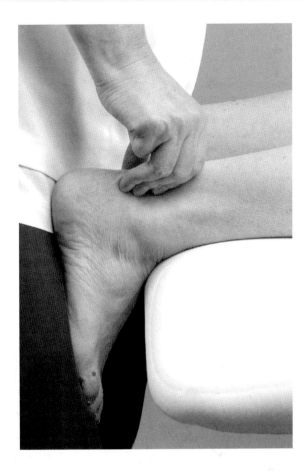

Figure 12.66   Transverse frictions at the insertion of the Achilles tendon into the calcaneum.

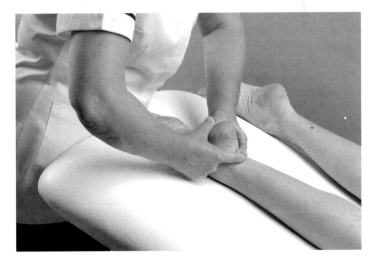

Relative rest is advised where functional movements may continue, but no overuse or stretching until the structure is pain-free on resisted testing.

Injection of the Achilles tendon

Controversy exists over the benefits and risks of corticosteroid injections and their relationship to tendon rupture (Kennedy & Baxter Willis 1976, Smart et al 1980, Kleinman & Gross 1983, Mahler & Fritschy 1992, Read & Motto 1992). Paavola et al (2002) suggest that the deleterious effects of peritendinous injections on human tendon properties is based solely on uncontrolled case studies, and that no well-controlled prospective clinical trials have been conducted to date. Corticosteroid injections tend to be used for chronic long-standing lesions in which it is difficult to assess the degree of degeneration present in the tendon and to qualify whether the complication of rupture occurred due to injection or the underlying degeneration. Uncomplicated early acute tendonitis may respond well to an early corticosteroid injection to relieve the inflammation if this is the true pathology, while tendinosis, i.e. focal degeneration of the tendon, may not benefit from corticosteroid injection. It seems that studies based on animal experiments show that intratendinous injections cause a reduction in the tensile strength of the Achilles tendon, while studies relating to peritendinous injections have not shown these adverse effects (Kleinman & Gross 1983, Mahler & Fritschy 1992, Read & Motto 1992).

Peritendinous* injection of the Achilles tendon (Cyriax & Cyriax 1983, Cyriax 1984)

Suggested needle size: 21G × 1¹/₂ in (0.8 × 40 mm) green needle
Dose: 20 mg triamcinolone acetonide in a total volume of 2 ml

*Note: the injection is peritendinous, aiming to bathe the sides of the tendon, and is not placed directly into the tendon.

Position the patient prone on the couch with the ankle resting in dorsiflexion. Bend the hub of the needle to facilitate entry alongside the tendon. Two insertions are made, one on each side of the tendon, renewing the needle in between. Advance the needle to its full length adjacent to the tendon and inject half of the solution as a bolus on each side, as the needle is withdrawn (Figs 12.67 and 12.68). The patient is advised to maintain a period of relative rest for approximately 2 weeks following injection.

Figure 12.67 Peritendinous injection of the Achilles tendon.

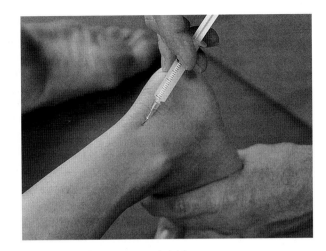

Figure 12.68 Peritendinous injection of the Achilles tendon showing direction of approach and needle position.

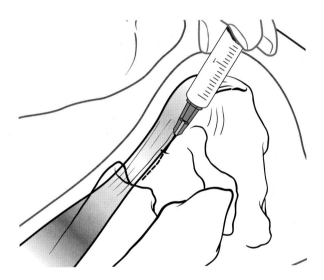

GASTROCNEMIUS MUSCLE BELLY

Strain of the gastrocnemius muscle belly often has an acute onset following a sudden sprinting action such as accelerating from a stationary position with the ankle in dorsiflexion, or lunging forward as in squash or tennis. Sudden eccentric overstretching of the muscle, such as missing your step on the kerb, is another mechanism (Brukner & Khan 2002). The lesion is sometimes called 'tennis leg' (Cyriax 1982). Patients feel as though they have been kicked or hit in the calf, the pain is acute and weight-bearing is difficult. The limb becomes swollen and bruising develops within 24–48 h. The diagnosis is conclusive from the history and palpation often localizes the lesion to the medial head of the gastrocnemius muscle belly or to the musculotendinous junction where a defect may be felt. Pain is reproduced by resisted plantarflexion and on passive dorsiflexion.

Deep vein thrombosis may be associated with calf injuries and may be difficult to exclude. Diagnosis is confirmed in the presence of constant pain, tenderness, heat, swelling and a positive Homan's sign involving pain on passive overpressure of dorsiflexion with the knee in extension (Brukner & Khan 2002).

A chronic strain of the gastrocnemius muscle belly may be the result of a past acute lesion or chronic overuse.

Treatment of acute gastrocnemius muscle belly lesion

Apply the principles of treatment for acute lesions, with protection, rest, ice, compression and elevation (PRICE) being applied as soon as possible after the onset. Gentle transverse frictions are given to the full extent of the lesion, at a depth judged to be appropriate for the irritability present, with the muscle belly in a relaxed position (Fig. 12.69). This imitates the normal function of the muscle belly fibres, which is to broaden as the muscle contracts. Transverse frictions are followed immediately by Grade A mobilizations. The patient is taught to maintain a normal heel–toe gait, with the aid of crutches if necessary. A heel raise takes the pressure off the muscle belly and can be gradually reduced as movement is regained.

The patient is seen ideally on a daily basis. An increasing depth of transverse frictions and greater range of Grade A mobilization is applied until full painless function is restored.

Treatment of chronic gastrocnemius muscle belly lesion

Deep transverse frictions are applied with the muscle belly in a relaxed position (Fig. 12.69), to facilitate the broadening of the fibres, having first gained analgesia with a more gently graded technique. Vigorous Grade A exercises are performed. The patient is treated until normal painless function is restored. Should the muscle need to be stretched, it is applied once the muscle is pain-free on resisted testing.

Figure 12.69 Transverse frictions for acute and chronic gastrocnemius muscle belly lesions.

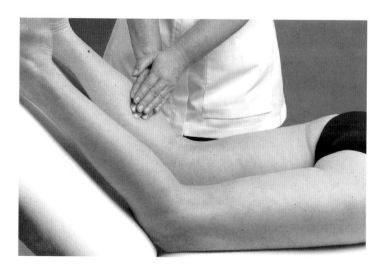

Treatment of gastrocnemius musculotendinous junction

If the lesion is in the musculotendinous junction it may be treated with transverse frictions. Locate the tender site and apply the principles with regard to depth, sweep and extent of the lesion and with consideration for the irritability of the lesion (Fig. 12.70).

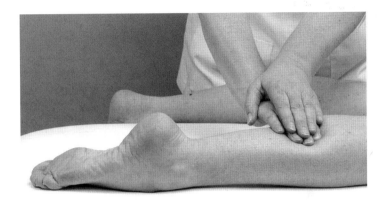

Figure 12.70   Transverse frictions to the gastrocnemius musculotendinous junction.

TIBIALIS POSTERIOR

The patient presents with a history of pain felt on the medial aspect of the ankle and the causative factors may not be known. It is often due to the repetitive microtrauma of overuse associated with overpronated foot postures and loss of the medial longitudinal arch. On inspection oedema may be present, thickening of the tendon along its course behind and below the medial malleolus may be obvious and heat may be felt on palpation. The positive sign is pain on resisted inversion and palpation for tenderness localizes the lesion. The lesion may be above, behind or below the medial malleolus or at the tendon insertion. Transverse frictions are applied with the tendon on the stretch in tenosynovitis, as the tendon is enclosed within a synovial sheath for its course around the malleolus. Alternatively, corticosteroid injection can be applied (apply the principles given above for the peroneal tendons).

References

Acus R W, Flanagan J P 1991 Perineural fibrosis of superficial peroneal nerve complicating ankle sprain: a case report. Foot and Ankle 11:233–235

Alfredson H, Pietilä T, Jonsson P et al 1998 Heavy-load eccentric calf muscle training for the treatment of chronic Achilles tendinosis. American Journal of Sports Medicine 26(3):360–366

Alfredson H, Lorentzon R 2000 Chronic Achilles tendinosis: recommendations for treatment and prevention. Sports Medicine 29(2):135–146

Anthony R J 1987 The functional anatomy of the running training shoe. Chiropodist 451–459

Auletta A G, Conway W F, Hayes C W et al 1991 Indications for radiography in patients with acute ankle injuries: role of the physical examination. American Journal of Roentgenology 157:789–791

Baxter D E 1994 The heel in sport. Clinics in Sports Medicine 13:683–693

Beumer A, van Hemert W L, Swierstra B A et al 2003 A biomechanical evaluation of clinical stress tests for syndesmotic ankle instability. Foot and Ankle International 24(4):358–363

Black H M, Brand R L, Eichelberger M R 1978 An improved technique for the evaluation of ligamentous injury in severe ankle sprains. American Journal of Sports Medicine 6:276–282

Blake R L, Anderson K, Ferguson H 1994 Posterior tibial tendinopathy. Journal of the American Podiatric Medical Association 84:141–149

Boruta P M, Bishop J O, Braly W G et al 1990 Acute lateral ankle ligament injuries: a literature review. Foot and Ankle 11:107–113

Boss A P, Hintermann B 2002 Anatomical study of the medial ankle ligament complex. Foot and Ankle International 23(6):547–553

Bottger B A, Schweitzer M E, El-Noueam K I et al 1998 MR imaging of the normal and abnormal retrocalcaneal bursae. American Roentgen Ray Society 170:1239–1241

Boytim M J, Fischer D A, Neumann L 1991 Syndesmotic ankle sprains. American Journal of Sports Medicine 19:294–298

Brooks S C, Potter B T, Rainey J B 1981 Treatment for partial tears of the lateral ligament of the ankle: a prospective trial. British Medical Journal 282:606–607

Brukner P, Khan K 2002 Clinical sports medicine, 2nd edn. McGraw-Hill, Sydney

Canoso J J 1981 Bursae, tendons and ligaments. Clinics in Rheumatic Diseases 7:189–221

Cetti R, Andersen I 1993 Roentgenographic diagnosis of ruptured Achilles tendons. Clinical Orthopaedics and Related Research 286:215–221

Chandler T J, Kibler W B 1993 A biomechanical approach to the prevention, treatment and rehabilitation of plantar fasciitis. Sports Medicine 15:344–352

Chandnani V P, Bradley Y C 1994 Achilles tendon and miscellaneous lesions. MRI Clinics of North America 2:89–96

Cornwall M W, Murrell P 1991 Postural sway following inversion sprain of the ankle. Journal of the American Podiatric Medical Association 81:243–247

Cyriax J 1982 Textbook of orthopaedic medicine, 8th edn. Baillière Tindall, London, vol 1

Cyriax J 1984 Textbook of orthopaedic medicine, 11th edn. Baillière Tindall, London, vol 2

Cyriax J, Cyriax P 1983 Illustrated manual of orthopaedic medicine. Butterworths, London

Dasgupta B, Bowles J 1995 Scintigraphic localization of steroid injection site in plantar fasciitis. Lancet 346:1400–1401

Edwards G S, DeLee J C 1984 Ankle diastasis without fracture. Foot and Ankle 4:305–312

Evans P 1990 Clinical biomechanics of the subtalar joint. Physiotherapy 76:47–81

Fox J M, Blanzina M E, Jobe F W et al 1975 Degeneration and rupture of the Achilles tendon. Clinical Orthopaedics and Related Research 107:221–224

Frey C, Shereff M J 1988 Tendon injuries about the ankle in athletes. Clinics in Sports Medicine 7:103–118

Frey C, Rosenberg Z, Shereff M J et al 1992 The retrocalcaneal bursa: anatomy and bursography. Foot and Ankle 13:203–207

Fujii T, Luo Z, Kitaoka H B et al 2000 The manual stress test may not be sufficient to differentiate ankle ligament injuries. Clinical Biomechanics 15:619–623

Gibbon W W, Cassar-Pullicino V N 1994 Heel pain. Annals of the Rheumatic Diseases 53:344–348

Grisogono V 1989 Physiotherapy treatment for Achilles tendon injuries. Physiotherapy 75:562–572

Hertel J 2002 Functional anatomy, pathomechanics, and pathophysiology of lateral ankle ligament instability. Journal of Athletic Training 37(4):364–375

Hocutt J E, Jaffe R, Rylander C R et al 1982 Cryotherapy in ankle sprains. American Journal of Sports Medicine 10:316–319

Hunter G 1998 Specific soft tissue mobilization in the management of soft tissue dysfunction. Manual Therapy 3(1):2–11

Hutson M A 1990 Sports injuries – recognition and management. Oxford Medical Publications, Oxford

Kannus V P A 1992 Evaluation of abnormal biomechanics of the foot and ankle in athletes. British Journal of Sports Medicine 26:83–89

Kannus P, Renstrom P 1991 Treatment for acute tears of the lateral ligaments of the ankle. Journal of Bone and Joint Surgery 73A:305–312

Kapandji I A 1987 The physiology of the joints: lower limb, 5th edn. Churchill Livingstone, Edinburgh, vol 2

Karlsson J, Lansingeer O 1992 Lateral instability of the ankle joint. Clinical Orthopaedics and Clinical Research 276:253–261

Karr S D 1994 Subcalcaneal heel pain. Orthopedic Clinics of North America 25:161–175

Kennedy J C, Baxter Willis R 1976 The effects of local steroid injections on tendons: a biomechanical and microscopic correlative study. American Journal of Sports Medicine 4:11–21

Kerkhoffs G M, Rowe B H, Assendelft W J et al 2002 Immobilization and functional treatment for acute lateral ankle ligament injuries in adults. Cochrane Review. In: Cochrane Library, Issue 2, Update Software, Oxford

Kesson M, Atkins A, Davies I 2003 Musculoskeletal injection skills. Butterworth Heinemann, Oxford

Kibler W B, Goldberg C, Chandler T J 1991 Functional biomechanical deficits in running athletes with plantar fasciitis. American Journal of Sports Medicine 19:66–71

Kim W, Voloshin A S 1995 Role of plantar fascia in the load bearing capacity of the human foot. Journal of Biomechanics 28:1025–1033

Kleinman M, Gross A E 1983 Achilles tendon rupture following steroid injection. Journal of Bone and Joint Surgery 65A:1345–1347

Kulthanan T 1992 Operative treatment of plantar fasciitis. Journal of the Medical Association of Thailand 75:337–340

Kumai T, Takakura Y, Rufai A et al 2002 The functional anatomy of the human anterior talofibular ligament in relation to ankle sprains. Journal of Anatomy 200(5):457–465

Lagergren C, Lindholm A 1958 Vascular distribution in the Achilles tendon. Acta Chirurgica Scandinavica 116:491–495

Lee T K, Maleski R 2002 Physical examination of the ankle for ankle pathology. Clinics in Podiatric Medicine and Surgery 19:251–269

Lentell G L, Latzman L L, Walters M R 1990 The relationship between muscle function and ankle stability. Journal of Orthopaedic and Sports Physical Therapy 11:605–611

Levangie P, Norkin C 2001 Joint structure and function, 3rd edn. F A Davis Co, Philadelphia

Litt J C B 1992 The sprained ankle: diagnosis and management of lateral ligament injuries. Australian Family Physician 21:447–457

Liu S H, Jason W J 1994 Lateral ankle sprains and instability problems. Clinics in Sports Medicine 13:793–809

McMinn R M H, Gaddum-Rosse P, Hutchings R T et al 1995 Functional and clinical anatomy. Mosby, London

Mahler F, Fritschy D 1992 Partial and complete ruptures of the Achilles tendon and local corticosteroid injections. British Journal of Sports Medicine 26:7–13

Marder R A 1994 Current methods for the evaluation of ankle ligament injuries. Journal of Bone and Joint Surgery 76A:1103–1111

Miller C A, Bosco J A 2002 Lateral ankle and subtalar instability. Hospital for Joint Diseases 60(3):143–149

Nordin M, Frankel V H 2001 Basic biomechanics of the musculoskeletal system, 3rd edn. Lippincott, Williams & Wilkins, Philadelphia

Norris C M 1998 Sports injuries: diagnosis and management for physiotherapists, 2nd edn. Butterworth Heinemann, Oxford

Ogilvie-Harris D J, Gilbart M 1995 Treatment modalities for soft tissue injuries of the ankle: a critical review. Clinical Journal of Sports Medicine 5:175–186

O'Hara J, Valle-Jones J C, Walsh H et al 1992 Controlled trial of an ankle support Malleotrain in acute ankle injuries. British Journal of Sports Medicine 26:139–142

Paavola M, Kannus P, Järvinen T A et al 2002 Current concepts review: Achilles tendinopathy. Journal of Bone and Joint Surgery 84A(11):2062–2076

Palastanga N, Field D, Soames R 2002 Anatomy and human movement, 4th edn Butterworth Heinemann, Oxford

Patterson M H, Cox W K 1999 Peroneus longus tendon rupture as a cause of chronic lateral ankle pain. Clinical Orthopaedics and Related Research 365:163–166

Read M T F, Motto S G 1992 Tendo Achillis pain: steroids and outcome. British Journal of Sports Medicine 26:15–21

Roberts C S, DeMaio M, Larkin J J et al 1995 Eversion ankle sprains. Sports Medicine Rehabilitation Series 18:299–304

Roycroft S, Mantgani A B 1983 Treatment of inversion injuries of the ankle by early active management. Physiotherapy 69:355–356

Sartoris D J 1994 Diagnosis of ankle injuries: the essentials. Journal of Foot and Ankle Surgery 33:102–107

Saw Y, Baltzopoulos V, Lim A et al 1993 Early mobilization after operative repair of ruptured Achilles tendon. International Journal of the Care of the Injured 24:479–484

Scranton P E, McDermott J E, Rogers J V 2000 The relationship between chronic ankle instability and variations in mortise anatomy and impingement spurs. Foot and Ankle International 21(8):657–664

Sellman J R 1994 Plantar fascia rupture associated with corticosteroid injection. Foot and Ankle International 15:376–381

Shrier I 1995 Treatment of lateral collateral sprains of the ankle: a critical appraisal of the literature. Clinical Journal of Sports Medicine 5:187–195

Smart G W, Taunton J E, Clement D B 1980 Achilles tendon disorders in runners – a review. Medicine and Science in Sports and Exercise 12:231–243

Stanley K L 1991 Ankle sprains are always more than 'just a sprain'. Postgraduate Medicine 89:251–255

Stephens M M 1994 Haglund's deformity and retrocalcaneal bursitis. Orthopedic Clinics of North America 25:41–46

Swain R A, Holt W S 1993 Ankle injuries: tips from sports medicine physicians. Postgraduate Medicine 93:91–100

Tropp H 2002 Commentary: functional ankle instability revisited. Journal of Athletic Training 37(4):512–515

Wilkerson L A 1992 Ankle injuries in athletes. Primary Care 19:377–392

Williams J G P 1986 Achilles tendon lesions in sport. Sports Medicine 3:114–115

Williams P L 1998 Gray's Anatomy: the anatomical basis of medicine and surgery, 38th edn. Churchill Livingstone, Edinburgh

Yu J S 2000 Pathologic and post-operative conditions of the plantar fascia: review of MR imaging appearances. Skeletal Radiology 29:491–501

Chapter **13**

The lumbar spine

SUMMARY

Low back pain presents a challenge to the clinician. Diagnosis is not simple and the clinical data collected may indicate complicated lesions, with several factors contributing to the signs and symptoms. One possible cause of back pain is lumbar disc lesion, the mechanism of which is still poorly understood. Mechanical, chemical and ischaemic factors are currently under investigation.

This chapter outlines the relevant anatomy to enable discussion of evidence for the causes of back pain and differential diagnosis. The clinical examination procedure will be outlined and interpreted, and the disc models used in orthopaedic medicine will be identified to act as a guide to treatment using this approach.

Emphasis will be placed on the selection of patients suitable for treatment and the contraindications to treatment will be discussed. Treatment techniques will be described and guidelines for safety in the application of treatment techniques will be suggested.

ANATOMY

There are five lumbar vertebrae, each with a large vertebral body designed for weight-bearing (Fig. 13.1). Each *vertebral body* consists of a shell of cortical bone surrounding a cancellous cavity of supporting struts and cross-beams called trabeculae. This provides a lightweight box with the strength to support longitudinally applied loads. The intervening *intervertebral disc* provides a mechanism for shock absorption, distribution of forces and movement (Jensen 1980).

The stabilizing function of the lumbar spine is achieved by the various bony processes that make up the posterior elements of the lumbar vertebrae, i.e. the pedicles and laminae, and the articular, spinous and transverse processes. The position and direction of the *articular processes* that form the synovial *zygapophyseal joints* prevent forward sliding and rotation of the vertebral bodies, while the *spinous and transverse processes* act as leverage and provide attachment for muscles.

The *vertebral foramen* is surrounded by the vertebral body in front and the posterior elements behind. It is triangular in the lumbar spine

Figure 13.1 Typical lumbar vertebra. From Anatomy and Human Movement by N Palastanga, D Field and R Soames. Reprinted by permission of Elsevier Ltd.

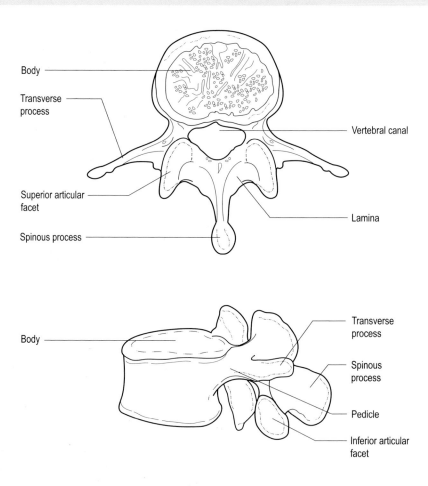

and is larger than that in the thoracic spine but smaller than that in the cervical spine. Together the vertebral foramina form the *vertebral canal* which contains the termination of the spinal cord opposite the L1–L2 disc, and the *cauda equina*. The vertebral canal can vary in shape and this may be relevant to pathology.

The *lumbar lordosis*, the posterior postural concavity, compensates for the inclination of the sacrum and maintains the upright posture. The wedge-shaped lumbosacral disc and vertebral body of L5 contribute to the lordosis as well as the antigravity effect of the constant activity in the erector spinae muscles that prevent the trunk from falling forwards (Oliver & Middleditch 1991).

THE INTERVERTEBRAL DISC

The intervertebral disc has special biomechanical requirements. It is strong to sustain weight and transmit loads while being able to deform to adjust to movement. The intervertebral disc has three parts: a central nucleus pulposus surrounded by a peripheral annulus fibrosus which blends above and below into vertebral end-plates.

The *nucleus pulposus* accommodates to movement and transmits compressive loads from one vertebral body to another. Its normal consistency has been likened to that of toothpaste. It is composed of irregularly arranged collagen fibres and cartilage cells scattered within amorphous ground substance. The collagen fibres are composed of type II collagen, suited to accept pressure and compression (see Ch. 2). The nucleus in particular has great water-binding capacity through its proteoglycan content. The fluid nature of the nucleus allows it to deform under pressure while the vertebral end-plates prevent its superior and inferior deformation. In this way the intervertebral disc supports and transmits loads.

Although it has long been recognized for its fluid properties, the nucleus also behaves as a viscoelastic solid under dynamic conditions. Iatridis et al (1996) investigated the viscoelastic properties of the healthy nucleus pulposus, showing it to be sensitive to different loading rates. The higher loading rates produced failure of the end-plate and vertebral body, while slower loading rates produced progressive failure of the annulus and disc herniation.

The *annulus fibrosus* consists of a geometrically organized arrangement of collagen and elastic fibres bound together by a proteoglycan gel, allowing it to support weight without buckling. Types I and II collagen exist in the annulus fibrosus, but the majority of fibres are type I, suited to withstand tensile forces. The fibres are arranged in concentric lamellae around the central nucleus. These tightly packed lamellae are arranged circumferentially at the periphery and can sustain high compressive loads. Adams et al (2002) suggest an analogy to the stiffness of a telephone directory wrapped into a cylinder and stood on its end. In each lamella, the collagen fibres lie parallel to each other, inclined at an angle of approximately 65–70° to the vertical (Fig. 13.2). The direction of fibres alternates in adjacent lamellae (Bogduk 1997). Marchand & Ahmed (1990) noted a number of irregularities within the laminate structure of the annulus, particularly at the posterolateral corners, where a number of incomplete layers were seen. Increased stresses applied to the annulus in this region could produce fissuring and provide the nuclear material with an escape route.

The annulus fibrosus acts like a ligament, restraining excessive movement to stabilize the intervertebral joint while allowing flexibility to permit normal movement. The alternating oblique annular fibres resist horizontal and vertical forces, allowing the annulus to oppose movement in all directions (Bogduk 1991).

The outer half of the annulus at least is known to have a nerve supply (Cavanaugh et al 1995, Coppes et al 1997). The main source of the supply is believed to be the sinuvertebral nerve and branches of the sympathetic trunks and its grey rami communicantes (Adams et al 2002). The sinuvertebral nerve supplies the disc at one level and the disc above (Bogduk 1997).

The *vertebral end-plates* are thin layers of cartilage, approximately 1 mm thick, covering the superior and inferior surfaces of the discs. They form a permeable barrier for diffusion, mainly between the nucleus and

Figure 13.2 Laminate structure of the disc. Reprinted from Clinical Anatomy of the Lumbar Spine and Sacrum. N Bogduk © 1998. by permission of Elsevier.

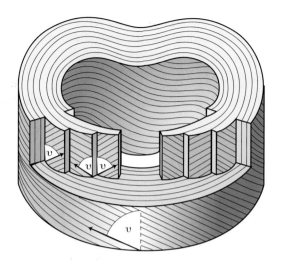

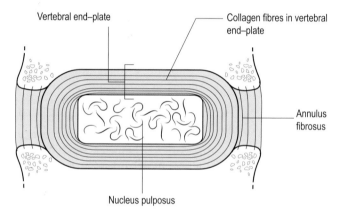

Vertebral end–plate

Collagen fibres in vertebral end–plate

Annulus fibrosus

Nucleus pulposus

the cancellous bone of the vertebral bodies. They fail relatively easily under excessive compressive loading.

Properties of the intervertebral disc

The intervertebral disc at rest possesses an intrinsic pressure due to the compressive effect of the elastic ligamentum flavum (Oliver & Middleditch 1991). This preloaded or prestressed state provides it with an intrinsic stability to resist applied forces such as body weight (Jensen 1980). The resting pressure is affected by posture and loading, being lowest in the lying position and highest in the sitting position, with a further increase if external loading is applied (Nachemson 1966). In the sitting position the spine usually rests in a degree of flexion and the activity in psoas major contributes a compressive effect on the disc as it stabilizes the spine.

Clinically, somatic back pain and radicular pain are affected by movements and posture, as well as being increased by straining, coughing or laughing. An increase in intradiscal pressure of about 50% was noted when straining was performed in standing, due to the increase in loading produced by muscle activity (Nachemson & Elfstrom 1970). The chart originating from the investigations of Nachemson (1966) has been reproduced in several publications as a useful guide to the variation in intradiscal pressure with different postures and activities (Fig. 13.3).

Figure 13.3 Discal pressures. Relative change in pressure (or load) in the third lumbar disc: (a) in various positions; (b) in muscle-strengthening exercises. From Nachemson A 1976 The lumbar spine: an orthopaedic challenge. Spine 1:59–71, with permission.

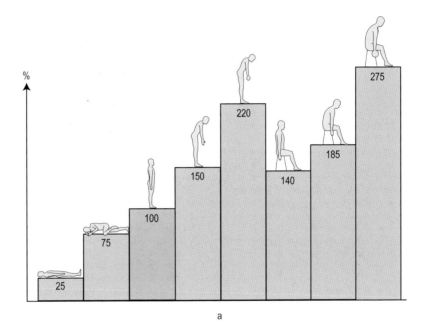

a

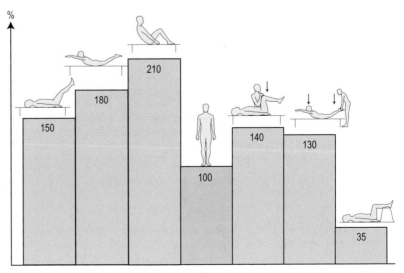

b

Movement of the spine involves simultaneous tension, compression and shear at different locations of the disc affecting intradiscal pressure and fluid flow. Flexion, extension and side flexion produce tension resulting in stretching of the annulus on one side, and compression on the other side through body weight (Jensen 1980). Flexion includes a component of forward translation that is stabilized by the zygapophyseal joints, while extension is limited by bony impaction of the inferior articular processes against the lamina of the vertebra below. Axial rotation produces torsion in the intervertebral discs, with tension in half of the annular fibres that are inclined towards the direction of the rotation, and impaction of the zygapophyseal joints. Side flexion is a composite movement which includes side flexion and rotation (Bogduk 1997).

As a viscoelastic material, the intervertebral disc is subjected to the phenomena of creep, hysteresis and set (Twomey & Taylor 1982, Bogduk 1997, Oliver & Twomey 1995), as discussed in Chapter 2. The creep behaviour of flexion and extension is similar, with the amount of creep increasing with load and progressing with time. Creep also increases with age when hysteresis recovery is slower. Flexion creep, in particular, has implications for occupations that require a constant flexed posture, e.g. manual workers. It may also be responsible for fatigue in the disc, making it vulnerable to a sudden applied force – the 'straw that breaks the camel's back'.

Nutrition of the intervertebral disc

The lumbar discs have a relatively poor blood supply since no arteries enter the disc (Adams et al 2002). Nutrition of the intervertebral disc occurs through two routes: the blood vessels situated around the peripheral annulus and those in the central portion of the vertebral end-plate. The mechanisms involved are diffusion and fluid flow and are interrelated. Both are affected by posture and motion (Adams & Hutton 1986).

The water content of the disc varies and represents a balance between two opposing osmotic and hydrostatic pressures, i.e. a swelling pressure (imbibition) which hydrates the disc and a mechanical pressure (posture, movement, loading and creep) which dehydrates the disc. Diurnal decrease in the total length of the spine is offset by its recovery in the supine position overnight (Parke & Schiff 1971, Porter 1995). Flexion postures cause a larger fluid outflow from the disc than erect or lordotic postures, with this outflow being further reduced when the spine is unloaded by lying down. Alternating between rest and activity will enhance fluid flow (Adams & Hutton 1983, 1986). Factors that influence the nutrition of the disc are increased loading, vibration or spinal deformity. Factors that compromise the vascular supply include smoking, vascular disease and diabetes (Buckwalter 1995).

ZYGAPOPHYSEAL JOINTS (FACET JOINTS)

The zygapophyseal joints are synovial joints that provide stability of the spine, control of movement and protection of the intervertebral discs (Fig. 13.4) (Taylor & Twomey 1994). The articular facets are covered with articular cartilage and the joints are surrounded by a fibrous capsule

Figure 13.4 Intra-articular structures of the lumbar zygapophyseal joints. (a) Coronal section of a left zygapophyseal joint showing fibroadipose meniscoids projecting into the joint cavity from the capsule over the superior and inferior poles of the joint.
(b) Lateral view of a right zygapophyseal joint, in which the superior articular process has been removed to show intra-articular structures projecting into the joint cavity across the surface of the inferior articular facet. The superior capsule is retracted to reveal the base of a fibroadipose meniscoid (FM) and an adipose tissue pad (AP). Another fibroadipose meniscoid at the lower pole of the joint is lifted from the surface of the articular cartilage. A connective tissue (CT) rim has been retracted along the posterior margin of the joint. Reprinted from Clinical Anatomy of the Lumbar Spine and Sacrum. N Bogduk © 1998 by permission of Elsevier.

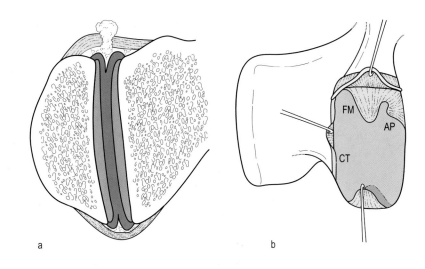

and lined with synovium. The **superior articular facets** face posteromedially and grasp onto the **inferior articular facets** of the vertebra above, which face anterolaterally. The resultant plane of the joint facilitates flexion and extension movements, but prevents rotation. It also restricts translation in healthy joints, helping to protect the lumbar disc from the shearing forces responsible for fissuring (Bogduk 1991, Taylor & Twomey 1994).

The **fibrous capsule** consists of an outer layer of regularly arranged connective tissue and an inner layer of yellow elastic fibres. Anteriorly the capsule is replaced by the **ligamentum flavum**, while some of the deep fibres of **multifidus** give the capsule reinforcement medially (Yamashita et al 1996). The superior and inferior aspects of the capsules are loose and contain **intra-articular structures** consisting of fat and meniscoid structures (Bogduk 1997). Fine nerve fibres thought to conduct nociceptive and proprioceptive sensations have been found (Yamashita et al 1996).

The zygapophyseal joints cannot be discounted as a cause of back pain since, as synovial joints, they may be subjected to trauma or arthritis. Degenerative changes usually coexist in the intervertebral joint of the same segment.

Authors have looked at the pattern of pain referral of the zygapophyseal joints in an attempt to establish a recognized syndrome and pain referral patterns (Mooney & Robertson 1976, Bogduk 1994). Schwarzer et al (1994a) acknowledged this joint as a possible source of pain, but questioned the existence of a facet syndrome. Some authors suggest that the zygapophyseal joint is responsible for the acute locked back, as the intra-articular structures become trapped between the articular surfaces (Bogduk 1997, Twomey & Taylor 1994), while Kuslich et al (1991) demonstrated that stimulation of the zygapophyseal joint capsule very rarely generated back pain. In a study of the relative contributions of the disc and zygapophyseal joint in chronic low back pain, pain was noted to arise more commonly from the disc than the zygapophyseal joint (Schwarzer et al 1994b).

Laslett & van Wijmen (1999) suggest that the symptomatic zygapophyseal joint presents with pain that settles well on lying down and four of the following criteria: age greater than 65; pain not increased by coughing; no pain on flexion in standing; pain not increased in rising from flexion; pain not increased by extension/rotation; or pain not increased by extension in standing.

The authors of this text accept the lack of evidence to attribute the cause of low back pain to one specific structure and that will also apply to the symptomatic zygapophyseal model presented above. Orthopaedic medicine treatments have traditionally been based on the discal model but it may be more clinically relevant to apply treatments selected on the basis of a particular set of signs and symptoms rather than to attempt to be too pedantic with regard to pathology (see below). It must be acknowledged that a lesion in any structure within a spinal segment will influence neighbouring structures and similarly treatment cannot be directed to one anatomical structure in isolation.

LIGAMENTS

Anterior and posterior longitudinal ligaments are well-developed in the lumbar region where both stabilize the vertebral bodies and control movement (Fig. 13.5). The *anterior longitudinal ligament* is widest in the lumbar spine where it covers most of the anterior and lateral surfaces of the vertebral bodies and intervertebral discs. The *posterior longitudinal ligament* is relatively weaker and has a denticulate arrangement that permits the passage of vascular structures. Superficial fibres bridge several vertebrae while deeper fibres pass over two joints and have lateral extensions intimately related to the intervertebral disc (Parke & Schiff 1971). The strong central portion of the posterior longitudinal ligament provides resistance to central disc displacement, deflecting it laterally where the lateral extensions are deficient and offer a space for posterolateral displacement.

The *ligamentum flavum* consists of predominantly yellow elastic fibres and connects adjacent laminae. It controls lumbar flexion by 'braking' the separation of the laminae and assisting the return to the upright posture. The elastic fibres also restore the ligament to its normal length after stretching, to prevent buckling into the spinal canal and compression of the spinal cord. Such pathology may arise in the degenerate ligament and contribute to stenosis.

The *iliolumbar ligament* provides stability for the lumbosacral junction (Yamamoto et al 1990), attaching the L5 transverse process to the pelvis. Sometimes a band also passes from the transverse process of L4. This anchorage of L5 to the pelvis may restrict the amount of accommodation possible for disc herniation. Disc herniation at the L5, S1 level may produce severe pain with the patient fixed in flexion, whereas herniation above this level, usually L4–L5, may be accommodated more readily by a lateral shift that will reduce pain.

Figure 13.5   The ligaments of
the lumbar spine.

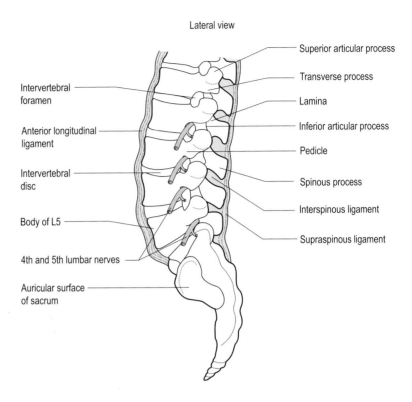

Lateral view

Superior articular process

Transverse process

Intervertebral
foramen

Lamina

Anterior longitudinal
ligament

Inferior articular process

Pedicle

Intervertebral
disc

Spinous process

Body of L5

Interspinous ligament

Supraspinous ligament

4th and 5th lumbar nerves

Auricular surface
of sacrum

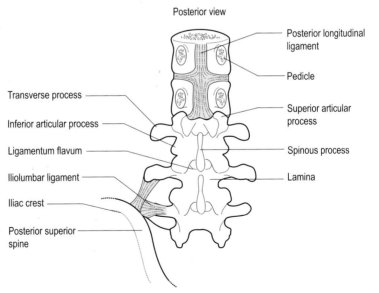

Posterior view

Posterior longitudinal
ligament

Pedicle

Transverse process

Inferior articular process

Superior articular
process

Ligamentum flavum

Spinous process

Iliolumbar ligament

Lamina

Iliac crest

Posterior superior
spine

LUMBAR SPINAL NERVES

The termination of the *spinal cord* lies approximately level with the L1–L2 disc, and the lumbar and sacral nerve roots descend vertically in the *cauda equina*, surrounded by the dural sac, to exit via their appropriate lumbar or sacral intervertebral foramina.

Dorsal (sensory) and ventral (mainly motor) nerve roots join to form the relatively short *spinal nerve* that is situated in the intervertebral foramen, together with the dorsal root ganglion. The *dorsal root ganglion* is the collected cell bodies of all sensory nerve fibres related to that segment. The cell bodies of the motor axons are located in the anterior horns of the grey matter in the spinal cord. In the intervertebral foramen the spinal nerve is surrounded by the dural nerve root sleeve, which eventually blends with the epineurium of the nerve. Immediately after leaving the intervertebral foramen the spinal nerve divides into *dorsal and ventral rami*.

Spinal nerves do not possess the same protective connective tissue sheaths as peripheral nerves and are therefore said to be vulnerable to direct mechanical injury (Rydevik & Olmarker 1992).

There are five pairs of lumbar nerves, five pairs of sacral nerves and one pair of coccygeal nerves. Their dorsal and ventral nerve roots pass in the cauda equina in an inferolateral direction to reach their appropriate level, before joining to emerge through the intervertebral foramina as the spinal nerves. Until the coccygeal level is reached there are several nerve roots passing vertically in the cauda equina (Fig. 13.6).

The clinical implications of this should be recognized as it is possible for a lumbar disc herniation to encroach on more than one nerve root. It also explains how a lumbar disc herniation could compress the S4 nerve root to affect bladder function.

DEGENERATIVE CHANGES IN THE LUMBAR SPINE

There is a suggestion that the intervertebral discs degenerate first and the subsequent reduction in the ability of the disc to equally distribute loads in all directions causes secondary degenerative changes in the zygapophyseal joints and ligaments (Acaroglu et al 1995, Prescher 1998). The degenerative process has been noted to be most predominant in the L4, L5 and L5, S1 levels but affects all levels of the lumbar spine, resulting in an overall reduction in spinal mobility (Prescher 1998).

The most marked ageing or degenerative changes occur in the nucleus of the intervertebral disc. There is a reduction in the water and proteoglycan content and a change in the number and nature of the collagen fibres, with the typical type II fibres of the nucleus changing to resemble the type I fibres of the annulus (Umehara et al 1996, Bogduk 1997). The water content of the nucleus reduces from 90% at birth to approximately 65–71% by the age of 75 and reduces the preloaded state of the disc (Jensen 1980, Taylor & Twomey 1994, Bogduk 1997). In section

Figure 13.6   The cauda equina and emerging nerve roots. From Functional Anatomy of the Spine by J Oliver and A Middleditch. Reprinted with permission of Harcourt Education Ltd.

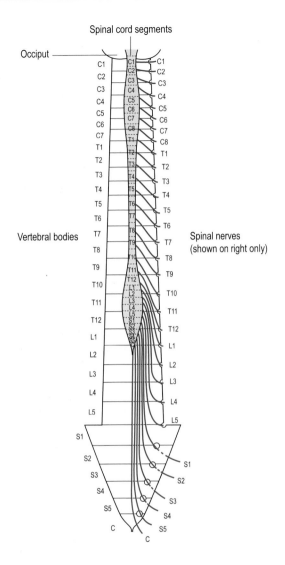

the ageing nucleus pulposus develops the appearance of a dry, crumbling mass, changing in colour from the normal glassy greyish-blue towards yellow and brown – an observation that is sometimes referred to as 'brown degeneration' (Prescher 1998).

The nucleus, in losing some of its fluid properties, is less able to exert a radial pressure on the annulus. Therefore, a greater portion of vertical load is supported by the annulus and the greater stresses contribute to circumferential tears and radial fissures. The lumbar discs become stiffer and less resilient and overall there is reduced mobility in the lumbar spine.

Degeneration affects the structure of the annulus, with a decrease in the number of lamellae. Individual lamellae become thicker and there is fraying, splitting and breakdown of the laminate structure with less evidence of a transitional zone between annulus and nucleus (Marchand

& Ahmed 1990, Bernick et al 1991, Holm 1993, Acaroglu et al 1995). This degenerative process causes a change in the tensile properties of the annulus that affect its mechanical properties, as well as rendering it vulnerable to failure at lower stresses (Acaroglu et al 1995).

Three types of annular defects are noted (Osti & Cullum 1994):

- *Rim lesions* – discrete defects between the outer annulus and the vertebral body
- *Circumferential tears* – more common in the lateral and posterior layers
- *Radial fissures* – commonly seen in degenerating discs, extending from the nucleus

Prescher (1998) explores the results of degeneration of the intervertebral disc material, suggesting that 'dislocation' of the annulus and/or the nucleus can occur, which may help in rationalizing the disc as a possible cause of spinal pain. The 'dislocation' may present as a *'disc protrusion'* – a bulging of the disc in a posterior, lateral or anterior direction, which mainly involves nuclear material pushing outwards and stretching or 'bulging' the annular fibres. Since annular fibres contain nociceptive nerve endings, stimulation of these may produce primary discal symptoms.

If annular fibres tear, the pressurized nuclear tissue pushes outward through the defect, resulting in *'disc prolapse'* where it may be responsible for compression or irritation of other pain-sensitive structures, resulting in secondary discal symptoms. The prolapsed tissue may be directed posteriorly, posterolaterally and anteriorly. If it detaches completely, it is referred to as *'sequestrated'*, when it may be directed further, either cranially or caudally. Posterolateral disc prolapse may encroach into the intervertebral canal and may compromise the emerging spinal nerve root, since the intervertebral disc is located at the same level as the emerging spinal nerve in the lumbar spine.

Bone density in the vertebral bodies reduces with age, causing weakening of the trabecular system, a loss of the horizontal trabeculae and a gradual collapse of the vertebral end-plate (Taylor & Twomey 1994, Prescher 1998). This results in the intervertebral disc bowing into the concavity of the weakened end-plate, with consequences for the nutrition of the disc via this route. A loss of overall height with ageing may not be due to a loss in disc height therefore, but a loss in vertebral body height due to the collapse of the vertebral end-plate and subsequent migration of the discal material into the vertebral body (Taylor & Twomey 1994, Bogduk 1997). However, Prescher (1998) suggests that a pronounced decrease in disc height may result in adjacent spinous processes coming into contact with one another ('kissing spines') causing grinding, sclerotic changes and even pseudoarthroses.

Prescher (1998) also discusses degeneration, i.e. spondyloarthrosis of the zygapophyseal joints, suggesting that this particularly affects lumbar joints in patients over 30. Loss of disc height would appear to be the trigger, causing caudal migration of the inferior articular processes and a posterior displacement (or retrolisthesis) of the vertebral body. Advanced spondyloarthrosis may result in anterior displacement of the vertebral bodies, particularly L4, which occurs with the pars interarticularis intact.

This phenomenon was noticed by Junghanns (cited in Prescher 1998) and was termed a pseudospondylolisthesis, occuring more frequently in females. This is a separate entity to a spondylolisthesis which affects L5 predominantly and occurs more commonly in males.

LUMBAR DISC LESIONS

Any structures in the lumbar region that receive a nerve supply can be a primary source of somatic pain. Congenital or acquired disorders of a single component of the motion segment cannot exist without affecting the functions of other components of the same segment and the functions of other segmental levels of the spine (Parke & Schiff 1971). However, Schwarzer et al (1994b) consider zygapophyseal joint pain to be uncommon, with discogenic pain a singular, independent disorder.

The zygapophyseal joints, as synovial joints, can be affected by arthritis and the presence of intra-articular structures makes derangement of the joint a possibility. The intervertebral disc is known to degenerate and since the outer annulus receives a nerve supply it can be a primary source of pain. Herniations of discal material are well-recognized and are a secondary cause of pain, affecting other pain-sensitive structures.

Traction exerted on the dura and noxious stimulation of the back muscles, ligaments and lumbar zygapophyseal joints have both provoked a pain response (Bogduk 1994). Compression of normal nerves does not provoke a pain response while stimulation of swollen, stretched or compressed nerve roots has been shown to produce leg pain, with the dorsal root ganglion tending to be more tender than other parts of the nerve (Kuslich et al 1991). In the same study, stimulation of the outer annulus fibrosus and the posterior longitudinal ligament produced back pain while there was tenderness on stimulation of the capsule of the zygapophyseal joint, also associated with localized back pain. Pain may be produced in any pain-sensitive structure through chemical, mechanical or ischaemic mechanisms, although it seems more than likely that all factors coexist in disc pathology or herniation.

Chemical pain is the result of irritation of the nociceptive nerve endings by the products of inflammation, generally following tissue damage. The products of inflammation can either sensitize nerve endings so that they respond to a lower threshold of stimulus, or activate silent nociceptors (see below) to provoke a response.

Mechanical pain occurs through stretching, compression or distortion of connective tissue structures stimulating the intervening nociceptors. Mechanical stress ultimately produces vascular changes and ischaemia, which activates nociceptors.

While acknowledging the existence of all pain-sensitive structures within the spinal joints, the discal model is central to the concepts of treatment in orthopaedic medicine. With evidence from scans more readily available, the disc would seem to be a major contributor to spinal pain, but the mechanisms of internal derangement, disc herniation and the recovery from disc pathology, often spontaneously, remain unknown. More recent work has concentrated on the chemical effects of displaced nuclear material, while the exact mechanism of pain produced by mechanical compression is unclear.

Primary disc pain

The outer part of the annulus fibrosus receives a nerve supply, some of which is thought to be nociceptive. Pressure exerted on the outer annulus and injection of contrast medium into the disc have each provoked a pain response (Bogduk 1994). Roberts et al (1995) found sensory nerve endings in the form of mechanoreceptors in intervertebral discs and the posterior longitudinal ligament. Golgi tendon organs were the most frequently seen. These may directly elicit pain or modulate muscle activity, perhaps in the form of muscle spasm that is often associated with lumbar lesions. Coppes et al (1997) established a more extensive disc innervation in severely degenerative human lumbar discs, when compared with normal discs, that invaded deeper than the outer third of the annulus. The nociceptive properties of some of the nerves were suggestive of substance P immunoreactivity.

As with all connective tissue structures, the elastic property of the collagen fibres in the annulus, enhanced by 'crimp', allows it to tolerate tensile forces. When placed under excessive mechanical tension the annulus deforms and may directly squeeze or distort pain-sensitive nerve endings, producing pain of mechanical origin. Once forces exceed normal limits microtrauma occurs, producing pain of chemical origin. The most vulnerable position for the annulus is when it is placed under rotational strains in flexion, ultimately resulting in circumferential splits (Bogduk 1997). Shear and tensile forces initiate damage at the peripheral portion of the disc but not at the centre, since fibre strain is always minimal at the centre and maximal at the periphery (Brinckmann 1986).

With consideration for the chemical contribution to low back pain, substance P causes the release of inflammatory mediators that affect the local environment and may sensitize nociceptors, resulting in chronic pain (Zimmermann 1992, Beaman et al 1993, Palmgren et al 1996). Substance P immunoreactive nerve fibres have been identified in the zygapophyseal joint capsule and synovial folds, the supraspinous ligament, posterior longitudinal ligament and the annulus fibrosus. Some fine unmyelinated and small myelinated fibres in the annulus are thought to serve as a type of pain fibre – termed silent nociceptor – that is not excited by mechanical stress, but responds to algesic chemicals produced at times of tissue damage or inflammation (Cavanaugh 1995).

There is no evidence as yet to support a nerve supply to the nucleus pulposus and pathological processes are thought to occur internally within the nucleus without provoking a pain response.

Secondary disc pain

Mixter & Barr (1934) suggested that a displaced fragment of the intervertebral disc into the vertebral canal causes mechanical compression of the lumbar nerve roots and sensory root ganglia. However, the mechanism by which back or leg pain is produced by this mechanical compression is still not fully understood. Kuslich et al (1991) demonstrated that stimulation of a normal nerve root did not produce a pain response, while stimulation of an already swollen, stretched or compressed nerve root produced leg pain. However, no suggestion was made for how much, or for how long, mechanical stress should be applied to a previously undamaged nerve root before changes occur to make it sensitive.

The extruded disc material in disc prolapse may consist of nuclear material, sometimes with end-plate material and occasionally elements of the annulus (Bogduk 1991, Brock et al 1992). However, normal disc material does not usually rupture and the nucleus is thought to undergo some process of deterioration or degradation, in order for it to be displaced (Bogduk 1991). Hormonal, nutritional or viral factors, or simply an acceleration of the degenerative process, have been proposed as possible reasons for the degradation of the nucleus.

Bogduk (1997) offers a plausible explanation of mechanical trauma together with an autoimmune reaction within the nucleus. Proteins in the nucleus may act as an antigen which, when exposed to the circulation for the first time, trigger an autoimmune response. Intrinsically, this can occur via contact with the circulatory plexus associated with the vertebral end-plate through microfracture due to compressive loading. The provoked autoimmune inflammatory response causes degradation of the nucleus which continues once the microfractures heal. Degrading the nuclear material in this way renders it capable of herniation. Changes must also occur within the annulus since herniation of nuclear material can only occur through a radial fissure in a weakened annular wall (Brinckmann 1986).

The posterolateral corners of the annulus are irregular, thin and potentially weak (Umehara et al 1996). Radial fissures and circumferential splits commonly develop here, providing an escape route for the degraded nuclear material, when a force is applied sufficient to expel it. Flexed postures, especially combined with rotation, trigger backwards herniation of the nuclear material through a weakened annular wall (Bogduk 1997).

As well as being a primary source of pain, the prolapsed disc can have a secondary effect on any pain-sensitive structure lying within the vertebral canal or intervertebral foramen. This effect can be mechanical through compression and distortion, chemical through the inflammatory process and ischaemic through the pressure of oedema.

Once discal material enters the vertebral canal it may again be treated as foreign and stimulate an extrinsic autoimmune inflammatory response as it comes into contact with the circulation in the vertebral canal. The resulting chemical mediators affect adjacent pain-sensitive structures. If the prolapsed fragment is small, it will be dealt with by the macrophage system; if large, the inflammatory process continues until the fragment is eventually organized into scar tissue (Hirabayashi et al 1990).

Both mechanical and inflammatory mechanisms can produce ischaemia. The inflammatory mediators produced are thought to have a role in somatic pain (McCarron et al 1987, Bogduk 1994) and in radicular pain (Doita et al 1996, Kang et al 1996, Takahashi et al 1996).

The quality of pain seems to be instrumental in distinguishing somatic and radicular pain. Somatic and somatic referred pain is produced when any sensitive structure is stimulated and is deep, aching and hard to localize. Radicular pain is produced when a nerve root is compressed and was described by Smyth & Wright, cited in Bogduk (1997), as shooting, lancinating pain felt in a relatively narrow band, approximately 4 cm wide, into the limb.

Compression of undamaged nerves produces numbness, paraesthesia and muscle weakness. Under some circumstances, which are not well-understood, compression alters nerve root conduction and compromises their nutritional support, causing them to become pain-sensitive through inflammation, ischaemia or both (Garfin et al 1995). Studies suggest that the products of the autoimmune inflammatory process stimulated by the displaced discal material may increase the sensitivity of the nerve root to bradykinin and be involved in the pathophysiology of radiculopathy (Saal 1995, Kang et al 1996, Takahashi et al 1996).

The mechanical effects of compression of a nerve root may be direct or more probably indirect through ischaemia. A sequence of events may be induced involving impairment of nutrition and increased microvascular permeability, leading to intraneural oedema, blockage of axonal transport and altered function (Rydevik & Olmarker 1992). For referred leg pain to be radicular in origin, arising from compression of a nerve root, it must be accompanied by other signs of compression – paraesthesia and muscle weakness. If these are absent, pain referred to the limb must be somatic in origin (Bogduk 1997).

However, in clinical practice, signs and symptoms of somatic and radicular pain coexist since, for a disc protrusion to compress a nerve root, it must first compress and stimulate nerve endings in its dural nerve root sleeve. Thus the dural nerve root sleeve produces somatic referred pain, either mechanical or chemical in origin, while the nerve root may produce radicular pain and other signs and symptoms of nerve compression.

In studies on peripheral nerves, a critical level of pressure is significant for structural and functional changes to occur and longer periods of compression would seem to be responsible for more damage. Prolonged compression may produce changes in axonal transport impairing the transport of proteins from the nerve cell body to the distal parts of the body and resulting in compression-induced effects in the distal axonal segment (double crush syndrome).

The trauma evoked by compression may alter the permeability of the intraneural vessels, resulting in oedema. The oedema usually persists after removal of the compression and therefore may adversely affect the nerve root for longer. The presence of intraneural oedema is thus related to intraneural fibrosis and adhesion formation.

Unfortunately, at the time of writing, there do not appear to have been many experimental studies on spinal nerves, but they are known to be more susceptible to compression than peripheral nerves since they do not have the same protective connective tissue sheaths. The critical pressure levels for compression to induce impairment of nerve nutrition or function are not known, or the length of time that compression needs to be applied before changes occur and they become pain-sensitive.

DIFFERENTIAL DIAGNOSIS AT THE LUMBAR SPINE

The mechanism by which the lumbar intervertebral disc produces pain is probably complicated, with several factors contributing to the diagnosis. It is important to understand the anatomy and the possible mechanisms for pain production, as discussed above.

Patients with non-mechanical causes of back pain can present with signs and symptoms that mimic those of disc pathology. It is important to recognize those features that allow them to be identified as 'red flags' (indicators of serious spinal pathology), since manual techniques are either contraindicated or not appropriate, and the patient needs to be referred to the appropriate specialist. The following section is divided into two parts. The first covers lumbar disc lesions; the second covers the non-mechanical causes of back pain and associated signs and symptoms.

A recap of the terminology used to describe disc herniation is provided below to add clarity to the following discussion. In contrast to the cervical spine, where the degenerate disc tends to displace as a central bar-like protrusion of the annulus, the degenerate lumbar disc involves degradation and herniation of nuclear material through a weakened annular wall. This herniation may occur as a protrusion into the weakened annulus where it may produce primary disc pain, or as a prolapse where nuclear material moves into the vertebral canal. Here it can have a secondary effect on any pain-sensitive structure by mechanisms involving compression, inflammation and ischaemia.

A central prolapse affects central structures, in particular the posterior longitudinal ligament and the dura mater. Pain arising from compression of the dura mater is multisegmental in nature (see Ch. 1). A posterolateral prolapse affects unilateral structures, mainly the dural nerve root sleeve and nerve root, which tend to produce segmental pain.

A disc herniation, either protrusion or prolapse, produces a pattern of signs and symptoms that are progressive, with a history of increasing, worsening episodes. Often the precipitating factor is trivial. The dural nerve root sleeve and nerve root are vulnerable in the lumbar spine to posterolateral prolapse, with pain and other associated symptoms referred into the leg. A classification of clinical models has been established to aid diagnosis and to establish treatment programmes. These are outlined in the treatment section later in this chapter, since they relate directly to treatment selection.

Disc protrusion

- Degenerate disc material bulges into the weakened laminate structure of the annulus, where it can produce primary disc pain since the outer annulus receives a nerve supply.

Disc prolapse

- Discal material passes through a radial or circumferential fissure in the annulus which provides it with an escape route into the vertebral canal where it has a secondary effect on the pain-sensitive structures in the vertebral canal. The sequela of this is sequestration of the disc.

OTHER CAUSES OF BACK PAIN, LEG PAIN AND ASSOCIATED SIGNS AND SYMPTOMS

Capsular pattern of the lumbar spine
- Limitation of extension.
- Equal limitation of side flexions.
- Usually full flexion.

Non-mechanical lesions, including serious pathology, have features that do not 'fit'. Since they represent contraindications to manual orthopaedic medicine treatments, they must be recognized and the patients referred appropriately.

Arthritis, in any form, presents with the capsular pattern which is demonstrated by the lumbar spine as a whole.

- *Degenerative osteoarthrosis* affects the intervertebral joint and the zygapophyseal joint. The consequences of degeneration and degradation of the intervertebral disc lead to increased possibility of disc herniation. Disruption of the intervertebral joint affects the zygapophyseal joint, causing the joint surfaces to bear increased weight
- *Osteophytes* may form at the peripheral margins of the disc, possibly in association with rim lesions of the annulus, as well as at the zygapophyseal joints. Overall the degenerative changes may lead to spinal stenosis
- *Spinal stenosis* is a term that has become synonymous with *neurogenic* or *spinal claudication*. It should be used to define any symptomatic condition in which limited space in the vertebral canal is a significant factor (Porter 1992). Lateral stenosis affects the nerve root; central stenosis affects the spinal cord or cauda equina and may coexist with lateral stenosis

Some patients have a developmental abnormality where the spinal canal has a trefoil shape in cross-section (Vernon-Roberts 1992) and spinal stenosis is particularly prevalent in this group. Narrowing can also occur as a result of degenerative changes through ageing, injury, disease, or as a result of surgery (Lee et al 1995). Irrespective of cause, a small vertebral canal can have clinical significance for back pain (Porter & Oakshot 1994).

Degenerative spinal stenosis can be associated with osteophyte formation at the vertebral body or zygapophyseal joints, with reactive proliferation of capsular and soft tissues, and fibrous scarring around the nerve roots. The vertebral canal can be compromised by thickening of the ligamentum flavum which shows a 50% increase in thickness with ageing over a normal lifespan (Twomey & Taylor 1994). Degenerative spondylolisthesis may also narrow the canal (Osborne 1974, Rauschning 1993).

A disc prolapse may significantly reduce the size of both the vertebral and intervertebral foramina and Porter et al (1978) noted that the risk of developing disabling symptoms from disc prolapse is inversely related to the size of the spinal canal. The anterior margin of the canal can be indented to compress the cauda equina by a lax posterior longitudinal ligament overlying degenerate prolapsed discs. Cyriax (1982) termed this the 'mushroom phenomenon'.

Spinal stenosis can produce neurogenic or spinal claudication which was recognized by Verbiest, in 1954, as due to structural narrowing of the vertebral canal compressing the cauda equina and producing claudication symptoms (Porter 1992). Men over the age of 50 with a lifestyle that has involved heavy manual work may be affected. The entire cauda equina can be compressed centrally causing bilateral symptoms, or the emerging nerve root can be affected (Osborne 1974). The patient complains of discomfort, pain, paraesthesia and heaviness in one or both legs while standing or walking. There may be night cramps and restless legs. A long history of back pain may be present and the patient may have undergone back surgery at some time. The symptoms are usually of several months' duration. There is usually a threshold distance when the symptoms develop and a tolerance when they have to stop; the tolerance distance is about twice the threshold (Porter 1992). These symptoms are similar to those of the ischaemic pain associated with intermittent claudication of peripheral vascular disease and with the age group affected; the two conditions can coexist, making diagnosis difficult.

With neurogenic claudication, stooping or bending forwards relieves the symptoms and allows the patient to continue. Flexion increases the space in the canal and tightens the ligaments, straightening out the buckling that tends to occur with degeneration. The patient can usually walk uphill, which involves a flexed posture, easier than walking downhill, which involves an extended posture.

On examination, the patient often stands with a stooped posture, with flexed hips and knees and a flattened lumbar spine with loss of the lordosis. This posture becomes more evident on walking. The capsular pattern is present with marked loss of spinal extension. Extension may produce the pain as it decreases the calibre of the spinal canal while, conversely, flexion relieves the pain (Osborne 1974). Dynamic variations in flexion and extension are related to changes in the buckling of the ligamentum flavum and the herniation of the intervertebral discs (Rauschning 1993). The rest of the examination may be unremarkable and back pain itself may not be a feature. Neurological signs are often absent.

Management may involve spinal decompressive surgery or advice on how to live with the condition. Symptoms do not usually resolve, but they do not always get worse.

- *Rheumatoid arthritis* can affect the spinal joints and this has been covered in Chapter 8. Ankylosing spondylitis is discussed in Chapter 14

Structural abnormalities can be completely asymptomatic or may produce pain, inflammation and neurological signs, or coexist with disc herniation.

- *Spondylolysis* is a defect in the pars interarticularis (the neural arch between the lamina and the pedicle) of L5 and sometimes L4
- *Spondylolisthesis* is an anterior shift of one vertebral body on another, usually involving slippage of L5 on S1. It may be congenital, acquired through degeneration, trauma, or as a sequela to spondylolysis. It is commonly associated with over-training in such sports as gymnastics, involving hyperextension, and the rotational stresses involved in fast bowling (Bush 1994). If symptomatic, the

main symptom is back pain that may be referred to the buttocks. The pain is aggravated by exercise and standing and is eased by sitting. Inspection may reveal excessive skin folds above the defect and a step defect may be felt on palpation (Norris 1998). On examination, extension is limited and painful and passive overpressure of the affected vertebra produces the pain. Diagnosis is confirmed by oblique X-rays that show the typical 'Scottie dog' with its collar representing fracture of the pars articularis

X-ray assesses the degree of spondylolisthesis which is measured by the distance the slipped upper vertebra moves forward on its lower counterpart. Slippage is divided into four degrees, progressing from a first-degree slip, which is a forward displacement of one quarter of the anteroposterior diameter of the vertebral body, to a fourth-degree slip with a full anteroposterior diameter displacement (Corrigan & Maitland 1983).

A particular feature of **serious non-mechanical conditions** is an unwell patient with possible weight loss. Neoplasm of the lumbar spine, although relatively uncommon, should be considered as a possible cause of low back and leg pain. Metastases may be secondary to carcinoma of the bronchus, breast, ovary, prostate, thyroid or kidney. Metastatic invasion may involve bone or may be intradural. Primary bone tumours occasionally affect the posterior elements of the vertebrae and multiple myeloma can produce backache due to vertebral involvement.

- **Neoplasm** involving the lumbar spine may be clinically silent or may produce pain in isolation or cause associated neurological deficit (Findlay 1992). The pain may be due to compression or distortion of pain-sensitive structures and/or to destructive changes in the bone. Neurological deficit is usually of a lower motor neuron type and it may begin either at the same time as the pain or prior to it

  The pain of neoplastic disease has characteristic features. It is usually deep-seated, boring, relatively constant, steadily worsening and often persistent at night. If there is collapse of the vertebral body, the pain will be associated with movement and activity due to the spinal instability (Findlay 1992). Aside from night pain, symptoms of weakness, fatigue and weight loss should be considered to be serious in a patient complaining of back pain.

  The signs and symptoms of a tumour can mimic a disc lesion. Palma et al (1994) reported three cases of neurinoma of the cauda equina initially misdiagnosed as a disc lesion. Pain which worsens during recumbency and improves in sitting and walking, together with bilateral, multiple root involvement, is more indicative of an expanding lesion in the cauda equina than sciatica. Unusual cases of a primary extraosseous Ewing sarcoma in a 15-year-old girl with a history of chronic back and leg ache (Allam & Sze 1994) and primary Hodgkin's disease of the bone presenting clinically with an extradural tumour (Moridaira et al 1994) exist in the literature.

- **Infection** may cause osteomyelitis or discitis and epidural abscess is possible. Pyogenic organisms, e.g. *Staphylococcus aureus*, *Myobacterium tuberculosis* or, rarely, *Brucella*, may be responsible (Kumar & Clark 2002). The clinical presentation of spinal infection varies from a complaint of back pain only, to being very ill, emaciated and febrile and with a raised erythrocyte sedimentation rate. On examination tenderness is elicited on percussion of the affected vertebra and widespread muscle spasm may be present. X-ray may show loss of bony contour, cavitation and collapse and possibly an associated paravertebral abscess (Kemp & Worland 1974)

- *Aortic aneurysms* are commonly abdominal (Kumar & Clark 2002). When they rupture they may present with epigastric pain that radiates through to the back. The patient is shocked and a pulsatile mass is felt. This situation is a medical emergency. Galessiere et al (1994) presented three cases of chronic, contained rupture of aortic aneurysms associated with vertebral erosion. The patients presented with a history of chronic backache

Non-organic back pain should be considered at the lumbar spine, although true psychogenic back pain is rare. Anxiety tends to be associated with acute back pain while depression is associated with chronic back pain; both are indicators of the patient's distress. Back pain may begin as a physical problem and, as such, is generally addressed by mechanical or physical treatments. If low back pain becomes chronic, psychosocial factors may be more obvious than physical signs, and illness behaviour becomes a relevant component. Illness behaviour is a normal phenomenon and a physical problem exists with varying degrees of illness behaviour (Waddell 1998). As clinicians, the physical and psychosocial factors that coexist in chronic pain must therefore be understood in order to provide total care. The interested reader is referred to the work of Waddell (1998) which includes the biopsychosocial model and describes non-organic or behavioural signs, the so called 'yellow flags', as indicators of pychological distress and risk of long-term disability.

COMMENTARY ON THE EXAMINATION

OBSERVATION

A general observation of the patient's *face, posture and gait* will alert the examiner to the seriousness of the condition. Patients in acute pain will generally look tired. They may have adopted an antalgic posture of flexion or lumbar scoliosis which is generally indicative of an acute locked back, possibly due to a disc lesion. A lumbar lateral shift is pathognomic of a disc lesion (Porter 1995). Patients may not be able to sit during the examination due to discomfort from this particular posture. Their gait may be uneasy with steps taken cautiously, obviously wary of provoking twinges of pain by sudden movements or pain on weight-bearing. A dropped foot may be evident on walking and will lead you to consider involvement of the L4 nerve root affecting the tibialis anterior muscle and interfering with function.

HISTORY (SUBJECTIVE EXAMINATION)

The history is particularly important at the spinal joints. Vroomen et al (1999) published a systematic review of the diagnostic value of the history and examination of patients with suspected sciatica, establishing that very little attention has been paid to the history of such events. Pain distribution was the only sensitive sign of the level of disc herniation, with straight leg raising seemingly a sensitive sign and crossed straight leg raise a strong indicator of nerve root compression. Disagreement exists in the literature with regard to the value of decreased muscle strength, sensory loss and altered reflexes as signs of nerve root involvement and it is unclear if the physical examination adds much to the diagnostic value of the history.

There is a close relationship between signs and symptoms from the lumbar spine, sacroiliac joint and hip joint. The history will help with the differential diagnosis but conditions at each of these areas can coexist. Major pathology can affect the spine, such as malignancy, infection, spondyloarthropathy or fracture, but these represent a small percentage of the problems compared with mechanical lesions of the lower back (Swezey 1993). X-ray findings can be misleading, particularly when showing the degenerative changes of osteoarthrosis which may or may not be painful. Similarly, spondylolysis progressing to spondylolisthesis occurs in approximately 5% of adults but is symptomatic in only half of them (Swezey 1993).

The *age, occupation, sports, hobbies and lifestyle* of the patient may give an indication of provoking mechanisms. Often the incident precipitating the episode of back pain may be relatively minor, though factors predisposing to the event may have been continuing for some time. While cure will be the initial aim of treatment for this presenting incident, ultimately the management of the condition and prevention of recurrence will become the patient's responsibility. Patients will require advice and guidance on management of their back condition to prevent chronicity.

Many occupations involve a flexion lifestyle, e.g. sedentary office work and brick-laying apply postural stress to the intervertebral joint. These patients require advice about changing postures to minimize the stress inflicted by work. Directives on the manual handling of loads are in existence and patients should receive advice about this in their place of work. The vibration of motor vehicle driving may have an influence, as well as the sitting posture involved, which is known to increase intradiscal pressure (Osti & Cullum 1994).

Assessment of patients with chronic low back pain presents a particular challenge to the clinician. Emotional, environmental and industrial factors may influence pain perception, while monotony or dissatisfaction at work or home is relevant (Osti & Cullum 1994). Distinction will need to be made between the true physical symptoms of the presenting condition and those relating to psychosocial factors that influence the way the patient reacts to the pain (see above). Inquiry should be made about the possibilities of secondary gain factors relating to disability, or the presence of psychological or social stresses that might predispose the patient to chronic pain disorders (Swezey 1993). Standard questions on quality of sleep, tiredness levels, concentration, appetite, etc. may establish whether the patient is depressed.

The *site* of the pain will give an indication of its origin (see Ch. 1). Lumbar pain is generally localized to the back and buttocks or felt in the limb in a segmental pattern. Sacroiliac pain may be unilateral, felt in the buttock, or more commonly in the groin, and occasionally referred into the leg. The hip joint may produce an area of pain in the buttock consistent with the L3 segment, pain in the groin, or pain referred down the anteromedial aspect of the thigh and leg to the medial aspect of the ankle. Dural pain is multisegmental and will be central or bilateral. Pressure on the dural nerve root sleeve will be referred segmentally to the relevant dermatome. Pressure on the nerve root will refer pain to the relevant limb with accompanying symptoms of paraesthesia at the distal end of the dermatome.

Vucetic et al (1995) considered the difficulty that patients have in giving a precise verbal description of pain. They support the use of a pain drawing, which may take a few minutes to obtain, but the result can be grasped at a glance. Waddell (1992) warns that how a patient draws pain is influenced by emotional distress and that non-anatomical, widespread and magnified drawings tell of the patient's distress rather than the physical characteristics of the pain.

The *spread* of pain will not only give an indication of its origin, but also the severity or irritability of the lesion. Generally, the more peripherally the pain is referred, the greater the source of irritation. A mechanical lesion due to a displaced lumbar disc produces central or unilateral back or buttock pain. If the pain shifts into the leg, it generally ceases or is reduced in the back. Pain of non-musculoskeletal origin does not follow this pattern and serious lesions produce an increasing spreading pain, with pain in the back remaining as severe as that felt peripherally.

The *onset and duration* of the pain can assist the choice of treatment (see below). In very general terms, a sudden onset of pain may respond to manipulation, while a gradual onset of pain may respond better to traction. The whole clinical picture will need to be reasoned through in order to make a decision about treatment which may contradict these rules of thumb.

The nature and mode of onset are important. The patient may remember the exact time and mode of onset which may have involved a flexed and rotated posture. If lifting was involved in the precipitating episode, it may only have been a trivial weight. If the patient reports a gradual onset of pain, it is worth questioning further for details of previous activity. A minor traumatic incident some time before the onset of back pain or the maintenance of a sustained flexion posture may have been sufficient to provoke the symptoms.

The gradual onset of degenerative osteoarthrosis is common in the zygapophyseal joints and hip joints, while a subluxation of the sacroiliac joint can occur with a sudden onset. Serious pathology develops insidiously.

If trauma is involved, the exact nature of the trauma should be ascertained and any possible fracture eliminated. Direct trauma may produce soft tissue contusions, while fracture may involve the spinous process, transverse process, pars interarticularis, vertebral body or vertebral end-plate. Compression fractures of the vertebral body are common in horse riders and those falling from a height, and involve the vulnerable cancellous bone of the vertebral body (Hartley 1995). Hyperflexion injuries may cause ligamentous lesions or involve the capsule of the zygapophyseal joint, while hyperextension injuries compress the zygapophyseal joints. Both forces can injure the intervertebral disc.

The *symptoms and behaviour* need to be considered. The behaviour of the pain will give an indication of the irritability of the patient's condition and provide clues to differential diagnosis. The pattern of all previous episodes of back pain should be ascertained, as in disc lesions a pattern of gradually worsening and increasing episodes of pain usually emerges.

The mechanisms whereby the disc herniation can cause pain have been discussed earlier in this chapter. The typical pattern of pain from disc herniation is usually one of a central pain which moves laterally. As the pain moves laterally, the central pain usually ceases or reduces. A gradually increasing central pain accompanied by an increasing leg pain is indicative of serious pathology and this pain is usually not altered by either rest or activity.

The daily pattern of pain is important and typically a disc lesion produces either a pattern of pain that is better first thing in the morning after rest, becoming worse as the day goes on, or, since the disc imbibes water overnight, the patient may experience increased pain on weight-bearing first thing in the morning due to increased pressure on sensitive tissues. Patients can sleep reasonably well at night as they are usually able to find a position of ease.

Mechanical pain can cause an on/off response through compression or distortion of pain-sensitive structures. This can involve the annulus itself or structures in the vertebral canal. The patient with a disc lesion usually complains of pain on movement easing with rest. Changing pressures in the disc affect the pain and it tends to be worse with sitting and stooping postures than when standing or lying down. In an acute locked back, small movements can create exquisite twinging pain.

Herniated disc material may produce an inflammatory response resulting in chemical pain. Chemical pain is characteristically a constant ache associated with morning stiffness. Sharper pain can also be associated with chemical irritation as the nerve endings become sensitized and respond to a lower threshold of stimulation. It is important to differentiate mechanical back pain from inflammatory arthritis and sacroiliac joint lesions through consideration of other factors, since they also produce pain associated with early-morning stiffness.

Radicular pain (see above) is generally a severe lancinating pain, often burning in nature, which is felt in the distribution of the dermatome associated with the nerve root. Sciatica is commonly associated with lumbar disc pathology and will occur if the L4–L5, S1 or S2 nerve roots are involved. If the higher levels are involved, pain will similarly be referred into the relevant segment.

The language used by patients to describe the quality of their pain will indicate the balance between the physical and emotional elements of their pain. Words such as 'throbbing', 'burning', 'twinging' and 'shooting' describe the sensory quality of the pain; emotional characteristics are expressed in such words as 'sickening', 'miserable', 'unbearable' and 'exhausting' or vocal complaints such as moans, groans and gasps (Waddell 1992, 1998).

The other symptoms described by the patient provide evidence for differential diagnosis, contraindications to treatment and the severity or irritability of the lesion. An increase in pressure through coughing, sneezing, laughing or straining can increase the back pain and this is the main dural symptom. Paraesthesia is usually felt at the distal end of the dermatome and is a symptom of nerve root compression. Confirmation of this is made through the objective compression signs of muscle weakness, altered sensation and reduced or absent reflexes.

Specific questions must be asked concerning pain or paraesthesia in the perineum and genital area as well as bladder and bowel function. The presence of any of these symptoms indicates compression of the S4 nerve root at the preganglionic extent which could produce irreversible damage, and indicates immediate referral for surgical opinion. Manipulation is absolutely contraindicated in these cases. The symptoms of difficulty in passing water, inability to retain urine or lack of sensation when the bowels are opened are important. It is not unusual to find urinary frequency or difficulty in defecating associated with effort in hyperacute lumbar pain.

Bilateral sciatica with objective neurological signs and bilateral limitation of straight leg raise suggest a massive central protrusion compressing the cauda equina through the posterior longitudinal ligament, with possible rupture of the ligament (Cyriax 1982). It is an absolute contraindication to manipulation, since a worsening of the situation could lead to irreversible damage to the cauda equina, as mentioned above. The symptoms of cauda equina compression should be distinguished from multisegmental, dural reference of pain into both legs, where there may be bilateral limitation of straight leg raise but no neurological signs.

Questioning the patient about *other joint involvement* will indicate whether inflammatory arthritis exists or if there is a tendency towards degenerative osteoarthrosis.

The *past medical history* and the patient's current general health will help to eliminate possible serious pathology, past or present. An unexplained recent weight loss may be significant in systemic disease or malignancy. Visceral lesions can refer pain to the back, e.g. kidney, aortic aneurysm or gynaecological conditions. Infections should be obvious, with an unwell patient showing a fever. Malignancy can affect the lumbar and pelvic region but the pattern of the pain behaviour does not generally fit that of musculoskeletal origin. Past history of primary tumour may indicate secondaries as a possible cause of back pain. Serious conditions produce an unrelenting pain; night pain is usually a feature and is responsible for the patient looking tired and ill.

The *medications* taken by the patient will indicate their current medical state as well as alerting the examiner to possible contraindications to treatment. Anticoagulant therapy and long-term oral steroids are contraindications to manipulation. It is useful to know what analgesics are being taken and how frequently. This gives an indication of the severity of the condition and can be used as an objective marker for progression of treatment, with the need for less analgesia indicating a positive improvement. If patients are currently taking antidepressant medication, this may indicate their emotional state and possibly exclude them from manipulation. Care is needed in making this decision, however, since antidepressants can be used in low doses as an adjunct to analgesics in back pain.

INSPECTION

The patient should be adequately undressed down to underwear and in a good light. The difficulty in undressing, especially of socks and shoes, is associated with disc pathology and indicates the irritability of the lesion. A general inspection from behind, each side, and in front will reveal any *bony deformity*. The general spinal curvatures are assessed, i.e. the cervical and lumbar lordosis and the thoracic kyphosis. The level of the shoulders, inferior angles of the scapulae, buttock and popliteal creases, the position of the umbilicus and the posture of the feet can all be assessed for relevance to the patient's present condition. Any structural or acquired scoliosis is noted. In disc pathology, the patient may have shifted laterally to accommodate the herniation and this is evident in standing. Small deviations can be noted by assessing the distance between the waist and the elbow in the standing position. In hyperacute back pain, the patient may be fixed in a flexed posture and unable to stand upright, and any attempt to do so produces twinges of pain.

The level of the iliac crests and the posterior and anterior superior iliac spines give an overall impression of leg length discrepancy or pelvic distortion (Fig. 13.7). If these are considered relevant, they can be investigated further. Postural asymmetry and malalignment are not necessarily indicative of symptoms. It is worth noting them, since imbalances can be explained to the patient and addressed in the final rehabilitation programme in an attempt to prevent recurrence. If structural abnormalities are considered responsible for the present condition, a full biomechanical assessment will need to be conducted.

Colour changes and *swelling* would not be expected in the lumbar spine unless there has been a history of direct trauma. Any marks on the skin, lipomata, 'faun's beards' (tufts of hair), birthmarks or café-au-lait spots may indicate underlying spinal bony or neurological defects (Hoppenfeld 1976, Hartley 1995). An isolated 'orange-peel' appearance of the skin that is tough and dimpled may indicate spondylolisthesis at

Figure 13.7   Inspection for
pelvic levels.

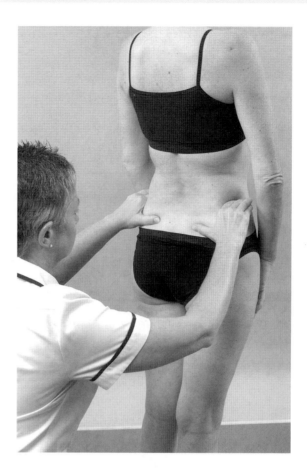

that level (Hartley 1995). Patients with low back pain often apply a hot
water bottle to the area, which produces an erythematous skin reaction
called erythema ab igne (redness from the fire). Swelling is not usually a
feature but muscle spasm may give the appearance of swelling,
especially to the patient.

Muscle wasting may not be obvious if the attack of low back pain is
recent. Chronic or recurrent episodes of pain may show wasting in the
calf muscles or possibly the quadriceps or gluteal muscles.

Palpation may be conducted to assess changes in skin temperature
and sweating suggestive of autonomic involvement. Palpation for swelling
is not usually necessary at the spinal joints. In standing, the lumbar spine
is palpated for a 'shelf' that would indicate spondylolisthesis.

STATE AT REST

Before any movements are performed, the state at rest is established to
provide a baseline for subsequent comparison.

The suggested sequence for the objective examination will now be
given, followed by a commentary including the reasoning in performing
the movements and the significance of the possible findings.

EXAMINATION BY SELECTIVE TENSION

Articular Signs

- Active lumbar extension (Fig. 13.8)
- Active lumbar right side flexion (Fig. 13.9a)
- Active lumbar left side flexion (Fig. 13.9b)
- Active lumbar flexion (Fig. 13.10)
- Resisted plantar flexion, gastrocnemius (Fig. 13.11): S1, 2

Supine Lying

- Passive hip flexion (Fig. 13.12)
- Passive hip medial rotation (Fig. 13.13)
- Passive hip lateral rotation (Fig. 13.14)
- Sacroiliac joint shear tests (Fig. 13.15a, b, c)
- FABER test (Fig. 13.16)
- Straight leg raise (Figs 13.17 and 13.18a, b): L4, 5, S1, 2

Resisted Tests for Objective Neurological Signs and Alternative Causes of Leg Pain; the Main Nerve Roots Involved are Indicated in Bold

- Resisted hip flexion, psoas (Fig. 13.19): L2
- Resisted ankle dorsiflexion, tibialis anterior (Fig. 13.20): L4
- Resisted big toe extension, extensor hallucis longus (Fig. 13.21): L5, S1
- Resisted eversion, peroneus longus and brevis (Fig. 13.22): L5, S1, 2

Skin Sensation (Fig. 13.23)

- Big toe only: L4
- First, second and third toes: L5
- Lateral two toes: S1
- Heel: S2

Reflexes

- Knee reflex (Fig. 13.24): L2, 3, 4
- Ankle reflex (Fig. 13.25): S1, 2
- Plantar response (Fig. 13.26)

Prone Lying

- Femoral stretch test (Figs 13.27, 13.28): L2, 3, 4
- Resisted knee extension, quadriceps (Fig. 13.29): L2, 3, 4
- Resisted knee flexion, hamstrings (Fig. 13.30): L5, S1, 2
- Static contraction of the glutei (Fig. 13.31): L5, S1, 2

Palpation

- Spinous processes for pain, range and end-feel (Fig. 13.32)

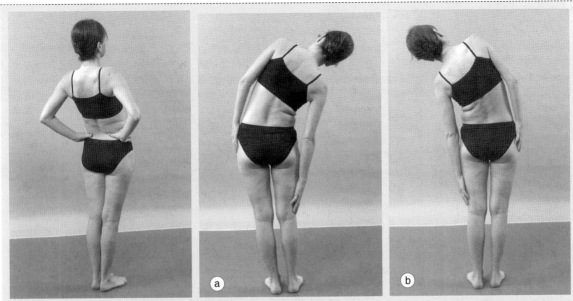

Figure 13.8   Active extension.

Figure 13.9   (a, b) Active side flexions.

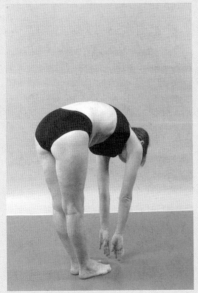

Figure 13.10   Active flexion.

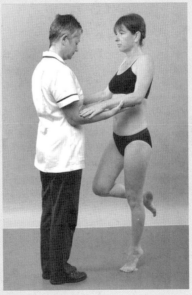

Figure 13.11   Resisted plantarflexion in standing.

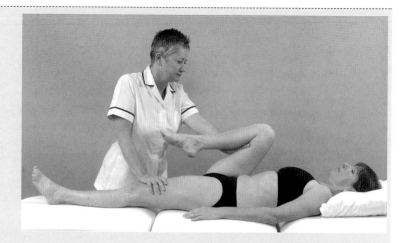

Figure 13.12   Passive hip flexion.

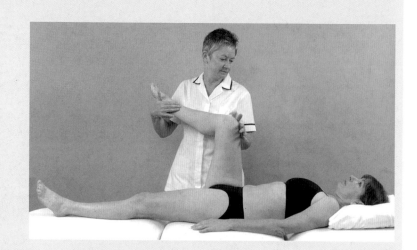

Figure 13.13   Passive hip medial rotation.

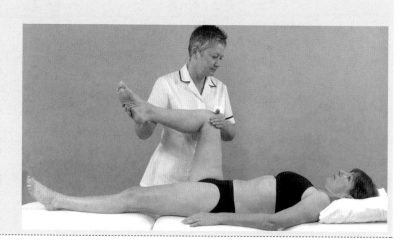

Figure 13.14   Passive hip lateral rotation.

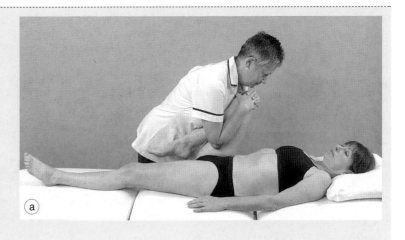

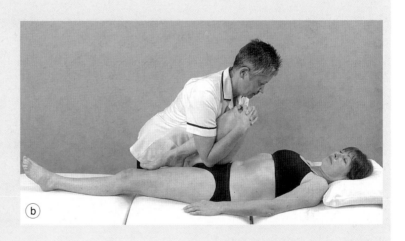

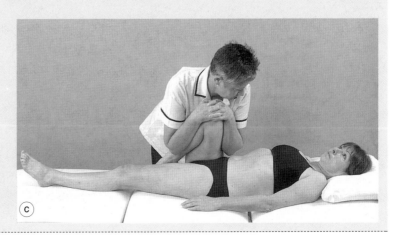

Figure 13.15 (a–c) Shear tests to assess the sacroiliac joint.

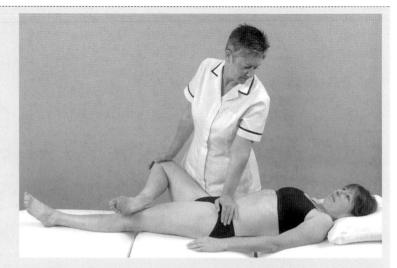

Figure 13.16   FABER test to assess the sacroiliac joint.

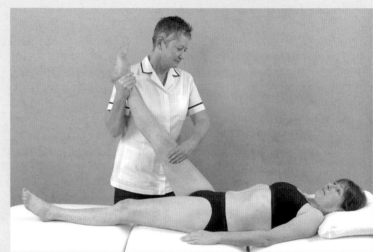

Figure 13.17   Straight leg raise.

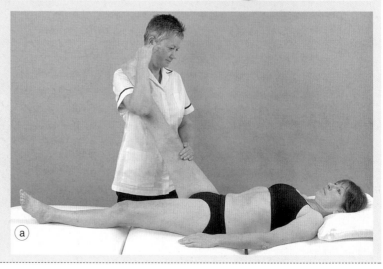

Figure 13.18   (a, b) Straight leg raise with sensitizing components.

ⓐ

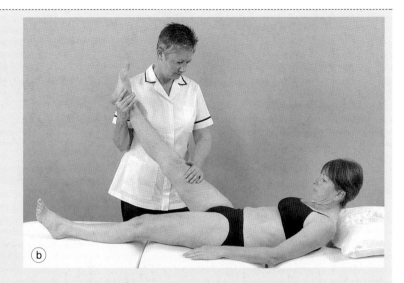

Figure 13.18   Cont'd

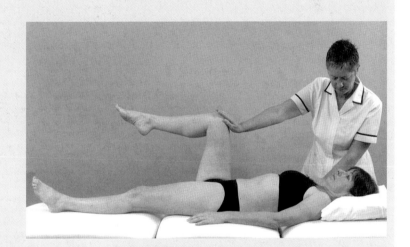

Figure 13.19   Resisted hip flexion.

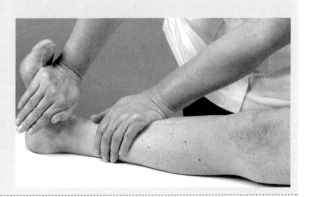

Figure 13.20   Resisted ankle dorsiflexion.

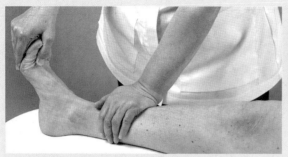

Figure 13.21   Resisted extension of the big toe.

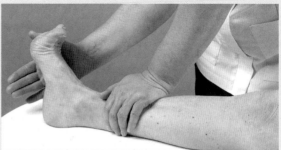

Figure 13.22   Resisted ankle eversion.

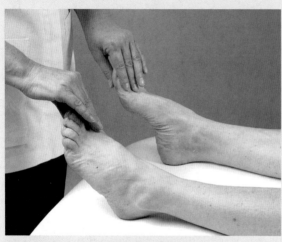

Figure 13.23   Checking skin sensation.

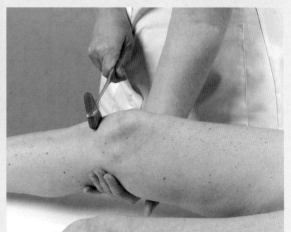

Figure 13.24   Knee reflex.

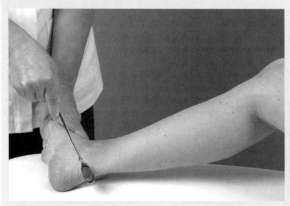

Figure 13.25   Ankle reflex.

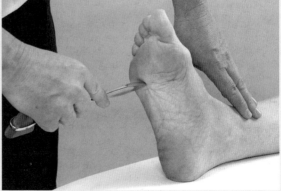

Figure 13.26   Plantar response.

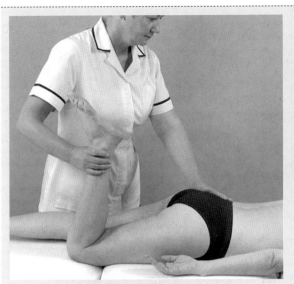

Figure 13.27 Femoral stretch test.

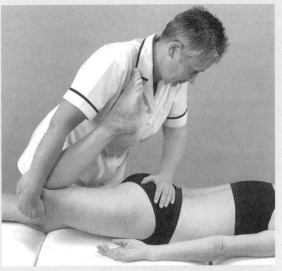

Figure 13.28 Femoral stretch test with sensitizing component.

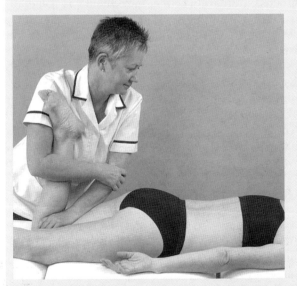

Figure 13.29 Resisted knee extension.

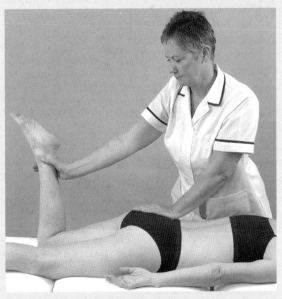

Figure 13.30 Resisted knee flexion.

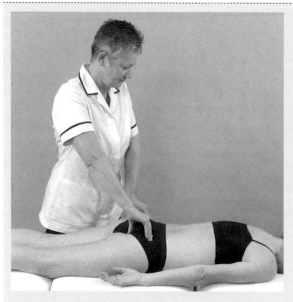

Figure 13.31   Gluteal contraction, squeezing muscle bulk to assess wasting.

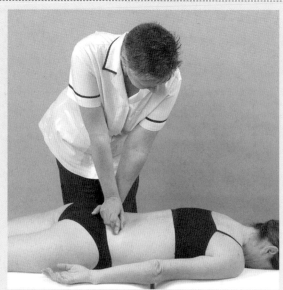

Figure 13.32   Palpation.

Capsular pattern of the lumbar spine
- Limitation of extension.
- Equal limitation of side flexions.
- Usually full flexion.

Active movements are tested in the lumbar spine since, in common with the other spinal regions and shoulders, it can be a focus for 'emotional' symptoms. The active movements indicate the 'willingness' to perform the movements as well as determining the presence of the capsular or non-capsular pattern. End-feel is not routinely assessed since the information gathered from the active movements is generally sufficient. The presence of a painful arc on any movement should be noted and Cyriax (1982) considered this to be pathognomic of disc lesion. Look for apprehension, guarding or exaggerated movements. The presence of the capsular pattern indicates arthritis and it is typically found in degenerative osteoarthrosis of the more mature spine.

An important finding is the non-capsular pattern, usually presenting as an asymmetrical limitation of lumbar movements, indicating a mechanical lesion. The hypothesis is that this is due to a lesion of the intervertebral disc, either as a disc protrusion where the nuclear material has passed into the weakened annulus causing primary disc pain, or as a disc prolapse which has herniated through an annular fissure into the vertebral canal to have a secondary effect on other pain-sensitive structures.

Gastrocnemius is assessed for objective signs of nerve root compression. Testing the muscle group against gravity in standing is convenient at this point, in terms of sequence, before lying the patient down.

The resisted tests are not part of the routine examination at the lumbar spine, but should be applied if there is a history of trauma, e.g. for a muscle lesion or suspected serious pathology, e.g. fracture, metastases or psychogenic pain (see Ch. 9).

In supine lying, other joints are eliminated from the examination to confirm that the site of the lesion is in the lumbar spine. Passive flexion, medial and lateral rotation are conducted at the hip, to assess the hip joint for the capsular pattern or other hip pathology. The sacroiliac joint is assessed by three provocative tests and the FABER test (see Ch. 14). To limit these tests to the hip and sacroiliac joint it may be necessary to place the patient's forearm under the lumbar spine to increase the lordosis and to stabilize the spine. If the lesion in the lumbar spine is very irritable, it may not be possible to conduct these tests adequately.

The straight leg raise is applied passively to each leg in turn, keeping the knee straight. If positive, this may be interpreted as a dural sign, or as an indicator of neural tension affecting the L4, 5, S1, 2 nerve roots. It is an important clinical test for assessing nerve root tension due to a disc lesion (Supik & Broom 1994, Jönsson & Strömqvist 1995). Increased pain on the addition of neck flexion incriminates the dura mater. Further sensitizing components such as passive ankle dorsiflexion, passive ankle plantarflexion and inversion, and passive hip medial rotation and adduction can also be added to explore the mobility of the nervous system further as appropriate.

The normal range of movement for the straight leg raise is between 60 and 120°, with movement being limited by tension in the hamstrings. The range of the straight leg raise should be consistent with the range of lumbar flexion, which is also limited to a certain degree by tension in the hamstrings. A disc prolapse does not always produce a positive sign on straight leg raise. If the nerve root exits high up in the intervertebral foramen, it may escape compression from a posterolateral disc prolapse.

The limited range of the straight leg raise is dependent upon the compression on the dura mater or dural nerve root sleeves and the greater the compression the greater the limitation. A painful arc may be found which is indicative of a small disc prolapse and is a 'useful' finding since, empirically, it usually implies that manipulation will be beneficial.

A bilateral limitation of straight leg raise is usually due to a central disc prolapse compressing the dura mater and is accompanied by an multisegmental distribution of pain.

Bilateral sciatica from the same level producing bilateral limitation of straight leg raise and objective neurological signs is indicative of cauda equina compression. It is an absolute contraindication to manipulation and requires urgent specialist opinion.

A 'crossed' or 'well leg raise' describes the production of the pain in the back or leg on the painful side on straight leg raise of the painless limb. The intensity of the pain induced by the crossed straight leg raise is usually less than that produced on the painful side (Karbowski & Dvorak 1995). Its explanation lies in the suggestion that if a posterolateral prolapse is sitting in the 'axilla' of the nerve root or directly anterior to the root, straight leg raising on the painless side will pull the root against the prolapse and give a positive sign. It usually occurs at the L4 level (Cyriax 1982, Khuffash & Porter 1989). Vroomen et al (1999) identified the crossed straight leg raise test as a specific test.

The patient is assessed for root signs and alternative causes of pain by the selective application of resisted tests. Objective signs of muscle weakness, altered skin sensation and absent or reduced reflexes will indicate compression of a nerve root.

The plantar response is assessed by stroking up the lateral border of the sole of the foot and across the metatarsal heads. The normal response is flexor with flexion of the big toe. The Babinski reflex (or Babinski sign) is extension of the big toe. This reflex is normal in infants under the age of 2 years but a sign of brain or spinal cord injury in older children and adults. The extensor plantar response is therefore indicative of an upper motor neuron lesion, although this is not likely to occur with lumbar lesions since the spinal cord ends at approximately the level of the L1, 2 disc.

The femoral stretch test (prone knee bending) is applied to assess the dura mater and the L2–L4 dural nerve root sleeves. The knee is passively flexed and, if positive, pain is usually produced at approximately 90°. A sensitizing component of hip extension can be added. Pain is usually felt in the back and the test is limited by tension in the quadriceps. If positive unilaterally it implicates the nerve roots, if positive bilaterally the dura mater is at fault. It is theoretically possible to produce a crossed or well leg femoral stretch test but this is not as commonly found in practice.

The remaining resisted tests for the quadriceps and hamstrings are conducted in prone lying. A static contraction of the gluteal muscles is performed to assess for muscle bulk and palpation is conducted, using the ulnar border of the hand on the spinous processes, for pain, range of movement and end-feel.

Any other tests can be added to this basic routine examination of the lumbar spine, including repeated, combined and accessory movements and neural tension testing as appropriate.

If serious pathology is suspected, further tests and specialist investigations will need to be implemented. Standard X-ray investigation provides little useful information for mechanical lesions over and above that gleaned from the clinical examination. However, if the patient fails to respond in the expected way further investigation may be indicated, including computed tomography or magnetic resonance imaging (MRI).

From the examination a working hypothesis is established and a treatment plan prepared.

MANAGEMENT OF BACK PAIN

Orthopaedic medicine aims to apply techniques of manipulation, traction and injections to lumbar disc lesions as appropriate. The choice of treatment will depend on the nature of the pain or the irritability of the lesion, the reference of pain and the mode of onset.

The report of the Clinical Standards Advisory Group (CSAG) (1994) gave management guidelines for back pain that have continued to be appropriate for clinical practice and the advice given to patients. The report emphasized the importance of early management of back pain, i.e. within the first 6 weeks from onset, since the establishment of chronic back pain makes any form of treatment difficult and less successful. The natural history of acute back pain is recovery, with a 90% chance of return to work within 6 weeks. However, 60% of these people will experience at least one recurrence of their pain within 1 year.

If back pain has not settled within 6 weeks it is at risk of becoming chronic and the longer patients are off work, the lower their chances of ever returning. Patients off work for 6 months have only a 50% chance of returning to their previous job. Once they have been off work for 2 years, or have lost their job because of back pain, they will have great difficulty in returning to any kind of work and any further treatment is unlikely to avoid chronic disability.

Following initial assessment the report encourages selection from a diagnostic triage that forms the basis for decisions about referral, investigation and further management. This diagnostic triage consists of:

- Simple backache in which a 90% recovery is expected within 6 weeks
- Nerve root pain with objective neurological signs in which a 50% recovery is expected within 6 weeks
- Possible serious pathology, e.g. cauda equina syndrome, which requires urgent referral for specialist opinion within hours, or infection, neoplasm and inflammatory arthritis which require relatively urgent referral depending on the condition

For more detailed information the reader is referred to the report itself.

LUMBAR DISC LESIONS: A CLASSIFICATION SYSTEM OF FOUR CLINICAL MODELS

In the past, treatment in orthopaedic medicine has been traditionally targeted at the disc, aiming to reduce displacement, relieve pain and restore movement. However, there is a lack of confidence in traditional pathoanatomical diagnostic labels such as this, and 'non-specific low back pain' has been used more recently as a description of the symptoms, since the cause of pain cannot be confidently localized to one specific structure (Laslett & van Wijmen 1999). Consequently, several authors have established classifications to determine treatment programmes and to assist prognosis. The reader is referred to the work of McKenzie (1981), Riddle (1998) and Laslett & van Wijmen (1999).

While not ideal, the presentation of signs and symptoms of lumbar lesions has been classified here into clinical models adapted from Cyriax's original theories to acknowledge the current lack of clear pathoanatomical diagnosis. These models are judgement-based and contribute to the clinical decision-making process to rationalize appropriate treatment programmes; they are not intended to be restrictive. The reader is encouraged to be inventive, to draw on other experiences and to implement the approach into their existing clinical practice when putting a treatment programme together for individual patients.

The treatment techniques described are by no means a cure-all for every case of back pain. However, uncomplicated lesions of recent onset may respond well to the manipulative techniques of orthopaedic medicine.

The key, as in the cervical spine, is the selection of appropriate patients for treatment.

For the purposes of the following classification of lesions, a lumbar lesion may present with the following features:

- An onset of back pain which may be in a multisegmental or segmental distribution (see Ch. 1)
- A typical mechanical history that describes pain aggravated by activity and certain postures, such as sitting, and relieved by rest and postures such as lying
- Symptoms such as a cough or sneeze increasing the pain
- Possible paraesthesia in a segmental pattern
- No significant 'red' or 'yellow flags' present in the history
- Examination revealing a non-capsular pattern of movement
- Limitation of straight leg raise and/or a positive femoral stretch test with possible objective neurological signs
- No contraindications to treatment

CLINICAL MODEL 1: LUMBAR LESION OF GRADUAL ONSET

Factors from the subjective examination

- Central, bilateral or unilateral pain (ideally not referred below the knee)
- Gradual onset
- Patient *cannot* recall the exact mode and time of onset
- May be precipitated by a period of prolonged flexion

Factors from the objective examination

- Non-capsular pattern of pain and limitation of movement
- *May* have increased pain on side flexion *towards* the painful side
- *No* neurological signs

Traction is the treatment of choice for a lumbar lesion of gradual onset. However, manipulation can be applied, providing there are no contraindications, since, if successful, the response is quicker. The manipulative techniques described below may be modified and applied as mobilizing techniques using manual distraction forces (see below).

CLINICAL MODEL 2: LUMBAR LESION OF SUDDEN ONSET

Factors from the subjective examination

- Central, bilateral or unilateral pain (ideally not referred below the knee)
- Sudden onset
- Patient *can* recall the exact mode and time of onset

Factors from the objective examination

- Non-capsular pattern of pain and limitation of movement
- *May* have increased pain on side flexion *away* from the painful side
- *No* neurological signs

Manipulation is the treatment of choice for lumbar lesions of sudden onset provided there are no contraindications to treatment.

CLINICAL MODEL 3: LUMBAR LESION OF MIXED ONSET

Factors from the subjective examination

- Central, bilateral or unilateral pain (ideally not referred below the knee)
- Patient *may* recall the exact mode and time of onset, but the initial pain settles
- Sometime later (hours or days) a gradual onset of pain occurs

Factors from the objective examination

- Non-capsular pattern of pain and limitation of movement
- *No* neurological signs

The treatment of choice is manipulation as it can achieve immediate results. If manipulation fails or is only partially successful, traction may be applied.

CLINICAL MODEL 4: LUMBAR LESION PRESENTING WITH REFERRED LEG SYMPTOMS

Factors from the subjective examination

- Initial presentation of central or unilateral back or buttock pain, followed by referred leg pain (the central pain usually ceasing or diminishing, see below)
- Sudden or gradual onset
- Often part of a history of increasing, worsening episodes, therefore usually a progression of the above models
- Patient may or may not recall the exact time and mode of onset
- Patient may complain of root symptoms, i.e. paraesthesia felt in a segmental distribution

- Non-capsular pattern of pain and limitation of movement reproducing back and/or leg symptoms
- Root signs may be present, i.e. sensory changes, muscle weakness, absent or reduced reflexes; consistent with the nerve root(s) involved

The hypothesis is more readily rationalized here, due to the nerve root involvement. A large secondary posterolateral prolapse of disc material has occurred, initially compromising central structures and moving posterolaterally to involve the exiting nerve root in the intervertebral foramen. Pain may be referred into the leg through compression of the dural nerve root sleeve or the nerve root itself. However, the mechanism of injury to the nerve may be more complicated than expressed here and may also involve chemical and ischaemic factors, all or some of which may affect the quality of the pain response (see above).

Pain, therefore, is segmental in distribution and if the nerve root is involved, there will be objective neurological signs. Since the nerve roots emerge obliquely in the lumbar spine, more than one nerve root may be involved in a disc lesion. Acute lumbar radiculopathy most commonly affects the L5 or S1 root and less commonly the L4 root. It is less common for the other roots to be affected (Caplan 1994).

Treatment is aimed at relieving pain. The limited evidence related to manipulation of patients with nerve root pain does not contraindicate its use but the CSAG report (1994) suggests that it should not be used in patients with severe or progressive neurological deficit to avoid the rare but serious risk of neurological complication. Manipulation may therefore be carefully applied provided the neurological signs are minimal and stable, i.e. non-progressive, and that no other contraindications exist.

The more peripheral the symptoms, the less likely manipulation is to be successful. Manipulation should not be attempted if the neurological deficit is severe and progressing, but other modalities, e.g. traction and mobilization, may provide pain relief. A caudal epidural of corticosteroid and local anaesthetic may be indicated (Cyriax & Cyriax 1983, Cyriax 1984, Vroomen et al 2000). Alternatively spontaneous recovery is likely and may be awaited with suitable reassurance and/or analgesia being given to the patient (see below).

A relatively rare presentation of referred leg symptoms was described by Cyriax (1982) as primary posterolateral prolapse of disc material where symptoms appear in the leg without prior presentation in the back or buttock. The hypothesis is that prolapsed disc material has moved posterolaterally to compress the dural nerve root sleeve while the central pain-sensitive structures have escaped compression such that back pain is never a feature.

It is an uncommon presentation and usually affects the younger adult patient. Relatively minor symptoms of unilateral leg pain are described in the absence of low back pain and the patient may consider the pain to be due to hamstring or calf strain. A non-capsular pattern of movement is present with lumbar movements provoking the leg symptoms. Treatment of choice is traction, in the absence of contraindications, although the condition usually recovers spontaneously over several weeks.

TREATMENT OF LUMBAR DISC LESIONS

Waddell (1998) reports on the evidence for manipulation which shows positive results of good short-term symptomatic relief for patients with acute back pain of less than 4–6 weeks' duration and without nerve root pain. Manipulation may also be effective in recurrent attacks.

Manipulation is the treatment of choice for uncomplicated back pain of recent onset. Ideal patients are those that fall into Clinical Models 2 and 3 but those that fall into Clinical Model 1 may also benefit (see above). Manipulation can be attempted for chronic back pain and for referred leg pain of somatic origin but is not indicated in patients with the severe lancinating pain of radicular origin or severe or progressive neurological deficit.

How manipulation works is not clear and many hypotheses are proposed, including mechanical, physiological and neurophysiological mechanisms (Twomey 1992). If successful, manipulation dramatically reduces pain and produces an increased range of movement. The principles of manipulation are described in Chapter 4.

The success of manipulation depends on the selection of suitable patients and indiscriminate manipulation will produce unsatisfactory results. Orthopaedic medicine spinal manipulation techniques aim to reduce the signs and symptoms of a lumbar disc lesion. In terms of expectations of treatment outcomes, the ideal patient for manipulation has, in summary:

- Mainly central or short unilateral back or buttock pain (the more distal the pain, the less likely manipulation is to succeed)
- Recent onset of pain, preferably within the last 6 weeks
- History of sudden onset of pain; the patient recalls the exact time and mode of onset
- Non-capsular pattern on examination
- Pain increased by side flexion away from the painful side
- No objective neurological signs
- No contraindications to manipulation

CONTRAINDICATIONS TO LUMBAR MANIPULATION

It is impossible to be absolutely definitive about all contraindications – the so called 'red flags' to lumbar manipulation – and nothing can substitute for a rigorous assessment of the presenting signs and symptoms and an accurate diagnosis of a mechanical lumbar lesion. Signs and symptoms of cauda equina syndrome including S4 symptoms of saddle anaesthesia and signs of bladder or bowel dysfunction require urgent neurosurgical referral (Lehmann et al 1991, O'Flynn et al 1992, Dinning & Schaeffer 1993). Bilateral sciatica from the same level with bilateral limitation of straight leg raise and bilateral objective neurological signs indicate a large, central disc prolapse threatening the cauda equina and each provides an absolute contraindication to manipulation (Dinning & Schaeffer 1993). This presentation must not be confused with multisegmental reference of bilateral pain in the absence of neurological signs, as these patients may benefit from the central treatment techniques suggested below.

Severe or progressive neurological deficit associated with Clinical Model 4 is too irritable for the treatment techniques suggested below. Similarly, hyperacute pain in which the patient has twinges and has difficulty even moving or assuming different postures is too irritable to manipulate. Manipulation may be an inappropriate technique for the patient with symptoms of neurogenic (spinal) claudication and associated spinal stenosis. The patient taking anticoagulant therapy, such as warfarin, is absolutely contraindicated due to the risk of intraspinal bleeding. The patient with blood-clotting disorders should also be considered at risk.

Through a thorough subjective and objective examination it should be possible to screen the patient presenting with their first episode of backache under 20 or over 50 and the patient with a past history of primary tumour to ensure that the back pain is mechanical in origin. Long-term systemic steroid use, inflammatory arthritis, known osteoporosis or HIV are all relative contraindications to manipulation. The systemically unwell patient or the patient experiencing constant, progressive non-mechanical pain or other signs of serious spinal pathology is not appropriate for manipulative techniques and fracture may need to be excluded in patients suffering recent traumatic incidents such as a road traffic accident.

Caution should be taken with the pregnant patient, although there is no evidence to suggest that manipulation is dangerous. Discussion with the patient of the risks and benefits will allow informed consent should the clinician judge the manipulation to be appropriate. 'Yellow flags' from the history and examination may highlight degrees of illness behaviour which make the patient inappropriate for manipulation.

The treatment regime discussed below is contraindicated in the absence of patient consent. The patient should be given all details of their diagnosis together with the proposed treatment regime and a discussion of the risks and benefits should ensue to enable them to give their informed consent. Consent is the patient's agreement, written or oral, for a health professional to provide care. It may range from an active request by the patient for a particular treatment regime to the passive acceptance of the health professional's advice. The process of consent, within the context of the orthopaedic medicine, is 'fluid' rather than one instance in time when the patient gives their consent. The patient is constantly monitored and feedback is actively requested. The treatment procedures can be progressed or stopped at the patient's request or in response to adverse reactions. Reassessment is conducted after each technique and a judgement made about proceeding. The patient has a right to refuse consent and this should be respected and alternative treatment options discussed. For further information on consent, the reader is referred to the Department of Health website: www.doh.gov.uk/consent.

Safety recommendations for spinal manipulative techniques are included in Appendix 2.

THE LUMBAR MANIPULATION PROCEDURE

It is recommended that a course in orthopaedic medicine is attended before the treatment techniques described are applied in clinical practice (see Appendix 1). Two types of manipulative techniques are used, the first incorporating a short or long lever arm according to the effect required:

- Rotational manoeuvres for unilateral pain
- Central manoeuvres for central pain

The techniques described below are conducted with the couch at a suitable height for the operator. Generally this should be as low as possible. The techniques may be easier to perform if the patient is asked to take in a small breath, with the technique being applied after the patient has breathed out. This encourages patient relaxation and will allow for the effective application of the overpressure with minimal tissue resistance.

Rotational manoeuvres

The following manoeuvres are described in a suggested order of progression for the novice manipulator but once experience is gained in the application of the techniques, any may be chosen as a starting point. The comparable signs are assessed after every manoeuvre and the next manoeuvre is chosen based on the outcome. As long as a technique is gaining an increase in range and/or a decrease in pain, it can be repeated. Improvement may reach a plateau or the feedback from the patient may become unclear. Only professional judgement will reliably dictate when treatment should be stopped in each treatment session. It is better to err towards the side of caution in the early stages of acquiring manipulative skill.

Distraction technique

Position the patient in side lying with the painful side uppermost. Flex the upper hip and knee with the knee just resting over the side of the bed to assist the rotational stress. Extend the lower leg. Pull the underneath shoulder firmly through such that the uppermost shoulder is positioned backwards and the pelvis positioned forwards. Stand behind the patient at waist level and place one hand over the greater trochanter, pointing down the long axis of the femur. Put your other hand comfortably on the patient's uppermost shoulder with your fingers pointing away from your other hand. Apply rotation with the hand on the greater trochanter until the pelvis lies just forwards of the midline and the patient's waist is upwards. Apply pressure equally through both hands to impart a distraction force; you will see the patient's waist crease stretch out as you lean through your arms (Fig. 13.33). Keep your arms straight as you apply a minimal amplitude, high velocity thrust once all of the slack has been taken up.

Short-lever rotation technique – pelvis forwards

Position the patient in supine lying with the hips and knees flexed (crook lying). Ask the patient to lift and rotate the hips so that they are lying with the painful side uppermost and the shoulders relatively flat. Position the

Figure 13.33   Distraction technique.

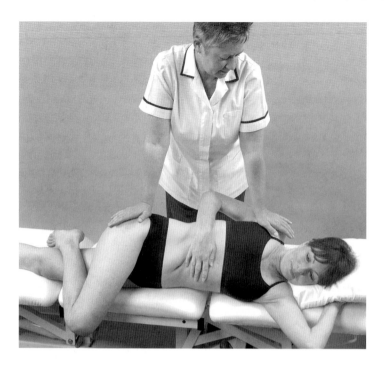

legs as for the distraction technique. Stand in front of the patient with one hand fixing the patient's shoulder while the other is placed with the heel of the hand on the blade of the ilium, with the forearm horizontal and your fingers pointing back towards you. Apply pressure through the hand on the ilium in a horizontal direction towards you to achieve a rotational strain (Fig. 13.34). Apply a minimal amplitude, high velocity thrust once all the slack has been taken up. If you find it difficult to apply the thrust with your hand against the ilium, slide your hand towards you to place the forearm against the bone to give you improved leverage.

Figure 13.34   Short-lever rotation technique – pelvis forwards.

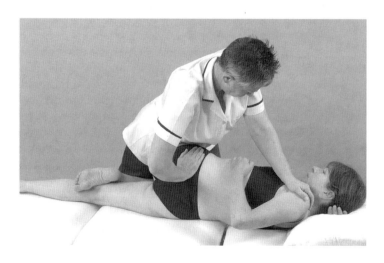

Short-lever rotation technique – pelvis backwards (Cyriax & Cyriax 1983, Cyriax 1984)

Position the patient in side lying with the painful side uppermost. Take the lower arm behind the patient and place the upper arm into elevation, resting in front of the patient's face. Extend the upper leg and flex the hip and knee of the lower leg. The shoulder will now be positioned forwards and the pelvis backwards. Stand behind the patient; place one hand on the scapula to give a little distraction to take up the slack. Place the other hand on the front of the pelvis with your forearm horizontal and pointing back towards you (Fig. 13.35). Apply a minimal amplitude, high velocity thrust once all of the slack is taken up.

Figure 13.35   Short-lever rotation technique – pelvis backwards.

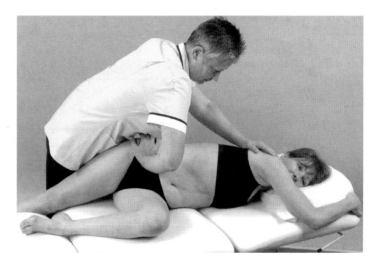

Long-lever rotation technique (Cyriax & Cyriax 1983, Cyriax 1984)

This is a stronger rotational manoeuvre and care is recommended in its application to older patients to avoid placing undue strain on the neck of the femur.

Position the patient as for the short-lever rotation – pelvis forwards technique. Stand in front of the patient at waist level, facing the patient's feet to allow the arms to be placed more vertically. Fix the shoulder with one hand and place the other hand behind the knee, with your thumb in the knee crease. Lean on the knee to produce a rotation strain (Fig. 13.36). Apply a minimal amplitude, high velocity thrust once all of the slack is taken up.

Figure 13.36 Long-lever rotation technique.

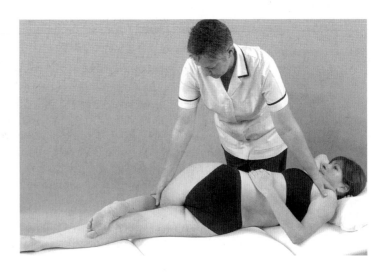

'Pretzel' technique

This is a strong, long-lever rotation technique when used as a manipulation. It can be broken down into its individual stages and used as a mobilizing technique for hyperacute pain in which the lesion is too irritable for manipulation (see below). It helps in both instances to be clear on the different stages of the technique. It may be useful for correcting a lateral shift (Cyriax & Cyriax 1983).

- Stand on the patient's painless side with the patient in supine lying. Flex the knees and cross the good leg over the bad (Fig. 13.37)
- Flex both hips (Fig. 13.38)
- Place your knee which is furthest from the patient's head at the patient's waist to act as a pivot point. Place your hands on the patient's knees and side flex the lumbar spine to gap the affected side (Fig. 13.39)
- Rotate the pelvis towards you until the patient's knees are resting on your thigh (Fig. 13.40)
- Gently lower your thigh, taking the pelvis further into rotation, ensuring that the other hand fixes the patient's shoulder flat on the couch (Fig. 13.41). Apply a minimal amplitude, high velocity thrust once all of the slack is taken up. Help the patient back to the starting position

Figure 13.37 'Pretzel' technique: starting position with knees flexed and 'good' leg placed over the 'bad'.

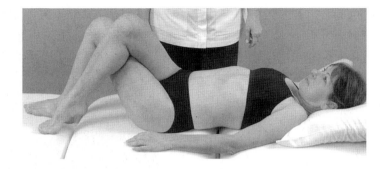

Figure 13.38 Both hips flexed.

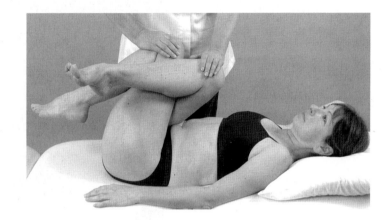

Figure 13.39 Spine side-flexed around pivot of caudal knee placed in patient's waist.

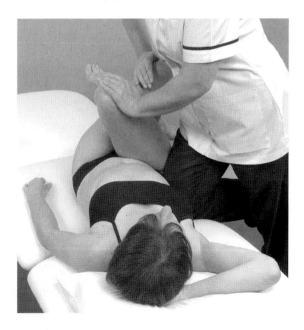

Figure 13.40 Pelvis rotated forwards to rest patient's knees against thigh.

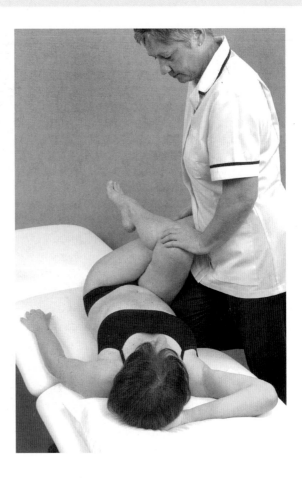

Figure 13.41 Lowering the patient's knees by removing the thigh, to take the pelvis into rotation, stabilizing the shoulder on the couch. Taking up the slack before applying the Grade C thrust.

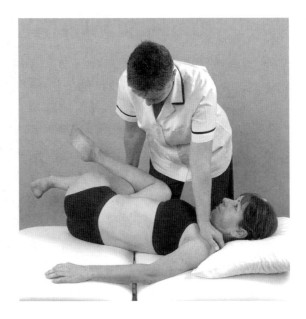

If the patient is large, an assistant may be required to fix the patient's shoulder.

For hyperacute pain, each step is conducted individually using Grade A mobilization, constantly monitoring for improvement before progressing to the next step. Progression through the steps is made cautiously and steadily and may take 5 or 10 min to achieve in the very irritable state. The end of range will not necessarily be reached before proceeding to the next step. The technique should not aggravate the pain and the patient should be firmly and comfortably supported throughout. This is not a manipulation as such and any other mobilizing modality may be applied at each stage.

Extension manoeuvres

Extension manoeuvres are used for central pain or pain that is referred unilaterally into the back only. They may be used as first-line treatment if a patient presents with central pain, or as a progression of the rotational manoeuvres as the pain centralizes.

Straight extension thrust technique (Cyriax & Cyriax 1983, Cyriax 1984)

This technique is indicated if a small central pain exists. Position the patient in prone lying and palpate the spinous processes to locate the painful level. Place the ulnar border of your hand over the tender spinous process and reinforce it with the other hand by placing the thumb web over your fingers. Apply pressure directly down onto the spinous process through straight arms (Fig. 13.42). Apply a minimal amplitude, high velocity thrust once all the slack is taken up by lifting and dropping your head down between your shoulders. Be careful not to lose the end of range by lifting your hands as you raise your head.

Figure 13.42 Straight extension thrust technique.

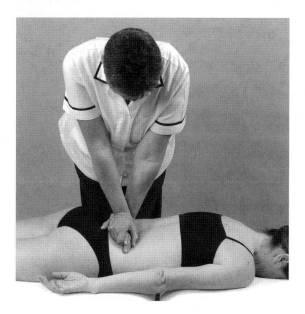

Unilateral extension thrust technique (Cyriax & Cyriax 1983, Cyriax 1984)

If the pain centralizes to a short unilateral pain, or the patient presents with a short unilateral pain, this technique may be applied. Position the patient in prone lying, stand on the painful side and palpate the spinous process to locate the painful level. Place the ulnar border of the hand over the transverse process at the tender level on the side furthest away from you. The pisiform should be adjacent to the spinous process and the pressure is applied through the paravertebral muscles for patient comfort. Stand close to the bed with your knees hooked onto the edge to enable you to lean over the patient. Apply pressure down onto the transverse process through arms as straight as possible, directing the pressure back towards your own knees (Fig. 13.43). Apply a minimal amplitude, high velocity thrust once all of the slack is taken up by lifting and dropping your head between your shoulders.

Figure 13.43 Unilateral extension thrust technique.

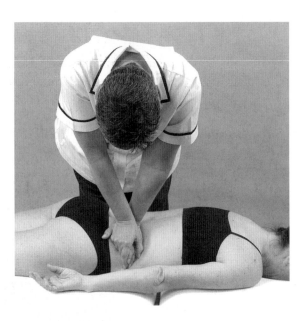

Extension technique with leverage (Cyriax & Cyriax 1983, Cyriax 1984)

If the above fails to clear unilateral pain, this technique is a little stronger. Position the patient in prone lying and stand on the painless side. Position one hand flat, just above the painful level. Wrap the other hand over and under the leg on the painful side just above the knee. Stand close to the couch, lift the leg on the painful side into full extension of the hip and lumbar spine and step backwards to apply side flexion, gapping the painful side (Fig. 13.44 a, b). Apply a minimal amplitude, high velocity thrust, continuing the direction of movement, once all of the slack is taken up.

Figure 13.44   (a, b) Extension technique with leverage.

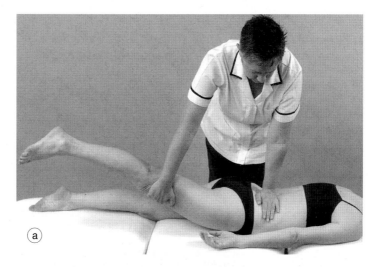

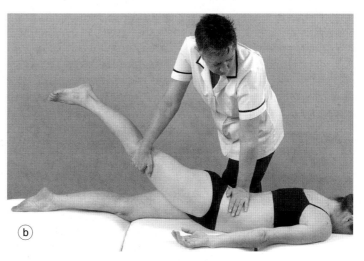

LUMBAR TRACTION

The major indication for lumbar traction is the presence of disc displacement of gradual onset or Clinical Model 1 (see above) which may be diagnosed following thorough assessment of the patient with consideration of the history and the presenting signs and symptoms. Traction may be applied to any of the other clinical models if other treatments have been unsuccessful or only partially successful, provided that there are no contraindications.

Contraindications to lumbar traction

- Patients with acute lumbago or sciatica usually associated with twinges and antalgic postures: the application of traction may be quite comfortable but as the traction is released the patient will be far worse and the pain and twinges will be agonizing. It may take some hours for the pain to subside sufficiently to allow the patient to get up and the whole experience is awful for both patient and therapist alike.

With patients with less irritable back pain, symptoms are often eased as traction is applied, but be particularly cautious if the history, signs and symptoms reveal an acute situation and the pain is completely relieved by traction

- Patients with severe cardiac or respiratory problems may not be able to tolerate either the straps or the supine lying position. A bad cough also contraindicates treatment since pain will be made much worse
- Patients with claustrophobia or other psychological disorders may become panic-stricken while undergoing traction, although such patients do not usually give consent to its application in the first place

While not absolute contraindications, there are several instances where traction is ill-advised or unlikely to be successful:

- S4 symptoms only, may theoretically respond to traction but it is always best to exercise caution in any situation that implies a large central protrusion, including bilateral sciatica from the same level (Cyriax 1982). Worsening of the situation could lead to increased compression on the cauda equina and possible permanent damage to bladder function
- The pain of disc protrusions with neurological deficit is unlikely to be relieved by traction since the protrusion is too large to be reduced. Manipulation is less likely still to be effective and the treatment of choice is epidural anaesthesia (see below)
- Sciatica which has lasted for more than 6 months is unlikely to respond to traction. The patient may be advised to await spontaneous recovery, to try epidural anaesthesia or to seek a surgical opinion, according to the severity of the symptoms and the patient's choice

Technique

Friction-free electrically operated traction beds have been designed which may be used in conjunction with electronically operated units that supply options for either rhythmical or static traction. Neither is an absolute necessity for the application of static traction as suggested by Cyriax & Cyriax (1983). The debate of sustained versus intermittent traction is considered in Chapter 4. Far less sophisticated apparatus may be used which is just as effective, but adjustments may then be needed to calculate the distracting force applied, on the basis of overcoming the friction forces created between the patient and the couch (see below).

A thoracic and a pelvic harness are affixed to either end of a couch and applied to the patient. Harnesses of modern design are usually comfortable and easy to readjust since they have Velcro™ fastenings. A simple device is required for taking up the slack and applying a continuous pull-down through the pelvic belt, so providing traction to the intervening lumbar spine.

The principle of application is that the pull should be as strong as is comfortable. In the early stages this was the only guideline provided and there was no way of knowing the exact poundage being applied. A spring balance was then introduced in series with the pelvic rope, which gave some indication of poundage. However, Judovitch & Nobel (1957) calculated the coefficient of friction to be 0.5 and, since half the body weight is distributed below the level of L3, then a force of $\frac{1}{2} \times 0.5 = \frac{1}{4}$ of the patient's body weight is required to overcome the friction between the body and the couch before the distracting force is applied to the spine. This is an important factor in calculating the actual poundages being applied when using a standard couch. When using a friction-free couch, the poundages registering on the accompanying machine are relatively faithful to the actual poundages being applied.

Feedback from the patient is just as important as in the days before a means of measuring poundages was devised and 'as strong as is comfortable' should still be the rule. An approximate estimate of the appropriate poundage may be made by assessing the size and weight of the patient, in the light of experience with other patients.

Before the commencement of treatment, a thorough explanation should be given to the patient on the reasons for applying the technique and the likely outcome, including any possible adverse effects such as stiffness or increased proximal pain. Consent should then be gained.

Before applying traction a selected comparable sign should be tested, such as the straight leg raise or particular lumbar movements in standing.

The patient does not need to be completely undressed for traction. Light clothing may be worn, being careful to remove belts, buckles, car keys, etc., and ensuring that clothing can separate in the middle. The patient is instructed to lie down sideways on the couch before rolling into supine lying.

The usual starting position is in supine lying but the number of pillows under head and knees may be adjusted for comfort. As the knees are lifted so the lumbar lordosis will flatten and a stool may be used to achieve Fowler's position (hips and knees flexed to 90°) if the patient is more comfortable with the spine completely flat.

Other positions such as prone lying may be tried if the patient is more comfortable in lumbar extension. Theoretically there are eight combinations of straps varying the patient's position between supine and prone, and choosing to place each of the thoracic and pelvic straps either underneath or on top of the patient. In practice, however, lying supine or prone, with the straps underneath the patient in both instances, are the two most popular and comfortable positions.

The thoracic belt should be tight enough to grip the chest to prevent it from sliding up towards the axillae, which is very uncomfortable and a little undignified for the well-endowed female. However, the grip should not be so tight as to restrict breathing, although patients will tend to find that they employ apical breathing more than diaphragmatic breathing while the traction is being applied.

The pelvic harness should sit comfortably above or around the iliac crests where it can pull down on the pelvis as the traction is applied but without slipping. The pelvic harness should not be so tight as to compress the abdomen uncomfortably and patients should be warned not to have a heavy meal before treatment.

If using a friction-free couch, ensure that the sliding lumbar section of the table is locked in its fixed position while the harnesses are being applied. The lumbar spine segment being treated should initially be placed over the division in the table.

The slack is taken up in the pelvic rope to apply tension to the system. This may be done by hand or through pulleys in the more rudimentary units, or by machine in an automatic unit. Traction is then applied steadily, either manually by releasing ropes, turning wheels, pumping down on handles, etc., or automatically.

At the first treatment, 20 min of traction is usually sufficient and provides enough time to be effective but not enough to overtreat, causing severe after-treatment stiffness or soreness. Feedback is encouraged from patients throughout treatment and it is essential to know if they become uncomfortable or if there is a marked increase in their pain. Simple adjustments can be made to lessen discomfort from the straps or to reduce the traction as necessary.

The patient should always be supplied with a means of summoning help such as a bell or buzzer. In subsequent treatments the time may be increased to 30 min. These timings are suggested on an empirical basis and little research has been done on this. Often the time allocated for treatment sessions in the appointment system is the limiting factor.

After treatment the traction should be released steadily and slowly, gaining feedback from the patient throughout, to be guided on the appropriate rate. The electrical units do not usually allow for this flexibility but do release steadily.

The traction belts are then released and patients are encouraged to wriggle for a minute or two. They are allowed to roll over but should not sit up until the residual stiffness following the application of traction has eased.

When ready, patients should be asked to turn onto their side, if they have not already done so, and to push themselves up sideways to avoid straining the back. Some patients need to sit for a moment or two until any dizziness or light-headedness arising from postural hypotension has subsided.

When dressing, patients should be advised to avoid bending, and should put tights or socks on by bringing the foot up towards them and doing shoes up by bringing the foot up onto a chair rather than by bending to the floor.

Patients should be encouraged to continue with their everyday activities within the limits of pain, but prolonged sitting or lifting should be avoided while the treatment is continuing.

In terms of treatment frequency and duration, ideally the patient should be seen daily, but the ideal is rarely attained due to the various time and financial constraints in both the National Health Service and the private sector. Traction is often perceived as an expensive use of resources that is not easily justified on the basis of its poor evidence base. However, evidence to demonstrate conclusively that it is ineffective is also wanting. In the authors' clinical experience it is still worth applying traction as frequently as possible and it will not necessarily fail if the ideal conditions are not available. Improvement should become apparent after three or four treatments and if no improvement is evident, modification of the traction position may be made before abandoning the modality altogether.

The physical treatment techniques of manipulation and traction have a limited use in the treatment of back pain. As has already been emphasized, the selection of suitable patients for such techniques is essential. The treatment programme for all patients should include a positive approach to the management of back pain with an emphasis on balanced activity and rest. Patients should be involved in the management of their condition and a home treatment regime should be implemented, including postural and ergonomic advice where appropriate. The reader is recommended to the McKenzie approach for the management of lumbar disc lesions, which particularly complements the orthopaedic medicine approach, although the hypotheses on pathology and explanation of effect differ.

LUMBAR INJECTIONS

Caudal epidural injections

Sicard in 1901 introduced local anaesthetic into the epidural space and this technique has continued, with the addition of corticosteroid in the 1950s, to be efficacious in the management of discogenic sciatica (Dilke et al 1973, Bush & Hillier 1991, Bush 1994). It is a well-tolerated procedure with a high patient satisfaction rate and relatively few side-effects. Recent adverse publicity of arachnoiditis is associated with the intrathecal rather than the epidural route (Bowman et al 1993).

Indications for caudal epidural injection

- Hyperacute pain which fails to settle with adequate analgesia and up to 3 days' bed rest, and is too irritable for manipulation or traction
- Radicular pain which has failed to respond to conservative management during the first 6 weeks from onset
- Chronic back or leg pain, with or without neurological deficit, which has failed to respond to conservative measures
- As a trial to treat pain before surgical intervention is considered

Bush & Hillier (1991) indicated that active intervention with caudal epidural injection of triamcinolone acetonide plus procaine improves signs and symptoms at the 4-week follow-up, with improvement maintained at 1-year follow-up.

The mechanism by which caudal epidural produces this improvement in pain relief is still debated and several hypotheses exist (Bush & Hillier 1991). Disc material can exert a mechanical effect through compression, a chemical effect through inflammation and an ischaemic effect through oedema. Introducing corticosteroid into the epidural space may directly affect the chemical and indirectly the ischaemic effects of pain. The introduction of fluid into a fluid-filled space can mechanically affect the relationship between the disc and the nerve root, while the introduction of local anaesthetic may have sufficient short-term effects to break the pain cycle.

Epidural injection via the caudal route can be carried out as an outpatient procedure. It is recommended that the procedure should only

Figure 13.45 Caudal epidural injection.

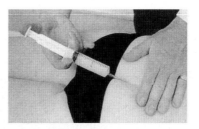

Figure 13.46 Caudal epidural injection, showing direction of approach and needle position.

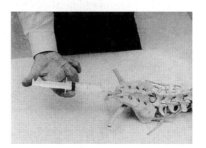

be conducted by an experienced medical practitioner, after appropriate training. The injection involves the introduction of 40–80 mg triamcinolone acetonide in 20–30 ml of 0.5% procaine hydrochloride via the sacral hiatus using a no-touch technique, with observation of blood or cerebrospinal fluid backflow (Figs 13.45 and 13.46) (Bush 1994).

SCLEROSANT THERAPY

Sclerosant or prolotherapy is used to treat chronic spinal instability and chronic pain. It involves the injection of a chemical irritant into the ligaments surrounding an unstable spinal or sacroiliac segment. The chemical irritant produces an inflammatory response, causing fibroblast hyperplasia and subsequent increase in strength of the supporting ligaments (Ongley et al 1987).

The patient undergoes manipulation first of all to ensure that a full range of movement is achievable and to reduce the disc displacement. An injection is given of a solution called P2G comprising phenol, dextrose and glycerine. Each osseoligamentous junction is infiltrated using a peppering technique (Fig. 13.47a, b, c). Injections are given at weekly intervals with a maximum of three or four injections. The patient is instructed to avoid flexion to allow the ligamentous tissue to contract sufficiently to stabilize the joints.

Orthopaedic medicine courses include the principles of sclerosant injections for medical practitioners but a period of supervised clinical practice is recommended.

MECHANISM OF SPONTANEOUS RECOVERY

Irrespective of treatment, the natural history of a disc prolapse is one of resolution (Bogduk 1991) and the possible mechanisms for this will now be discussed.

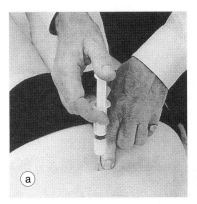
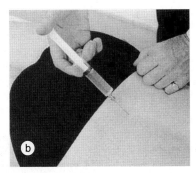
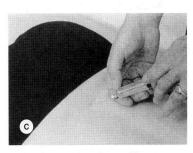

Figure 13.47 (a–c) Sclerosant injection, indicating needle placement to pepper the lumbosacral and sacroiliac ligaments.

Bush et al (1992) demonstrated that a high proportion of patients with discogenic sciatica made a good recovery together with resolution of the disc herniation in a significant number. They concluded that, with good pain control, nature can be allowed to run its course. Ellenberg et al (1993) prospectively studied 14 patients with definite radiculopathy and disc herniation on computed tomographic scan. They showed that the natural history of disc herniation with radiculopathy is improvement or complete recovery in 78% in 6–18 months, with non-surgical management.

Pople & Griffith (1994) suggested that a disc protrusion stretches the posterior longitudinal ligament, producing predominantly back pain, while a disc prolapse exiting through a tear in the posterior longitudinal ligament produces reduced tension. This explains why patients with an extruded fragment often experience a decrease or complete resolution of back pain as the root symptoms begin. According to Cyriax (1982), nerve root pain is expected to recover spontaneously provided the backache ceases when the pain shifts into the leg. This may take 8–12 months but the older the patient, the longer or less likely the spontaneous recovery. Cyriax (1982) considered recovery to occur through mechanisms of shrinkage of the prolapsed disc material or through its accommodation by vertebral erosion. Nerve root atrophy may occur with the patient losing pain through ischaemia of the nerve root, but the neurological signs tending to take longer to recover.

With advanced technology involving magnetic resonance imaging scans, the position of the prolapse can be seen and monitored. It may be seen to disappear completely, reduce or remain evident and is not necessarily indicative of symptomatology. In some cases the improvement in clinical findings is seen before recessive changes are observed on magnetic resonance imaging (Teplick & Haskin 1985, Delauche-Cavallier et al 1992, Komori et al 1996), or the prolapse can persist with no symptoms at all (Bush et al 1992). A prolapsed fragment of nuclear material may be reduced through a process of disc absorption that involves neovascularization and macrophage phagocytosis (Saal et al 1990, Doita et al 1996, Ito et al 1996).

References

Acaroglu E R, Iatridis J C, Setton L A et al 1995 Degeneration and ageing affect the tensile behaviour of human lumbar annulus fibrosus. Spine 20:2690–2701

Adams M A, Hutton W C 1983 The effect of posture on the fluid content of lumbar intervertebral discs. Spine 8:665–671

Adams M A, Hutton W C 1986 The effect of posture on diffusion into lumbar intervertebral discs. Journal of Anatomy 147:121–134

Adams M, Bogduk N, Burton K et al 2002 The biomechanics of back pain. Churchill Livingstone, Edinburgh

Allam K, Sze G 1994 MR of primary extraosseous Ewing sarcoma. American Journal of Neuroradiology 15:305–307

Beaman D N, Graziano G P, Glover R A et al 1993 Substance P innervation of lumbar spine facet joints. Spine 18:1044–1049

Bernick S, Walker J M, Paule W J 1991 Age changes to the annulus fibrosus in human intervertebral discs. Spine 16:520–524

Bogduk N 1991 The lumbar disc and low back pain. Neurosurgery Clinics of North America 2:791–806

Bogduk N 1994 Innervation, pain patterns and mechanisms of pain production. In: Twomey L T (ed) Clinics in physical therapy, physical therapy of the low back, 2nd edn. Churchill Livingstone, Edinburgh, pp 93–109

Bogduk N 1997 Clinical anatomy of the lumbar spine and sacrum, 3rd edn. Churchill Livingstone, Edinburgh

Bogduk N, Twomey L T 1991 Clinical anatomy of the lumbar spine. Churchill Livingstone, Edinburgh

Bowman S J, Wedderburn L, Whaley A et al 1993 Outcome assessment after epidural corticosteroid injection for low back pain and sciatica. Spine 18:1345–1350

Brinckmann P 1986 Injury of the annulus fibrosus and disc protrusions – an in vitro investigation on human lumbar discs. Spine 11:149–153

Brock M, Patt S, Mayer H 1992 The form and structure of the extruded disc. Spine 17:1457–1461

Buckwalter J A 1995 Aging and degeneration of the human intervertebral disc. Spine 20:1307–1314

Bush K 1994 Lower back pain and sciatica – how best to manage them. British Journal of Hospital Medicine 51:216–222

Bush K, Hillier S 1991 A controlled study of caudal epidural injections of triamcinolone plus procaine for the management of intractable sciatica. Spine 16: 572–575

Bush K, Cowan N, Katz D E et al 1992 The natural history of sciatica associated with disc pathology. Spine 17:1205–1212

Caplan L R 1994 Management of patients with lumbar disc herniations with radiculopathy. European Neurology 34:114–119

Cavanaugh J M 1995 Neural mechanisms of lumbar pain. Spine 20:1804–1809

Cavanaugh J M, Kallakuri S, Ozaktay A C 1995 Innervation of the rabbit lumbar intervertebral disc and posterior longitudinal ligament. Spine 20:2080–2085

Clinical Standards Advisory Group (CSAG) Report 1994 Back pain. HMSO, London

Coppes M, Enrico M, Ralph T, Gerbrand G 1997 Innervation of 'painful' lumbar discs. Spine 22(20):2342–2349

Corrigan B, Maitland G D 1983 Practical orthopaedic medicine. Butterworths, London

Cyriax J 1982 Textbook of orthopaedic medicine, 8th edn. Baillière Tindall, London, vol 1

Cyriax J 1984 Textbook of orthopaedic medicine, 11th edn. Baillière Tindall, London, vol 2

Cyriax J, Cyriax P 1983 Illustrated manual of orthopaedic medicine. Butterworths, London

Delauche-Cavallier M-C, Budet C, Laredo J-D et al 1992 Lumbar disc herniation. Spine 17:927–933

Dilke T W F, Burry H C, Grahame R 1973 Extradural corticosteroid injection in management of lumbar nerve root compression. British Medical Journal 2:635–637

Dinning T A R, Schaeffer H R 1993 Discogenic compression of the cauda equina – a surgical emergency. Australian and New Zealand Journal of Surgery 63:927–934

Doita M, Kanatani T, Harada T et al 1996 Immunohistologic study of the ruptured intervertebral disc of the lumbar spine. Spine 21:235–241

Ellenberg M R, Ross M L, Honet J C et al 1993 Prospective evaluation of the course of disc herniations in patients with proven radiculopathy. Archives of Physical Medicine and Rehabilitation 74:3–8

Findlay G F G 1992 Tumours of the lumbar spine. In: Jayson M (ed) The lumbar spine and back pain, 4th edn. Churchill Livingstone, Edinburgh, pp 355–369

Galessiere P F, Downs A R, Greenberg H M 1994 Chronic, contained rupture of aortic aneurysms associated with vertebral erosion. Canadian Journal of Surgery 37:23–28

Garfin S R, Rydevik B, Lind B et al 1995 Spinal nerve root compression. Spine 20:1810–1820

Hartley A 1995 Practical joint assessment: lower quadrant, 2nd edn. Mosby, London, pp 1–88

Hirabayashi S, Kumano K, Tsuiki T et al 1990 A dorsally displaced free fragment of lumbar disc herniation and its interesting histologic findings. Spine 15:1231–1233

Holm S 1993 Pathophysiology of disc degeneration. Acta Orthopaedica Scandinavica 64 (Suppl. 251):13–15

Hoppenfeld S 1976 Physical examination of the spine and extremities. Appleton Century Crofts, Philadelphia

Iatridis J C, Weidenbaum M, Setton L A et al 1996 Is the nucleus pulposus a solid or a fluid? Mechanical behaviour of the nucleus pulposus of the human intervertebral disc. Spine 21:1174–1184

Ito T, Yamada M, Ikuta F et al 1996 Histologic evidence of absorption of sequestration-type herniated disc. Spine 21:230–234

Jensen G M 1980 Biomechanics of the lumbar intervertebral disc: a review. Physical Therapy 60:765–773

Jönsson B, Strömqvist B 1995 The straight leg raising test and the severity of symptoms in lumbar disc herniation. Spine 20:27–30

Judovitch B, Nobel G R 1957 Traction therapy, a study of resistance forces. American Journal of Surgery 93:108–114

Kang J D, Georgescu H I, McIntyre-Larkin L et al 1996 Herniated lumbar intervertebral discs spontaneously produce matrix metalloproteinases, nitric oxide, interleukin-6, and prostaglandin E2. Spine 21:271–277

Karbowski K, Dvorak J 1995 Historical perspective: description of variations of the sciatic stretch phenomenon. Spine 20:1525–1527

Kemp H B S, Worland J 1974 Infections of the spine. Physiotherapy 60:2–6

Khuffash B, Porter R W 1989 Cross leg pain and trunk list. Spine 14:602–603

Komori H, Shinomiya K, Nakai O et al 1996 The natural history of herniated nucleus pulposus with radiculopathy. Spine 21:225–229

Kumar P, Clark M 2002 Clinical medicine, 5th edn. Baillière Tindall, London

Kuslich S D, Ulstrom C L, Michael C J 1991 The tissue origin of low back pain and sciatica. Orthopedic Clinics of North America 22:181–187

Laslett M, van Wijmen P 1999 Low back and referred pain: diagnosis and a proposed new system of classification. NZ Journal of Physiotherapy 27:5–14

Lee H-M, Kim N-H, Kim H-J et al 1995 Morphometric study of the lumbar spinal canal in the Korean population. Spine 20:1679–1684

Lehmann O J, Mendoza N D, Bradford R 1991 Beware the prolapsed disc. British Journal of Hospital Medicine 46:52

McCarron R F, Wimpee M W, Hudkins P G et al 1987 The inflammatory effect of the nucleus pulposus – a possible element in the pathogenesis of low back pain. Spine 12:760–764

McKenzie R A 1981 The lumbar spine: mechanical diagnosis and therapy. Spinal Publications, Waikanae, New Zealand

Marchand F, Ahmed A M 1990 Investigation of the laminate structure of the lumbar disc annulus fibrosus. Spine 15:402–410

Mixter W J, Barr J S 1934 Rupture of the intervertebral disc with involvement of the spinal canal. New England Journal of Medicine 211:210–215

Mooney V, Robertson J 1976 The facet syndrome. Clinical Orthopaedics and Related Research 115:149–156

Moridaira K, Handa H, Murakami H et al 1994 Primary Hodgkin's disease of the bone presenting with an extradural tumour. Acta Haematologica 92:148–149

Nachemson A 1966 The load on lumbar discs in different positions of the body. Clinical Orthopaedics 45:107–122

Nachemson A, Elfstrom G 1970 Intravital dynamic pressure measurements in lumbar discs, a study of common movements, manoeuvres and exercises. Scandinavian Journal of Rehabilitation Medicine 1 (Suppl.): 1–38

Norris C M 1998 Sports injuries: diagnosis and management for physiotherapists, 2nd edn. Butterworth Heinemann, Oxford

O'Flynn K J, Murphy R, Thomas D G 1992 Neurogenic bladder dysfunction in lumbar intervertebral disc prolapse. British Journal of Urology 69:38–40

Oliver J, Middleditch A 1991 Functional anatomy of the spine. Butterworth Heinemann, Oxford

Oliver M J, Twomey L T 1995 Extension creep in the lumbar spine. Clinical Biomechanics 10:363–368

Ongley M J, Klein R G, Dorman T A et al 1987 A new approach to the treatment of chronic low back pain. 2(8551):143–146

Osborne G 1974 Spinal stenosis. Physiotherapy 60:7–9

Osti O L, Cullum D E 1994 Occupational low back pain and intervertebral disc degeneration – epidemiology, imaging and pathology. Clinical Journal of Pain 10:331–334

Palastanga N, Field D, Soames R 2002 Anatomy and human movement, 4th edn. Butterworth Heinemann, Oxford

Palma L, Mariottini A, Muzii V F et al 1994 Neurinoma of the cauda equina misdiagnosed as prolapsed lumbar disc. Journal of Neurosurgical Sciences 38:181–185

Palmgren T, Gronblad M, Virri J et al 1996 Immunohistochemical demonstration of sensory and autonomic nerve terminals in herniated lumbar disc tissue. Spine 21:1301–1306

Parke W W, Schiff D C M 1971 The applied anatomy of the intervertebral disc. Orthopedic Clinics of North America 2:309–324

Pople I K, Griffith H B 1994 Prediction of an extruded fragment in lumbar disc patients from clinical presentations. Spine 19:156–158

Porter R W 1992 Spinal stenosis of the central and root canal. In: Jayson M (ed) The lumbar spine and back pain, 4th edn. Churchill Livingstone, Edinburgh, pp 313–332

Porter R W 1995 Pathology of symptomatic lumbar disc protrusion. Journal of the Royal College of Surgeons of Edinburgh 40:200–202

Porter R W, Hibbert C S, Wicks M 1978 The spinal canal in symptomatic lumbar disc lesions. Journal of Bone and Joint Surgery 60B:485–487

Porter R W, Oakshot G 1994 Spinal stenosis and health status. Spine 19:901–903

Prescher A 1998 Anatomy and pathology of the ageing spine. European Journal of Radiology 27:181–195

Rauschning W 1993 Pathoanatomy of lumbar disc degeneration and stenosis. Acta Orthopaedica Scandinavica 64(Suppl. 251):3–12

Riddle D L 1998 Classification and low back pain: a review of the literature and critical analysis of selected systems. Physical Therapy 78(7):708–737

Roberts S, Eisenstein S M, Menage J et al 1995 Mechanoreceptors in the intervertebral discs, morphology, distribution and neuropeptides. Spine 20:2645–2651

Rydevik B, Olmarker K 1992 Pathogenesis of nerve root damage. In: Jayson M (ed) The lumbar spine and back pain, 4th edn. Churchill Livingstone, Edinburgh, pp 89–90

Saal J S 1995 The role of inflammation in lumbar pain. Spine 20:1821–1827

Saal J A, Saal J S, Herzog J 1990 The natural history of lumbar intervertebral disc extrusions treated non-operatively. Spine 15:683–686

Schwarzer A C, Aprill C N, Derby R et al 1994a The relative contributions of the disc and zygapophyseal joint in chronic low back pain. Spine 19:801–806

Schwarzer A C, Aprill C N, Derby R et al 1994b Clinical features of patients with pain stemming from the lumbar zygapophyseal joints – is the lumbar facet syndrome a clinical entity? Spine 19:1132–1137

Supik L F, Broom M J 1994 Sciatic tension signs and lumbar disc herniations. Spine 19:1066–1068

Swezey R 1993 Pathophysiology and treatment of intervertebral disk disease. Rheumatic Disease Clinics of North America 19:741–757

Takahashi H, Suguro T, Okazima Y et al 1996 Inflammatory cytokines in the herniated disc of the lumbar spine. Spine 21:218–224

Taylor J, Twomey L 1994 The lumbar spine from infancy to old age. In: Twomey L, Taylor J (eds) Clinics in physical therapy, physical therapy of the low back, 2nd edn. Churchill Livingstone, Edinburgh, pp 1–56

Teplick J G, Haskin M E 1985 Spontaneous regression of herniated nucleus pulposus. American Journal of Roentgenology 145:371–375

Twomey L T 1992 A rationale for the treatment of back pain and joint pain by manual therapy. Physical Therapy 72:885–892

Twomey L, Taylor J 1982 Flexion creep deformation and hysteresis in the lumbar vertebral column. Spine 7:116–122

Twomey L T, Taylor J 1994 The lumbar spine: structure, function, age changes and physiotherapy. Australian Physiotherapy Journal, 40th Jubilee Issue, 72:19–30

Umehara S, Tadano S, Abumi K et al 1996 Effects of degeneration on the elastic modulus distribution in the lumbar intervertebral discs. Spine 21:811–820

Vernon-Roberts B 1992 Age-related and degenerative pathology of intervertebral discs and apophyseal joints. In: Jayson M (ed) The lumbar spine and back pain, 4th edn. Churchill Livingstone, Edinburgh, pp 17–41

Vroomen P, de Krom M, Knotternus J 1999 Diagnostic value of history and physical examination in patients suspected of sciatica due to disc herniation: a systematic review. Journal of Neurology 246:899–906

Vroomen P, de Krom M, Slofstra P, Knotternus J 2000 Conservative treatment of sciatica: a systematic review. Journal of Spinal Disorders 13(6):463–469

Vucetic N, Määttänen H, Svensson O 1995 Pain and pathology in lumbar disc hernia. Clinical Orthopaedics and Related Research 320:65–72

Waddell G 1992 Understanding the patient with backache. In: Jayson M (ed) The lumbar spine and back pain, 4th edn. Churchill Livingstone, Edinburgh, pp 469–485

Waddell G 1998 The back pain revolution. Churchill Livingstone, Edinburgh

Yamamoto I, Panjabi M M, Oxland T R et al 1990 The role of the iliolumbar ligament in the lumbosacral junction. Spine 15:1138–1141

Yamashita T, Minaki Y, Ozaktay A C et al 1996 A morphological study of the fibrous capsule of the human lumbar facet joint. Spine 21:538–543

Zimmermann M 1992 Basic neurophysiological mechanisms of pain and pain therapy. In: Jayson M (ed) The lumbar spine and back pain, 4th edn. Churchill Livingstone, Edinburgh, pp 43–59

Chapter 14

The sacroiliac joint

SUMMARY

Sacroiliac dysfunction describes a broad set of signs and symptoms associated with the sacroiliac joint and its surrounding structures (Dreyfuss et al 1996, Levangie 1999). Pain due to hypomobility, hypermobility, malalignment, fixation, joint subluxation and ligament strain can lead to structural changes in the joint and soft tissues (Freburger & Riddle 2001). Lesions tend to be long-standing and are difficult to diagnose, often mimicking pain of lumbar origin. This chapter begins with a presentation of the anatomy of the joint and links it with possible pathology and methods of differential diagnosis of its mechanical and non-mechanical lesions.

In general terms, treatment consists of mobilization, manipulation and/or exercise of hypomobile or subluxed joints, and stabilization through supportive belts, exercise and occasionally sclerosant injection for hypermobile joints. Intra-articular injections have also been discussed (Schmid 1984, Calvillo et al 2000). Contraindications to treatment are few and emphasis is placed on assessment strategies on which to base treatment selection and appropriate exercise programmes. The paucity of evidence to support current assessment methods is discussed.

ANATOMY

The pelvis is a unique osteoarticular ring consisting of the two innominate bones, which articulate anteriorly at the symphysis pubis, and posteriorly at the sacrum, which is suspended between the innominate bones by its ligaments. Since form follows function, small structural differences occur between the sexes, with women exhibiting greater mobility of the sacroiliac joints (Harrison et al 1997). The function of the bony pelvis is to support and transmit body weight from the trunk to the lower limbs and, vice versa, to dampen the distribution of ground reaction forces occurring during gait activities. It protects and provides support for the viscera and also provides attachment for ligaments and leverage for muscles.

The *sacrum* is a large triangular mass of bone formed by the fusion of the five sacral vertebrae (Fig. 14.1). The *sacral base* lies superiorly and

Figure 14.1 (a, b) Sacrum, showing bony landmarks.

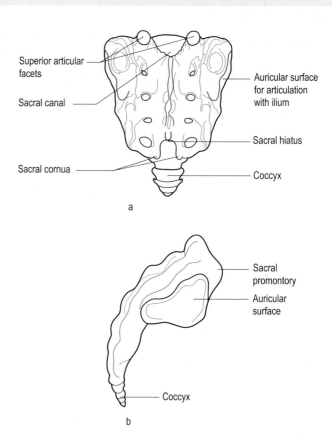

Superior articular facets

Sacral canal

Auricular surface for articulation with ilium

Sacral hiatus

Sacral cornua

Coccyx

a

Sacral promontory

Auricular surface

Coccyx

b

is angulated upwards and forwards, articulating with the fifth lumbar vertebra to form the lumbosacral angle. Its anterior border is the *sacral promontory*. The apex of the sacrum lies inferiorly and articulates with the coccyx, a small triangular bone formed by the fusion of approximately four small vertebrae.

The pelvic surface of the sacrum is relatively smooth while its dorsal surface is roughened and displays three distinct crests: a *median crest* represents the fused spinous processes, an *intermediate crest* the fused articular processes and a *lateral crest* the fused transverse processes of the sacral vertebrae. The lateral crest provides attachment for the posterior sacroiliac ligaments.

The laminae and spinous processes of the fourth and fifth sacral vertebrae are absent, forming an opening known as the *sacral hiatus*. Anatomical anomalies are common here and elements of the other vertebrae may be missing, making this a variably sized opening (Trotter 1947). The *sacral cornua* are the remnants of the articular processes of the fourth or fifth sacral vertebra projecting downwards on either side of the sacral hiatus. They provide palpable bony landmarks for the sacral hiatus which is clinically relevant in the placement of a caudal epidural injection. To palpate the sacral cornua, place the thumb and middle finger of one hand on the posterior superior iliac spines (PSIS) and use the index finger to make an equilateral triangle. The position of the index finger now gives the approximate position of the sacral cornua and hence the sacral hiatus.

The *sacral canal* is triangular in shape and formed by the fused sacral vertebral foramina. The dural sac usually terminates at the level of the lower border of the second sacral vertebra where it contracts into a filament and continues through the sacral canal to the coccyx, to become continuous with the periosteum (Trotter 1947). Four pairs of sacral foramina provide an exit for the sacral spinal nerves. The lateral surface of the sacrum is expanded superiorly and provides an articulating surface for the sacroiliac joint. This surface bears an auricular (ear-like) surface anteriorly, which is shaped more like an 'L' than an ear, and a pitted irregular surface posteriorly, for the attachment of the posterior and interosseous sacroiliac ligaments.

The *hip or innominate bone* is made up of the *ilium* above, the *pubis* in front and the *ischium* behind. The *acetabulum* is the cup shaped hollow on its outer surface at the junction of the three component bones.

The ilium possesses several palpable bony landmarks. Those relevant here are:

- The iliac crest which gives an approximate indication of the level of the spinous process of L4
- The anterior superior iliac spine (ASIS) which lies at the anterior end of the iliac crest
- The anterior inferior iliac spine (AIIS) which lies below the superior spine and is not so readily palpable
- The posterior superior iliac spine (PSIS), indicated by a dimple (dimple of Venus) approximately 4 cm lateral to the spinous process of S2.
- The posterior inferior iliac spine (PIIS) lying below the superior spine and difficult to palpate

The *iliac fossa* lies medially, its posterior aspect thickened, roughened and marked by the iliac tubercle for the attachment of the posterior and interosseous sacroiliac ligaments. In front of the roughened area lies an auricular-shaped articular surface corresponding to the articular surface of the sacrum. Laterally the blade of the ilium provides attachment for the gluteal muscles.

THE SACROILIAC JOINT

The sacroiliac joint is essentially a synovial joint with its surfaces covered by articular cartilage, lined with synovial membrane and surrounded by a fibrous capsule, reinforced by ligaments. The anterior third of the articulation between the sacrum and the ilium is considered to be a true synovial joint, with the remaining articulation supported by ligamentous attachments that convert the joint into a part syndesmosis (Harrison et al 1997). Due to its deep location, its position in the osteo-articular ring and the variability in anatomy between sides and individuals, the sacroiliac joint is a difficult joint to study (Zheng et al 1997).

The auricular-shaped articular facets on the ilium and the sacrum have reciprocally irregular joint surfaces which provide the joint with great stability. In basic terms, a bump or ridge on one surface will articulate with a pit or depression on the other. The joint surfaces are relatively planar in the young, but following puberty irregularities develop, more so in the male sacroiliac joint, making it inherently more stable. Two types of joint surface irregularities were described by Vleeming et al (1990a, 1990b) in a study of prepared human sacroiliac joints. Ridges on one joint surface had complementary depressions on the other, and areas of coarse and smooth texture existed. The irregularities in the joint surfaces appear to represent adaptations to stability promoted by increased body weight during the adolescent growth spurt. These irregularities also provide the joint surfaces with high coefficients of friction, further contributing to the joint's renowned stability. The irregularities continue to progress with age and fusion of the joint is said to develop in the elderly. However, Vleeming et al (1990a) suggest caution when interpreting X-rays of the sacroiliac joints since the ridges and depressions can be misinterpreted as osteophytes.

The way in which the joint surfaces interdigitate allows weight-bearing but restricts movement, contributing to the stability of the joint. Major subluxation of the joint is not commonly seen clinically, but the interdigitating articular surfaces make minor subluxation a possibility. Vleeming et al (1990b) surmise from friction experiments that, under abnormal loading conditions, it is possible to force sacroiliac joint surfaces into a new position in which the ridges and depressions are no longer complementary, suggesting a blocked joint or minor subluxation.

The suspension of the wedge-shaped sacrum between the two ilia provides it with a self-locking mechanism. This self-locking mechanism involves both form and force closure (Lee 2000). Form closure indicates stability due to the closely fitting joint surfaces, the friction coefficient of the roughened articular cartilage and the integrity of the strong sacroiliac ligaments, so that little or no external forces are required to maintain static stability. Force closure indicates the dynamic stability of the joint in which extra forces are needed to maintain stability. Movements occurring in the sacroiliac joint are small, but as the sacrum moves, activity in the surrounding muscle groups together with increased ligamentous tension enhances the compression forces on the joint to facilitate the force closure mechanism, making load transfer more efficient (Lee 2000). Increasing weight applied to the sacral base, such as the effects of gravity or the compression forces of the trunk, will also enhance the force closure mechanism, holding the sacrum more tightly in situ through tension in its ligaments (Fig. 14.2) (Kapandji 1974). This arrangement is thought to be similar to the keystone of an arch in which stability is created where the greater the force applied, the greater the resistance offered (Harrison et al 1997).

The fibrous capsule is reinforced by strong posterior ligaments and weaker anterior ligaments, while a set of accessory ligaments contributes a stabilizing effect on the joint. These strong ligaments prevent translation of the sacrum and separation of the joint. The *interosseous*

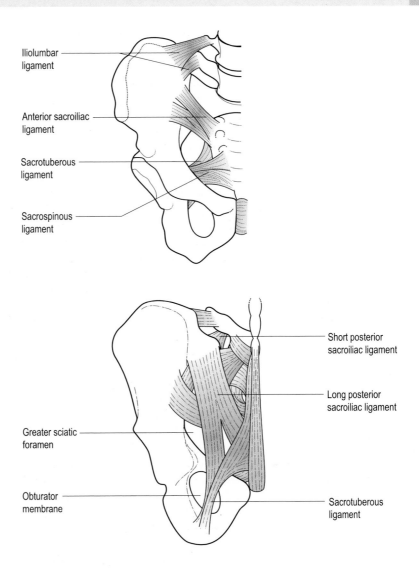

Figure 14.2   The sacroiliac joint and ligaments. From Anatomy and Human Movement by N Palastanga, D Field and R Soames. Reprinted by permission of Elsevier Ltd.

sacroiliac ligament forms the main union between the sacrum and ilium, filling the gap between the lateral sacral crest and the iliac tuberosity (Lee 2000). It strongly resists separation and translation forces and is a physical barrier to palpation of the sacroiliac joint which makes intra-articular injection difficult (Harrison et al 1997, Lee 2000).

The *posterior sacroiliac ligament* covers the interosseous ligament and has long and short fibres. Short horizontal fibres are placed superiorly where they resist forward movement of the sacral promontory. Longer vertical fibres, continuous with the sacrotuberous ligament, are more superficial and resist a downwards movement of the sacrum relative to the ilium. The long posterior fibres are said to be tense under counternutation, an upwards, backward, nodding movement of the sacrum (Vleeming et al 1996) (see below).

The *anterior sacroiliac ligament* forms a weak thickening of the anterior joint capsule.

Accessory ligaments exert a stabilizing effect on the joint:

The *sacrotuberous ligament* attaches by a broad base from the PSIS, the side of the sacrum and the coccyx, partially blending with the posterior ligaments. Its fibres converge to pass downwards and laterally, twisting and broadening again at its attachment to the ischial tuberosity where it blends with the tendon of biceps femoris and the lower fibres of gluteus maximus.

The *sacrospinous ligament* is thinner and triangular, lying anterior to the sacrotuberous ligament. It passes from the lower part of the sacrum and coccyx to the spine of the ischium and its pelvic surface blends with the coccygeus muscle.

The sacrotuberous and sacrospinous ligaments lie below and lateral to the joint, preventing the tendency for the apex of the sacrum to tilt upwards as body weight is directed down onto the base of the sacrum. The *iliolumbar ligaments* anchor the transverse processes of the fifth lumbar vertebra to the ilium (an attachment to the fourth lumbar vertebra may also be present), stabilizing the lumbosacral junction against the tendency for the sacral promontory to move forwards under the influence of gravity and body weight.

THE SACROCOCCYGEAL JOINT

This is a symphysis between S5 and the first coccygeal segment, but the joint is often obliterated in old age. Flexion and extension movements occur which are largely passive (Lee 2000, Palastanga et al 2002).

THE SYMPHYSIS PUBIS

The symphysis pubis is the joint between the medial surfaces of the two innominate bones. An interpubic fibrocartilaginous disc is situated within the joint and the surrounding joint capsule is supported by ligamentous thickenings. A *superior pubic ligament* is a thick fibrous band joining the pubic crests and tubercles, while an *arcuate pubic ligament* arches between the inferior pubic rami, blending with the intra-articular disc, to support the joint inferiorly (Palastanga et al 2002).

MOVEMENT OF THE SACROILIAC JOINT

Many strong muscles pass over the sacroiliac joint, but none directly affects it. However, the ligaments of the sacroiliac joint and lumbar spine fuse with the thoracolumbar fascia and as such provide attachments for the main trunk stabilizing muscles. Activity in these stabilizing muscles provide a 'self-bracing' mechanism which in turn contributes to stability at the sacroiliac joints (Harrison et al 1997). There seems to be a general agreement that some passive movement does occur at the sacroiliac joint, but how much and in which direction is still not certain. Movement descriptions applied to the sacroiliac joint include subluxation, upslip, downslip, outflare, inflare, anterior or posterior rotation or torsion, all of which describe movement of the ilium on the sacrum (Oliver & Middleditch 1991, Swezey 1998, Williams 1998, Cibulka 2002). Kapandji (1974) refers to the movements as nutation and counternutation (Latin, *nutare* = to nod) where movement of the sacrum on the ilium is described.

Cibulka (2002) questions the notion that all of these movements occur at the sacroiliac joint, arguing that in common with other synovial joints, the movement patterns at the sacroiliac joint are determined by the shape and orientation of the articular surfaces. Therefore, although structurally separate, they act together functionally as one bicondylar joint, and have two degrees of freedom.

The primary movement is considered to be an anterior or posterior sagittal tilt otherwise called torsion, rotation or nutation in the descriptions above. However, minor frontal and transverse movements of the joints also occur, dependent upon the individual's joint alignment, which possibly explains the observation of inflares and outflares. The secondary movement is an antagonistic innominate motion where movement on one side is accompanied by a correlative movement on the other, making the two sacroiliac joints interdependent on each other, and never independent.

During symmetrical activities such as sitting or standing, movement normally occurs simultaneously in the two sacroiliac joints with either an anterior or posterior innominate tilt or rotation that brings the two anterior and posterior superior iliac spines to lie in roughly the same horizontal plane. During asymmetrical activities such as walking or running, just as one hip flexes and the other extends, one innominate bone tilts posteriorly while the other tilts anteriorly. Cibulka (2002) suggests that the relationship between the right and left innominate bones should be observed, as patients with sacroiliac dysfunction demonstrate an antagonistic asymmetrical position even in symmetrical postures such as sitting and standing. This notion that movement of one innominate bone occurs with correlative movement of the opposite innominate can be applied to manipulative techniques which can be reversed and performed on the opposite side. Zheng et al (1997) produced an experimental biomechanical model of the pelvis to study the sacroiliac joint that emphasized this interdependence of the three joints of the pelvic ring, the two sacroiliac joints and the symphysis pubis.

In a study of healthy individuals between the ages of 20 and 50 years, the average total rotational movement in the sacroiliac joint between erect standing and standing on one leg was 2° (Jacob & Kissling 1995, Kissling & Jacob 1996). One subject, excluded from this analysis because of occasional symptoms, was found to have more than 6° of movement.

Functionally, movements at the sacroiliac joint occur in combination with the adjacent joints. Variations between the two joints and between individuals are common, making objective examination of these joints difficult.

Although the sacroiliac joints are relatively immobile and stable, they are susceptible to mechanical trauma. Joint sprain and minor subluxations occur and, symptomatically, patients respond well to manipulation. In the discussion that follows below the subjective judgements made on sacroiliac static or dynamic alignment are not reliable indicators of dysfunction; therefore correction of alignment is not necessarily indicative of cure. As synovial joints they are subject to the various forms of arthritis and the degenerative changes associated with the ageing process. Reduced mobility seems to occur through a process of fibrous bands or fibrocartilaginous adhesion formation rather than bony ankylosis (Cassidy 1992, Palastanga et al 2002).

Mechanical lesions are less common in the older age group as movements reduce. The ligaments of the female pelvis relax during pregnancy, increasing the range of movement and making the sacroiliac joint locking mechanism less effective. During this time the relative hypermobility of the sacroiliac joints makes them susceptible to strain and subluxation.

NERVE SUPPLY

The nerve supply is variable and differs between individuals and often between the two sacroiliac joints in the same person; a variety of explanations for this is offered by the various texts. In general terms, however, the sacroiliac joint and its surrounding ligaments receive a supply derived from L2–S3 nerve roots (Oliver & Middleditch 1991, Calvillo et al 2000, Lee 2000, Palastanga et al 2002). Some of the supply is directly from the sacral plexus and dorsal rami and some indirectly via the superior gluteal nerve and obturator nerve.

Fortin et al (1999a) conducted an anatomical study on cadavers determining that the joint itself is predominantly innervated by sacral dorsal rami (S1–S3). This observation was supported by the pain diagrams (see below) reported by asymptomatic volunteers upon direct capsular stimulation, and with reduced pain in symptomatic subjects treated by intra-articular injection of an anaesthetic. As well as revealing pain-sensitive nerve endings within the joint, observations revealed the presence of mechanoreceptors which, in addition to signalling pain, could inform the central nervous system of abnormal loading, excessive movement and inflammation.

This extensive segmental supply and variation means that pain patterns can be confusing and may mimic other conditions. In a case report, Dangaria (1998) described a female patient presenting with low back pain, frequency and urgency of micturition whose symptoms were completely relieved by manipulation of the sacroiliac joint. The relief of all symptoms was attributed to the common nerve supply between the bladder and sacroiliac joint.

DIFFERENTIAL DIAGNOSIS AT THE SACROILIAC JOINT

Manipulative techniques are appropriate for mechanical lesions of the sacroiliac joint, i.e. minor subluxations and ligamentous strain. Assessment for displacement of the joint may be attempted through palpation tests but, in clinical practice, the small amount of movement at the sacroiliac joint makes this assessment difficult. Other means of applying compression, shear and distraction to the joints will be suggested, to incriminate the joint as a cause of pain. This section will discuss the differential diagnosis at the sacroiliac joint to distinguish mechanical lesions from other pathology.

Mechanical lesions of the sacroiliac joint

Diagnosis is clinical, taking into account the history, palpation for asymmetry in static and dynamic postures and the pain provocation tests. Diagnosed sacroiliac joint sprain, with or without subluxation, usually responds well to manipulation. Although the ideal treatment is yet to be validated, Calvillo et al (2000) suggest that treatment should be directed at restoring joint homeostasis. With this in mind, the indications, contraindications and treatment techniques will be described later in this chapter.

OTHER CAUSES OF SACROILIAC PAIN AND ASSOCIATED SIGNS AND SYMPTOMS

Arthritis can affect the sacroiliac joint since it is a mobile, weight-bearing, part synovial joint and may develop the same problems as other synovial joints. Normally, as described throughout this text, arthritis will manifest itself as the capsular pattern. However, at the sacroiliac joint, movements of accessory glide and translation mean that establishing the capsular pattern as such is difficult. The joint undergoes degenerative changes, reducing the mobility still further and making mechanical lesions less likely in the older age group.

The spondyloarthropathies such as ankylosing spondylitis, psoriatic arthritis and Reiter's syndrome may manifest themselves initially as sacroiliitis in which the pain provocation tests described below will probably be positive, but the history will demonstrate an inflammatory rather than mechanical lesion.

- *Ankylosing spondylitis* is a chronic seronegative inflammatory arthritis affecting the axial skeleton in particular (Rai 1995, Kumar & Clark 2002). It affects men more commonly than women, although it may exist subclinically in women. It has an insidious onset in men under the age of 40, who complain of back and buttock pain, persisting for several months. The symptoms are typical of an inflammatory condition, with the pain and early-morning stiffness eased by movement and exercise. Sacroiliac joints are often the first target for the disease and sacroiliitis may be seen on X-ray. The later stages involve the whole spine, when the X-ray appearance is of a 'bamboo' spine. The disease is related to the presence of factor human leukocyte antigen (HLA)-B27 and blood tests will usually confirm clinical diagnosis. On examination there is loss of the lumbar lordosis, increased thoracic kyphosis and decreased chest expansion. Sacroiliitis gives severe pain when the sacroiliac joints are compressed
- *Reiter's syndrome* is a form of seronegative reactive arthritis that can follow gastrointestinal or genital tract infections (Keat 1995, Kumar & Clark 2002). The arthritis affects the lower limb joints, more readily the knees and ankles, but can also affect the sacroiliac joints. Non-specific urethritis and conjunctivitis may accompany the condition

Serious non-mechanical conditions, including tumour, sepsis and fracture, can affect the sacroiliac joint and need to be excluded before manipulation is applied. Serious conditions of the pelvis may produce the 'sign of the buttock' (see Ch. 9). Pain associated with the sacroiliac joint in the elderly should be viewed with suspicion until proven otherwise, since mechanical lesions are rare in the sacroiliac joints in this age group.

- *Malignant disease* can involve the sacroiliac joint directly or indirectly (Silberstein et al 1992). Metastases may be a cause of pain in the pelvis of older patients
- *Infection*, as in osteomyelitis in the pelvis or upper femur, produces severe pain felt in the pelvic region and the patient is unwell with a high fever and marked tenderness over the affected bone
- *Septic arthritis*, although uncommon in the sacroiliac joint, presents dramatically with pain, heat and swelling. The patient is unwell and febrile
- *Fracture* of the sacrum or pelvic bones is suspected if the patient presents with a history of trauma, severe pain and much bruising

Other musculoskeletal lesions can produce pain felt in the region of, or referred to, the sacroiliac joint. Differential diagnosis is difficult because the signs and symptoms overlap considerably. Muscle imbalances may need to be addressed, particularly weakness of gluteus medius, within the main hip abductors. Weakness of gluteus medius can cause a pelvic drop on the stance phase of gait, resulting in a compensatory hip hiking brought about by quadratus lumborum (Chen et al 2002).

- *Lumbar disc lesions* produce pain felt in one or both buttocks. Distinguishing features of the history may help exclude it as a cause of pain, but lesions commonly coexist. Disc lesions are aggravated by posture and movement, eased by rest, and often better in the early morning. Dural involvement produces pain on coughing, sneezing and straining; radicular involvement produces objective neurological signs and sensory neurological symptoms
- *Hip joint* pathology refers pain to the L3 dermatome and may involve unilateral low back and upper buttock pain. Examination of the hip produces positive signs
- *Trochanteric bursitis* may produce lateral hip and thigh pain
- *Myofascial pain* due to trigger points in piriformis, gluteus maximus or quadratus lumborum may refer pain into the area of the sacroiliac joint (Chen et al 2002)
- *Coccydynia* is pain in the region of the coccyx which can arise following direct trauma such as a fall directly onto the bottom. The lumbar spine can also refer pain to the area of the coccyx

COMMENTARY ON THE EXAMINATION

OBSERVATION

A general observation is made, including the patient's *face, posture and gait*. Serious conditions of the pelvis may produce severe pain, of which night pain is a feature, and this may be evident in the face of the patient, who looks tired and drawn from lack of sleep. The posture and gait may show abnormalities and these need careful assessment to ascertain if they are relevant to the patient's presenting condition. Generally, a mechanical lesion of the sacroiliac joint rarely alters the gait pattern while sacroiliitis can be very painful, and the patient may not like to weight-bear on the affected side.

HISTORY (SUBJECTIVE EXAMINATION)

A careful history is taken because the differential diagnosis of mechanical lesions, subluxation or strain of the sacroiliac joint is particularly reliant on features of the history.

The patient's *age* is relevant as mechanical lesions of all joints in this region tend to present as a condition of middle age. Caution is required in the elderly and the young who seemingly present with a mechanical sacroiliac joint lesion, as this is uncommon. Younger patients may show postural asymmetry which may need correction to avoid later problems.

Occupation, sports, hobbies and lifestyle may all have relevance to a sacroiliac mechanical lesion. Any occupation or sport that involves increased weight-bearing through one leg may place abnormal stresses on the sacroiliac joint, e.g. driving, ballet, hurdling.

Mechanical lesions of the sacroiliac joint affect both sexes, but they are more common in women. The irregularities in the articular surfaces are more predominant in the male sacroiliac joint, giving it a greater inherent stability. During pregnancy, the ligaments of the pelvis soften to allow more movement and the joints are more susceptible to injury and subluxation. If subluxation occurs during this time and is not reduced, the abnormality remains once the ligaments tighten in the postpartum phase and the patient may encounter long-term problems.

The nature of the nerve supply to the sacroiliac joint and its surrounding ligaments makes the *site and spread* of the pain difficult to relate to specific diagnosis. The site and spread could be equally indicative of lumbar spine or hip pathology or mimic other conditions. Commonly a localized buttock pain is present, often centred around the PSIS. The spread of pain from the sacroiliac joint may be into the groin and front of the thigh, into the buttock and posterior thigh, and possibly into the calf. Fortin et al (1994a, 1994b) looked at patterns of pain referral using anaesthetic injections to map an area of hypaesthesia (a reduced sensibility to touch) in normal subjects and provocative injections followed by injection of anaesthetic in symptomatic subjects. All subjects felt hypaesthesia or pain locally over the sacroiliac joint, with variable referral to the lateral aspect of the buttock, to the greater trochanter and into the upper lateral thigh. This variation in pain response is consistent with the variable and extensive nerve root supply to the sacroiliac joint. Fortin et al (1994a, 1994b) felt it important to limit the pain mapping pattern to the area common to each subject and therefore most likely to represent sacroiliac joint symptoms. This was established as an area 3 × 10 cm just inferior to the PSIS. They concluded that the use of pain diagrams is a worthwhile preliminary diagnostic tool in conjunction with the history and complete physical examination.

Derby (1994) challenged Fortin et al's results, suggesting that although the first study mapped a consistent area of pain in asymptomatic volunteers, the second failed to report detailed pain relief information or to control for a placebo response. Slipman et al (2000) attempted to develop the work of Fortin et al in a retrospective study and identified 18 potential areas of pain referral based on fluoroscopically guided diagnostic sacroiliac joint blocks on 50 consecutive patients. A total of 72% reported pain in the lower lumbar region, 94% in the buttock and 14% in the groin; 50% of the patients in this study reported symptoms in the lower limb, with younger patients more likely to describe pain below the knee. The authors give an honest appraisal of the limitations of their study and it is clear that more work is required to provide credible evidence.

Schwarzer et al (1995) found no conventional predictive features of sacroiliac joint pain except for a strong association with groin pain. Dreyfuss et al (1996) suggest that a distinguishing feature for sacroiliac joint pain syndrome may be the absence of pain felt above the L5 level, while Freburger and Riddle (2001), in reviewing the published evidence to guide examination of the sacroiliac joint, found some support for the following pain descriptions: absence of pain in the lumbar region, pain felt below L5 and pain in the region of the PSIS.

Fortin et al (1999b) expanded their studies on pain referral patterns by observing the pattern of contrast fluid movement during sacroiliac arthrography to determine whether any communication existed between the sacroiliac joint and adjacent neural structures. They established five principal patterns of extracapsular contrast fluid movement, three of which suggested a potential pathway of communication into the dorsal sacral foramina, into the fifth lumbar epiradicular sheath and into the lumbosacral plexus. They hypothesize that if the joint capsule is disrupted, intra-articular contents such as inflammatory chemical mediators, in symptomatic patients, could leak and irritate adjacent neural structures which could produce lower limb symptoms similar to those seen in discogenic and facet joint pain.

Therefore, best practice currently relies on studies which provide the clinician with a model of possible pain referral which should not be taken in isolation but should encompass a full differential diagnosis.

The mode of *onset and duration* of the symptoms of sacroiliac mechanical lesions can be helpful. Sacroiliac pain syndrome or dysfunction may have a sudden onset, when it is usually associated with some form of trauma, e.g. a fall from a height, slipping down the stairs jarring the leg, or a motor vehicle accident where the foot was placed heavily on the brake. A torsional strain is common and the mechanism of injury may involve straightening up from the stooped position (Leblanc 1992). Sporting activities which exert repetitive lower intensity forces or a single strong force, such as running, jumping and squatting, may produce excessive movement or stress in the sacroiliac joint and surrounding tissues, leading to overload injuries and soft tissue failure (Chen et al 2002).

A gradual strain of the sacroiliac joint may occur through repeated minor trauma, which is often related to occupation, e.g. constant driving over rough ground or persistent pressure being exerted through one sacroiliac joint.

If female, the patient should be questioned about any significant events during pregnancy that may have provoked symptoms. Gynaecological surgery and obstetric delivery often require the use of the lithotomy position, when the woman is positioned lying on her back with her hips and knees flexed to 90°. This tilts the pelvis posteriorly and may place undue stress on the sacroiliac joints.

The duration is also relevant. Patients have usually had their problem for a long time since it produces a dull ache, which may be tolerated more than the pain of acute onset, or severe sciatica, associated with lumbar pathology. The duration of symptoms also gives a prognostic indicator. Adaptive shortening occurs in chronic subluxation and the chance of correction using manipulative techniques after a long duration is slim. However, manipulation may help the pain even without correction of the deformity.

The *symptoms and behaviour* need to be considered. The behaviour of the pain indicates the nature of the condition and should distinguish it from a lumbar or hip joint pathology. Typically the patient complains of early-morning stiffness and pain, relieved by movement and made worse with rest, which may be due to the presence of inflammation. Sleep can be disturbed as the pain wakes the patient when turning at night. The pain may also be worse when lying on the affected side. Twinges of pain are common, especially after a period of rest, when the patient takes time to 'get going' again. Sit to stand movements may reproduce symptoms and patients commonly point to the sacral sulcus, which is tender to palpation (Cibulka 2002).

Patients may complain of other symptoms which are typical of mechanical sacroiliac pain and distinguish it from other lesions. They cannot sit still or stand for long periods and the joint likes to be moved and exercised. Sunbathing, for example, is extremely uncomfortable, since they do not like lying flat with legs outstretched and find it hard to lie prone while reading a book. They cannot balance very well on the affected leg.

The absence of certain symptoms is also relevant in distinguishing sacroiliac joint problems from pain of lumbar origin, particularly arising from nerve root compression. There should be no paraesthesia and no bladder or bowel symptoms. A cough and sneeze may provoke a little pain, but this should always be in the back and not in the leg.

Symptoms of serious pathology, such as night pain and sweats, fever, feeling generally unwell or unexplained recent weight loss, should be excluded.

Other joint involvement will alert the examiner to possible inflammatory arthritis. However, the initial presentation of ankylosing spondylitis in the sacroiliac joints is common, without other joint signs or symptoms.

Past medical history will give information concerning conditions that may be relevant to the patient's current complaint, always with the possible presence of serious illness in mind. An indication of the general health of the patient will indicate any systemic illness and it may be pertinent to take the patient's temperature. Recent pregnancy may be a less sinister element of medical history that could be relevant to sacroiliac joint problems. A mechanical lesion of the sacroiliac joint is a common cause of pain in pregnancy, particularly in the later stages. The increase in weight, change in posture and release of the hormone relaxin all contribute to mechanical instability of the pelvis. Manipulation is indicated in these patients and the pregnancy is not a contraindication in itself (Golighty 1982, Daly et al 1991).

The *medications* currently being taken by the patient should be listed. This may provide further indication of the patient's past medical history or alert the examiner to possible serious pathology, contraindications to treatment, and indications of past history of primary tumour, e.g. tamoxifen, an anti-oestrogen medication which is used in the treatment of some forms of breast cancer (Rang et al 2003). Anticoagulants and the use of long-term steroids should also be considered. The use of regular analgesia is worth noting as this may provide an objective marker for reassessment.

INSPECTION

Position the patient in standing, undressed to underwear and in a good light. Assessment for *bony deformity* and overall posture is made with particular attention to pelvic asymmetry.

Pelvic asymmetry in the static posture:

- Level of iliac crests (Fig. 14.3)
- Level of ASIS (Fig. 14.3)
- Level of PSIS (Fig. 14.4)
- Leg length
- General spinal curvatures
- Increased or decreased lordosis

Be aware that these signs cannot be considered in isolation as anomalies and leg length discrepancies commonly exist. The presence or absence of obvious asymmetry without associated appropriate symptoms is not necessarily relevant to mechanical dysfunction of the sacroiliac joint.

The assessment for positional alignment of various landmarks around the pelvis to establish asymmetry in either static or dynamic postures is a popular assessment tool, but is not without controversy. It must be recognized that this method lacks reliability and validity and is a subjective interpretation based on the examiner's eye and experience. Freburger & Riddle (1999) tested a method for measuring sacroiliac alignment using handheld calipers and an inclinometer in 73 symptomatic patients, but their results did not prove any more reliable than the observations mentioned above. Such studies rely on skillful therapists who are assumed to have a high level of knowledge of anatomy and are able accurately to palpate bony landmarks. However, Koran & McConnell (cited in O'Haire & Gibbons 2000) suggest that this is not necessarily the case, and Lewitt & Rosina (1999) suggest that palpating bone through soft tissue can produce a palpatory illusion due to changes in the soft tissue that occur as the result of pain. A further source of error could be the difficulty in accurately palpating bony landmarks in obese patients.

Figure 14.3   Assessing level of iliac crests and anterior superior iliac spines.

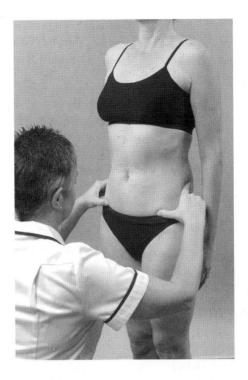

Figure 14.4   Assessing level of posterior superior iliac spines.

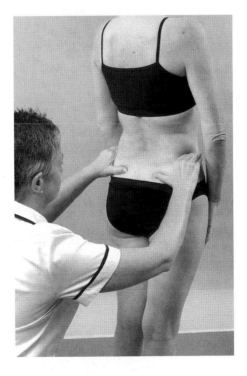

Riddle & Freburger (2002) were unsuccessful in demonstrating inter-tester reliability of a composite of four tests of pelvic symmetry and sacroiliac joint movement using a large group of patients. It was concluded that the individual tests had slightly higher reliability and that provocative, rather than alignment or movement, tests may have more support.

Colour changes, muscle wasting and swelling are unusual unless there is a history of trauma. In sacroiliac joint strain or subluxation, an area of apparent swelling is sometimes present over the sacrum, usually associated with muscle spasm.

STATE AT REST

Before any movements are performed, the state at rest is established to provide a baseline for subsequent comparison.

The suggested sequence for the objective examination will now be given, followed by a commentary including the reasoning in performing the movements and the significance of the possible findings.

EXAMINATION BY SELECTIVE TENSION (OBJECTIVE EXAMINATION)

Eliminate the Lumbar Spine

- Active lumbar extension (Fig. 14.5)
- Active right lumbar side flexion (Fig. 14.6a)
- Active left lumbar side flexion (Fig. 14.6b)
- Active lumbar flexion (Fig. 14.7)

Eliminate the Hip

- Passive hip flexion (Fig. 14.8a)
- Passive hip medial rotation (Fig. 14.8b)
- Passive hip lateral rotation (Fig. 14.8c)

Provocative Shear Tests for the Posterior Sacroiliac Ligaments (Saunders 2000)

- Hip flexion towards the ipsilateral shoulder (Fig. 14.9)
- Hip flexion towards the contralateral shoulder (Fig. 14.10)
- Hip flexion towards the contralateral hip (Fig. 14.11)

Pain Provocation Test for the Anterior Ligaments

- FABER test (Fig. 14.12)

Palpation

- For tenderness

Dynamic Asymmetry Palpation Test to Determine Treatment Technique

- The 'walk' test (Fig. 14.13a, b)

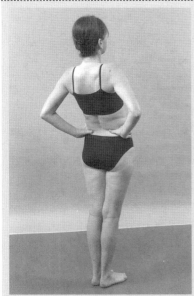

Figure 14.5   Active lumbar extension.

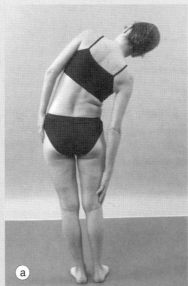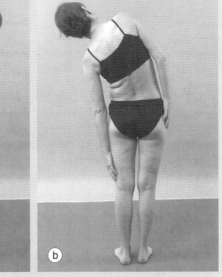

Figure 14.6   (a, b) Active lumbar side flexions.

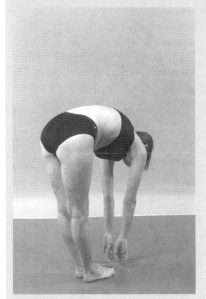

Figure 14.7   Active lumbar flexion.

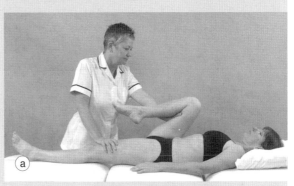

Figure 14.8   Passive hip movements: (a) flexion; (b) medial; and (c) lateral rotation.

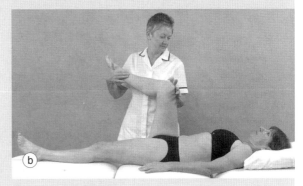

Figure 14.8   Cont'd.

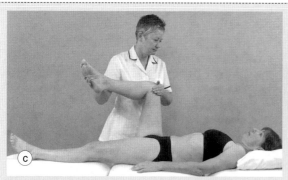

Figure 14.8   Cont'd.

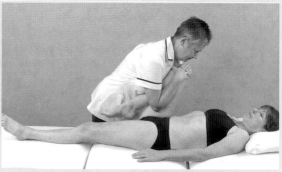

Figure 14.9   Shear test with the femur pointing towards the ipsilateral shoulder.

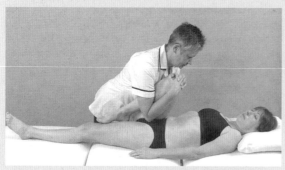

Figure 14.10   Shear test with the femur pointing towards the contralateral shoulder.

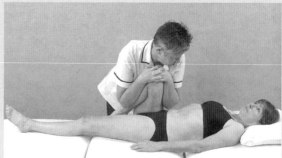

Figure 14.11   Shear test with the femur pointing towards the contralateral hip.

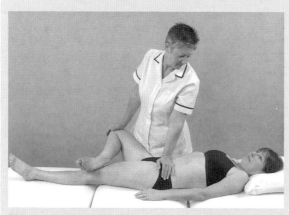

Figure 14.12   FABER or 4-test.

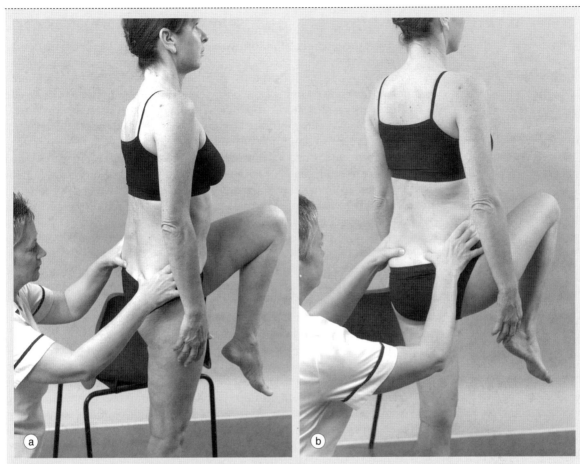

Figure 14.13   (a, b) The 'walk' test.

Examination of the sacroiliac joint must include elimination of the lumbar spine and hip joint as possible alternative causes of pain. The active movements of the lumbar spine and passive hip movements are assessed for range of movement and provocation of pain. If the symptoms are arising from the sacroiliac joint, pain is more commonly felt at the end of range of these movements, especially lumbar extension and passive hip lateral rotation. A unilateral reduction of hip lateral rotation has been associated with sacroiliac dysfunction (Chen et al 2002). The gross limitation of movement associated with lumbar lesions is not expected. Cited in Cibulka (2002), Mennell & Stoddard are credited with suggesting that in sacroiliac dysfunction, palpation of the lumbar vertebrae in a posterior/anterior direction does not provoke the patient's pain, whereas the patient may have pain on springing the sacrum or compression of the sacroiliac joints.

PAIN PROVOCATION TESTS

Pain provocative tests for the posterior sacroiliac ligaments include the 'posterior thigh thrust test' (known as the 'POSH', i.e. 'posterior shear', test in Broadhurst & Bond 1998; the 'posterior shear', 'posterior glide' or 'thigh thrust' test in Laslett & Williams 1994; and the 'thigh thrust' or 'femoral shear' test in Kokmeyer et al 2002).

The aim of this test is to apply a posterior shearing force to the sacroiliac joint via the femur but it relies on the lumbar spine and hip first being excluded as a cause of pain. The patient lies supine with the ipsilateral knee flexed to approximately 90° and the contralateral leg extended. The examiner adducts the femur to the midline and applies axial pressure along the length of the femur. A similar test has also been described by Saunders (2000) and has been modified to include two additional provocative testing positions:

- Hip flexion towards the ipsilateral shoulder (Fig. 14.9)
- Hip flexion towards the contralateral shoulder (Fig. 14.10)
- Hip flexion towards the contralateral hip (Fig. 14.11)

With the above tests, care should be taken not to excessively adduct the femur as this is uncomfortable in the normal state and may contribute to false-positive results.

For the purposes of assessment in orthopaedic medicine, the three pain provocation tests for the posterior ligaments, and one pain provocation test, the FABER test for the anterior ligaments, will be described. Reproduction of the patient's pain on the provocation tests constitutes a positive result.

THREE PAIN PROVOCATION TESTS FOR THE POSTERIOR SACROILIAC LIGAMENTS

The tests are applied as a thrust through the shaft of the femur to assess the posterior ligaments. All three tests are performed on the pain-free side first for subsequent comparison with the painful side.

(1) Place the patient in supine lying, flex the hip to approximately 90° and adduct the femur towards the ipsilateral shoulder. Grasp the patient's knee with linked hands and apply a thrust down through the line of the

shaft of the femur to stress the posterior sacroiliac joint ligaments. Pain in the buttock on the affected side denotes a positive test (Fig. 14.9).

The test is then repeated twice, but using in turn: (2) hip flexion towards the contralateral shoulder (Fig. 14.10); and (3) hip flexion and adduction towards the contralateral hip (Fig. 14.11) as the starting positions. Take care to release some pressure from the hip joint flexion and adduction before applying the downward thrust.

PAIN PROVOCATION TEST FOR THE ANTERIOR LIGAMENTS

The *FABER test* (Fig. 14.12) assesses mainly the anterior ligaments and derives its name from the combination of movements applied, being Flexion, ABduction and External Rotation of the hip. It is also known as Patrick's test or the '4-test' because of the resultant position of the limb.

Perform the test on the pain-free side first for subsequent comparison. With the patient in supine lying, the foot of one leg is placed on the knee of the other and the leg allowed to rest in lateral rotation and abduction. An assessment is made of the range of movement which is usually limited in sacroiliac joint problems. Pain reported at this stage is more likely to be indicative of hip joint pathology. Stabilize the opposite side of the pelvis and stress the sacroiliac joint by placing gentle downward pressure on the flexed knee. Pain now reported in the back incriminates the sacroiliac joint as a cause of symptoms (Hoppenfeld 1976).

Most authors agree that pain provocation tests are more reliable than palpation tests for sacroiliac joint dysfunction (Kokmeyer et al 2002). However, no individual pain provocation test has sufficient reliability or validity, leaving this a controversial topic. A battery of tests is used in clinical practice and it is commonplace to select three or four individual tests (Broadhurst & Bond 1998, Chen et al 2002).

Dreyfuss et al (1996) attempted to validate 12 commonly used tests by intra-articular diagnostic blocks using a stringent criterion of 90% relief of pain on re-assessment. The tests assessed failed to show diagnostic value, but four tests proved the most sensitive in this study in the following order: (1) sacral sulcus tenderness; (2) pain over the sacroiliac joint; (3) buttock pain; (4) patient pointing to the posterior superior iliac spine.

Broadhurst & Bond (1998) included the FABER test in their study, determining it to have a high degree of sensitivity and specificity. Van der Wurff et al (2000) present a systematic methodological review of reliability studies for pain provocation and motion palpation tests, identifying nine studies with acceptable methodological scores. The thrust test using the femur as a lever and Gaenslen's test (see below) seem to have the greatest reliability. However, the results were not shown to be uniformly reliable and van der Wurff et al (2000) suggest that upgrading the methodology of the tests would not have improved the results.

Laslett & Williams (1994) assessed the reliability of various provocation tests and found that the distraction, compression, posterior thigh thrust and pelvic torsion tests (Gaenslen's test) have the greatest inter-therapist reliability out of seven tests assessed, but that these need to be studied further in order to establish their diagnostic power.

Freburger & Riddle (2001) found some support in the literature for the following pain provocation tests: FABER test, palpation over the sacral sulcus, thigh thrust or posterior shear test, resisted hip abduction, iliac compression and gapping. They suggest that in the absence of stronger evidence, positive pain provocation tests together with the patient's descriptive information on pain referral patterns are used towards diagnosis of sacroiliac joint dysfunction.

Kokmeyer et al (2002) recruited 78 subjects in a study to determine the reliability of a multitest regimen of five sacroiliac joint pain provocation tests for dysfunction. They describe the tests, but suggest that they have been modified, which raises the issue of standardization. They conclude that better statistical reliability could have been achieved by using the five tests in combination, rather than the individual tests themselves, and advocate a regimen of three positive indicators in the five tests. Levin et al (1998, 2001) also raised standardization issues by examining the consistency of force variation and force distribution during pain provocation tests and their importance to pain response. They concluded that force registration would be a step towards standardizing the pain provocation tests.

The controversial issues discussed above mean that a number of different tests are described in various sources, many of them variations on a common theme. In order to apply current evidence, the thrust tests using the thigh as a lever, the FABER test and Gaenslen's test are currently supported by some evidence. Other tests should be recognized as a guide until reliability and validity are confirmed. It must also be acknowledged that the pain provocation tests are non-specific because they stress a number of adjacent structures around the hip, the lower lumbar spine and the sciatic and femoral nerves (Chen et al 2002). Diagnostic injection under fluoroscopic guidance is considered to be the gold standard for diagnosis, but has the disadvantage of being an invasive procedure and is not therefore used as a first line assessment tool (Calvillo et al 2000, Chen et al 2002).

PALPATION

Palpation may be conducted for tenderness which is often located over the PSIS, sacral sulcus and surrounding area and is absent on the unaffected side. However, such tenderness is also often present in lumbar pathology and should not be taken by itself as a positive sign of sacroiliac joint involvement.

DYNAMIC ASYMMETRY PALPATION TESTS TO DETERMINE TREATMENT TECHNIQUE

Dynamic palpation tests assess symmetry and movement of the pelvis and are applied to determine the choice of treatment technique. Like the pain provocation tests above, these tests are also a source of controversy within the literature. O'Haire & Gibbons (2000) demonstrated a greater intra-tester reliability than inter-tester, stating that the reliability of palpation requires validation. One might expect that the examiner's level of experience would be reflected in their palpation skills but this is not supported by the literature and disappointing results may be due to examiners failing to palpate the same structures.

Levangie (1999) assessed the association between innominate torsion and four movement tests and concluded that the tests were not useful in identifying innominate torsion, warning clinicians to be cautious in their use until more reliable data are available.

Palpation tests to detect joint mobility will be included here, but at the time of writing no evidence was found in the literature to support them. It is also worth considering that in assessing the standing forward flexion test (see below), Egan et al (1996) found a positive result in asymptomatic patients, which questions the belief in a cause–effect relationship between asymmetry and symptoms.

The *'walk' test* (Saunders 2000) (Fig. 14.13a, b) may be applied. The patient stands with both hands on a wall or chair to balance themselves. Crouch down so that you are at eye level with the sacrum and the PSISs. Tuck each thumb up and under the PSIS on either side to firmly locate their position. Ask the patient to flex alternate hips without tilting the pelvis, as if taking a marching step, and note the movement of one PSIS in relation to the other. If normal, the clinician would expect the PSIS on the non-weight-bearing leg to rotate posteriorly. In order for the test to be significant and imply hypomobility, a comparison between the two sides is made. If the symptomatic side rotates less posteriorly or more posteriorly than the asymptomatic side a clue is given to aid treatment choice.

The authors have observed clinically that in conducting the 'walk' test, balance on the standing leg may be difficult, and that juddering of the abdominal muscles and/or hip flexors of the non-weight-bearing leg may occur, possibly indicating poor core stability.

The test may provide a clue for the application of treatment techniques in that if the PSIS on the painful side appears to rotate more posteriorly in relation to the other, then a technique, and appropriate exercises, will be selected to produce anterior rotation, and vice versa. If no movement abnormality is detected, a more general technique will be applied.

An alternative is the *Gillet test*, also known as the ipsilateral kinetic test or ipsilateral rotation test, (Fowler 1994, Dreyfuss et al 1996, Levangie 1999, Lee 2000) which may also be applied to assess symmetry on movement. With the patient in standing, supported against a wall, place your right thumb on the right PSIS. Place your left thumb on the median sacral crest at the level of S2, or the sacral base, keeping thumbs parallel. Ask the patient to flex the right hip and knee. The right innominate bone should rotate posteriorly relative to the fixed sacrum and therefore the movement of the right thumb should be caudal. The test is positive and demonstrates hypomobility if the right thumb fails to move posteriorly relative to the sacrum. Repeat the test on the other side to compare.

The *pelvic torsion test (Gaenslen's test)* may be applied. Place the patient in supine lying with one hip and knee fully flexed to the chest and the other fully extended over the edge of the couch. This position applies opposing torsional stresses to the sacroiliac joints. Repeat the test by moving the patient to the other edge of the couch and reversing the position of the legs. A position which reproduces the patient's back pain may be a useful guide for the development of home exercises to achieve and maintain mobility (see below).

To recap, diagnosis at the sacroiliac joint relies on the history (subjective examination) and positive pain provocation tests. The dynamic asymmetry palpation tests provide clues to treatment.

Having completed the examination, an hypothesis is established relating to the patient's signs and symptoms. If a diagnosis of a mechanical lesion of the sacroiliac joint is made, manipulation is the treatment of choice provided no contraindications exist.

MECHANICAL LESIONS OF THE SACROILIAC JOINT

Diagnosis at the sacroiliac joint is challenging due to varied and overlapping symptoms, a rich and varied nerve supply and because symptoms may be due to a distant manifestation of injury in other parts of the kinetic chain (Chen et al 2002). It must be recognized that until supported by evidence, diagnosis depends on the clinician's interpretation of a number of factors including the subsequent response to treatment. Progression of treatment is based on the process of constant re-examination. As examination of the sacroiliac joint is not usually conducted in isolation, the recommended guidelines for safe practice of manipulation are the same as that covered in the lumbar spine (see Ch. 13). The clinician must take all due care when applying the treatment techniques.

Indications for sacroiliac joint manipulation are as follows:

- History of a mechanical lesion of the sacroiliac joint, implying hypomobility on the symptomatic side due to subluxation or sprain
- Absence of signs in the lumbar spine and hip
- At least one positive pain provocation test
- Static and dynamic palpation tests can indicate a pelvic rotation or asymmetry that may help with choice of treatment technique after clinical diagnosis

CONTRAINDICATIONS TO SACROILIAC JOINT MANIPULATION

These are few and will be determined by 'red flags' highlighted during the history and examination procedures. An absence of dural, cauda equina and radicular signs and/or symptoms would be expected. The clinician should be alert to indications of serious pathology and any drug history requiring caution. Sacroiliac dysfunction in the elderly is an uncommon cause of pain and caution is suggested before proceeding with the manipulative techniques described below. Occasionally the patient may present with a highly irritable lesion and it may not be possible to apply the manipulative techniques. In such a case, for the reasons suggested above, it may be possible to reverse the technique and apply it to the asymptomatic side.

SACROILIAC MANIPULATION PROCEDURE

It is recommended that a course in orthopaedic medicine is attended before the treatment techniques described are applied in clinical practice (see Appendix 1). For all sacroiliac techniques, the height of the couch is a matter of personal choice. As a suggestion, placing the couch at the level of your mid-thigh gives you the opportunity to assist the technique by gapping/distraction of the joint. However, the position will ultimately be determined by the relative sizes of the clinician and the patient – in general, the larger the patient, the lower the bed.

Sacroiliac joint gapping/distraction technique (Saunders 2000)

The indication for this technique is diagnosis of sacroiliac joint hypomobility with no observable pelvic asymmetry or difference in movement of the PSIS during the dynamic palpation tests.

Position the patient in side lying, painful side uppermost, pulling the underneath shoulder well through to stabilize the patient. Flex the upper leg so that the hip is in a neutral position with the knee over the edge of the bed. Stand in front of and facing the patient and take your forearm that is closest to the patient's head and place it comfortably in the patient's waist under the ribs, to fix the lumbar spine, while allowing the pelvis to fall slightly backwards. Apply downwards pressure along the line of the femur to gap/distract the sacroiliac joint and maintain this by resting your caudal knee against the patient's flexed knee (Fig. 14.14a). Place your other forearm on the blade of the ilium, to be at right angles with your forearm in the patient's waist.

Figure 14.14   (a, b) Sacroiliac joint-gapping technique.

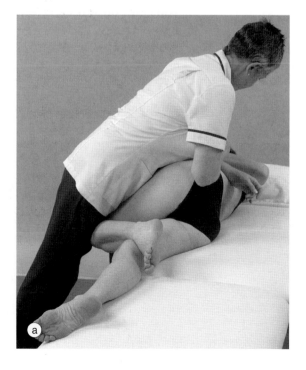

Figure 14.14 Cont'd.

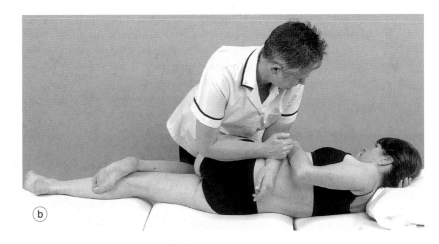

Continue to take up the slack by drawing the forearm on the ilium towards you and apply a minimal amplitude, high velocity thrust at the end of range (Fig. 14.14b).

Rotation of the pelvis down/posteriorly on the painful side (Saunders 2000)

The indication for this technique is diagnosis of sacroiliac joint hypomobility with either static or dynamic palpation tests, indicating that the PSIS is rotated up or anteriorly on the painful side in relation to the other PSIS. Position the patient as above and fix under the rib cage with the forearm as before. Place the patient's flexed hip and knee towards more hip flexion to assist rotation of the pelvis posteriorly on the painful side. Gap/distract the sacroiliac joint as described above. Place the medial epicondyle of your other elbow on the patient's ischial tuberosity. Once all the slack has been taken up by rotating your body and arms to pull the ischial tuberosity towards you, apply a minimal amplitude, high velocity thrust (Fig. 14.15).

Figure 14.15 Rotation of the pelvis posteriorly or downwards on the painful side.

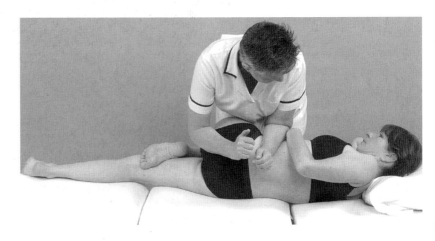

Rotation of the pelvis up/anteriorly on the painful side (Saunders 2000)

The indication for this technique is diagnosis of sacroiliac joint hypomobility with the palpation tests indicating that the PSIS is rotated down or posteriorly on the painful side in relation to the other PSIS.

Position the patient as above and fix under the rib cage with one forearm. Place the flexed hip and knee towards hip extension to assist rotation of the pelvis anteriorly on the painful side. Gap/distract the sacroiliac joint as described above. Place the forearm of your other arm to apply pressure just behind the iliac crest, but keep your forearms parallel. Pull your arm on the iliac crest towards you and under your other arm and, once all the slack has been taken up, apply a minimal amplitude, high velocity thrust (Fig. 14.16).

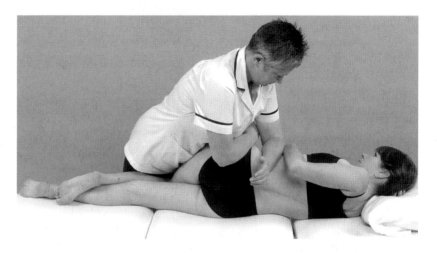

Figure 14.16 Rotation of the pelvis anteriorly or upwards on the painful side.

Leg tug

The indication for this technique is any diagnosis of sacroiliac joint hypomobility; it is particularly useful during the later stages of pregnancy. Position the patient comfortably in supine lying with the couch at about knee height. Hold the patient's ankle of the symptomatic side and place your knee against the patient's foot on the good side, to prevent the patient slipping down the bed. Apply a degree of distraction together with a circumduction movement of the hip. Once the patient relaxes, apply a sharp caudal tug (Fig. 14.17).

Reducing hypomobility due to a sacroiliac subluxation or relieving stress on the ligaments can be very successful. Following treatment, attention should be given to the prevention of recurrence. Discussions with the patient will allow advice to be given about lifestyle habits that may be contributing to the condition and any imbalances and postural problems can be addressed. Following reduction of subluxation in the later stages of pregnancy, a supportive brace may be helpful. The following exercises may be useful in a maintenance programme:

Figure 14.17   Leg tug.

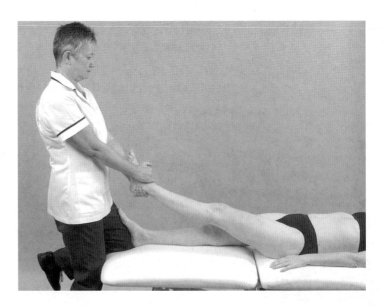

- In supine lying, ask the patient to flex one knee to the chest while the other leg hangs over the edge of the couch. Anterior or upwards rotation is encouraged in the extended leg and posterior or downwards rotation in the flexed leg (Fig. 14.18)
- Standing with one leg on a stool, ask the patient to make a lunging movement forwards, involving flexion at the hip and extension at the lumbar spine. Anterior or upwards rotation of the PSIS is encouraged on the side of the standing, extended leg, and posterior or downwards rotation of the PSIS is encouraged on the side of the flexed leg (Fig. 14.19 a, b)

Figure 14.18   Exercise in supine lying, encouraging movement of the posterior superior iliac spine.

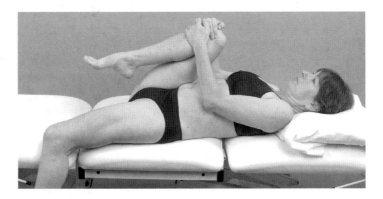

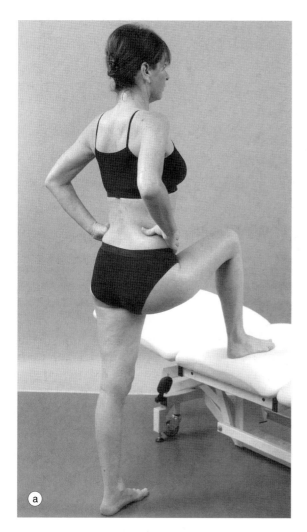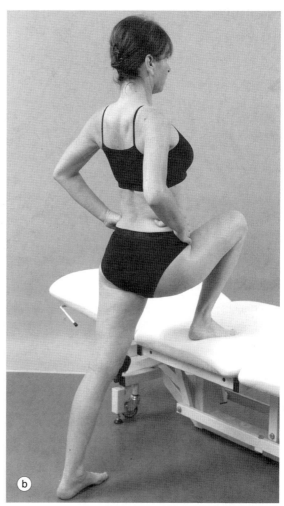

Figure 14.19   (a, b) Exercise in standing, encouraging movement of the posterior superior iliac spine.

SACROILIAC HYPERMOBILITY

Hypermobility or instability of one sacroiliac joint may be due to a traumatic incident, repetitive microtrauma or secondary to hormonal changes (Lee 2000). Diagnosis will again be clinical depending on the history and the pain provocation tests. The static and dynamic palpation tests will demonstrate asymmetry while objectively the joint will give an impression of hypomobility when the pain provocation tests are applied. Applying the manipulative techniques (see above) may successfully correct the malalignment of the symptomatic sacroiliac joint. Once reduction has been effected, stability tests reveal the excessive range of movement and this will need the support of a pelvic belt and correction of any muscle imbalances. This topic is outside the scope of this text, however, and the reader is referred to other texts. Sclerosant injections have also been described (see below).

SACROILIAC TRACTION

The use of traction is not indicated with a sacroiliac joint problem. Where the differential diagnosis is uncertain between a lumbar or sacroiliac joint problem, the latter may be suspected if the application of traction makes the pain worse, since the position of the pelvic harness over the ilia applies stress through the sacroiliac joints when the traction is applied.

SCLEROSANT INJECTIONS

In cases of extreme laxity of the sacroiliac joints, associated with frequent episodes of subluxation, sclerosant injections may be used to induce scarring in the ligaments, so tightening the tissues to support the joint (see Ch. 13). It is important that the subluxation is reduced before the injections are given. Sclerosants would not be appropriate in pregnancy but, in any event, the ligamentous softening is likely to resolve spontaneously within 4–5 months of delivery.

References

Broadhurst N A, Bond M J 1998 Pain provocation tests for the assessment of sacroiliac dysfunction. Journal of Spinal Disorders 11(4):341–345

Calvillo O, Skaribas I, Turnipseed J 2000 Anatomy and pathophysiology of the sacroiliac joint. Current Review of Pain 4(5):356–361

Cassidy J D 1992 The pathoanatomy and clinical significance of the sacro-iliac joints. Journal of Manipulative and Physiological Therapeutics 15:41–42

Chen Y C, Fredericson M, Smuck M 2002 The sacroiliac joint pain syndrome in active patients: a look behind the pain. Physician and Sports Medicine 30(11):30–37

Cibulka M T 2002 Understanding sacroiliac joint movement as a guide to the management of a patient with unilateral low back pain. Manual Therapy 7(4):215–221

Daly K M, Frame P S, Rapaza P A 1991 Sacro-iliac subluxation: a common, treatable cause of low back pain in pregnancy. Family Practice Research Journal 11:149–159

Dangaria T R 1998 A case report of sacroiliac joint dysfunction with urinary symptoms. Manual Therapy 3(4):220–221

Derby R 1994 Point of view. Spine 19:1489

Dreyfuss P, Michaelsen M, Pauza K, McLarty J, Bogduk N 1996 The value of medical history and physical examination in diagnosing sacroiliac joint pain. Spine 21:2594–2602

Egan D, Cole J, Twomey L 1996 The standing forward flexion test: an inaccurate determinant of sacroiliac joint dysfunction. Physiotherapy 82(4):236–242

Fortin J D, Dwyer A P, West S et al 1994a Sacro-iliac joint – pain referral maps upon applying a new injection/arthrography technique, part I. Asymptomatic volunteers. Spine 19(13): 1475–1482

Fortin J D, Aprill C N, Ponthieux B et al 1994b Sacroiliac joint – pain referral maps upon applying a new injection/arthrography technique, part II. Clinical evaluation. Spine 19(13):1483–1489

Fortin J D, Kissling R O, O'Connor B L et al 1999a Sacroiliac joint innervation and pain – a review paper. American Journal of Orthopaedics 28(12):687–690

Fortin J D, Washington W J, Falco F J E 1999b Three pathways between the sacroiliac joint and neural structures. American Journal of Neuroradiology 20(8):1429–1434

Fowler C 1994 Muscle energy techniques for pelvic dysfunction. In: Boyling J D, Palastanga N (eds) Grieve's Modern manual therapy, 2nd edn. Churchill Livingstone, Edinburgh, pp 781–791

Freburger J K, Riddle D L 1999 Measurement of sacroiliac joint dysfunction: a multicentre intertester reliability study. Physical Therapy 79(12):1134–1141

Freburger J K, Riddle D L 2001 Using published evidence to guide the examination of the sacroiliac joint. Physical Therapy 81(5):1135–1143

Golighty R 1982 Pelvic arthropathy in pregnancy and the puerperium. Physiotherapy 68:216–220

Harrison D E, Harrison D D, Troyanovich S J 1997 The sacroiliac joint: a review of anatomy and biomechanics with clinical implications. Journal of Manipulative and Physiological Therapeutics 20(9):607–617

Hoppenfeld S 1976 Physical examination of the spine and extremities. Appleton Century Crofts, Philadelphia

Jacob H A C, Kissling R O 1995 The mobility of the sacro-iliac joints in healthy volunteers between 10 and 50 years of age. Clinical Biomechanics 10:352–361

Kapandji I A 1974 The physiology of the joints, the trunk and the vertebral column. Churchill Livingstone, Edinburgh, vol 3

Keat A 1995 Reiter's syndrome and reactive arthritis. In: Collected Reports on the Rheumatic Diseases. Arthritis and Rheumatism Council for Research, London, pp 61–64

Kissling R O, Jacob H A C 1996 The mobility of the sacroiliac joints in healthy subjects. Bulletin Hospital for Joint Diseases 54(3):158–164

Kokmeyer D J, van der Wurff P, Aufdemkampe G et al 2002 The reliability of multitest regimens with sacroiliac pain provocation tests. Journal of Manipulative and Physiological Therapeutics 25(1):42–48

Kumar P, Clark M 2002 Clinical medicine, 5th edn. Baillière Tindall, London

Laslett M, Williams M 1994 The reliability of selected pain provocation tests for sacro-iliac joint pathology. Spine 19(11):1243–1249

Leblanc K 1992 Sacro-iliac sprain: an overlooked cause of back pain. American Family Physician November: 1459–1463

Lee D 2000 The pelvic girdle. Churchill Livingstone, Edinburgh

Levangie P K 1999 Four clinical tests of sacroiliac dysfunction: the association of test results with innominate torsion among patients with and without low back pain. Physical Therapy 79(11):1043–1057

Levin U, Nilsson-Wikmar L K, Stendtröm C H 1998 Reproducibility of manual pressure force on provocation of the sacroiliac joint. Physiotherapy Research International 3(1):1–14

Levin U, Nilsson-Wikmar L, Harms-Ringdahl K et al 2001 Variability of forces applied by experienced physiotherapists during provocation of the sacroiliac joint. Clinical Biomechanics 16:300–306

Lewitt K, Rosina A 1999 Why yet another diagnostic sign of sacro-iliac movement restriction? Journal of Manipulative and Physiological Therapeutics 22(3):154–160

O'Haire C, Gibbons P 2000 Inter-examiner and intra-examiner agreement for assessing sacroiliac anatomical landmarks using palpation and observation: a pilot study. Manual Therapy 5(1):13–20

Oliver J, Middleditch A 1991 Functional anatomy of the spine. Butterworth Heinemann, Oxford

Palastanga N, Field D, Soames R 2002 Anatomy and human movement, 4th edn. Butterworth Heinemann, Oxford

Rai A 1995 Ankylosing spondylitis. In: Collected Reports on the Rheumatic Diseases. Arthritis and Rheumatism Council for Research, London, pp 65–68

Rang H P, Dale M M, Ritter J M et al 2003 Pharmacology, 5th edn. Churchill Livingstone, Edinburgh

Riddle D, Freburger J K 2002 Evaluation of the presence of sacroiliac joint region dysfunction using a combination of tests: a multicentre intertester reliability study. Physical Therapy 82(8):772–781

Saunders S 2000 Orthopaedic medicine course manual. Saunders, London

Schmid H J A 1984 Sacroiliac diagnosis and treatment. Manual Medicine 1:33–38

Schwarzer A C, Aprill C N, Bogduk N 1995 The sacro-iliac joint in chronic low back pain. Spine 20:31–37

Silberstein M, Hennessy O, Lau L 1992 Neoplastic involvement of the sacroiliac joint – MR and CT features. Australasian Radiology 36:334–338

Slipman C W, Jackson H B, Lipetz J S et al 2000 Sacroiliac joint pain referral zones. Archives of Physical Medicine and Rehabilitation 81(3):334–338

Swezey R L 1998 The sacroiliac joint. Physical Medicine and Rehabilitation Clinics of North America 9(2):515–519

Trotter M 1947 Variations of the sacral canal: their significance in the administration of caudal analgesia. Current Researches in Anesthesia and Analgesia 26:192–202

van der Wurff P, Hagmeijer R H M, Meyne W 2000 Clinical test of the sacroiliac joint, part I. Reliability. Manual Therapy 5(1):30–36

Vleeming A, Stoeckart R, Volkers C W et al 1990a Relation between form and function in the sacro-iliac joint, part I. Clinical anatomical aspects. Spine 15(2):130–132

Vleeming A, Stoeckart R, Volkers C W et al 1990b Relation between form and function in the sacro-iliac joint, part II. Biomechanical aspects. Spine 15(2):133–135

Vleeming A, Pool-Goudzwaard L, Hammudoghlu D et al 1996 The function of the long dorsal sacro-iliac ligament. Spine 21(5):556–562

Williams P L 1998 Gray's Anatomy: the anatomical basis of medicine and surgery, 38th edn. Churchill Livingstone, Edinburgh

Zheng N, Watson L G, Yong-Hing K 1997 Biomechanical modelling of the human sacroiliac joint. Medical and Biological Engineering and Computing 35(2):77–82

Appendix 1

COURSES IN ORTHOPAEDIC MEDICINE

Courses in orthopaedic medicine are held at a variety of venues both nationally and internationally. The course design usually consists of distance learning packages, modular taught blocks, intermodular projects and a final practical and theoretical examination. The educational aims of the courses include the development of clinical reasoning skills, critical analysis of outcomes and self-evaluation.

The course content includes clinical examination and diagnosis, applied anatomy, soft tissue treatment techniques of manipulation and mobilization, and injection techniques. Much of the course is devoted to practical work in small groups with close supervision and feedback. The courses are supported by a comprehensive illustrated manual.

The course acts as an introduction to injection techniques and leads into an advanced module to teach injection skills. A separate module in advanced clinical practice in orthopaedic medicine may also be accessed following successful completion of the basic course.

For more details of the courses available please contact the following organizations:

Society of Orthopaedic Medicine (registered charity no 802164)

Administrative director
Amanda Sherwood
PO Box 223
Patchway
Bristol
BS32 4XD

www.soc-ortho-med.org

AFFILIATED ORGANIZATIONS

Cyriax Organisation

Contact
Nigel Hanchard
School of Health and Social Care
University of Teesside
Middlesbrough
Tees Valley
TS1 3BA

nigel.hanchard@ntlworld.com

European Teaching Group of Orthopaedic Medicine

Contact
Steven De Coninck
ETGOM
Lepelemstraat 4
B 8421 De Haan
Belgium

www.etgom.be
info@etgom.be

Irish Society of Orthopaedic Medicine

Course organizer
Dr Pierce Molony
Johnstownbridge
Enfield
Co Meath
Ireland

www.isom.ie

Orthopaedic Medicine International

Course administrator
Pauline Hill
3 Garden Court
Birkrigg Park
High Carley
Ulverston
Cumbria
LA12 6UF

Orthopaedic Medicine Seminars

Course organizer
Mrs S Saunders FCSP
20 Ailsa Road
Twickenham
TW1 1QW

Association of Chartered Physiotherapists in Orthopaedic Medicine (ACPOM)

Details of the specific interest group, ACPOM, are available from:
The Chartered Society of Physiotherapy
14 Bedford Row
London
WC1R 4ED

Appendix 2

SAFETY RECOMMENDATIONS FOR SPINAL MANIPULATIVE TECHNIQUES

Following the recommendations given below will help to ensure maximum safety and preparation for the unexpected. The practitioner must take all due care while applying the treatment techniques and ensure appropriate education and competence in the techniques to be applied.

ENSURE THAT

- A full history and examination have been completed and recorded, sufficient to establish indications and to exclude contraindications to treatment.
- Specific questions have been asked relating to the following, and the result recorded:

In the cervical spine

drop attacks
dizziness (vertigo), nausea
past history of trauma
cardiovascular disease
anticoagulant therapy
blood clotting disorders
inflammatory arthritis

The history may steer the clinician to ask further questions relating to:

visual disturbances
difficulty in speaking or swallowing
unsteadiness in gait or general feelings of weakness
past medical history
medications
general health

At the time of writing, prior to application of cervical manipulation a recognized vertebrobasilar artery test should be conducted in each session which includes manipulation and should be negative.

In the thoracic spine

unexplained weight loss
bilateral paraesthesia in the hands and feet
anticoagulant therapy
long-term oral steroids
inflammatory arthritis
past history of trauma
bladder or bowel symptoms
past medical history
medications
general health

In the lumbar spine

bladder and bowel symptoms
saddle anaesthesia
anticoagulant therapy
blood clotting disorders
inflammatory arthritis
past history of trauma
past medical history
medications
general health

ENSURE THAT

- From the examination, the following factors are present:
  a non-capsular pattern of limited movement
  a normal plantar response
  no increase in reflexes.
- There are no contraindications to manipulation. The more peripheral the symptoms, the less likely manipulation is to work, but it may be attempted if minimal neurological signs exist. If neurological deficit is severe and progressing, manipulation should not be attempted but other modalities may be more effective, e.g. traction and mobilization.
- You have provided sufficient information, including possible risks and advice, if manipulation is indicated, so that the patient can give informed consent. You must respect the right of the patient to refuse manipulation.
- You re-examine the patient after the application of each technique and base decisions to continue on the outcome of the previous technique.
- Any significant adverse response to treatment is reported immediately to the patient's doctor.

Manipulation produces immediate results, therefore treatment should be progressed following a constant reassessment and clinical reasoning process. If a technique helps, it is repeated; if it is unsuccessful, another technique or alternative modality may be chosen according to professional judgement.

Glossary

Allodynia   Pain produced by a stimulus which is not normally painful.

Anomalous cross-links   An abnormal number of cross-links (adhesions), developing as a result of a stationary attitude of collagen fibres; responsible for the toughness and resilience of scar tissue.

Capsular pattern   A limitation of movement in a specific pattern which is peculiar to each joint and indicates the presence of an arthritis.

Close packed   The position in which a joint is most stable, when the joint surfaces fit closely together and are maximally congruent.

Compression   A squashing or pushing force resulting in the structure becoming shortened and broadened.

Corticosteroids   Potent anti-inflammatory drugs. In orthopaedic medicine: injections used to treat chronic inflammatory soft tissue lesions, acute episodes of degenerative osteoarthrosis and inflammatory arthritis.

Creep   A property of viscoelastic structures which consists of a small, almost imperceptible movement, occurring when a constant stress is applied for a prolonged period of time.

Cross-links   Either weak intramolecular hydrogen bonds connecting molecules or stronger covalent intermolecular bonds connecting collagen fibrils and fibres. The links provide connective tissue structures with tensile strength and the greater the number of cross-links, the stronger the structure.

Deformation   A change in length or shape due to the application of a stress, represented as strain on the stress–strain diagram.

Distraction/traction   A force applied in opposite directions across a joint causing the joint surfaces to separate.

Dysaesthesia   Damage to any of the senses, especially touch, but not to the point of anaesthesia.

Elasticity   The property of a material or a structure which allows it to deform when a force is applied. The change is temporary and the original form is restored when the deforming force is removed.

Elastic range   Represented on the stress–strain diagram as the range of loading within which a material or structure remains elastic, i.e. it can resume its original form after the deforming force is removed.

End-feel   A specific sensation imparted through the examiner's hands at the extreme of passive movement.

Enthesis   The point at which a tendon inserts into bone.

Enthesopathy   A lesion at the teno-osseous junction, e.g. tennis elbow at the common extensor origin.

Fatigue   A process by which a structure fails when subjected to repetitive low loading cycles.

Force   An action which produces movement by pushing or pulling, known as mechanical stress and expressed as the force per unit area.

Force couple   The application of equal, but opposite, parallel forces.

Glycosaminoglycans (GAGs)   Long-chain molecules, the building blocks for proteoglycans.

Grade A mobilization   A passive, active or active/assisted mobilization performed within the patient's pain-free range at peripheral joints.

Grade A movement   A mid-range pain-free movement applied to spinal joints.

Grade B mobilization   A mobilization applied at the end of available range. A sustained stretching technique aimed to produce permanent lengthening of connective tissue structures.

Grade B movement   A movement to the end of range at the spinal joints.

Grade C mobilization   A manipulation involving a minimal amplitude, high velocity thrust applied at the end of range once all of the slack has been taken up. It can be applied to certain peripheral or spinal lesions.

Hysteresis   A property of viscoelastic structures in which the resumption of its original length occurs more slowly than the deformation.

Load A general term describing the application of a force and/or moment (torque) to a structure.

Local anaesthetic A pain-inhibiting drug. In orthopaedic medicine injections, used for diagnostic and therapeutic effects.

Macrofailure Occurs when there is rupture of a structure and it is unable to sustain further load. Represented by a rapid fall in the stress–strain curve.

Microfailure Occurs when a structure reaches its elastic limit with progressive failure of cross-links and fibrils.

Moment A force that produces bending or torque.

Motion segment A functional spinal segment consisting of two adjacent vertebral bodies together with their joints and surrounding soft tissues.

Non-capsular pattern A pattern of limited and/or painful movements which does not fit the capsular pattern of that particular joint.

Paraesthesia Numbness, tingling, 'pins and needles'.

Plasticity The property of a structure which permits it to undergo permanent deformation when the distorting force is large enough to load the structure beyond its elastic range.

Plastic range Represented on the stress–strain diagram as the range of loading within which a material or structure cannot resume its original form once the deforming force is removed, i.e. the elastic range of the structure is exceeded.

Pressure phenomenon Pain and paraesthesia occurring as the pressure is applied.

Proteoglycans Protein-carbohydrate complex consisting of GAGs covalently bound to protein.

Release phenomenon The sensation of deep painful paraesthesia occurring as pressure is released from a nerve trunk.

Selective tension The application of appropriate stress to soft tissue structures in order to test function.

Set The difference between the original and final length or shape of a structure once the deforming force is removed.

Shear A force applied parallel to the surface of the structure, causing angular deformation.

Sign of the buttock Pain on straight leg raise which increases on flexing the knee and hip. It is a sign of serious pathology.

Stiffness The resistance of a structure to the deforming force.

Strain The deformation or change in dimension of a material or structure in response to an externally applied load or force.

Stress The load or force applied to a structure resulting in strain or deformation.

Stress–strain curve A diagrammatic representation of the mechanical behaviour of a material or structure. Stress is plotted on the y axis and represents the tensile, compressive, shear or torsional force applied. Strain is plotted on the x axis and represents the deformation or elongation of the material.

Tendinitis Inflammation of a tendon.

Tendinopathy General term for any pathology in a tendon.

Tendinosis Degenerative tendon changes.

Tenosynovitis Inflammation between a tendon and its sheath.

Tensile strength The maximum stress or load sustained by a material.

Tension A force of equal and opposite loads which results in lengthening and narrowing of the fibres of a material or structure.

Torsion A combination of shear, tensile and compressive force or load applied to a structure causing it to rotate about an axis. The load is called the torque.

Traction/distraction A force applied in opposite directions across a joint causing the joint surfaces to separate.

Translation Parallel movement of two opposing surfaces causing them to slide across one another.

Transverse frictions A specific type of massage applied to connective tissue structures to produce therapeutic movement, traumatic hyperaemia, pain relief and improved function.

Viscoelasticity The property of a material to change when under constant deformation.

Viscosity The property of a fluid which resists flowing.

Wolff's law   A law that states that bone is laid down where it is needed along the lines of stress, and reabsorbed when not needed.

Yield point   The point of the stress–strain curve at which appreciable deformity occurs, without any appreciable increase in load.

Index